Figures available in three downloadable sizes (resolutions)

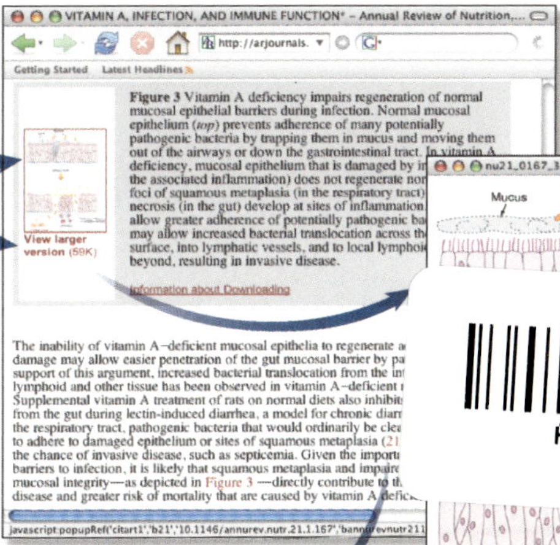

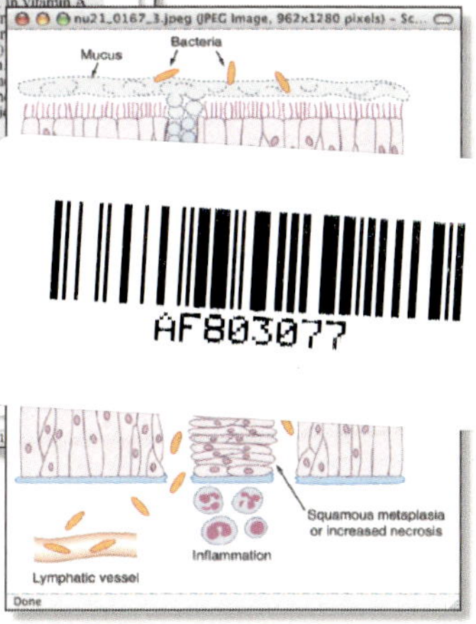

Citations in text link to references in bibliography

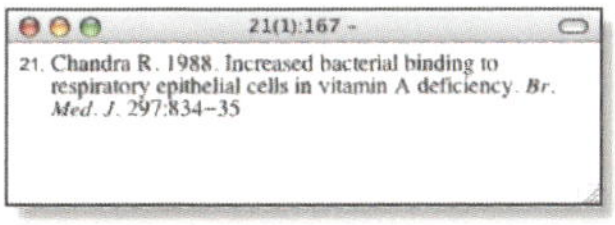

References in Annual Reviews chapter bibliography link out to sources of cited articles online

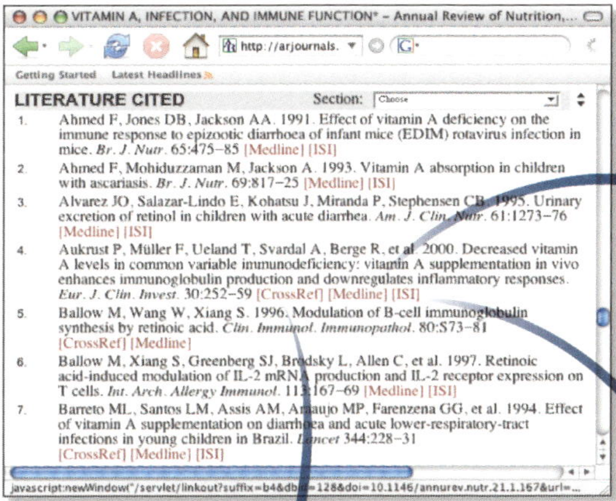

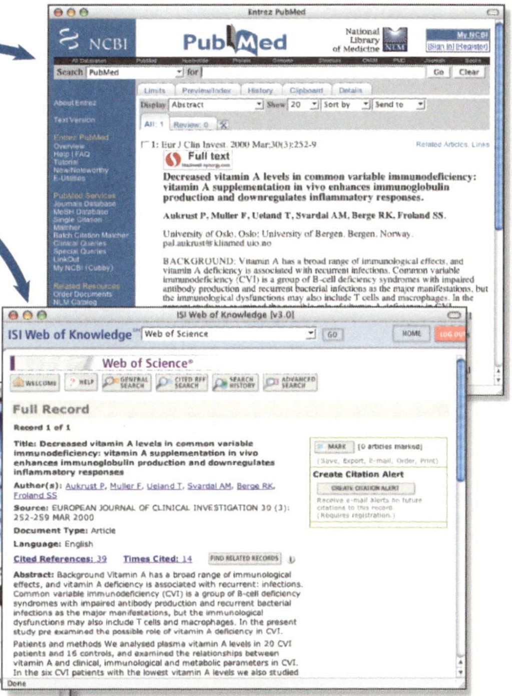

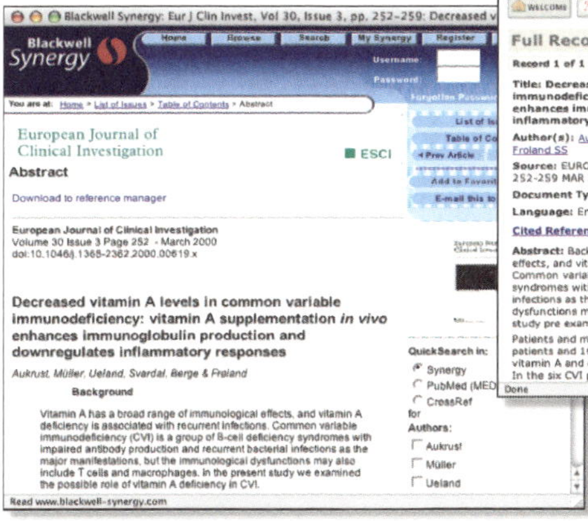

Annual Review of Nutrition

PREFACE

Volume 25 of the *Annual Review of Nutrition* is my first as editor. Equally sharing editorial duties for this volume were Dennis Bier and Barbara Bowman as associate editors. The extremely high ISI® ranking of the *Annual Review of Nutrition* is due to standards established by past editors Don McCormick, Bob Olson, and Bill Darby. Throughout its 25-year history, this Annual Reviews series has adhered to the mission of providing "critical authoritative reviews" that cover the spectrum of nutrition research from molecules to populations. Suggestions for topics are generated by an editorial committee, which includes term and ad hoc members. For volume 25, this committee was composed of Raymond Burk, Stephen Goodman, Dale Romsos, Steven Zeisel, former editor Don McCormick, and the current editors.

The prefatory chapter in this *Annual Review of Nutrition* volume is by David Kritchevsky. Rather than taking an autobiographical approach, Kritchevsky, with coauthor Martin Eastwood, describes evolution in the understanding of dietary fiber. McGuinness describes how glucose metabolism dysregulates during infection, and Newburg and coauthors discuss the relationship between milk glycans and protection against enteric pathogens. Dietary approaches to the treatment of insulin-resistance syndrome are reviewed by Reaven, and pediatric obesity and insulin resistance are discussed by Cruz and colleagues. Developmental roles of essential fatty acids are discussed by Heird and Lapillonne; how fatty acids regulate genes of lipid metabolism is described by Sampath and Ntambi; Corella and Ordovas discuss how diet influences genes of lipid metabolism that have single nucleotide polymorphisms; and Dark describes how lipid cycles influence physiology and behavior in hibernators. The neurobiology of energy intake and meal frequency is presented by Mattson, and the cow as a model of food intake regulation is described by Allen and coworkers. Nutrition-genomic approaches have been described by Kilberg and coauthors to define how cells respond to amino acid limitation; Shay and Banz describe how some botanicals regulate gene transcription; and a discussion of *Drosophila* as a model for human gene-nutrient effects is presented by Ruden et al. Mechanisms of vitamin A absorption are reviewed by Harrison, and regulation of vitamin C transport is discussed by Wilson. Reviews are also presented by Berkner on vitamin K-dependent carboxylase; by Zempleni on noncarboxylase roles of biotin; and by Singh et al. on vitamin E oxidative stress and inflammation. How phosphorus homeostasis is regulated via a Na-phosphate cotransporter is discussed by Tenenhouse; and Burk and Hill review the influence of selenoprotein P on selenium metabolism. Nutrient effects on redox regulation in cancer cells is presented by McEligot et al., and developmental determinants of blood pressure is reviewed by Adair and Dahly.

Finally, we need to thank the entire staff at Annual Reviews, but particularly Lisa Dean, our Production Editor, for her work throughout the year, and Sam Gubins, Annual Reviews President.

Robert J. Cousins
Editor

Annual Review of Nutrition
Volume 25, 2005

CONTENTS

ERRATA

An online log of corrections to *Annual Review of Nutrition* chapters may be found at http://nutr.annualreviews.org/

Related Articles

From the ***Annual Review of Biochemistry***, Volume 74, 2005

Applications of DNA Microarrays in Biology, Roland B. Stoughton

NOD-LRR Proteins: Role in Host-Microbial Interactions and Inflammatory Disease, Naohiro Inohara, Mathias Chamaillard, Christine McDonald, and Gabriel Nuñez

Structure and Function of Fatty Acid Amide Hydrolase, Michele K. McKinney and Benjamin F. Cravatt

Monitoring Energy Balance: Metabolites of Fatty Acid Synthesis as Hypothalamic Sensors, Paul Dowell, Zhiyuan Hu, and M. Daniel Lane

Structure and Physiologic Function of the Low-Density Lipoprotein Receptor, Hyesung Jeon and Stephen C. Blacklow

Gene Therapy: Twenty-First Century Medicine, Inder M. Verma and Matthew D. Weitzman

The Structural Biology of Type II Fatty Acid Biosynthesis, Stephen W. White, Jie Zheng, Yong-Mei Zhang, and Charles O. Rock

Structural Studies by Electron Tomography: From Cells to Molecules, Vladan Lučić, Friedrich Förster, and Wolfgang Baumeister

From the ***Annual Review of Cell and Developmental Biology***, Volume 21, 2005

Docosahexaenoic Acid, Fatty Acid-Interacting Proteins, and Neuronal Function: Breastmilk and Fish Are Good for You, Joseph R. Marszalek and Harvey L. Lodish

From the ***Annual Review of Genomics and Human Genetics***, Volume 6, 2005

Disease Gene Recovery Through Integrative Genomics, Vamsi Mootha

Evolution of the ATP-Binding Cassette (ABC) Transporter Superfamily in Vertebrates, Michael Dean and Tarmo Annilo

The Patterns of Natural Variation in Human Genes, Dana C. Crawford, Dayna T. Akey, and Deborah A. Nickerson

From the ***Annual Review of Medicine***, Volume 56, 2005

G Protein Polymorphisms in Hypertension, Atherosclerosis, and Diabetes, Winfried Siffert

Metabolic Syndrome: A Clinical and Molecular Perspective, David E. Moller and Keith D. Kaufman

Monogenic Obesity in Humans, I. Sadaf Farooqi and Stephen O'Rahilly

From the ***Annual Review of Physiology***, Volume 67, 2005

Intracellular Calcium Release and Cardiac Disease, Xander H.T. Wehrens, Stephan E. Lehnart, and Andrew R. Marks

Endocrinology of the Stress Response, Evangelia Charmandari, Constantine Tsigos, and George Chrousos

Novel Renal Amino Acid Transporters, Francois Verrey, Zorica Ristic, Elisa Romeo, Tamara Ramadan, Victoria Makrides, Mital H. Dave, Carsten A. Wagner, and Simone M.R. Camargo

Renal Tubule Albumin Transport, Michael Gekle

From the ***Annual Review of Public Health***, Volume 26, 2005

Competing Dietary Claims for Weight Loss: Finding the Forest Through Truculent Trees, David L. Katz

Water and Bioterrorism: Preparing for the Potential Threat to U.S. Water Supplies and Public Health, Patricia L. Meinhardt

Economic Causes and Consequences of Obesity, Eric A. Finkelstein, Christopher J. Ruhm, and Katherine M. Kosa

Magnitude of Alcohol-Related Mortality and Morbidity Among U.S. College Students Ages 18–24: Changes from 1998 to 2001, Ralph Hingson, Timothy Hereen, Michael Winter, and Henry Wechsler

Declining Rates of Physical Activity in the United States: What are the Contributors?, Ross C. Brownson, Tegan K. Boehmer, and Douglas A. Luke

Primary Prevention of Diabetes: What Can Be Done and How Much Can Be Prevented?, Matthias B. Schulze and Frank B. Hu

ANNUAL REVIEWS is a nonprofit scientific publisher established to promote the advancement of the sciences. Beginning in 1932 with the *Annual Review of Biochemistry*, the Company has pursued as its principal function the publication of high-quality, reasonably priced *Annual Review* volumes. The volumes are organized by Editors and Editorial Committees who invite qualified authors to contribute critical articles reviewing significant developments within each major discipline. The Editor-in-Chief invites those interested in serving as future Editorial Committee members to communicate directly with him. Annual Reviews is administered by a Board of Directors, whose members serve without compensation.

Annu. Rev. Nutr. 2005. 25:1–8
doi: 10.1146/annurev.nutr.25.121304.131658

DIETARY FIBER: How Did We Get Where We Are?

Martin Eastwood
Gastrointestinal Unit, Department of Medicine, Western General Hospital, University of Edinburgh, Edinburgh EH43XU Scotland; email: martin.eastwood@btinternet.com

David Kritchevsky*
Wistar Institute, Philadelphia, Pennsylvania 19104; email: kritchevsky@wistar.org
**Corresponding author*

Key Words colon cancer, breast cancer, cardiovascular heart disease, diverticulosis, fermentable fiber metabolism

■ **Abstract** Dietary fiber has been a topic of considerable interest among nutritionists and clinicians for the past 50 years. Many studies on fiber have concentrated on fiber isolates, resulting in findings that have ignored fiber as a component of fruits, vegetables, nuts, cereals, and legumes in the general diet. The principle actions of fiber are to alter the nature of the contents of the gastrointestinal tract and to modify the absorption of other nutrients and chemicals. Fiber is but one component of plant food, and to neglect the other components—be they proteins, lipids, vitamins, minerals, antioxidants, or the secondary metabolites—is to seriously limit our understanding. Much of the effort expended in defining fiber and studying the fiber isolate would have been better focused using this whole-plant-food approach. Greater progress in our understanding of the relevance of fiber in the etiology of disease would have been achieved if a more holistic approach had been followed.

CONTENTS

EVOLUTION IN THE UNDERSTANDING OF DIETARY FIBER

Nutritionists and the public have not been consistent in their regard of fiber in the diet. Some have considered fiber as an integral part of the diet. For others, refinement of food, cereals in particular (especially in bread), and extraction of fruit juices, which are then fermented and even distilled to form alcoholic drinks, implies sophistication.

0199-9885/05/0714-0001$20.00

Throughout recorded history, the merit of whole foods has been emphasized by various writers beginning with Hippocrates, then Stubs and Tyron in the sixteenth century, and onto the nineteenth century with Graham (24) in the United States and Allinson (5) and Hurst (27) in Great Britain. In the United States, Kellogg (28) taught that whole cereal foods were important for health, whereas Alvarez (3) viewed humans as carnivores and condemned the use of extra roughage. Few of these strongly held opinions were supported by experimentation; exceptions include McCarrison (34), who served in the Indian Medical Service.

During the nineteenth and early twentieth century, advances were made in the analytical methodology of food components, including water, nitrogenous materials, and lipids, which leave a carbohydrate residue. Nutritionists required a more precise breakdown, and a crude fiber analysis, using acid and alkaline digestion-simulating events in the upper gastrointestinal tract, was developed by the Weende Experimental Station in Germany. This method was subsequently refined by Rubner and his colleagues (39). Atwater (8), at the turn of the twentieth century, showed that foods containing crude fiber increased fecal energy losses but crude fiber itself did not contribute to the metabolizable energy of the body. In their treatise, "The Chemical Composition of Foods," McCance & Widdowson (33) tackled the problem of analyzing food composition. They considered dietary carbohydrates as either available or unavailable. Available carbohydrates were absorbed in the foregut and were glucogenic. Unavailable carbohydrates (or roughage) were the indigestible structural carbohydrates (nonstarch polysaccharides and lignin) from the plant cell wall. Animal metabolic studies had shown that this unavailable carbohydrate was fermented in the colon, yielding short-chain fatty acids. Williams & Olmsted (47) also developed methods for analyzing available carbohydrates and the indigestible polysaccharides, hemicelluloses, cellulose, and lignin. Hellendoorn (26) emphasized the importance in colonic physiology of short-chain fatty acids released by fermentation in the colon.

Subsequent research on fiber has followed two paths, one physiological, the other committed to etiology and epidemiology. An early experiment was to measure the distribution of bile acids along the small intestine of the rat; contrary to expectations, the greatest amount was found in the ileum, where bile acids are absorbed (20). Increasing the fiber content of the diet of rats increased the pool of bile acids and the amount of these acids in the ileum. Subsequently, fiber—particularly lignin—was shown to adsorb bile acids (21). This led to two experiments in human male subjects, one conducted in a Trappist Cistercian monastery, and the other with volunteers. Each failed to show any hypocholesterolemic influence of increased dietary fiber or wheat bran (17, 22). The latter experiment was of additional interest: The length of each trial period was three weeks, which was the time available between a medical faculty ball and Christmas. This period has since been used in a number of experiments.

In separate studies, Kritchevsky & Tepper (31) showed that the protective effect of a commercial chow diet against the development of atheroma was not due to the small amount of unsaturated fat present but rather to the presence of fiber in the chow. Subsequent experiments with other polysaccharides (29) showed a consistent influence of fiber on lipid metabolism in animals. This finding led to experiments that showed fiber's ability to adsorb bile acids (30).

Cleave (16) argued lucidly that many of the diseases that are a product of civilization were secondary to those resulting from the consumption of refined or fiber-depleted carbohydrate foods, including sugar as well as white flour. Independently, Burkitt (13), Painter (36), Trowell (43), and Walker (45) convinced nutritionists and the public that fiber deficiency was a real problem.

While investigating his eponymous tumor, Burkitt had traveled widely in Africa to establish the peculiar geographical distribution of this cancer. He became puzzled by the apparent rarity of many surgical and medical diseases in black Africans, disorders that were common in Europe and in white Africans (13). Soon Burkitt started to diverge from the major point of Cleave's hypothesis by relating appendicitis, colorectal cancer, hemorrhoids, and varicose veins to low fiber intakes rather than to high sugar consumption. In the 1970s, Burkitt was joined by Trowell (43), Painter (36), and Walker (45) in declaiming that the low prevalence in developing countries of diabetes, gall stones, ischemic vascular disease, obesity and diverticular disorder, large bowel cancer, appendicitis, hiatal hernia, varicose veins, and hemorrhoids—all of which are commonly seen in Western countries—was due to diet, particularly to the greater amount of fiber consumed. Painter et al. (37) made the important observation that increased dietary fiber, particularly wheat bran, alleviated the symptoms of patients with diverticulosis, a condition that had long been treated with low-residue diets. This observation did much to stimulate the present intensive study of dietary fiber because it was based on objective evidence rather than extrapolations from observations and epidemiological evidence. Interest in fiber burgeoned, and fiber became important as a nutritional debating point and as a topic for research.

To study dietary fiber, two requirements had to be met. First, the definition of fiber had to be agreed upon. The debate over the definition of dietary fiber began before the publication of Trowell's paper in 1972 (43). His definition was viewed by some as too imprecise to be used to develop the quantitative studies that were essential for testing the epidemiological elements of the hypothesis (41, 42). Trowell's various definitions always contained three criteria for dietary fiber: a physiological, a botanical, and a chemical. Of these, only the first criterion, i.e., the resistance of dietary fiber against human digestive enzymes, has remained unchanged throughout the years. The botanical description changed from "skeletal remains of plant cells," to "remnants of plant cells," to "remnants of the plant cell wall," to "structural polymers of the plant cell wall." Trowell's chemical descriptions of dietary fiber were not precise and changed repeatedly. The American Association of Cereal Chemists' Fiber Definition Committee presented its definition of dietary fiber under the title "All Dietary Fiber is Fundamentally Functional." The committee defined dietary fiber as "functional, and if a fiber exhibits the requisite functionality(ies), it is dietary fiber, no matter what its source or history" (4).

The debate over developing a comprehensive definition for fiber continues today, and no single analytical strategy is fully able to incorporate all requirements. This is because both fiber and starch are omnipresent together in plant foods, and the physiological status of both dietary fiber and starch, e.g., resistant starch, is variable (23a, 40). Englyst & Cummings (23) proposed replacing the term "dietary fiber" with "non-starch polysaccharides." Heaton and colleagues (25) stressed the importance of the physical state of fiber, which is not usually emphasized in fiber definitions.

Second, methods of analysis had to be determined to study fiber. These methods of analysis have developed along two principle and different pathways (23, 35, 38, 42, 44): (*a*) gravimetric methods, in which the fiber is isolated and weighed, and (*b*) component analysis methods, in which dietary fiber constituents are determined more or less specifically.

Burkitt, Trowell, Painter, and Walker enthusiastically promoted the virtues of increasing the fiber content of the diet, and based their recommendations on what they perceived to be a self-evident fact, not a hypothesis (14, 36, 45). Although appealing to many, their lectures were not well received by all. They were clinicians, not nutritionists and, as most professionals with a medical clinical training, did not welcome polypharmacy. They preferred to focus on a single entity in the diet. They developed a reductionist approach, in contrast to the nutritionist's view of a rounded, complete diet in which all components are adequately represented. Perhaps Cleave's hypothesis (16) was closer to the view with which nutritionists currently would feel most comfortable.

Thirty-two years have passed since the British Nutrition Society hosted the first conference on dietary fiber in Edinburgh. Approximately 10,000 papers have been published since the 1950s on the topic of dietary fiber. Once attributed to a low-fiber diet, duodenal ulceration has been shown to be caused by *helicobacter pylorus*, and researchers have found other etiologies for hypertension, hiatus hernia, deep vein thrombosis, and diabetes.

What would have happened if Burkitt and Trowell had emphasized the value of plant foods? The epidemiology of the value of fruits, vegetables, and cereal grains (6), as opposed to only fiber, has proved to be much more consistent. The value of eating plant food, which incorporates dietary fiber and plant metabolites, might have been the focus of attention rather than fiber as one specific isolate (16, 18, 19).

Dietary fiber has never been formally accepted or proposed as an essential component of the diet. However, a diet containing little fiber has been blamed for many of the chronic diseases of modern society. The assumed importance of dietary fiber has been in its putative role in preventing a number of chronic and sometimes mortal conditions. This assumption led to discoveries relating to dietary fiber being accorded comparable significance to those of the discovery of vitamins, essential amino acids, and fatty acids. The influences of dietary fiber on a number of diseases (including heart disease, colonic diverticulosis, and cancer) are discussed at length in chapters in a recent compendium on fiber (15). It is evident that few indisputable effects of fiber alone have been identified. It is possible that the only condition with a clear etiological association with a low fiber-containing diet is the development of colonic diverticulosis (46).

THE METABOLIC FATE OF FERMENTABLE FIBERS: NEW DIRECTIONS

Dietary fiber has been described as a substance impervious to degradation by our endogenous enzymes. Fermentable fibers are degraded by the intestinal flora to yield short-chain fatty acids. However, when ^{14}C-labeled fiber is fed to rats, ^{14}C is incorporated into tissues in several forms. How these products affect overall metabolism remains to be elucidated. Uniformly labeled primary cells walls (^{14}C-PCW) were obtained by growing spinach cultures in a medium containing D-[U^{14}C-glucose]. The preparation yielded ^{14}C-homogalacturonan (30% of recovered ^{14}C), ^{14}C-rhamnogalacturonan (23% of recovered ^{14}C), other hemicelluloses (3% of recovered ^{14}C), and cellulose (21% of recovered ^{14}C). There were small amounts (<3%) of ^{14}C-protein and ^{14}C-starch. Recovered lignan was unlabeled. The pectic fraction of the plant cell walls was preferentially degraded completely in the gastrointestinal tract. Of the total ^{14}C dose, 22% was recovered in the host liver, adipose tissue, and skin; 26% was excreted as $^{14}CO_2$; and 18% appeared in the feces. ^{14}C was found in all tissues of the body, but it was particularly concentrated in the adrenal glands, colon, and cecum. ^{14}C was also recovered from the liver, where it was present predominantly in phospholipid, and in the skin, where it was present in protein and in fatty acids esterified into cholesterol.

When spinach cultures were incubated with D-[6-^{14}C] glucuronic acid, more than 85% of the label appeared at the C6 position of pectic galaturonic residues. A second preparation contained ^{14}C in the pectic methyl ester group. Rats fed uronate-labeled pectin excreted 37% of the label as $^{14}CO_2$, and those fed methyl-labeled pectin excreted 18%. In both studies, ^{14}C was recovered from the liver, mainly as protein (principally alanine), and in fatty acids esterified to cholesterol. In rats fed ^{14}C-labeled gelatinized starch, 25% of the ^{14}C was expressed as $^{14}CO_2$. When rats were fed resistant starch, ^{14}C was accumulated in muscle, skin, liver, and intestinal tissues.

These studies demonstrate both bacterial fermentation and host metabolism of the fermentation products. The study of pectin and starch metabolism under any number of physiological circumstances is now possible (1, 2, 9–12).

CONCLUSIONS

Dietary fiber has been and continues to be an exciting topic to explore. In retrospect, it was a mistake—possibly a necessary mistake—to isolate fiber from the overall field of plant food nutrition. One possible explanation for this is that clinicians

TABLE 1 Specific anticarcinogenic phytochemicals

Allium components	Isothiocyanates
Carotenoids	Limonene
Coumarins	Phenols
Flavonoids	Plant sterols
Folic acid	Saponins
Glucosinolates	Selenium
Indoles	Thiocyanates
Inositol hexaphosphate	Vitamin C
Isoflavones	Vitamin E

who were active in this field had medical training that emphasizes single-treatment regimes. As a result, research was focused on a single item. One bullet is enough, and more confuses.

The principle actions of fiber are to alter the nature of the contents of the gastrointestinal tract and to modify the absorption of other nutrients and chemicals. Plant whole foods are of fundamental importance in our diet. Although fiber is found in fruits, vegetables, nuts, cereals, and legumes, it is but one component of that plant food. Neglecting the other components, whether they be proteins, lipids, vitamins, minerals, antioxidants, or secondary metabolites, limits our understanding. Much of the effort on defining fiber and studying the fiber isolate would have been better applied to a whole-plant-food approach (see Table 1).

The mantra of five fruits and vegetables a day is an attempt to be holistic in approach. However, the value of this recommendation is blunted by not specifying which five, and whether they should be roots, stalks, red, green, or yellow. What components of these fruits, vegetables, nuts, and legumes are important? Our belief is that the list of important components of plant foods is only just beginning to be made, and in the future, secondary metabolites will be recognized as important. When they are identified, they should be fitted into this holistic nutritional approach rather than heralded, as with fiber, as an isolate that does everything. To complicate things further is the finding that, coincidental with intensive farming, the nutrient content of plants may vary (32). Another unexplored element is the possibility that individual needs may vary depending on the genetic makeup of the individual.

Nutrition is about food. Interest in a single component may further our understanding of the whole, but should not suggest supremacy of any one item. An analogy is the orchestra: It is important to discuss and understand each instrument, yet we must also recognize how the instruments interrelate. In the study of food, the nutritionist is the conductor, not the composer.

The *Annual Review of Nutrition* is online at http://nutr.annualreviews.org

LITERATURE CITED

1. Abia R, Fry SC, Eastwood MA. 1996. Fate of U-14C-gelatinized and U-14C-retrograded bean starch in the rat. *J. Food Sci. Agric.* 44:2316–23
2. Abia R, Fry SC, Eastwood MA. 1996. Metabolic transformation of U-14C-resistant and U-14C-gelatinized bean starch in the rat. *J. Food Sci. Agric.* 44:2324–29
3. Alvarez WC. 1931. *An Introduction to Gastro-Enterology*. London: Heinemann
4. Am. Assoc. Cereal Chemists Dietary Fiber Definition Comm. 2003. All dietary fiber is fundamentally functional. *Cereal Foods World* 48:128–31
5. Allinson TR. 1885. *The Advantages of Wholemeal Bread*. London: Allinson Publ.
6. Anderson JW. 2003. Whole grains protect against cardiovascular disease. *Proc. Nutr. Soc.* 62:13542
7. Deleted in proof
8. Atwater WO. 1900. Discussion of the terms digestibility, availability and fuel value. *Twelfth Annu. Rep. Storrs Agric. Exper. Station*, Storrs, Conn., p. 69
9. Buchanan CJ, Fry SC, Eastwood MA. 1994. Metabolism and fate of dietary (U-14C)-labelled spinach cell walls in the rat. *J. Sci. Food Agric.* 64:135–40
10. Buchanan CJ, Fry SC, Eastwood MA. 1994. The metabolism and fate of [methyl-14C] and [uronate-6-14C] pectin-labelled dietary plant cell walls in the rat. *J. Sci. Food Agric.* 66:163–73
11. Buchanan CJ, Fry SC, Eastwood MA. 1995. Metabolism of dietary (acetyl-1-14C)-plant cell walls in the rat intestine. *J. Sci. Food Agric.* 67:367–74
12. Buchanan CJ, Wallace G, Fry SC, Eastwood MA. 1996. In vivo release of 14C-labelled phenolic groups from intact dietary spinach cell walls during passage through the rat intestine. *J. Sci. Food Agric.* 71:459–46
13. Burkitt DP. 1969. Related disease—related cause? *Lancet* ii:1229–31
14. Burkitt DP, Trowell HC, eds. 1975. *Refined Carbohydrate Foods and Disease. Some Implications of Dietary Fibre*. London: Academic
15. Cho SS, Dreher ML, eds. 2001. *Handbook of Dietary Fiber*. New York: Marcel Dekker
16. Cleave TL. 1974. *The Saccharine Disease*. Bristol: Wright
17. Eastwood MA. 1969. Dietary fibre and serum lipids. *Lancet* ii:1222–24
18. Eastwood MA. 1999. Interaction of dietary antioxidants in vivo: how fruit and vegetables prevent disease? *Q. J. Med.* 92:527–30
19. Eastwood MA. 2001. A molecular biological basis for the nutritional and pharmacological benefits of dietary plants. *Q. J. Med.* 94:45–48
20. Eastwood MA, Boyd GS. 1968. Studies on the quantitative distribution of bile salts along the rat small intestine under varying dietary regimes. *Biochim. Biophys. Acta* 152:159–64
21. Eastwood MA, Hamilton D. 1968. Studies on the adsorption of bile salts to non-absorbed components of diet. *Biochim. Biophys. Acta* 152:159–66
22. Eastwood MA, Kirkpatrick J, Mitchell WD, Bone A, Hamilton T. 1973. Effects of dietary supplements of wheat bran and cellulose on faeces and bowel function. *Br. Med. J.* 4:392–94
23. Englyst HN, Cummings JH. 1990. Non-starch polysaccharides (dietary fiber) and resistant starch. In *New Developments of Dietary Fiber*, ed. I Furda, CJ Brine, pp. 205–25. New York: Plenum

23a. Food Nutr. Board, Inst. Health, Natl. Acad. Sci. 2001. *Dietary Reference Intakes; Proposed Definitions of Dietary Fiber*. Washington, DC: Natl. Acad. Press

24. Graham SA. 1837. *A Treatise on Bread and Bread Making*. Boston
25. Haber GB, Heaton KW, Murphy D, Burroughs L. 1977. Depletion and disruption of dietary fiber. Effects on satiety, plasma-glucose and serum-insulin. *Lancet* ii:679–82
26. Hellendoorn EW. 1983. Fermentation as the principal cause of the physiological activity of indigestible food residue. In *Topics in Dietary Fiber Research*, ed. GA Spiller, pp. 127–68. New York: Plenum
27. Hurst AF. 1909. *Constipation and Allied Intestinal Disorders*. London: Oxford Univ. Press
28. Kellogg JH. 1923. *New Dietetics: A Guide to Scientific Feeding in Health and Disease*. Battle Creek, MI: Modern Med. Publ.
29. Kritchevsky D. 1986. Dietary fiber and atherosclerosis. In *Dietary Fiber, Basic and Clinical Factors*, ed. GV Vahouny, D Kritchevsky, pp. 265–74. New York: Plenum
30. Kritchevsky D, Story JA. 1974. Binding of bile salts in vitro by non-nutritive fiber. *J. Nutr.* 104:458–62
31. Kritchevsky D, Tepper SA. 1968. Experimental atherosclerosis in rabbits fed cholesterol-free diets: influence of chow components. *J. Atheroscler. Res.* 8:357–69
32. Mayer A-M. 1997. Historical changes in the mineral content of fruits and vegetables. *Br. Food J.* 99:207–11
33. McCance RA, Widdowson EM. 1940. The chemical composition of foods. *Spec. Rep. Ser. Med. Res. Council*, No. 235. London: HMSO
34. McCarrison RA. 1926. A good diet and a bad one: an experimental contrast. *Indian J. Med. Res.* 14:649–57
35. McLeary BV. 2003. Dietary fibre analysis. *Proc. Nutr. Soc.* 62:3–9
36. Painter NS. 1975. *Diverticular Disease of the Colon*. London: Heinemann
37. Painter NS, Almeida AZ, Colebourne KW. 1972. Unprocessed bran in treatment of diverticular disease of the colon. *Br. Med. J.* 2:137–40
38. Prosky L, Asp N-G, Schweizer TF, DeVries JW, Furda I. 1988. Determination of insoluble, soluble and total dietary fiber in foods and food products: inter-laboratory study. *J. Assoc. Off. Anal. Chem.* 71:1017–23
39. Rubner M. 1917. Untersuchungen uber Vollkornbrot. *Arch. Anat. Physiol.* 74: 245–37
40. Southgate DAT. 1982. Definitions and Terminology of Dietary Fiber. In *Dietary Fiber in Health and Disease*, ed. Vahouny GV, Kritchevsky D, pp. 1–8. New York. Plenum
41. Southgate DAT. 1992. The dietary fibre hypothesis: a historical perspective in dietary fibre—a component of food. In *Nutritional Function in Health and Disease*, ed. TF Schweizer, CA Edwards, pp. 3–20. London: Springer-Verlag
42. Southgate DAT, Englyst HN. 1985. Dietary fibre: chemistry, physical properties and analysis. In *Dietary Fibre, Fibre-Depleted Foods and Disease*, ed. H Trowell, D Burkitt, K Heaton, pp. 31–55. London: Academic
43. Trowell HC. 1972. Ischemic heart disease and dietary fiber. *Am. J. Clin. Nutr.* 25:926–32
44. Van Soest PJ. 1963. Use of detergents in the analysis of fibrous feeds. II. A rapid method for the determination of fiber and lignin. *J. Assoc. Off. Anal. Chem.* 46:829–35
45. Walker ARP. 1974. Dietary fibre and the patterns of disease. *Ann. Intern. Med.* 80: 663–64
46. Wess L, Eastwood M, Busuttil A, Edwards C, Millar ER. 1996. An association between maternal diet and colonic diverticulosis in an animal model. *Gut* 39:423–27
47. Williams RD, Olmsted WH. 1936. The effects of cellulose, hemicellulose and lignans on the weight of the stool: a contribution to the study of laxation in man. *J. Nutr.* 11:433–39

Annu. Rev. Nutr. 2005. 25:9–35
doi: 10.1146/annurev.nutr.24.012003.132159

First published online as a Review in Advance on April 22, 2005

DEFECTIVE GLUCOSE HOMEOSTASIS DURING INFECTION

Owen P. McGuinness
Department of Molecular Physiology and Biophysics, Vanderbilt University School of Medicine, Nashville, Tennessee 37232-0615; email: owen.mcguinness@vanderbilt.edu

Key Words glucagon, insulin resistance, sepsis, nutritional support, enteral nutrition, parenteral nutrition, hyperglycemia, gluconeogenesis, lactate

■ **Abstract** Infection leads to profound alterations in whole-body metabolism, which is characterized by marked acceleration of glucose, fat and protein, and amino acid flux. One of the complications of infection, especially in the nutritionally supported setting, is hyperglycemia. The hyperglycemia is caused by peripheral insulin resistance and alterations in hepatic glucose metabolism. The defects in hepatic glucose metabolism include overproduction of glucose and a failure of the liver to appropriately adapt when nutritional support is administered. Investigators have suggested that multiple factors contribute to the observed defects. In this review, I focus primarily on alterations in carbohydrate metabolism, examining both the metabolic response to infection and inflammatory stress, the role of the accompanying neuroendocrine and inflammatory responses in the metabolic response, and the interaction between the endocrine response to infection and nutritional support.

CONTENTS

INTRODUCTION

Infection leads to profound alterations in whole-body metabolism, which is characterized by marked acceleration of glucose, fat and protein, and amino acid flux. This acceleration of flux per se is not detrimental except that it is accompanied by net protein loss and diabetic-like hyperglycemia. These two accompanying metabolic side effects, along with a number of other factors, influence the morbidity and mortality of the individuals with accompanying infections. Many of these patients receive nutritional support. Yet until recently the threshold for correcting hyperglycemia has been rather high (~200 mg/dl). Recent clinical trials indicate that aggressive management of glucose levels in the ICU setting (~100 mg/dl) has marked beneficial effects on morbidity and mortality (48, 56, 152, 159, 160). The primary option for management of hyperglycemia is the administration of exogenous insulin. While exogenous insulin can be a panacea in correcting hyperglycemia, recent evidence suggests that it may also modulate the underlying inflammatory response.

In this review, I focus primarily on alterations in carbohydrate metabolism. I begin with a discussion of the general metabolic response to infection and inflammatory stress and the factors that contribute to the acceleration of glucose flux. The neuroendocrine response is a major mediator of the changes in glucose flux during infection. To better understand how these hormones can contribute to the overall metabolic response to inflammation I first discuss how these hormones regulate hepatic metabolism both acutely and chronically in the absence of inflammation. This is followed by a discussion of how the presence of inflammation alters their normal interaction and the ability of insulin to modulate their action. In fact, inflammation impairs the responsiveness of the liver and other tissues to both anabolic and catabolic hormones. The net interaction of the underlying defects in hormonal responsiveness and the accompanying hormonal response determines the overall response, which is generally catabolic. Finally, I discuss the unique response of the body to nutritional support. The liver switches from a site of glucose production in the fasted state to a major site of glucose consumption during nutritional support, and inflammation blocks the liver's normal response. The failure of the liver to consume glucose efficiently during nutritional support aggravates the hyperglycemia that is seen.

OVERALL CHANGES IN GLUCOSE FLUX DURING INFLAMMATION

One of the characteristic effects of infection is hyperglycemia (13). The magnitude of the hyperglycemia is influenced by the fasting state and the severity of the illness. Glucose utilization is increased during infection due to the combined increase in glucose clearance and glucose levels (mass action). In spite of the increase in glucose utilization, hyperglycemia occurs due to a combined increase in glucose production and a failure of peripheral glucose clearance to increase in proportion to the increase in glucose production (49).

Hypoglycemia can be observed during inflammatory stress. A potent stimulator of the inflammatory response is endotoxin. Following the acute injection of endotoxin in humans there is a rapid rise in splanchnic glucose release and a gradual rise in arterial glucose levels (49). With increasing doses of endotoxin in other species, the increase in glucose production (two- to threefold) is more robust and is persistent (91). However, despite this increase, hypoglycemia can develop after a period of hyperglycemia. In fact, with very high doses of endotoxin the progression to hypoglycemia can be very rapid and can be accompanied by a fall, rather than a rise, in glucose production. The mechanism for this is discussed below.

During prolonged infection, as is seen in the intensive care unit, basal glucose production is increased [twofold (134, 143, 155)] after a brief fast in the presence or absence of hyperglycemia (Figure 1). This increase is seen in animal models as well (90, 106). The contribution of glycogenolysis and gluconeogenesis to the increase in glucose production is dependent upon the duration of the stress. Following the acute administration of endotoxin, glycogenolysis is the primary source of the glucose carbon (119), but during chronic infections, if glycogen stores are depleted, an increase in gluconeogenesis contributes to the enhancement of glucose production (90, 106). Although gluconeogenesis has not been directly measured in glycogen-replete states, both processes are likely increased.

In some ways, it is surprising that gluconeogenesis can increase during an inflammatory stress; however, this is dose and possibly species dependent. It is well known that prior exposure to endotoxin or infection decreases the capacity of the liver to synthesize glucose in vitro (14, 29, 47, 67, 123, 149, 162). Increases in gluconeogenic precursor supply and hormones that are known to enhance gluconeogenesis are ineffective in livers isolated from infected animals. Yet in vivo, except following very severe inflammatory stress where hypoglycemia can develop, gluconeogenesis is either maintained at baseline or increased. Presumably, the infection-induced increase in gluconeogenic substrate supply and the elevated levels of stress hormones combine to sustain, and in some cases augment, the gluconeogenic rate in vivo.

GLUCONEOGENESIS AND SUBSTRATE AVAILABILITY DURING INFLAMMATION

Substrate availability has been promoted as a primary mechanism for the increase in glucose production during inflammatory stress. While adequate substrate availability is required to support elevated gluconeogenic rates, enhanced substrate delivery alone does not translate into an increase in glucose production. Acute increases in lactate or alanine do not increase glucose production (28, 38, 109), even in a glycogen-depleted setting where glucagon is markedly increased (110,

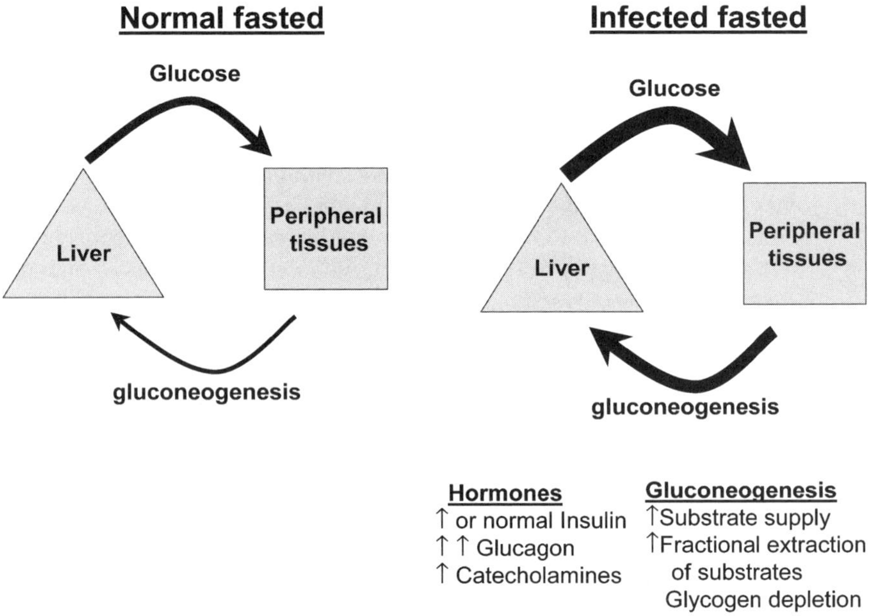

Figure 1 Impact of inflammation on gluconeogenesis and hepatic glucose production in the fasted state.

167). An increase in gluconeogenic precursor availability, even in stressed states, does not impair insulin suppression of liver glucose production (155). Thus, gluconeogenic precursor availability per se is not an important determinant of glucose production.

Fatty acid availability and the hormonal environment can dictate the effectiveness of the increase in substrate supply. Combined increases in gluconeogenic precursor supply and fatty acids will increase hepatic glucose production (109). Increases in fatty acids impair insulin suppression of hepatic glucose production (147). They suppress the glycogenolytic and enhance the gluconeogenic effects of both glucagon and epinephrine (24, 61). Given that fatty acid availability is increased during infection and inflammatory stress (166, 169), this may help contribute to any observed increase in gluconeogenesis.

A reciprocal fall in net glycogen breakdown buffers the effect of a rise in gluconeogenic precursor supply on hepatic glucose production. Gluconeogenic precursor uptake increases as substrate supply increases. In a setting of fixed hormone levels, physiologic increases in alanine concentration proportionally increase net hepatic alanine uptake (38). Increases in lactate concentration increase net hepatic lactate uptake, but this is not a linear function of substrate delivery (28). Investigators who decreased substrate supply in septic rats and humans using dichloroacetic acid (DCA) (59, 86) observed a fall in lactate and a concomitant fall in glucose production, which suggests substrate supply helps drive the rise in glucose production. In humans, infusion of DCA (73) will modulate glucose production in a setting where glycogen stores are depleted. Unfortunately, DCA may exert effects on the liver and peripheral tissues, which makes interpretations of the effects of substrate supply on liver glucose production suspect (39).

Although increased lactate production does contribute to the elevated lactate levels during inflammatory stress, this is not the only story. In fact, whole-body lactate flux increases to a lesser extent than lactate levels in septic patients, suggesting that lactate clearance falls. To address the potential role of hypoxia in the elevated lactate levels, DCA was administered to enhance pyruvate dehydrogenase activity in muscle (59). Using radiolabeled glucose and pyruvate, the investigators observed that DCA enhanced the fraction of pyruvate oxidized, despite a marked lowering of lactate and pyruvate levels, which suggests that anaerobic glycolysis may not be a significant contributor to elevated lactate levels during sepsis. That tissue hypoxia is not the primary mechanism for the lactic acidosis is supported by the fact that tissue levels of adenosine triphosphate, as assessed with phosphorus nuclear magnetic resonance in animals, are not decreased (71).

The two determinants of the gluconeogenic response are the delivery of gluconeogenic substrates to the liver (product of liver blood flow and substrate concentration) and the ability of the liver to extract the gluconeogenic precursors. Depending upon the magnitude of the stress and the specific gluconeogenic precursor, one or both may determine the gluconeogenic response in a given species. Although it is often stated that gluconeogenic precursor supply increases during infection, in fact this is not true for all gluconeogenic precursors. In humans (49), following a very low dose of endotoxin, gluconeogenic precursor delivery increased primarily because of a rise in lactate concentration, as the levels of other gluconeogenic precursors (alanine and glutamine) fell. This increase in lactate concentration, combined with the 50% increase in splanchnic blood flow, resulted in an increase in hepatic lactate delivery. The rise in lactate delivery primarily dictated the change in lactate uptake by the splanchnic bed, since splanchnic fractional extraction of lactate did not increase. Despite a fall in alanine and glutamine levels, net splanchnic uptake of both precursors increased because of a rise in fractional extraction by the splanchnic bed and the rise in splanchnic blood flow. The rise in gluconeogenic precursor uptake could account for approximately 50% of the endotoxin-induced rise in liver glucose production in the human after a very low dose of endotoxin. In other species where higher doses of endotoxin can be given, the rise in lactate is due in part to a decrease in whole-body lactate clearance (138); however, increases in lactate turnover contribute as well (165). Adrenergic blockade attenuated the rise in lactate concentration (64). Nevertheless, it is difficult to evaluate the role of the catecholamines, since hypoglycemia and hypotension developed during adrenergic blockade. With higher doses of endotoxin in a canine model, glycogen breakdown was the primary source of the increase in glucose production, despite the fact that the levels of lactate and alanine rose (119). The actual uptake of these substrates by the liver does not increase markedly in endotoxemia.

In the glycogen-depleted setting, the liver is a net consumer of lactate. However, following the administration of endotoxin, the net uptake of lactate decreases and in fact, the liver transiently switches to lactate release, in spite of a rise in arterial lactate levels. The switch to lactate release occurs because of a robust increase in hepatic glycolysis driven by a concomitant rise in hepatic glycogenolysis. In the case of alanine, arterial levels rise progressively. Yet the fractional extraction of alanine tends to fall, minimizing the rise in net hepatic alanine uptake. When combined with the fact that net hepatic uptakes of the other gluconeogenic amino acids (threonine, glutamine, serine, and glycine) do not rise, net hepatic uptake of gluconeogenic precursors [an index of gluconeogenesis (119)] does not rise following the administration of endotoxin.

With chronic infections, gluconeogenesis is likely increased. An increase in gluconeogenesis has been directly assessed in animal models (106). Although it likely increased in humans (143), gluconeogenesis has not been accurately quantified. The method used to assess gluconeogenesis (tracer-determined alanine conversion to glucose) is prone to errors and does not yield a quantifiable measure of gluconeogenesis (81). Moreover, this method does not separate the contributions of the kidney and the liver to whole-body gluconeogenesis. Normally renal gluconeogenesis is a minor contributor to whole-body glucose flux (20). However, the kidney can be a significant site of lactate removal in stressful settings (6). As with an acute inflammation, the relationship between increases in lactate levels and net splanchnic lactate uptake in chronic infection are not straightforward. In severely septic patients, the splanchnic bed is not a significant producer or consumer of lactate (32) despite marked elevations in lactate levels. The net balance of lactate in patients who were consumers of lactate could at most account for less than 1% (0.01 mg/kg/min) of the predicted net splanchnic glucose output (~2 mg/kg/min). With lethal doses of endotoxin, the impairment in gluconeogenic capacity of the liver is so marked that total glucose production rapidly falls and hypoglycemia ensues once hepatic glycogen stores are depleted. In that setting, the liver is not a significant consumer or producer of lactate (23). Thus, despite the increased availability of lactate and in many cases other gluconeogenic substrates during infection and inflammation, the relative importance of gluconeogenesis and glycogenolysis to the total rate of glucose production is difficult to predict.

NORMAL INTERACTION BETWEEN COUNTERREGULATORY HORMONES AND HEPATIC METABOLISM

The alteration in metabolism that accompanies inflammation represents an integration of three separate but interrelated biological responses: (*a*) activation of the neuroendocrine system, (*b*) release of cytokines from the activated immune system, and (*c*) release of lipid mediators from multiple cell types (84). The differing metabolic responses to acute endotoxin administration and chronic infection can be explained in part by the differing acute and chronic responses of the liver to stress hormones.

Since Shamoon et al. (139) conducted their original studies, it has been hypothesized that many of the metabolic responses observed during infection could be explained by a synergistic interaction between the accompanying hormonal responses to inflammation. In these seminal studies, Shamoon and colleagues demonstrated that the hyperglycemic response to a hormone could be amplified if other counterregulatory hormones were also infused. In those studies (139), it was observed that over the course of 5 to 7.5 hours of hormone infusion, epinephrine (13x basal)-amplified glucagon stimulated glucose turnover. The addition of cortisol (4x basal) further enhanced stimulation of glucose turnover, such that the response was greater than the sum of their individual effects. Unfortunately, defining how these hormones interact acutely as well as chronically to control the metabolic response is complex. Moreover, it is even more complex, given that during infection these hormones have to interact with the immune response. To explain how these hormones might interact, the discussion below first describes some of the known effects of these hormones when they are infused acutely in isolation, and then relates what is known about how some of them interact.

Glucagon is a potent stimulator of glucose production; its effect wanes with time (19, 21). The effect of glucagon on glucose production has been shown to result primarily from a rapid, potent, time-dependent effect on glycogenolysis, and to a lesser extent, from a less potent, slower effect on gluconeogenesis (22, 104). In fact, glucagon has been shown to acutely increase hepatic gluconeogenic efficiency in vivo (154), yet the contribution of the rise in gluconeogenesis to the increase in glucose production was small. This paradox may be explained by the fact that glucagon has little effect on gluconeogenic substrate mobilization from muscle or fat. Thus, any enhancement of gluconeogenic flux would initially increase gluconeogenesis, but then the gluconeogenic substrate levels in blood would fall and the gluconeogenic contribution to glucose production would return toward its basal rate.

Epinephrine can also increase glucose production in a rapid, time-dependent manner, albeit with a decreased sensitivity on a molar basis compared with glucagon (26, 153). The effect of epinephrine on glucose production results from a stimulation of both gluconeogenesis and glycogenolysis. The increase in gluconeogenesis is due to the indirect action of the hormone on peripheral substrate release, whereas enhancement of glycogenolysis is due to the direct action of epinephrine on the liver (25, 27). Subsequent studies (61) demonstrated that when the hormone increased the gluconeogenic precursor supply, it caused a compensatory decrease in its glycogenolytic action, implying a reciprocal relationship between the two processes. Increasing the gluconeogenic precursor supply to the liver increased gluconeogenesis but did not increase total glucose production, thereby implying a decrease in glycogenolysis. Studies examining the interaction between epinephrine, cortisol, and glucagon clearly demonstrate that they can have an additive effect on glucose production (60, 61, 100), with little evidence of synergy. Moreover, the mobilization of gluconeogenic substrates by epinephrine only increases the contribution of gluconeogenesis to whole-body glucose production.

In summary, although the studies of Shamoon et al. (139) would suggest potential synergy between counterregulatory hormones in the acute setting, in subsequent well-controlled studies there was little evidence of synergy. Moreover, although these hormones may differentially regulate gluconeogenic precursor supply and consequently the contribution of gluconeogenesis to total glucose production, gluconeogenic precursor supply does not determine the overall rate of glucose production.

For many types of inflammatory stressors, the endocrine response persists for multiple days. The metabolic response to a chronic elevation in hormones may differ markedly from that seen in the acute setting. Studies (7, 54) in humans observed that a combined infusion of glucagon, epinephrine, and cortisol (5- to 20-fold and 4-fold, respectively) for three days could lead to sustained hyperglycemia and elevated glucose production. Subsequent studies in dogs (111), using a three-day infusion of glucagon, epinephrine, norepinephrine, and cortisol, produced a metabolic response similar to that in humans. The sustained increase in liver glucose production was due primarily ($\sim$70%) to an increase in gluconeogenesis.

Additional studies examined the contribution of the individual hormones to the overall response to chronic (three days) stress hormone infusion (SHI). Initial studies examined the impact of the acute discontinuation of a specific hormone after a chronic SHI. Acute removal of glucagon (three hours) markedly decreased net hepatic glucose output and hepatic glycogenolysis (115). Net hepatic gluconeogenic precursor uptake was not altered; the majority of the gluconeogenic carbon was diverted to glycogen synthesis. A similar response was observed when the chronic epinephrine infusion was discontinued (117). Net hepatic glucose output was completely suppressed, whereas net hepatic gluconeogenic precursor uptake was minimally affected. These data could be interpreted to suggest that both epinephrine and glucagon have no impact on gluconeogenesis and primarily affect hepatic glycogen metabolism. Thus, another hormone (e.g., cortisol or norepinephrine) must drive the rise seen in gluconeogenesis during chronic SHI. Yet chronic infusion of cortisol alone has only modest effects on gluconeogenesis (58), and acute removal of norepinephrine had little, if any, impact. The impact of acute removal of a hormone may not reflect its role in a chronic process such as SHI.

The impact of the absence of a chronic elevation of a single hormone on the overall metabolic response to SHI was also evaluated. The absence of an increase in glucagon during SHI nearly completely prevented the SHI-induced increase in net hepatic glucose output (107). Interestingly, despite chronic elevations in cortisol and catecholamines, futile cycling of glucose into and out of the liver was enhanced, which suggests that glucagon can serve as a brake to limit hepatic glucose entry in a setting of hyperglycemia and thus sustain the hyperglycemia. Moreover, the rise in gluconeogenesis was absent despite marked elevations in gluconeogenic substrate (e.g., lactate and alanine) concentrations. The most dramatic effects were a failure of the liver to revert to lactate consumption despite elevated lactate concentrations and a failure of net hepatic alanine fractional extraction to increase. Conversely, the absence of an increase in epinephrine also blunted the hyperglycemia, but it had little impact on gluconeogenesis or gluconeogenic precursor supply (116). This is in marked contrast to the acute effects of epinephrine, which enhances gluconeogenic supply and gluconeogenesis. In contrast to epinephrine, the lack of a rise in norepinephrine had little impact on the overall metabolic response to SHI. Interestingly, the absence of a rise in cortisol eliminated the SHI-induced increase in gluconeogenesis, primarily by decreasing substrate supply (51). The enhanced extraction of gluconeogenic substrates by the liver persisted. Moreover, hepatic glycogen stores, which in fact tended to rise during SHI, were markedly depleted by SHI when a rise in cortisol was absent. This is consistent with the observed increase in hepatic glycogen content when cortisol was increased chronically in the absence of a rise in the other counterregulatory hormones (58).

Thus, in the context of elevations in multiple counterregulatory hormones, these hormones work in concert to maintain hyperglycemia by increasing hepatic glucose production (both glycogenolysis and gluconeogenesis; Figure 1). The synergy that can occur between the hormones in augmenting net hepatic glucose production is accomplished by targeting one of four cellular processes: (*a*) substrate supply, (*b*) the capacity of the liver to take up gluconeogenic precursors, (*c*) mobilization of glycogen stores, or (*d*) facilitation of glucose release by the liver while minimizing hepatic glucose entry.

HORMONAL CONTROL OF THE METABOLIC RESPONSE TO INFLAMMATION

The metabolic response to inflammation is complex. The alterations that accompany infection represent an integration of three separate but interrelated biological responses: (*a*) activation of the neurohumoral system, (*b*) production of cytokines, and (*c*) release of lipid mediators from multiple cell types. The intertwining of these systems has made it difficult to differentiate between the primary and the secondary events, which direct the metabolic response to infection.

Activation of the adrenergic system appears to be one of the primary mechanisms for the rapid increase in hepatic glucose production that occurs following acute endotoxin administration (64). Combined (α and β) adrenergic blockade prevented the increase in hepatic glucose production in the conscious rat. Interestingly, blockade of either α or β adrenergic receptors did not completely attenuate the response to endotoxin.

The rise in glucagon may also contribute to the rise in hepatic glucose production. Glucagon is markedly elevated during infection and inflammation (8, 12, 30, 49, 88). The increase in glucagon levels is generally greater than one might see during hypoglycemia (9). Moreover, although the rise in glucagon secretion has not been directly measured during inflammation, it is substantially greater than the rise in the arterial levels (70). The glucagon assay detects both the biologically active glucagon and a large molecular-weight glucagon that is thought to be derived from the intestine (161). As much as 50% of the basal immunoreactive glucagon is not biologically active. Consequently, a doubling of immunoreactive glucagon levels (50 to 100 pg/ml) can represent a more than fourfold rise in glucagon secretion.

The rise in glucagon may also contribute to the rise in hepatic glucose production following endotoxin administration. The endotoxin-induced rise in glucagon persisted in the presence of adrenergic blockade, yet an increase in hepatic glucose production was absent (64). This led the authors to conclude that the rise in glucagon does not contribute to the endotoxin-induced rise in hepatic glucose production. In a normal setting, the rise in glucagon observed during endotoxemia would markedly increase hepatic glucose metabolism (154). It is likely that if glucagon had not increased, hepatic glucose production would have fallen below basal rates because of the concomitant rise in insulin or more likely because of an underlying impairment in hepatic metabolism. As a result, hypoglycemia would have developed. In fact, one of the hallmarks of a rise in glucagon is a rise in the fractional extraction of alanine by the liver (154). Following endotoxin administration, hepatic fractional extraction of alanine did not increase, consistent with an impairment in glucagon action during endotoxemia (119). At present, no studies have assessed the role of glucagon in the response to endotoxin.

A number of investigators have examined the role of catecholamines and glucagon in the overall hepatic response to chronic stress. In one of the first studies (72), which was done in burn patients, somatostatin was infused with replacement of insulin with or without glucagon replacement. When glucagon was not replaced, endogenous glucose production and arterial glucose concentration decreased markedly. Exogenous glucose had to be infused to prevent hypoglycemia. Subsequent studies in dogs (113, 168) and rats (88) with an infection also demonstrated that acute correction of the hyperglucagonemia decreased hepatic glucose production due to a fall in hepatic glycogenolysis.

We (113) observed, using a combination of tracer and arterio-venous difference techniques, that suppression of the hyperglucagonemia did not alter net hepatic gluconeogenic precursor uptake. In the specific case of alanine, the fall in net hepatic fractional extraction of alanine after lowering the glucagon concentration was offset by a gradual elevation of arterial alanine concentration. This is consistent with the known potent effect of glucagon on hepatic amino acid transport (75). The fall in glucose production was due to a diversion of the gluconeogenic carbon to glycogen rather than release as glucose. In many ways, this is reminiscent of the effects observed when glucagon was acutely discontinued during SHI (115). The lack of a detectable effect on the gluconeogenic process may indicate that the impact of the acute removal of glucagon does not reflect its chronic role during an infection. If the glucagon response was simulated in noninfected animals, liver glucose production was not augmented (114). However, when the chronic glucagon infusion was acutely discontinued, a comparable fall in hepatic glucose output was observed and hepatic gluconeogenic precursor uptake was unaltered

(114). The chronic hyperglucagonemia markedly augmented the capacity of the liver to take up gluconeogenic precursors. Yet this did not enhance net hepatic gluconeogenic precursor uptake and glucose output, presumably because the arterial gluconeogenic substrate concentrations decreased (109). In fact, this up-regulation in the capacity to take up gluconeogenic precursors (specifically alanine) far exceeded that seen when an infection accompanied the hyperglucagonemia (106). Thus, a defect in glucagon action may limit glucagon effectiveness in augmenting the gluconeogenic process when an infection is present.

Catecholamines also contribute to the increase in hepatic glucose production during infection; however, their importance is dependent upon the severity of the stress. Following a mild infection in which basal catecholamines were minimally elevated, combined adrenergic blockade had no effect on hepatic glucose production (63). When sympathetic outflow was markedly elevated, combined adrenergic (α and β) blockade prevented the sepsis-induced (168) as well as the endotoxin-induced (64, 82) increase in hepatic glucose production. The elevated lactate levels seen during chronic infection were not altered by adrenergic blockade (82). However, they were attenuated following an acute administration of endotoxin (64).

Glucocorticoids increase markedly following endotoxemia (46, 119, 136, 156). Their acute role in sustaining liver glucose production is likely modest. Adrenalectomy increases the susceptibility to hypoglycemia (105). Acute elevations in cortisol have minimal effects on hepatic glucose production or gluconeogenesis (57). As mentioned above, cortisol may amplify the effects of the other counterregulatory hormones.

Interpreting the roles of the endocrine hormones is difficult in a setting where insulin is ever changing and its ability to antagonize the hormones may be modified by the accompanying illness. Thus, quantifying the role of a given classical counterregulatory hormone in the overall metabolic response of the liver is difficult. Moreover, as is discussed below, since the accompanying cytokine response to inflammatory stress interacts with and may actually blunt the effectiveness of the stress hormones as well as insulin, defining the specific role of a hormone may be difficult.

INSULIN RESISTANCE AND INFLAMMATION

Insulin resistance is characteristic of sepsis and inflammation. It is reversible once the injury or inflammation has been resolved. Many tissues are involved, including the muscle, liver, and adipose, and the inflammatory cells themselves. Because of the multiple cellular targets and the difficulty in controlling for variables such as duration of fasting, age, glycemia, severity of injury, and drug treatment, quantifying the extent of the glucose intolerance was initially difficult (103). An additional confounding response was that of endotoxemia, where hypoglycemia can occur, and initially investigators suggested either insulin action was enhanced or endotoxin induced insulin-like effects (47, 96).

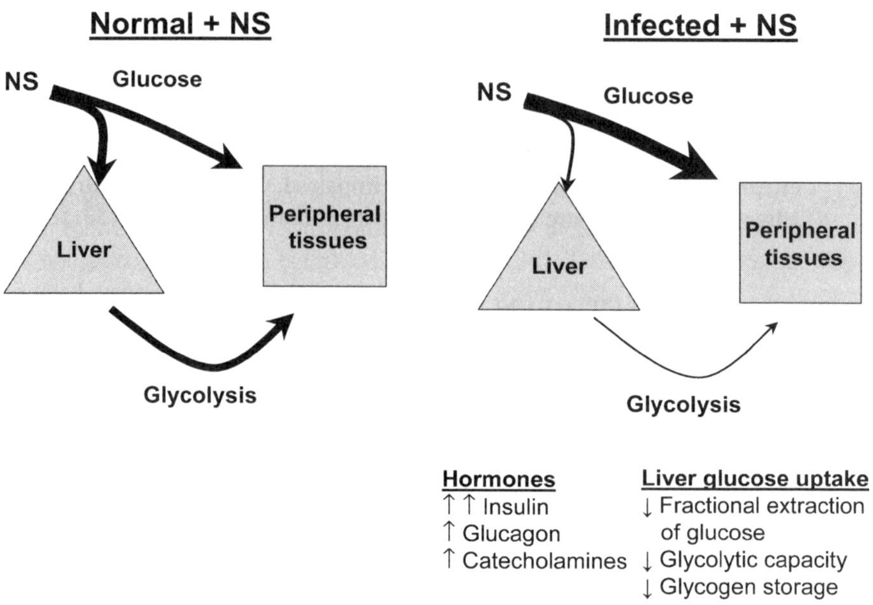

Figure 2 Impact of inflammation on glucose uptake by hepatic and peripheral tissues during nutritional support (NS).

75% of the glucose taken up was released as lactate and delivered to peripheral tissues (i.e., reverse Cori cycle). Since removal of lactate by peripheral tissues is more efficient than glucose and is not dependent upon insulin (28), the response of the liver limits the severity of the hyperglycemia and hyperinsulinemia that otherwise would occur (Figure 2). Clearly then, any defect in hepatic glucose uptake during TPN would predispose the individual to hyperglycemia and/or hyperinsulinemia.

Interestingly, the rate of glucose uptake by the liver during chronic TPN is greater than that which would have been predicted based upon acute studies. The liver of the normal animal receiving chronic TPN consumes a substantial net quantity of glucose (~4.5 mg/kg^{-1}/min^{-1}) in the presence of normal glucose levels (120 mg/dl) and only mild hyperinsulinemia (15 μU/ml) (108). In the acute setting, these levels of insulin and glucose would not initiate net hepatic glucose uptake (NHGU). Three factors regulate NHGU acutely: the hepatic glucose load (blood flow $\times$ glucose level), the hormonal milieu (insulin and glucagon levels), and the route of glucose delivery (portal signal). Physiologic increases in glucose alone will not induce NHGU. However, in the presence of elevated glucose, insulin increases NHGU in a dose-dependent manner. It is enhanced further if the glucose is administered into the portal vein (which activates the portal signal) (125, 127). To induce NHGU of the magnitude seen in the normal animal during TPN (~4 mg/kg^{-1}/min^{-1}), the arterial plasma glucose levels would have to be greater than 200 mg/dl and the arterial insulin levels would have to exceed 170 μU/ml (125). In fact, to obtain substantial NHGU with more physiologic insulin levels (~30 μU/ml), the glucose would have to be infused into the portal vein to activate the portal signal and the arterial glucose levels would have to exceed 200 mg/dl. Thus, the liver of the TPN-adapted dog increased its capacity to consume glucose. A potential explanation is an increase in glucokinase activity (5, 126), possibly initiated by the prolonged exposure to mild hyperinsulinemia and to the very low glucagon levels seen during TPN. However, this likely is not the sole explanation.

The acute versus chronic modulation of liver glucose uptake in the setting of continuous nutritional support varies markedly. Glycogen synthesis is the primary fate of glucose taken up by the liver following a meal (127). Surprisingly, despite the large activation of glycolysis following TPN, acute increases in glucose and insulin or direct activation of glucokinase primarily divert the additional glucose carbon to glycogen rather than to lactate (17, 41). The preferential diversion of glucose carbon to glycogen may be explained by a property of glucokinase (i.e., hexokinase IV). Overexpression of glucokinase, but not hexokinase I, diverts glucose to glycogen. In contrast, overexpression of hexokinase I diverts the glucose to glycolysis (137). The fact that acute manipulation of glucose and insulin, as well as glucokinase, diverts glucose away from a very active glycolytic pathway during TPN is consistent with this observation. Thus, glycogen synthesis is the preferred site for glucose disposal when acute manipulations are made, irrespective of the liver's metabolic state.

The mechanism whereby glycogen is no longer a major metabolic fate during TPN is unknown. Overexpression of glucokinase improves hepatic glucose utilization (137). Because glucokinase preferentially diverts glucose to glycogen, this casts doubt on activation of glucokinase as the sole explanation for the increased rate of glucose uptake and lactate release during TPN. Glycogen synthesis may be suppressed by accumulating glycogen stores (37). However, glycogen synthase activity does not decrease in glycogen-replete rats (53), and acute activation of glucokinase is very effective in augmenting liver glucose uptake (42) in the TPN-adapted state. Glycogenolysis may increase to equal the rate of glycogen synthesis, leading to rapid cycling of glucose through glycogen. Consistent with this, while 75% of NHGU is released as lactate during TPN, only 30% of U-^{14}C glucose taken up by the liver is diverted to lactate. The remainder of the U-^{14}C glucose either accumulates in glycogen or is oxidized. However, a net decrease in glycogen synthesis alone likely will not explain the preferential diversion to lactate. A specific activation of glycolysis, possibly mediated by a rise in fructose 2,6-bisphosphate, an activator of phosphofructokinase, and pyruvate kinase, likely contributes (131).

In response to infection, the ability of the liver to remove an exogenous glucose load acutely delivered into a peripheral vein is decreased (112). We have observed a similar response in infected animals adapted to TPN (108). The infection-induced decrease in NHGU during an acute peripheral glucose infusion was due to both an impaired stimulation of hepatic glucose uptake and an impaired suppression of hepatic glucose production (112). The impaired suppression of glucose production is a characteristic of infection in humans (11, 142). In the TPN-adapted animal, an impairment in hepatic glucose uptake (Figure 2) is the primary contributor to the defect during infection; however, glucose production would be elevated as well were it not for the compensatory hyperinsulinemia (40). The mechanism(s) for this is (are) unknown.

Elevated glucagon concentrations likely contribute to the impaired net liver glucose uptake during infection. Chronic elevations in glucagon may also explain the need for additional insulin to restrain hepatic glucose production. Acute increases in glucagon antagonize liver glucose uptake by stimulating hepatic glucose production and inhibiting glycogen synthesis (66). However, the acute and chronic effects of glucagon are markedly different. Acutely, glucagon regulates glycogen metabolism, but chronically it regulates gluconeogenesis (107, 115). As mentioned above, chronically it can limit cortisol-induced enhancement in liver glucose uptake and facilitate glucose production (51). It is most effective in increasing gluconeogenesis when an adequate supply of gluconeogenic amino acids and lipids, both of which are supplied in TPN, are present (102, 112). One possible mechanism by which glucagon could limit liver glucose uptake is inhibition of glucokinase (129, 130). However, chronic activation of glucokinase (chronic fructose infusion) alone cannot correct the infection-induced impairment in liver glucose uptake (43). This suggests that the infection-induced impairment in liver glucose uptake may be due to defects at multiple sites. Glucagon is a potent inhibitor of phosphofructokinase and pyruvate kinase (129, 130). Thus, combined decreases in glucokinase, phosphofructokinase, and pyruvate kinase could explain the decrease in liver glucose uptake and the lactate release seen during infection. A host of other factors (including cytokines, prostaglandins, and nitric oxide) may contribute to the alterations in hepatic glucose production. However, many of their effects on glucose metabolism are mediated both directly and indirectly via their activation of the neuroendocrine system (3, 87, 92, 94, 150). Inhibition of nitric oxide does not alter liver glucose uptake during infection (16). Catecholamines can inhibit liver glucose uptake (108), but significant impairment in the hepatic response to TPN is seen in models with very little elevation in catecholamine levels.

Correction of the infection-induced hyperglycemia by administration of insulin may not necessarily improve liver glucose uptake. Although administering insulin can facilitate NHGU, the concomitant lowering of glucose levels will counteract this effect. As mentioned above, two of the three major determinants of NHGU are the insulin and glucose levels. Increases in insulin not only improve NHGU, they also increase muscle glucose uptake (170). Based upon the studies of Myers et al. (125) in 42-hour fasted dogs, $\sim$15% of the exogenous glucose delivered into a peripheral vein was disposed of by the liver in the presence of acute moderate elevations of insulin and glucose levels. Further increases in the insulin level did not alter this percentage. This is in marked contrast with the response seen following TPN in the normal dog, where the liver removed 45% of the exogenous glucose in the absence of hyperglycemia (15). Interestingly, when glucose levels in

42-hour fasted dogs were increased in a stepwise manner in the presence of fixed elevated insulin levels (~33 μU/ml), the glucose disposed by the liver increased progressively from 14% to 29% (124). Thus, acute hyperglycemia tends to shift glucose carbon to the liver and away from the periphery. In fact, our data indicate that acute increases in arterial glucose levels in the TPN-adapted state have a much greater impact on liver glucose uptake than do proportional increases in insulin (17, 41).

Predicting the impact of correcting infection-induced hyperglycemia on liver glucose uptake is difficult; infection impairs both insulin- and glucose-dependent liver glucose uptakes. Infection impairs the slope of the relationship between glucose levels and NHGU (↓ ~45%). Despite this impairment, NHGU is still more responsive to increases in glucose concentration than to insulin concentrations (40), and increases in insulin above the already elevated insulin level did not improve liver glucose uptake. Thus, in the clinical setting, correction of hyperglycemia by exogenous infusion of insulin could decrease net liver glucose uptake in individuals who are already able to mount an insulin response, even if it is inadequate to maintain euglycemia. If the liver's contribution to whole-body glucose disposal decreases as insulin levels are increased and glucose levels are decreased, glucose utilization by peripheral tissues becomes the predominant mechanism for the lowering of glucose levels. Individuals with pre-existing insulin resistance are at greatest risk for the complications of hyperglycemia during nutritional support, especially when an infection is present (18, 31, 34). The combination of the infection-induced peripheral insulin resistance and the unresponsiveness of the liver to additional insulin contribute to the very high insulin requirements in these populations (118). Thus, these studies suggest that the acute correction of infection-induced hyperglycemia by administering exogenous insulin does not improve, and may even exacerbate, the infection-induced impairment in liver glucose uptake.

A body of evidence suggests that total enteral nutrition (TEN) may be more efficacious than TPN in reducing secondary infections and decreasing mortality (80). One proposed benefit of TEN is the preservation of the gut "barrier." TEN is reported to prevent translocation of bacteria into the portal and possibly the systemic circulation (35, 135). During TPN, gut atrophy occurs (4), which may allow translocation (62, 101). Support for the "translocation hypothesis" in animal models has been documented; however, there is no direct or convincing indirect evidence that it modifies or prevents bacterial translocation in humans (146). TEN may modify the gut inflammatory response, which in turn alters the general response to injury (36). TEN is beneficial to the gut; whether this is the sole mechanism by which it improves patient outcome is unclear.

One possible benefit of TEN, especially on hepatic function, is the direct delivery of the nutrients into the portal circulation. In fact, infusion of nutrients into the portal circulation was more effective in improving plasma protein levels in stressful situations than was the peripheral route (36, 128, 171). However, in nonstressed animals, portal nutrition was no more beneficial than was a peripheral route (45, 77). The improvement in hepatic metabolism following portal nutrient delivery in stress situations indicates that factors in addition to improved gut function contribute to the improved outcome of enterally fed patients. The accretion of hepatic glycogen may help protect the liver from periods of hepatic microcirculatory ischemia commonly seen during infection (2). In addition, increased amino acid delivery to the liver may also be beneficial in meeting the increased protein synthetic needs of the liver. In normal animals, acute delivery of glucose via the portal vein amplifies hepatic glucose uptake and glycogen repletion (127). Thus, we expected that during TEN, liver glucose uptake would be higher than during TPN; however, that was not the case (15). In fact, when identical nutrient solutions were given to dogs as TEN and TPN, the liver removed a similar amount of glucose. However, insulin levels were higher with TEN than TPN, and peripheral glucose uptake was lower in TEN. Since the portal signal inhibits peripheral glucose uptake in addition to stimulating NHGU (52), it may explain the impaired peripheral glucose uptake and higher insulin requirements seen during TEN. The possible explanations as to why TEN did not enhance NHGU further include (*a*) portal delivery of nonglucose substrates (amino acids) inhibits the effect of the portal signal on NHGU (122), (*b*) the portal signal is ineffective at the liver in the chronic nutritionally supported state (52), and (*c*) endocrine alterations, such as elevated glucagon levels, during TEN limit the rise in NHGU. Amino acids delivered enterally directly enter the portal circulation and may inhibit liver glucose uptake. Portal, but not peripheral, delivery of gluconeogenic amino acids inhibits the effect of the portal signal (122). Another possibility is that the portal signal is ineffective in the background of the large adaptations seen during TPN. This is likely, given that an acute, but not chronic, increase in fructose is effective (42, 43), and fructose is thought to act on the same enzymes as the portal signal.

SUMMARY

Infection and inflammation result in profound activation of the glucoregulatory system. In many other types of acute stressors, such as exercise and hypoglycemia, the tissue responses to hormones are generally amplified or at least sensitized, allowing rapid adjustments to be made during the stress. By contrast, in the setting of inflammation nearly all organs become hyporesponsive, shifting the body to a state of metabolic inflexibility. The root cause of this inflexibility is unclear but is likely dependent upon the inflammatory response rather than simply the neuroendocrine response. One consequence of this metabolic inflexibility is hyperglycemia, especially during nutritional support.

ACKNOWLEDGMENTS

This work was supported by NIH Grant DK-43748 (P.I., Owen McGuinness), Clinical Nutrition Research Unit Grant P30-DK-26657, and the Vanderbilt Diabetes Training and Research Center Grant (DK-20593).

LITERATURE CITED

1. Aguirre V, Werner ED, Giraud J, Lee YH, Shoelson SE, White MF. 2002. Phosphorylation of Ser307 in insulin receptor substrate-1 blocks interactions with the insulin receptor and inhibits insulin action. *J. Biol. Chem.* 277:1531–37
2. Asher EF, Garrison RN, Ratcliff EJ, Fry DE. 1983. Endotoxin, cellular function, and nutrient blood flow. *Arch. Surg.* 118:441–45
3. Bagby GJ, Lang CH, Skrepnik N, Spitzer JJ. 1992. Attenuation of glucose metabolic changes resulting from TNF-alpha administration by adrenergic blockade. *Am. J. Physiol.* 262:R628–35
4. Barber AE, Jones WG 2nd, Minei JP, Fahey TJ 3rd, Lowry SF, Shires GT. 1991. Bacterial overgrowth and intestinal atrophy in the etiology of gut barrier failure in the rat. *Am. J. Surg.* 161:300–4
5. Barzilai N, Rossetti L. 1993. Role of glucokinase and glucose-6-phosphatase in the acute and chronic regulation of hepatic glucose fluxes by insulin. *J. Biol. Chem.* 268:25019–25
6. Bellomo R. 2002. Bench-to-bedside review: lactate and the kidney. *Crit. Care* 6: 322–26
7. Bessey PQ, Aoki TT, Wilmore DW. 1985. Fuel utilization following injury: relationship to hormonal environment. *J. Surg. Res.* 38:484–93
8. Bessey PQ, Lowe KA. 1993. Early hormonal changes affect the catabolic response to trauma. *Ann. Surg.* 218:476–89
9. Biggers DW, Myers SR, Neal D, Stinson R, Cooper NB, et al. 1989. Role of brain in counterregulation of insulin-induced hypoglycemia in dogs. *Diabetes* 38:7–16
10. Buday AZ, Lang CH, Bagby GJ, Spitzer JJ. 1986. Glycogen synthase and phosphorylase activities during glycogen repletion in endotoxemic rats. *Circ. Shock* 19:149–63
11. Carlson GL. 2004. Hunterian Lecture. Insulin resistance in human sepsis: implications for the nutritional and metabolic care of the critically ill surgical patient. *Ann. R. Coll. Surg. Engl.* 86:75–81
12. Caruana JA, Camara DS, Schneeberger GJ, Nolan JP. 1984. The clearance capacity of the canine liver for a portal vein endotoxin infusion. *J. Surg. Res.* 37:197–201
13. Cely CM, Arora P, Quartin AA, Kett DH, Schein RM. 2004. Relationship of baseline glucose homeostasis to hyperglycemia during medical critical illness. *Chest* 126:879–87
14. Ceppi ED, Knowles RG, Carpenter KM, Titheradge MA. 1992. Effect of treatment in vivo of rats with bacterial endotoxin on fructose 2,6-biphosphate metabolism and L-pyruvate kinase activity and flux in isolated liver cells. *Biochem. J.* 284:761–66
15. Chen SS, Donmoyer C, Zhang Y, Hande SA, Lacy DB, McGuinness OP. 2000. Impact of enteral and parenteral nutrition on hepatic and muscle glucose metabolism. *J. Parenter. Enteral Nutr.* 24:255–60
16. Chen SS, Donmoyer CM, Ejiofor J, McCay J, Archuletta R, et al. 2002. Impact of intraportal N(omega)-nitro-L-arginine infusion on hepatic glucose metabolism in total parenteral nutrition-adapted dogs: interaction with infection. *Metabolism* 51: 274–83
17. Chen SS, Donmoyer CM, Pearson DA, Poole A, Zhang Y, et al. 2004. Impact of infection on glucose-dependent liver glucose uptake during TPN: interaction with insulin. *Am. J. Physiol.* 286:E286–95
18. Chen Y-D, Swislocki ALM, Hellenbeck CB, Wu M-S, Reaven GM. 1988. Relationship between plasma glucose and insulin concentration, glucose production and glucose disposal in normal subjects

and patients with non-insulin-dependent diabetes. *J. Clin. Invest.* 67:1084–89
19. Cherrington AD, Diamond MP, Green DR, Williams PE. 1982. Evidence for an intrahepatic contribution to the waning effect of glucagon on glucose production in the conscious dog. *Diabetes* 31:917–22
20. Cherrington AD, Wasserman DH, McGuinness OP. 1994. Renal contribution to glucose production after a brief fast: fact or fancy? *J. Clin. Invest.* 93:2303
21. Cherrington AD, Williams PE, Shulman GI, Lacy WW. 1981. Differential time course of glucagon's effect on glycogenolysis and gluconeogenesis in the conscious dog. *Diabetes* 30:180–87
22. Chhibber VL, Soriano C, Tayek JA. 2000. Effects of low-dose and high-dose glucagon on glucose production and gluconeogenesis in humans. *Metabolism* 49:39–46
23. Chrusch C, Bands C, Bose D, Li X, Jacobs H, et al. 2000. Impaired hepatic extraction and increased splanchnic production contribute to lactic acidosis in canine sepsis. *Am. J. Respir. Crit. Care Med.* 161:517–26
24. Chu CA, Galassetti P, Igawa K, Sindelar DK, Neal DW, et al. 2003. Interaction of free fatty acids and epinephrine in regulating hepatic glucose production in conscious dogs. *Am. J. Physiol.* 284:E291–301
25. Chu CA, Sindelar DK, Neal DW, Allen EJ, Donahue EP, Cherrington AD. 1997. Comparison of the direct and indirect effects of epinephrine on hepatic glucose production. *J. Clin. Invest.* 99:1044–56
26. Chu CA, Sindelar DK, Neal DW, Cherrington AD. 1996. Direct effects of catecholamines on hepatic glucose production in conscious dog are due to glycogenolysis. *Am. J. Physiol.* 271:E127–37
27. Chu CA, Sindelar DK, Neal DW, Cherrington AD. 1997. Portal adrenergic blockade does not inhibit the gluconeogenic effects of circulating catecholamines on the liver. *Metabolism* 46:458–65
28. Connolly CC, Stevenson RW, Neal DW, Wasserman DH, Cherrington AD. 1993. The effects of lactate loading on alanine and glucose metabolism in the conscious dog. *Metabolism* 42:154–61
29. Cornell RP, Filkins JP. 1974. Characterization of gluconeogenesis in enzymatically isolated parenchymal cells of rat liver. *Proc. Soc. Exp. Biol. Med.* 145:203–9
30. Dahn MS, Lange P. 1982. Hormonal changes and their influence on metabolism and nutrition in the critically ill. *Intensive Care Med.* 8:209–13
31. Davis SN, McGuinness OP, Cherrington AD. 1990. Insulin action in vivo. In *Diabetes Annual IV*, ed. KGMM Alberti, LP Krall, pp. 585–602. Amsterdam: Elsevier Sci.
32. De Backer D, Creteur J, Silva E, Vincent JL. 2001. The hepatosplanchnic area is not a common source of lactate in patients with severe sepsis. *Crit. Care Med.* 29:256–61
33. Defalque D, Brandt N, Ketelslegers JM, Thissen JP. 1999. GH insensitivity induced by endotoxin injection is associated with decreased liver GH receptors. *Am. J. Physiol.* 276:E565–72
34. Defronzo RA, Ferrannini E, Simonson DC. 1989. Fasting hyperglycemia in non-insulin dependent diabetes mellitus: contribution of excessive hepatic glucose production and impaired tissue glucose uptake. *Metabolism* 38:387–91
35. Deitch EA. 1992. Multiple organ failure pathophysiology and potential future therapy. *Ann. Surg.* 216:117–34
36. Deitch EA, Xu D, Franko L, Ayala A, Chaudry IH. 1995. Evidence favoring the role of the gut as a cytokine-generating organ in rats subjected to hemorrhagic shock. *Shock* 1:141–46
37. DeWulf H, Hers HG. 1968. The interconversion of liver glycogen synthase a and b in vitro. *Eur. J. Biochem.* 6:552–57

38. Diamond MP, Rollings RC, Steiner KE, Williams PE, Lacy WW, Cherrington AD. 1988. Effect of alanine concentration independent of changes in insulin and glucagon on alanine and glucose homeostasis in the conscious dog. *Metabolism* 37:28–33
39. Diamond MP, Suhrer JH Jr, Williams PE, Lacy WW, Cherrington AD. 1982. Contribution of the liver and extrasplanchnic tissues to the hypoglycemic action of dichloroacetate in the conscious dog. *Diabetes* 31:(Pt 1):326–32
40. Donmoyer CM, Chen S-S, Hande SA, Lacy DB, Ejiofor J, McGuinness OP. 2000. Hyperinsulinemia compensates for infection-induced impairment in net hepatic glucose uptake during TPN. *Am. J. Physiol.* 279:E235–43
41. Donmoyer CM, Chen S-S, Lacy DB, Pearson DA, Poole A, et al. 2003. Infection impairs insulin-dependent hepatic glucose uptake during total parenteral nutrition. *Am. J. Physiol.* 284:E574–82
42. Donmoyer CM, Ejiofor J, Lacy DB, Chen S-S, McGuinness OP. 2001. Fructose augments infection-impaired net hepatic glucose uptake during TPN administration. *Am. J. Physiol.* 280:E703–11
43. Donmoyer CM, Lacy DB, Zhang Y, Chen S-S, McGuinness OP. 2002. Impact of chronic fructose infusion on hepatic metabolism during TPN administration. *Am. J. Physiol.* 283:E1151–58
44. Engelman JA, Berg AH, Lewis RY, Lisanti MP, Scherer PE. 2000. Tumor necrosis factor alpha-mediated insulin resistance, but not dedifferentiation, is abrogated by MEK1/2 inhibitors in 3T3-L1 adipocytes. *Mol. Endocrinol.* 14:1557–69
45. Fairman RM, Crosby LO, Stein TP, Buzby GP, Mullen JL. 1983. Prehepatic total parenteral nutrition in the chair-adapted primate. *J. Parenter. Enteral Nutr.* 7:237–43
46. Feuerstein G, Hallenbeck JM, Vanatta B, Rabinovici R, Perera PY, Vogel SN. 1990. Effects of gram-negative endotoxin on levels of serum corticosterone, TNFα, circulating blood cells, and the survival of rats. *Circ. Shock* 30:265–78
47. Filkins JP, Cornell RP. 1974. Depression of hepatic gluconeogenesis and the hypoglycemia of endotoxin shock. *Am. J. Physiol.* 227:778–81
48. Finney SJ, Zekveld C, Elia A, Evans TW. 2003. Glucose control and mortality in critically ill patients. *JAMA* 290:2041–47
49. Fong YM, Marano MA, Moldawer LL, Wei H, Calvano SE, et al. 1990. The acute splanchnic and peripheral tissue metabolic response to endotoxin in humans. *J. Clin. Invest.* 85:1896–904
50. Frost RA, Nystrom GJ, Lang CH. 2002. Lipopolysaccharide regulates proinflammatory cytokine expression in mouse myoblasts and skeletal muscle. *Am. J. Physiol. Regul. Integr. Comp. Physiol.* 283: R698–709
51. Fujiwara T, Cherrington AD, Neal DW, McGuinness OP. 1996. Role of cortisol in the metabolic response to stress hormone infusion in the conscious dog. *Metabolism* 45:571–78
52. Galassetti P, Shiota M, Zinker BA, Wasserman DH, Cherrington AD. 1998. A negative arterial-portal venous glucose gradient decreases skeletal muscle glucose uptake. *Am. J. Physiol.* 275:E101–11
53. Gannon MC, Nuttall FQ. 1997. Effect of feeding, fasting, and diabetes on liver glycogen synthase activity, protein, and mRNA in rats. *Diabetologia* 40:758–63
54. Gelfand RA, Matthews DE, Bier DM, Sherwin RS. 1984. Role of counterregulatory hormones in the catabolic response to stress. *J. Clin. Invest.* 74:2238–48
55. Gibson FA, Hinds CJ. 1997. Growth hormone and insulin-like growth factors in critical illness. *Int. Care Med.* 23:369–78
56. Golden SH, Peart-Vigilance C, Kao WH, Brancati FL. 1999. Perioperative glycemic control and the risk of infectious complications in a cohort of adults with diabetes. *Diabetes Care* 22:1408–14

57. Goldstein R, Palmer B, Liu R, Massillon D. 1995. The effects of chronic hypercortisolemia on gluconeogenesis assessed using two independent methods in vivo. *Diabetes* 44(Suppl. 1):201
58. Goldstein RE, Wasserman DH, McGuinness OP, Lacy DB, Cherrington AD, Abumrad NN. 1993. Effects of chronic elevation in plasma cortisol on hepatic carbohydrate metabolism. *Am. J. Physiol.* 264:E119–27
59. Gore DC, Jahoor F, Hibbert JM, DeMaria EJ. 1996. Lactic acidosis during sepsis is related to increased pyruvate production, not deficits in tissue oxygen availability. *Ann. Surg.* 224:97–102
60. Gustavson SM, Chu CA, Nishizawa M, Farmer B, Neal D, et al. 2003. Interaction of glucagon and epinephrine in the control of hepatic glucose production in the conscious dog. *Am. J. Physiol. Endocrinol. Metab.* 284:E695–707
61. Gustavson SM, Chu CA, Nishizawa M, Farmer B, Neal D, et al. 2003. Glucagon's actions are modified by the combination of epinephrine and gluconeogenic precursor infusion. *Am. J. Physiol. Endocrinol. Metab.* 285:E534–44
62. Hadfield RJ, Sinclair DG, Houldsworth PE, Evans TW. 1995. Effects of enteral and parenteral nutrition on gut mucosal permeability in the critically ill. *Am. J. Respir. Crit. Care Med.* 152:1545–48
63. Hargrove DM, Bagby GJ, Lang CH, Spitzer JJ. 1988. Adrenergic blockade does not abolish elevated glucose turnover during bacterial infection. *Am. J. Physiol.* 254:E16–22
64. Hargrove DM, Bagby GJ, Lang CH, Spitzer JJ. 1988. Adrenergic blockade prevents endotoxin-induced increases in glucose metabolism. *Am. J. Physiol.* 255: E629–35
65. Hellerstein MK. 1999. De novo lipogenesis in humans: metabolic and regulatory aspects. *Eur. J. Clin. Nutr.* 53(Suppl. 1):53–65
66. Holste LC, Connolly CC, Moore MC, Neal DW, Cherrington AD. 1997. Physiological changes in circulating glucagon alter hepatic glucose disposition during portal glucose delivery. *Am. J. Physiol.* 273:E488–96
67. Horton RA, Knowles RG, Titheradge MA. 1994. Endotoxin causes reciprocal changes in hepatic nitric oxide synthesis, gluconeogenesis, and flux through phosphoenolpyruvate carboxykinase. *Biochem. Biophys. Acta* 204:659–65
68. Hotamisligil GS. 2003. Inflammatory pathways and insulin action. *Int. J. Obes. Relat. Metab. Disord.* 27(Suppl. 3):53–55
69. Hotamisligil GS, Murray DL, Choy LN, Spiegelman BM. 1994. Tumor necrosis factor-α inhibits signaling from the insulin receptor. *Proc. Natl. Acad. Sci. USA* 91:4854–58
70. Ishida T, Lewis RM, Hartley CJ, Entman ML, Field JB. 1978. Comparison of hepatic extraction of insulin and glucagon in conscious dogs. *Endocrinology* 112:1098–109
71. Jacobs DO, Maris J, Fried R, Settle RG, Rolandelli RR, et al. 1988. In vivo phosphorus 31 magnetic resonance spectroscopy of rat hind limb skeletal muscle during sepsis. *Arch. Surg.* 123:1425–28
72. Jahoor F, Herdon DN, Wolfe RR. 1986. Role of insulin and glucagon in the response of glucose and alanine kinetics in burn-injured patients. *J. Clin. Invest.* 78:807–14
73. Jahoor F, Peters EJ, Wolfe RR. 1990. The relationship between gluconeogenic substrate supply and glucose production in humans. *Am. J. Physiol.* 258:E288–96
74. Johnson TS, O'Leary M, Justice SK, Maamra M, Zarkesh-Esfahani SH, et al. 2001. Differential expression of suppressors of cytokine signalling genes in response to nutrition and growth hormone in the septic rat. *J. Endocrinol.* 169:409–15
75. Kilberg MS, Stevens BR, Novak DA. 1993. Recent advances in mammalian

amino acid transport. *Annu. Rev. Nutr.* 13: 137–65
76. Kim HJ, Higashimori T, Park SY, Choi H, Dong J, et al. 2004. Differential effects of interleukin-6 and -10 on skeletal muscle and liver insulin action in vivo. *Diabetes* 53:1060–67
77. King WWK, Boelhouwer RU, Kingsworth AN, Ross JS, Young VR, Malt RA. 1983. Nutritional efficacy and hepatic changes during intragastric, intravenous and prehepatic feeding in rats. *J. Parenter. Enteral Nutr.* 7:443–46
78. Klover PJ, Zimmers TA, Koniaris LG, Mooney RA. 2003. Chronic exposure to interleukin-6 causes hepatic insulin resistance in mice. *Diabetes* 52:2784–89
79. Krogh-Madsen R, Moller K, Dela F, Kronborg G, Jauffred S, Pedersen BK. 2004. Effect of hyperglycemia and hyperinsulinemia on the response of IL-6, TNF-alpha, and FFAs to low-dose endotoxemia in humans. *Am. J. Physiol. Endocrinol. Metab.* 286:E766–72
80. Kudsk KA, Whitnal M, Abrams JS, Mougey EH. 1993. Enteral and tumor necrosis factor in normal rats. *J. Trauma* 132:946–52
81. Landau BR. 1999. Quantifying the contribution of gluconeogenesis to glucose production in fasted human subjects using stable isotopes. *Proc. Nutr. Soc.* 58:963–72
82. Lang CH. 1992. Sepsis-induced insulin resistance in rats is mediated by a beta-adrenergic mechanism. *Am. J. Physiol.* 263:E703–11
83. Lang CH. 1993. Beta-adrenergic blockade attenuates insulin resistance induced by tumor necrosis factor. *Am. J. Physiol.* 264:R984–91
84. Lang CH. 2001. Sepsis-induced changes in pancreatic hormone secretion. In *Handbook of Physiology: The Endocrine Pancreas and Regulation of Metabolism*, ed. LS Jefferson, AD Cherrington, pp. 999–1014. New York: Oxford Univ. Press
85. Lang CH, Bagby GJ, Blakesley HL, Spitzer JJ. 1987. Fever is not responsible for the elevated glucose kinetics in sepsis. *Proc. Soc. Exp. Biol. Med.* 185:455–61
86. Lang CH, Bagby GJ, Blakesley HL, Spitzer JJ. 1987. Glucose kinetics and pyruvate dehydrogenase activity in septic rats treated with dichloroacetate. *Circ. Shock* 23:131–41
87. Lang CH, Bagby GJ, Blakesley HL, Spitzer JJ. 1987. Inhibition of eicosanoid production by BW755C does not attenuate sepsis-induced alterations in glucose kinetics. *Circ. Shock* 22:105–13
88. Lang CH, Bagby GJ, Blakesley HL, Spitzer JJ. 1989. Importance of hyperglucagonemia in eliciting the sepsis-induced increase in glucose production. *Circ. Shock* 29:181–91
89. Lang CH, Bagby GJ, Buday AZ, Spitzer JJ. 1987. The contribution of gluconeogenesis to glycogen repletion during glucose infusion in endotoxemia. *Metabolism* 36:180–87
90. Lang CH, Bagby GJ, Spitzer JJ. 1984. Carbohydrate dynamics in the hypermetabolic septic rat. *Metabolism* 33:959–63
91. Lang CH, Bagby GJ, Spitzer JJ. 1985. Glucose kinetics and body temperature after lethal and nonlethal doses of endotoxin. *Am. J. Physiol.* 248:R471–78
92. Lang CH, Blakesley HL, Bagby GJ, Spitzer JJ. 1988. Lipoxygenase and cyclooxygenase blockade by BW755C prevents endotoxin-induced hypotension but not changes in glucose metabolism. *Horm. Metab. Res.* 20:551–54
93. Lang CH, Dobrescu C. 1989. In vivo insulin resistance during nonlethal hypermetabolic sepsis. *Circ. Shock* 28:165–78
94. Lang CH, Dobrescu C. 1989. Interleukin-1 induced increases in glucose utilization are insulin mediated. *Life Sci.* 45:2127–34
95. Lang CH, Dobrescu C. 1989. Sepsis-induced changes in in vivo insulin action in diabetic rats. *Am. J. Physiol.* 257(Pt. 1): E301–8

96. Lang CH, Dobrescu C. 1991. Gram-negative infection increases noninsulin-mediated glucose disposal. *Endocrinology* 128:645–53
97. Lang CH, Dobrescu C, Bagby GJ. 1992. Tumor necrosis factor impairs insulin action on peripheral glucose disposal and hepatic glucose output. *Endocrinology* 130:43–52
98. Lang CH, Dobrescu C, Meszaros K. 1990. Insulin-mediated glucose uptake by individual tissues during sepsis. *Metabolism* 39:1096–107
99. Lang CH, Obih JA, Bagby GJ, Bagwell JN, Spitzer JJ. 1991. Endotoxin-induced increases in regional glucose utilization by small intestine: a TNF-independent effect. *Am. J. Physiol.* 260(Pt. 1):G548–55
100. Lecavalier L, Bolli G, Gerich J. 1990. Glucagon-cortisol interactions on glucose turnover and lactate gluconeogenesis in normal humans. *Am. J. Physiol.* 258:E569–75
101. Lipman TO. 1998. Grains or veins: Is enteral nutrition really better than parenteral nutrition? A look at the evidence. *J. Parenter. Enteral Nutr.* 22:167–82
102. Long CL, Kinney JM, Geiger JW. 1976. Nonsuppressability of gluconeogenesis by glucose in septic patients. *Metabolism* 25:193–201
103. Long CL, Spencer JL, Kinney JM, Geiger JW. 1971. Carbohydrate metabolism in man: effect of elective operations and major injury. *J. Appl. Physiol.* 31:110–16
104. Magnusson I, Rothman DL, Gerard DP, Katz LD, Shulman GI. 1995. Contribution of hepatic glycogenolysis to glucose production in humans in response to a physiological increase in plasma glucagon concentration. *Diabetes* 44:185–89
105. McCallum RE, Seale TW, Stith RD. 1983. Influence of endotoxin treatment on dexamethasone induction of hepatic phosphoenolpyruvate carboxykinase. *Infect. Immun.* 39:213–19
106. McGuinness OP. 1994. The impact of infection on gluconeogenesis in the conscious dog. *Shock* 2:336–43
107. McGuinness OP, Burgin K, Moran C, Bracy D, Cherrington AD. 1994. Role of glucagon in the metabolic response to stress hormone infusion in the conscious dog. *Am. J. Physiol.* 266:E438–47
108. McGuinness OP, Donmoyer CM, Ejiofor J, McElligott S, Lacy DB. 1998. Hepatic and muscle glucose metabolism during total parenteral nutrition: impact of infection. *Am. J. Physiol.* 275:E763–69
109. McGuinness OP, Ejiofor J, Audoly LP, Schrom N. 1998. Regulation of glucose production by NEFA and gluconeogenic precursors during chronic glucagon infusion. *Am. J. Physiol.* 275:E432–39
110. McGuinness OP, Ejiofor J, Lacy DB, Schrom N. 2000. Hepatic glucose metabolism during intraduodenal glucose infusion: impact of infection. *Am. J. Physiol.* 279:E108–15
111. McGuinness OP, Fujiwara T, Murrell S, Bracy D, Neal D, et al. 1993. Impact of chronic stress hormone infusion on hepatic carbohydrate metabolism in the conscious dog. *Am. J. Physiol.* 265:E314–22
112. McGuinness OP, Jacobs J, Moran C, Lacy DB. 1995. Impact of infection on hepatic disposal of a peripheral glucose infusion in the conscious dog. *Am. J. Physiol.* 269:E199–207
113. McGuinness OP, Lacy DB, Anderson J. 1995. Effect of acute glucagon removal on metabolic response to infection in conscious dog. *Am. J. Physiol.* 268:E92–99
114. McGuinness OP, Lacy DB, Eliasson KE. 1996. Hyperglucagonemia and hepatic glucose metabolism during infection in the conscious dog. *Am. J. Physiol.* 270: E580–86
115. McGuinness OP, Murrell S, Moran C, Bracy D, Cherrington AD. 1994. The effect of acute glucagon removal on the metabolic response to stress hormone infusion in the conscious dog. *Metabolism* 43:1310–17
116. McGuinness OP, Shau V, Benson EM,

Lewis M, Snowden RT, et al. 1997. Role of epinephrine and norepinephrine in the metabolic response to stress hormone infusion in the conscious dog. *Am. J. Physiol.* 273:E674–81

117. McGuinness OP, Snowden RT, Moran C, Neal DW, Fujiwara T, Cherrington AD. 1999. Impact of acute epinephrine removal on hepatic glucose metabolism during stress hormone infusion. *Metabolism* 48:910–14
118. McMahon MM, Rizza RA. 1996. Nutrition support in hospitalized patients with diabetes mellitus. *Mayo Clin. Proc.* 71:587–94
119. Meinz HM, Lacy DB, Ejiofor J, McGuinness OP. 1998. Alterations in hepatic gluconeogenic amino acid uptake and gluconeogenesis in the endotoxin-treated conscious dog. *Shock* 9:296–303
120. Meszaros K, Lang CH, Bagby GJ, Spitzer JJ. 1987. Contribution of different organs to increased glucose consumption after endotoxin administration. *J. Biol. Chem.* 262:10965–70
121. Meszaros K, Lang CH, Bojta J, Spitzer JJ. 1989. Early changes in glucose utilization of individual tissues after endotoxin administration. *Circ. Shock* 29:107–14
122. Moore MC, Hsieh PS, Flakoll PJ, Neal DW, Cherrington AD. 1999. Differential effect of amino acid infusion route on net hepatic glucose uptake in the dog. *Am. J. Physiol.* 276:E295–302
123. Morikawa S, Inubushi T, Takahashi K, Ishii H, Ozawa K. 1998. Gluconeogenesis and phosphoenergetics in rat liver during endotoxemia. *J. Surg. Res.* 74:179–86
124. Myers SR, Biggers DW, Neal DW, Cherrington AD. 1991. Intraportal glucose delivery enhances the effects of hepatic glucose load on net hepatic glucose uptake in vivo. *J. Clin. Invest.* 88:158–67
125. Myers SR, McGuinness OP, Neal DW, Cherrington AD. 1991. Intraportal glucose delivery alters the relationship between net hepatic glucose uptake and the insulin concentration. *J. Clin. Invest.* 87:930–39
126. Neimeyer H, Ureta T, Clark-Turri L. 1975. Adaptive character of liver glucokinase. *Mol. Cell Biochem.* 6:109–26
127. Pagliassotti MJ, Cherrington AD. 1992. Regulation of net hepatic glucose uptake in vivo. *Annu. Rev. Physiol.* 54:847–60
128. Piccone VA, LeVeen HH, Glass P, Berlyne G, Lundin AP. 1980. Prehepatic hyperalimentation. *Surgery* 87:263–70
129. Pilkis SJ. 1970. Hormonal control of hexokinase activity in animal tissues. *Biochim. Biophys. Acta* 215:461–76
130. Pilkis SJ, el-Maghrabi MR, Claus TH. 1988. Hormonal regulation of hepatic gluconeogenesis and glycolysis. *Annu. Rev. Biochem.* 57:755–83
131. Pilkis SJ, Granner DK. 1992. Molecular physiology of the regulation of hepatic gluconeogenesis and glycolysis. *Annu. Rev. Physiol.* 54:885–909
132. Pittner RA, Spitzer JA. 1993. Shift from alpha- to beta-type adrenergic receptor-mediated responses in chronically endotoxemic rats. *Am. J. Physiol.* 264:E650–54
133. Reithmann C, Hallstrom S, Pilz G, Kapsner T, Schlag G, Werdan K. 1993. Desensitization of rat cardiomyocyte adenylyl cyclase stimulation by plasma of noradrenaline-treated patients with septic shock. *Circ. Shock* 41:48–59
134. Saeed M, Carlson GL, Little RA, Irving MH. 1999. Selective impairment of glucose storage in human sepsis. *Br. J. Surg.* 86:813–21
135. Saito H, Trocki O, Alexander JW, Kopcha R, Heyd T, Joffe SN. 1987. The effect of route of nutrient administration on the nutritional state, catabolic hormone secretion, and gut mucosal integrity after burn injury. *J. Parenter. Enteral Nutr.* 11:1–7
136. Santos AA, Scheltinga MR, Lynch E, Brown EF, Lawton P, et al. 1993. Elaboration of interleukin 1-receptor antagonist is not attenuated by glucocorticoids after endotoxemia. *Arch. Surg.* 128:138–43

137. Seoane J, Barbera A, Telemaque-Potts S, Newgard CB, Guinovart JJ. 1999. Glucokinase overexpression restores glucose utilization and storage in cultured hepatocytes from male Zucker diabetic fatty rats. *J. Biol. Chem.* 274:31833–38
138. Severin PN, Uhing MR, Beno DW, Kimura RE. 2002. Endotoxin-induced hyperlactatemia results from decreased lactate clearance in hemodynamically stable rats. *Crit. Care Med.* 30:2509–14
139. Shamoon H, Hendler R, Sherwin RS. 1981. Synergistic interactions among antiinsulin hormones in the pathogenesis of stress hyperglycemia in humans. *J. Clin. Endocrinol. Metab.* 52:1235–41
140. Shangraw RE, Jahoor F, Wolfe RR, Lang CH. 1996. Hunterian lecture: insulin resistance in human sepsis-induced insulin resistance. *Crit. Care Med.* 24:75–81
141. Shangraw RE, Jahoor F, Wolfe RR, Lang CH. 1996. Pyruvate dehydrogenase inactivity is not responsible for sepsis-induced insulin resistance. *Crit. Care Med.* 24:566–74
142. Shaw JH, Wolfe RR. 1985. Response to glucose and lipid infusions in sepsis: a kinetic analysis. *Metabolism* 34:442–49
143. Shaw JHF, Klein S, Wolfe RR. 1985. Assessment of alanine, urea and glucose interrelationships in normal subjects and in patients with sepsis with stable isotopes. *Surgery* 97:557–67
144. Sidossis LS, Mittendorfer B, Chinkes D, Walser E, Wolfe RR. 1999. Effect of hyperglycemia-hyperinsulinemia on whole body and regional fatty acid metabolism. *Am. J. Physiol.* 276:E427–34
145. Sidossis LS, Mittendorfer B, Walser E, Chinkes D, Wolfe RR. 1998. Hyperglycemia-induced inhibition of splanchnic fatty acid oxidation increases hepatic triacylglycerol secretion. *Am. J. Physiol.* 275:E798–805
146. Sigurdsson GH. 1995. Is translocation of bacteria and endotoxin from the gastrointestinal tract a source of sepsis in critically ill patients? *Acta Anaes. Scand.* 39:11–19
147. Sindelar DK, Chu CA, Rohlie M, Neal DW, Swift LL, Cherrington AD. 1997. The role of fatty acids in mediating the effects of peripheral insulin on hepatic glucose production in the conscious dog. *Diabetes* 46:187–96
148. Soop M, Duxbury H, Agwunobi AO, Gibson JM, Hopkins SJ, et al. 2002. Euglycemic hyperinsulinemia augments the cytokine and endocrine responses to endotoxin in humans. *Am. J. Physiol.* 282: E1276–85
149. Spitzer JA, Nelson KM, Fish RE. 1985. Time course of changes in gluconeogenesis from various precursors in chronically endotoxemic rats. *Metabolism* 34:842–49
150. Spitzer JJ, Bagby GJ, Hargrove DM, Lang CH, Meszaros K. 1989. Alterations in the metabolic control of carbohydrates in sepsis. *Prog. Clin. Biol. Res.* 308:545–61
151. Spolarics Z, Bagby GJ, Lang CH, Spitzer JJ. 1991. Up-regulation of glucose metabolism in Kupffer cells following infusion of tumour necrosis factor. *Biochem. J.* 278:515–19
152. Stagnaro-Green A, Barton MK, Linekin PL, Corkery E, deBeer K, Roman SH. 1995. Mortality in hospitalized patients with hypoglycemia and severe hyperglycemia. *Mt. Sinai J. Med.* 62:422–26
153. Stevenson RW, Steiner KE, Connolly CC, Fuchs H, Alberti KG, et al. 1991. Dose-related effects of epinephrine on glucose production in conscious dogs. *Am. J. Physiol.* 260:E363–70
154. Stevenson RW, Steiner KE, Davis MA, Hendrick GK, Williams PE, et al. 1987. Similar dose responsiveness of hepatic glycogenolysis and gluconeogenesis to glucagon in vivo. *Diabetes* 36:382–89
155. Tappy L, Cayeux M, Schneiter P, Schindler C, Temler E, et al. 1995. Effect of lactate on glucose metabolism in healthy subjects and severely injured hyperglycemic patients. *Am. J. Physiol.* 268:E630–35

156. Thompson WA, Coyle S, Van Zee K, Oldenburg H, Trousdale R, et al. 1994. The metabolic effects of platelet-activating factor antagonism in endotoxemic man. *Arch. Surg.* 129:72–79
157. Ueki K, Kondo T, Kahn CR. 2004. Suppressor of cytokine signaling 1 (SOCS-1) and SOCS-3 cause insulin resistance through inhibition of tyrosine phosphorylation of insulin receptor substrate proteins by discrete mechanisms. *Mol. Cell Biol.* 24:5434–46
158. Ueki K, Kondo T, Tseng YH, Kahn CR. 2004. Central role of suppressors of cytokine signaling proteins in hepatic steatosis, insulin resistance, and the metabolic syndrome in the mouse. *Proc. Natl. Acad. Sci. USA* 101:10422–27
159. Umpierrez GE, Isaacs SD, Bazargan N, You X, Thaler LM, Kitabchi AE. 2002. Hyperglycemia: an independent marker of in-hospital mortality in patients with undiagnosed diabetes. *J. Clin. Endocrinol. Metab.* 87:978–82
160. van den Berghe G, Wouters P, Weekers F, Verwaest C, Bruyninckx F, et al. 2001. Intensive insulin therapy in the critically ill patients. *N. Engl. J. Med.* 345:1359–67
161. Vranic M, Engerman R, Doi K, Morita S, Yip CC. 1976. Extrapancreatic glucagon in the dog. *Metabolism* 25:1469–73
162. Wang K, Deutschman CS, Clemens MG, De Maio A. 1995. Reciprocal expression of phosphoenolpyruvate carboxykinase and acute phase genes during acute inflammation. *Shock* 3:204–9
163. White RH, Frayn KN, Little RA, Threlfall CJ, Stoner HB, Irving MH. 1987. Hormonal and metabolic responses to glucose infusion in sepsis studies by the hyperglycemia glucose clamp technique. *J. Parenter. Enteral Nutr.* 11:345–53
164. Wolfe RR. 1999. Sepsis as a modulator of adaptation to low and high carbohydrate and low and high fat intakes. *Eur. J. Clin. Nutr.* 53:S136–42
165. Wolfe RR, Elahi D, Spitzer JJ. 1977. Glucose and lactate kinetics after endotoxin administration in dogs. *Am. J. Physiol.* 232:E180–85
166. Wolfe RR, Herndon DN, Jahoor F, Miyoshi H, Wolfe M. 1987. Effect of severe burn injury on substrate cycling by glucose and fatty acids. *N. Engl. J. Med.* 317:403–8
167. Wolfe RR, Jahoor F, Shaw JH. 1987. Effect of alanine infusion on glucose and urea production in man. *J. Parenter. Enteral Nutr.* 11:109–11
168. Wolfe RR, Shaw JH. 1985. Glucose and FFA kinetics in sepsis: role of glucagon and sympathetic nervous system activity. *Am. J. Physiol.* 248:E236–43
169. Wolfe RR, Shaw JH, Durkot MJ. 1983. Energy metabolism in trauma and sepsis: the role of fat. *Prog. Clin. Biol. Res.* 111:89–109
170. Yki-Jarvinen H. 1993. Action of insulin on glucose metabolism in vivo. *Baillieres Clin. Endocrinol. Metab.* 7:903–27
171. Ziegler TR, Gatzen C, Wilmore DW. 1994. Strategies for attenuating protein-catabolic responses in the critically ill. *Annu. Rev. Med.* 45:459–80

Annu. Rev. Nutr. 2005. 25:37–58
doi: 10.1146/annurev.nutr.25.050304.092553

First published online as a Review in Advance on May 3, 2005

HUMAN MILK GLYCANS PROTECT INFANTS AGAINST ENTERIC PATHOGENS

David S. Newburg
Division of Pediatric Gastroenterology and Nutrition, Massachusetts General Hospital, Charlestown, Massachusetts 02129-4404; email: dnewburg@partners.org

Guillermo M. Ruiz-Palacios
Departamento de Infectologia, Instituto Nacional de Ciencias Medicas y Nutricion, Mexico City DF 14000, Mexico; email: gmrps@servidor.unam.mx

Ardythe L. Morrow
Center for Epidemiology and Biostatistics, Cincinnati Children's Hospital Medical Center, Cincinnati, Ohio 45229-3039; email: ardythe.morrow@cchmc.org

Key Words oligosaccharides, breastfeeding, diarrhea, mucosal immunity

■ **Abstract** Breastfed infants have lower morbidity and mortality due to diarrhea than those fed artificially. This had been attributed primarily to the secretory antibodies and prebiotic factors in human milk. Oligosaccharides are the third largest component of human milk. They were initially considered to be functionless by-products of glycoprotein and glycolipid synthesis during milk production. However, in the past few decades it has become apparent that the human milk oligosaccharides are composed of thousands of components, at least some of which protect against pathogens. Oligosaccharide protection against infectious agents may result in part from their prebiotic characteristics, but is thought to be primarily due to their inhibition of pathogen binding to host cell ligands. Most human milk oligosaccharides are fucosylated, and their production depends on enzymes encoded by the genes associated with expression of the Lewis blood group system. The expression of specific fucosylated oligosaccharides in milk thus varies in relation to maternal Lewis blood group type, and is significantly associated with the risk of infectious disease in breastfed infants. Specific fucosylated moieties of oligosaccharides and related glycoconjugates (glycans) are able to inhibit binding and disease by specific pathogens. This review presents the argument that specific glycans, especially the oligosaccharides, are the major constituent of an innate immune system of human milk whereby the mother protects her infant from enteric and other pathogens through breastfeeding. The large input of energy expended by the mother in the synthesis of milk oligosaccharides is consistent with the human reproductive strategy of large parental input into rearing relatively few offspring through a prolonged period of maturation. These protective glycans may prove useful as a basis for the development of novel prophylactic and therapeutic agents that inhibit diseases caused by mucosal pathogens.

CONTENTS

INTRODUCTION: PROTECTION BY BREASTFEEDING

A relationship between breastfeeding and health of the infant has been noted from the times of the first recorded use of human milk substitutes, going back thousands of years (61). A more recent example is a study in Chicago in the 1930s in which more than 20,000 mother-infant dyads were systematically studied to determine disease incidence in infants in relation to mode of infant feeding (15). Infants consuming their mother's milk were found to have a several-fold lower risk of diarrheal disease, and a lower risk of respiratory infections as well as other types of infectious disease, including otitis media. The findings of this large, early study were generally replicated by subsequent studies conducted over several decades. Recent randomized clinical trials of breastfeeding promotion demonstrate that when breastfeeding rates increase, there is a proportional decrease in infant diarrhea (24, 30).

MECHANISMS OF BREASTFEEDING PROTECTION

Prebiotics

In the 1950s, based on advances in understanding of infant nutrition, many thought the improved composition of milk substitutes justified a shift to the use of artificial feeding. This perspective was reinforced by the reports that formula-fed infants typically gained more weight than did breastfed infants (25). However, the higher morbidity and mortality due to diarrhea and respiratory infections observed in artificially fed infants suggested a potent ability of breastfeeding to protect infants against infectious disease. This observation naturally led to heightened interest in identifying mechanisms whereby breastfeeding might protect against disease, including psychosocial factors, avoidance of contaminated food and water, superior nutrition, and human milk components that might directly or indirectly protect breastfed infants.

In 1905 (56), the difference in the composition of intestinal microflora was documented between breastfed and precociously weaned infants. Breastfed infants were noted to have predominance of lactobacilli, and, in particular, *Lactobacillus bifidus* (now known as *Bifidobacterium bifidum*), which was cultured from the feces of breastfed infants. In contrast, adults and precociously weaned infants had a predominance of *Escherichia coli*. Breastfeeding was hypothesized to mediate protection of the infant through milk components that specifically supported colonization by *L. bifidus*. *L. bifidus*, in turn, acidified the gut, bound to potential sites for colonization, and thereby inhibited pathogens from colonizing the gut and causing disease. It was not until 1974 that a glycan from human milk that stimulated the growth of *L. bifidus* was isolated and posited to be the heretofore undefined "bifidus factor" (17). Other types of indigestible oligosaccharides from other sources have since been found to stimulate colonization by *B. bifidum* and several lactobacilli. When fed in the diet, such materials stimulate gut colonization by beneficial microbes, presumably promoting health, and are known as prebiotics. Beneficial microorganisms that are introduced directly in the diet are known as probiotics. Human milk, through its oligosaccharides, acts as a prebiotic. Breastfeeding may also introduce probiotics into the digestive tract of the nursing infant, thereby protecting the infant from infectious disease (17).

Secretory Antibodies

In 1892, the ability of milk to transfer immunity from the mother to her offspring was reported (11), and in 1903 this property was attributed to milk antibodies (49). When significant amounts of secretory antibodies (sIgA) were found in human milk in 1961 (18), they were assumed to be the major agents whereby milk protected nursing infants. The very high concentrations of sIgAs in colostrum seemed consistent with human milk being a medium through which the maternal adaptive immune system could transmit mucosal protection to the infant gut, augmenting the gift of maternal antibody through prenatal transfer of serum antibodies across the human placenta. This seemed an effective mechanism to protect infants from pathogens to which the mother had prior exposure. However, upon exposure of the mother-infant dyad to a new pathogen, the prolonged lag between exposure and the appearance of the sIgA in the milk seemed enough time for the pathogen to establish a profound infection in the infant. Thus, other forms of interim protection seemed necessary to fully account for protection of infants by breastfeeding.

Multifunctional Agents

Other protective components found in human milk include multifunctional agents. These are milk constituents that function as a source of nutrients and that also function, either directly or through partial digestion products, as pathogen inhibitors. For example, lysozyme and lactoferrin, major sources of protein, are bacteriostatic or bacteriolytic. Free fatty acids and monoglycerides released from human milk triglycerides in the stomachs of breastfed infants and peptides released upon partial digestion of lactoferrin and other milk proteins exhibit a wide array of antibacterial, antiviral, and antiprotozoal activities (35). These multifunctional agents in human milk had been thought to slow the process of infection in nursing infants until sufficient sIgA appeared in the milk they were consuming, after which the multifunctional agents could act synergistically with antibody protection.

Multifunctional components may affect disease processes other than acute diarrhea. For example, a different form of multifunctional component from milk that inhibits tumors was recently described. The major protein found in human milk, α-lactalbumin, under acidic conditions in the presence of oleic acid, conditions that occur in the stomachs of breastfed infants, forms an alternate structural conformer. This α-lactalbumin-oleic acid complex, named HAMLET (<u>h</u>uman <u>α</u>-lactalbumin <u>m</u>ade <u>le</u>thal to <u>t</u>umor cells), seems to inhibit a wide array of tumors by triggering an apoptosis-like event (54). Current understanding of protective components of milk is that each may have a very specific mode of inhibition with regard to pathogens, location in the infant gut, host state, and timing. Some may exist only transiently or conditionally. However, the multiplicity of agents and their synergy result in potent protection by milk (16, 22, 32, 35, 45, 48).

Oligosaccharides and Other Glycans

The human milk oligosaccharides are complex carbohydrate structures attached to a lactose moiety at the reducing end. Human milk also contains glycoconjugates in which complex carbohydrate structures are attached at their reducing end to lipid to form glycolipids, or are attached to macromolecules to form glycopeptides, glycoproteins, glycosaminoglycans, or mucins. All of these are glycans. Recently, the oligosaccharides and other glycans of human milk have been gaining increasing attention as a major class of anti-infective agents in human milk. This review presents the argument that these milk glycans, by inhibiting the ability of pathogens to bind to their host cell receptors, represent a heretofore-underappreciated major mechanism whereby human milk affords robust protection to the nursing infant.

HUMAN MILK OLIGOSACCHARIDES AND OTHER GLYCANS

Although lactose was first isolated from milk in 1633, it was 1933 before the nonlactose carbohydrate fraction of human milk was isolated and the 1950s before the oligosaccharides were systematically characterized (40). Most human milk oligosaccharides are derived from 12 core structures made up of glucose, galactose, and *N*-acetylglucosamine. Four types of terminal fucose linkages and three types of sialic acid linkages can give rise to a vast array of compounds. Hundreds, and perhaps many thousands, of human milk oligosaccharides are thought to exist (51). Of these, well over a hundred structures have now been isolated and characterized. Almost all have lactose on the reducing end, and most have at least one fucose or sialic acid on the nonreducing terminus. Because these glycan structures are analogous to glycan moieties of the more complex glycoconjugates, such as glycolipids, glycoproteins, mucins, and glycosaminoglycans, it was originally thought that the milk oligosaccharides were an accidental by-product of having large amounts of active glycosyltransferases needed for glycoconjugate synthesis. This notion was reinforced by the resistance of glycans to digestion (breastfed baby stool was a known rich source of human milk glycans) and by the lack of any known biological functions. However, over the course of lactation, the production of milk represents a major commitment of maternal resources. A milk component that represents significant maternal calories but with no nutritional or other biological role would be inconsistent with the biological frugality that usually ensues from many generations of intermittent marginal nutritional status. That these milk oligosaccharides and glycoconjugates, that is, these human milk glycans, had a function seemed a reasonable hypothesis (38). Furthermore, because the milk oligosaccharides and glycans are made by the same types of glycosyltransferases that are responsible for the synthesis of human cell surface glycans, they would be expected to have structural moieties in common. Most enteric pathogens use cell surface glycans to identify and bind to their target cells as the critical first step in pathogenesis. Thus, soluble glycans from milk could competitively inhibit the ability of pathogens to bind to receptors in the gut and thereby protect the breastfed infant from diarrhea (Figure 1).

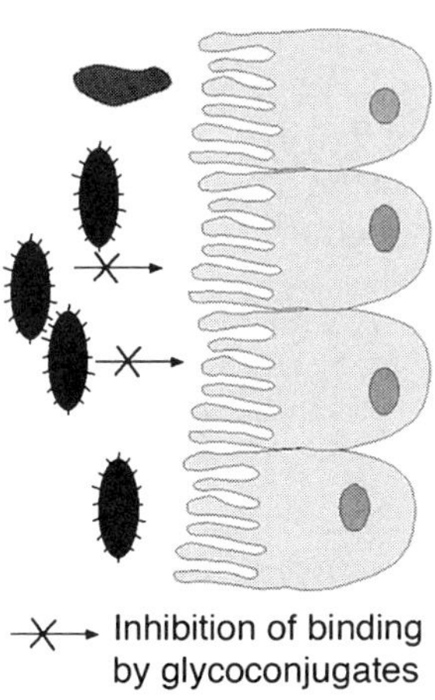

Figure 1 If human milk glycoconjugates contain epitopes that bind to specific pathogens, they can compete for the pathogen binding sites and block pathogens from binding to their host cell receptors in the mucosa.

In 1983, two observations suggested that human milk glycans could serve to protect against disease. In one, the human milk ganglioside fraction was reported to inhibit the activity of labile toxin of *E. coli*, as well as that of cholera toxin (44). Both of these toxins were known to bind to the ganglioside GM1, a monosialylated glycosphingolipid. These data implied that a human milk glycolipid that binds to a pathogen might inhibit the ability of the pathogen to bind to the intestinal mucosa of infants, thereby protect nursing infants from the diarrhea induced by the pathogen, in this case, labile toxin of *E. coli* or its homologue, cholera toxin. The other observation was that a factor in human milk inhibited the ability of stable toxin (ST) of *E. coli* to induce diarrhea in vivo. This human milk component did not partition into organic solvents, was dialyzable, was stable to heat, protease, acid or alkaline pH, but was destroyed by strong acid digestion that hydrolyzes glycosidic linkages, which suggested that the protective molecule could be an oligosaccharide or glycoconjugate, i.e., a glycan. Other indications that the human milk glycans might participate in the protection of breastfed infants included reports in 1986 that human milk glycans inhibit *Streptococcus pneumoniae* binding to human cells (1), and in 1991 that they inhibit binding by enteropathogenic *E. coli* (9).

FUCOSYLATED INHIBITORS OF PATHOGENS

Many enteric pathogens are inhibited by human milk, and for several, fucosylated glycans proved to be the active components.

Stable Toxin of *Escherichia coli*

To investigate whether the factor in human milk that inhibits ST was an oligosaccharide, fractions of human milk were tested, at the concentrations found in milk, for their ability to inhibit ST in vivo. The ST-protective factor was isolated and characterized as follows: Pooled human milk was separated into its components, and the only component that inhibited ST was the oligosaccharide fraction. Of the subfractions, only the neutral oligosaccharides inhibited (Table 1). The activity was specific to the neutral oligosaccharides that bound *Ulex europaeus; U. europaeus*

TABLE 1 Stable toxin (ST) protective activity: charcoal fraction separated by charge

ST	Lethality	Percent
ST + saline	32/50	61
ST + acidic oligosaccharides	34/60	57
ST + neutral oligosaccharides	13/59*	22
ST + milk aq_4	14/52*	27

*Value differs significantly from control value, $p < 0.0003$.

lectin avidly binds α1,2-linked fucose structures, which strongly suggested that the ST-protective factor in milk was a fucosylated oligosaccharide. Diluted to the volume of milk from which it was isolated, the Ulex-adherent fucosylated oligosaccharide fraction was as effective as human milk itself in preventing mortality in suckling mice due to ST-induced diarrhea (41).

The mechanism whereby the oligosaccharide inhibits ST was studied in T84 cells, an immortal line of human enterocytes. These cells express guanylate cyclase, whose extracellular domain is the receptor for ST, and whose intracellular activity produces cyclic GMP. Elevated cyclic GMP causes loss of chloride and bicarbonate transport, ultimately leading to the efflux of fluid and electrolytes. In vivo, the result is secretory diarrhea. In the presence of the protective fucosyloligosaccharides of human milk, ST is unable to stimulate production of cyclic GMP, either in intact T84 cells or in isolated membrane preparations. The mechanism of this protection appears to be binding by the oligosaccharide to the T84 extracellular domain of guanylate cyclase, thereby blocking its binding by ST. This prevents the ST-induced loss of chloride ion homeostasis and secretory diarrhea (8).

The *U. europaeus*–binding fucosyloligosaccharide fraction was resolved into more than 30 components by semipreparative high-performance liquid chromatography. Of these fractions, only one displayed consistent, robust activity at the concentration found in human milk. This fraction was further subfractionated into seven components; when purified to homogeneity only one of these inhibited the diarrheagenic activity of stable toxin in the suckling mouse. We estimate that this subfraction is active at a concentration of approximately 30 parts per billion (0.000003%), the concentration at which it is found in human milk (37).

Campylobacter

Campylobacter is a bacterium carried by birds, including domestic fowl, and is the single largest cause of bacteria-induced diarrhea worldwide. In nitrocellulose-immobilized neoglycoproteins, campylobacter has high avidity for the fucosylated antigen H-2 (Fucα1,2Galβ1,4GlcNAc); this specificity is confirmed by inhibition of campylobacter binding by monoclonal antibodies against the H-2 epitope. *Campylobacter jejuni*, which normally does not bind to Chinese hamster ovary cells, bound avidly when the cells were transfected with a human α1,2-fucosyltransferase gene that caused overexpression of the H-2 fucosylated antigen (Figure 2, see color insert, main panel).

This binding was inhibited by ligands that bind to H-2, e.g., *Ulex europaeus* agglutinin, *Lotus tetragonolobus* lectins, and anti-H-2 mAbs, or by H-2 soluble mimetics, e.g., H-2 neoglycoproteins, human milk fucosylated oligosaccharides, and 2′-fucosyllactose (2′-FL) (Table 2), which compete with cell receptors (Figure 2, upper right inset). Thus, the fucosylated H-2 antigen was established as the host cell surface antigen that is the determinant of susceptibility to campylobacter infection, and human milk oligosaccharides inhibit campylobacter binding to this critical determinant (46).

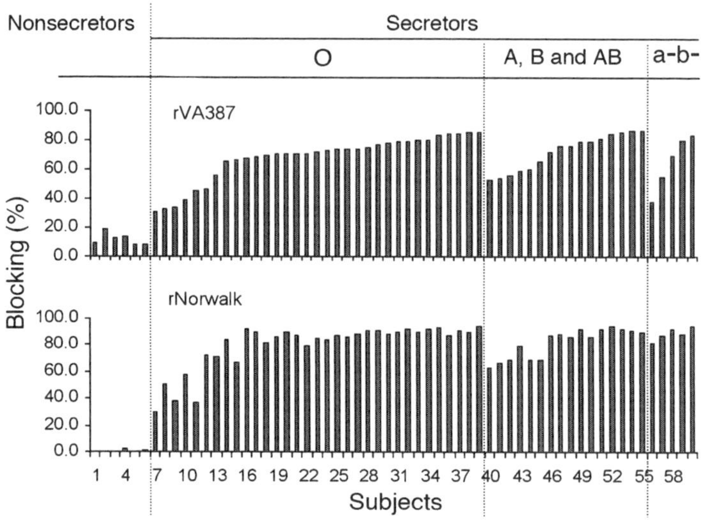

Figure 3 Inhibition of norovirus binding by human milk. Milk of secretors of all blood group types was effective at blocking binding, whereas milk from nonsecretors did not block binding. [Adapted from (23) and reprinted with permission from The University of Chicago Press]

most human milks contain glycans that specifically block NV binding to histo-blood group antigen receptors, which may provide protection to infants from NV infection.

INNATE IMMUNITY

We hypothesize that these fucosylated glycans are an essential part of the innate immune system of human milk whereby the mother protects her infant. If this were so, three characteristics are expected: (*a*) The glycans would be constitutively expressed in milk independently of the history of maternal exposure to pathogens. (*b*) The active glycans would need to be resistant to digestion in the gut so that they could be present at the site of infection. (*c*) Variation in the presence of these fucosylated glycans in milk should have a measurable consequence on the risk of disease by the relevant pathogens in breastfed infants. Each of these three criteria was investigated.

Constitutive Expression

Secretor and nonsecretor individuals are defined by the presence or absence of α1,2-linked fucosylated epitopes in their secretions, including saliva, tears, and milk. Thus, variation in milk glycan expression was typically thought of in terms of homozygous recessive (nonsecretors, no glycans with α1,2-linked fucose), homozygous dominant (secretors, high levels of α1,2-fucosylated glycans), and heterozygotes (secretors, intermediate levels of α1,2-linked fucosylated glycans) (14, 58). To this was added a fourth phenotype (55). The distribution of these phenotypes differs among populations (12), and oligosaccharide expression changes over the course of lactation (7, 12).

When individual oligosaccharides are measured in milk from a population of lactating mothers over the entire course of lactation, yet more complexity emerges (4). Nonsecretors do indeed produce milk that lacks α1,2-linked fucosyloligosaccharides, but after approximately a half-year of lactation, 2-linked fucosyloligosaccharides gradually become a significant component of the milk. Secretors produce milk that contains 2-linked fucosyloligosaccharides over the entire course of lactation, but the absolute and relative amounts of the individual oligosaccharides change over the course of lactation: The ratio of α1,2-linked fucosyloligosaccharides to α1,3- and α1,4-linked fucosyloligosaccharides declines exponentially (from a fivefold ratio in the first month to about 1:1 at the end of one year). However, among secretors, mothers who produce the highest amount of α1,2-linked oligosaccharides at any point in lactation tend to produce the highest amounts at other points of lactation, and likewise those who produce the lowest amounts tend to do so throughout the course of lactation. Thus, the pattern of oligosaccharide expression relative to the rest of the population tends to remain constant. This is consistent with genetic variation as the basis of variable expression of oligosaccharides in milk. In secretors, expression of the α1,2-linked fucosyloligosaccharides decreases over the course of lactation, with a reciprocal increase in expression of α1,3/4-linked fucosyloligosaccharides. In nonsecretors, expression of α1,3/4-linked oligosaccharides decreases over the course of lactation with a reciprocal increase in α1,2-linked oligosaccharides late in lactation. This inverse relationship implies reciprocal control of synthesis of these oligosaccharides, perhaps through reciprocal control of expression of fucosyltransferase genes, such as the secretor and Lewis genes that control the individual differences in expression of Lewis blood group type.

Synthesis of Oligosaccharides in Mammary Gland

All secretors express the secretor gene (*FUT2*) for the production of α1,2-fucosyltransferase. Of these, those of the Lewis a−b− blood group phenotype (Le^{a-b-}) do not express the Lewis gene (*FUT3*), which encodes the α1, 3/4-fucosyltransferase, while individuals of Le^{a-b+} blood group phenotype express the *FUT3* as well as *FUT2* genes. Just as differences in the expression of these two genes are invoked to explain the Lewis blood group system of fucosylated glycolipid expression in erythrocytes, the expression of those same genes may also explain the variation in expression of fucosylated oligosaccharides in milk. If so, the Lewis blood group type of the mother should strongly relate to fucosyloligosaccharide expression in her milk. The data are consistent with this prospectively studied from birth to two years of age with infant feeding and diarrhea data collected weekly. A single milk sample collected from mothers 1–5 weeks postpartum was analyzed for oligosaccharide content. Infants who developed diarrhea associated with ST of *E. coli* were consuming milk with significantly lower 2-linked to 3/4-linked oligosaccharide ratios than those of the remaining infants. Similarly, campylobacter diarrhea occurred less often in infants whose mother's milk contained high levels of 2′-FL, the specific 2-linked fucosyloligosaccharide that inhibits campylobacter. Norovirus diarrhea occurred less often in infants whose mother's milk contained high levels of lacto-*N*-difucohexaose (LDFH-I), a 2-linked fucosyloligosaccharide that contains an epitope that inhibits NV binding in vitro. Moderate-to-severe diarrhea of all causes occurred less often in infants whose milk contained high levels of total 2-linked fucosyloligosaccharide as a percent of milk oligosaccharide (Figure 6).

Host cell receptors for other pathogens can be glycans whose terminal moieties contain nonfucosylated epitopes. Binding by these pathogens likewise may be inhibited by milk glycans whose terminal moieties resemble their gut glycan receptors. Rotavirus is an example.

Rotavirus Inhibition by Human Milk Lactadherin

Infection by rotavirus is responsible for much of the diarrhea in infants around the world, and especially for diarrhea of young children in developed countries. The ability of rotavirus to infect MA-104 cells in culture is inhibited by human milk, and this inhibition is due to a mucin-associated 46 kDa milk glycoprotein named lactadherin. As shown in Figure 7 (see color insert), the inhibition is dose-dependent; furthermore, after sialic acid is removed from lactadherin, its ability

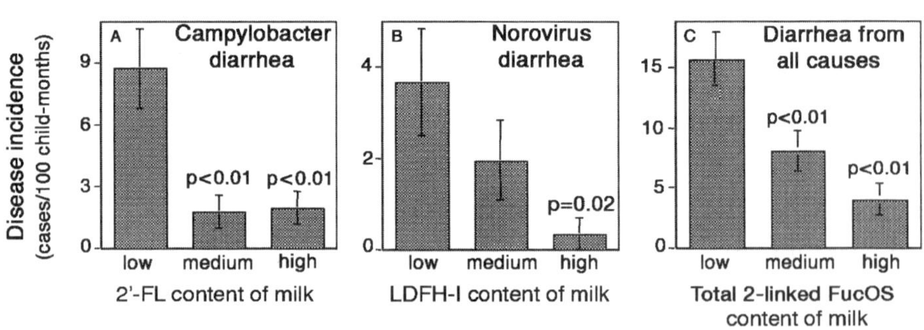

Figure 6 Diarrhea in nursing infants and content of 2′-fucosylated oligosaccharides in the milk consumed. *Panels A–C*: Content of milk refers to specific oligosaccharides as a percent of total oligosaccharide; low, medium, and high groups are tertiles of n = 31 infants each. *Panel C*: Diarrhea from all causes refers to all moderate-to-severe diarrhea. 2′-FL, 2′-fucosyllactose; LDFH-I, lacto-*N*-difucohexaose I; FucOS, fucosylated oligosaccharides. [Adapted from (31), with permission from Elsevier]

to inhibit rotavirus is essentially lost, which suggests that the glycan portion of the molecule may be responsible for inhibition and that a specific terminal sialic acid may be required for inhibition to occur. Lactadherin from human milk also inhibits rotavirus (EDIM strain) gastroenteritis in mice. Most pathogenic strains of rotavirus bind to a host cell glycoprotein receptor that contains a terminal sialic acid, and inhibition of this binding is thought to be the mechanism whereby lactadherin inhibits rotavirus (62).

The clinical relevance of variable expression of lactadherin in maternal milk was examined in a study conducted on rotavirus diarrhea in 200 infants in Mexico City (34). Infants were enrolled from birth, monitored regularly by enzyme immunoassay for rotavirus in stools, serology for induction of antirotavirus antibody in serum, and for feeding and stool patterns. Milk samples were obtained from the mothers weekly until four weeks post partum and monthly thereafter. The sample collected immediately before an episode of rotavirus infection was assayed for lactadherin, butyrophilin, mucin, and sIgA. Thirty-one infants were infected with rotavirus in the absence of other confounding pathogens. Of these, 15 infants exhibited symptoms of diarrhea, while 16 had no symptoms. The median concentration of lactadherin in maternal milk samples obtained 4–41 days before the infection was 48 μg/ml in the asymptomatic group and 29 μg/ml in the symptomatic group. Although these medians did not differ significantly, logistic regression analysis adjusted for age at infection and sIgA concentration revealed a significant difference between the groups in regard to concentration of milk lactadherin levels (Figure 8). Thus, variation in the concentration of the glycan, lactadherin, that inhibits rotavirus in vitro and in vivo is a determinant in the risk of diarrhea in nursing infants who are infected with rotavirus. This inhibition by lactadherin during nursing provides the dual purpose of preventing diarrhea when the infant is most vulnerable while still permitting the infant to raise antibodies to rotavirus, allowing for protection from rotavirus after weaning. No significant association between symptom status and concentrations of butyrophilin, mucin, or sIgA was found. This suggests that the milk glycans make a major contribution to the protection of breastfed infants from diarrheal disease that, in some cases, is at least as important as the secretory antibodies. We conclude that the human milk glycans are a major component of an innate immune system of human milk that plays a significant role in the ability of the mother to confer protection to her infant against disease.

Milk Glycan Inhibition of Other Pathogens

The human milk glycans that inhibit specific pathogens described above are representative of a growing family of such milk glycans that have been found to inhibit key steps of pathogenesis of individual pathogens in vitro, ex vivo, or in vivo (Table 4). In most cases, the detailed chemical structure of the specific inhibitor has not been fully defined. Although each of these milk glycans is capable of inhibiting only a specific pathogen or family of pathogens, their presence in the

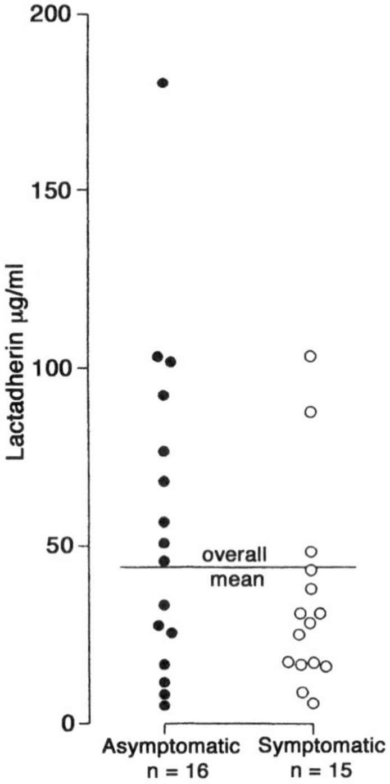

Figure 8 Breastfed infants infected with rotavirus but who remained asymptomatic were consuming milk with significantly higher content of lactadherin than milk consumed by infants who were infected and exhibited diarrhea; $p = 0.01$. [Reprinted from (34), with permission from Elsevier]

aggregate may represent an armamentarium that may be able to protect infants from many, and perhaps most, of the common enteric diseases, and perhaps many other diseases, of childhood.

PERSPECTIVE

In the arts, the mother/infant nursing dyad represents the essence of human kindness. Viewed through the lens of sociobiology, breastfeeding is considered the apex of altruism in the animal kingdom, wherein the mother gives of her own body to protect and nurture her progeny, but for the purpose of maximizing her own reproductive potential (19, 60). Two defining features of humans are a large brain and slow maturation; this combination optimizes the efficiency and duration of learning, allowing transmission across generations of large amounts of information needed for maintaining a complex culture. For this to occur, the optimum

TABLE 4 Human milk glycoconjugates that inhibit pathogens

Glycoconjugate	Pathogen	Reference	Typical concentration[a]
GM1	Labile toxin, cholera toxin	(44)	180 μg/liter
GM3	Enteropathogenic *Escherichia coli*	(20)	13 mg/liter
Gb_3	Shiga toxin	(36)	100–150 μg/liter
Sulfatide	Human immunodeficiency virus	(59)	100 μg/liter
Chondroitin sulfate	Human immunodeficiency virus	(39)	6 mg/liter
Lactadherin	Rotavirus	(62)	100 μg/liter
Mucin	S-fimbriated *E. coli*	(50)	1 g/liter
Mannosylated glycopeptide	Enterohemorrhagic *E. coli*	(2)	60 mg/liter
Oligosaccharides	*Streptococcus pneumoniae*	(1)	0.2–10 g/liter
	Enteropathogenic *E. coli*	(9)	3 g/liter
	Listeria monocytogenes	(6)	3 g/liter
Fucosylated oligosaccharides	*Campylobacter jejuni*	(46)	1–25 mg/liter
	Vibrio cholerae	(46)	1–25 mg/liter
	Stable toxin	(41)	40 μg/liter
Macromolecule-associated glycans	Noroviruses	(23)	370 mg/liter
	Pseudomonas aeruginosa	(26)	370 mg/liter
Sialyllactose	Cholera toxin	(21)	200 mg/liter
	E. coli	(53, 57)	200 mg/liter
	P. aeruginosa	(10)	200 mg/liter
	Aspergillus fumigatus conidia	(3)	200 mg/liter
	Influenza virus	(13, 29)	200 mg/liter
	Polyomavirus	(52)	200 mg/liter
	Helicobacter pylori	(33)	200 mg/liter

[a]Typical concentration of active fraction or component of milk; calculated by D.S.N. from published and unpublished data.

reproductive strategy is to rear relatively few offspring who are intensively nurtured by the parents over this extended maturation. Perhaps the most significant component of this huge parental investment in the survival of their offspring is the protection afforded by breasts that, in addition to providing balanced nutrients, are optimized to provide both innate and adaptive immune products that synergistically protect the infant from a vast array of virulent and often lethal pathogens that emerge from the environment.

in carbohydrate composition in human milk over 4 months of lactation. *Pediatrics* 91:637–41
8. Crane JK, Azar SS, Stam A, Newburg DS. 1994. Oligosaccharides from human milk block binding and activity of the *Escherichia coli* heat-stable enterotoxin (STa) in T84 intestinal cells. *J. Nutr.* 124:2358–64
9. Cravioto A, Tello A, Villafan H, Ruiz J, del Vedovo S, Neeser J-R. 1991. Inhibition of localized adhesion of enteropathogenic *Escherichia coli* to HEp-2 cells by immunoglobulin and oligosaccharide fractions of human colostrum and breast milk. *J. Infect. Dis.* 163:1247–55
10. Devaraj N, Sheykhnazari M, Warren WS, Bhavanandan VP. 1994. Differential binding of *Pseudomonas aeruginosa* to normal and cystic fibrosis tracheobronchial mucins. *Glycobiology* 4:307–16
11. Ehrlich P, Hubner W. 1892. Uber die Ubertragung von Immunitat durch Milch [On the transfer of immunity by milk]. *Deutsch Med. Wochenschr.* 18:393
12. Erney RM, Malone WT, Skelding MB, Marcon AA, Kleman-Leyer KM, et al. 2000. Variability of human milk neutral oligosaccharides in a diverse population. *J. Pediatr. Gastroenterol. Nutr.* 30:181–92
13. Gambaryan AS, Tuzikov AB, Piskarev VE, Yamnikova SS, Lvov DK, et al. 1997. Specification of receptor-binding phenotypes of influenza virus isolates from different hosts using synthetic sialylglycopolymers: non-egg-adapted human H1 and H3 influenza A and influenza B viruses share a common high binding affinity for 6′-sialyl(N-acetyllactosamine). *Virology* 232:345–50
14. Grollman EF, Kobata A, Ginsburg V. 1969. An enzymatic basis for Lewis blood types in man. *J. Clin. Invest.* 48:1489–94
15. Grulee CG, Sanford HN, Herron PH. 1934. Breast and artificial feeding. *JAMA* 103:735–38
16. Gustafsson L, Boiers C, Hallgren O, Mossberg A-K, Pettersson J, et al. 2005. HAMLET kills tumor cells by apoptosis: structure, cellular mechanisms, and therapy. *J. Nutr.*(Suppl.)135:1301–5
17. Gyorgy P, Jeanloz RW, Von Nicolai H, Zilliken F. 1974. Undialyzable growth factors for *Lactobacillus bifidus* var. pennsylvanicus. Protective effect of sialic acid bound to glycoproteins and oligosaccharides against bacterial degradation. *Eur. J. Biochem.* 43:29–33
18. Hanson L. 1961. Comparative immunological studies of the immune globulins of human milk and blood serum. *Int. Arch. Allergy Appl. Immunol.* 18:241–67
19. Hrdy SB. 1999. *Mother Nature*. New York: Random House
20. Idota T, Kawakami H. 1995. Inhibitory effects of milk gangliosides on the adhesion of *Escherichia coli* to human intestinal carcinoma cells. *Biosci. Biotechnol. Biochem.* 59:69–72
21. Idota T, Kawakami H, Murakami Y, Sugawara M. 1995. Inhibition of cholera toxin by human milk fractions and sialyllactose. *Biosci. Biotechnol. Biochem.* 59:417–19
22. Isaacs C. 2005. Human milk inactivates pathogens individually, additively, and synergistically. *J. Nutr.* (Suppl.)135:1288–90
23. Jiang X, Huang P, Zhong W, Tan M, Farkas T, et al. 2004. Human milk contains elements that block binding of noroviruses to human histo-blood group antigens in saliva. *J. Infect. Dis.* 190:1850–59
24. Kramer MS, Chalmers B, Hodnett ED, Sevkovskaya Z, Dzikovich I, et al. 2001. Promotion of Breastfeeding Intervention Trial (PROBIT): a randomized trial in the Republic of Belarus. *JAMA* 285:413–20
25. Kramer MS, Guo T, Platt RW, Shapiro S, Collet JP, et al. 2002. Breastfeeding and infant growth: biology or bias? *Pediatrics* 110:343–47
26. Lesman-Movshovich E, Lerrer B, Gilboa-Garber N. 2003. Blocking of *Pseudomonas aeruginosa* lectins by human milk glycans. *Can. J. Microbiol.* 49:230–35
27. Lindesmith L, Moe C, Marionneau S,

Ruvoen N, Jiang X, et al. 2003. Human susceptibility and resistance to Norwalk virus infection. *Nat. Med.* 9:548–53
28. Marionneau S, Ruvoen N, Le Moullac-Vaidye B, Clement M, Cailleau-Thomas A, et al. 2002. Norwalk virus binds to histo-blood group antigens present on gastroduodenal epithelial cells of secretor individuals. *Gastroenterology* 122:1967–77
29. Matrosovich MN, Gambaryan AS, Tuzikov AB, Byramova NE, Mochalova LV, et al. 1993. Probing of the receptor-binding sites of the H1 and H3 influenza A and influenza B virus hemagglutinins by synthetic and natural sialosides. *Virology* 196:111–21
30. Morrow AL, Guerrero ML, Shults J, Calva JJ, Lutter C, et al. 1999. Efficacy of home-based peer counselling to promote exclusive breastfeeding: a randomised controlled trial. *Lancet* 353:1226–31
31. Morrow AL, Ruiz-Palacios GM, Altaye M, Jiang X, Guerrero ML, et al. 2004. Human milk oligosaccharides are associated with protection against diarrhea in breast-fed infants. *J. Pediatr.* 145:297–303
32. Morrow AL, Ruiz-Palacios GM, Jiang X, Newburg DS. 2005. Human milk glycans that inhibit pathogen binding protect breastfeeding infants against infectious diarrhea. *J. Nutr.* (Suppl.)135:1306–9
33. Mysore JV, Wigginton T, Simon PM, Zopf D, Heman-Ackah LM, Dubois A. 1999. Treatment of *Helicobacter pylori* infection in rhesus monkeys using a novel antiadhesion compound. *Gastroenterology* 117: 1316–25
34. Newburg D, Peterson J, Ruiz-Palacios G, Matson D, Morrow A, et al. 1998. Role of human-milk lactadherin in protection against symptomatic rotavirus infection. *Lancet* 351:1160–64
35. Newburg DS. 2005. Innate immunity and human milk. *J. Nutr.* (Suppl.)135:1310–14
36. Newburg DS, Ashkenazi S, Cleary TG. 1992. Human milk contains the Shiga toxin and Shiga-like toxin receptor glycolipid, Gb_3. *J. Infect. Dis.* 166:832–36
37. Newburg DS, Chaturvedi P, Crane JK, Cleary TG, Pickering LK. 1995. Fucosylated oligosaccharide(s) of human milk inhibits stable toxin of *Escherichia coli*. In *Complex Carbohydrates and Advances in Biosciences*, ed. VP Agrawal, CB Sharma, A Sah, MD Zingde, pp. 199–226. Muzaffarnagar, India: Society Biosci.
38. Newburg DS, Daniel PF, O'Neil NE, McCluer RH. 1986. High performance liquid chromatography of oligosaccharides from human milk and colostrum. In *Human Lactation 2: Maternal and Environmental Factors*, ed. M Hamosh, AS Goldman, pp. 581–88. New York: Plenum
39. Newburg DS, Linhardt RJ, Ampofo SA, Yolken RH. 1995. Human milk glycosaminoglycans inhibit HIV glycoprotein gp120 binding to its host cell CD4 receptor. *J. Nutr.* 125:419–24
40. Newburg DS, Neubauer SH. 1995. Carbohydrates in milk. In *Handbook of Milk Composition*, ed. RG Jensen, pp. 273–349. San Diego: Academic
41. Newburg DS, Pickering LK, McCluer RH, Cleary TG. 1990. Fucosylated oligosaccharides of human milk protect suckling mice from heat-stabile enterotoxin of *Escherichia coli*. *J. Infect. Dis.* 162:1075–80
42. Newburg DS, Ruiz-Palacios GM, Altaye M, Chaturvedi P, Meinzen-Derr J, et al. 2004. Innate protection conferred by fucosylated oligosaccharides of human milk against diarrhea in breastfed infants. *Glycobiology* 14(3):253–63; erratum 14(5):13G
43. Obermeier S, Rudloff S, Pohlentz G, Lentze MJ, Kunz C. 1999. Secretion of ^{13}C-labelled oligosaccharides into human milk and infant's urine after an oral [^{13}C]galactose load. *Isotopes Environ. Health Stud.* 35:119–25
44. Otnaess AB, Laegreid A, Ertresvag K. 1983. Inhibition of enterotoxin from *Escherichia coli* and *Vibrio cholerae* by gangliosides from human milk. *Infect. Immun.* 40:563–69
45. Phadke SM, Deslouches B, Hileman SE, Montelaro RC, Wiesenfeld HC, Mietzner

TA. 2005. Antimicrobial peptides in mucosal secretions: the importance of local secretions in mitigating infection. *J. Nutr.* (Suppl.)135:1291–95
46. Ruiz-Palacios GM, Cervantes LE, Ramos P, Chavez-Munguia B, Newburg DS. 2003. *Campylobacter jejuni* binds intestinal H(O) antigen (Fucα1,2Gal β1,4GlcNAc), and fucosyloligosaccharides of human milk inhibit its binding and infection. *J. Biol. Chem.* 278:14112–20
47. Ruvoen-Clouet N, Ganiere JP, Andre-Fontaine G, Blanchard D, Le Pendu J. 2000. Binding of rabbit hemorrhagic disease virus to antigens of the ABH histo-blood group family. *J. Virol.* 74:11950–54
48. Salminen SJ, Gueimonde M, Isolauri E. 2005. Probiotics that modify disease risk. *J. Nutr.* (Suppl.)135:1296–300
49. Schlossman A, Moro E. 1903. Zur Kenntniss der Arteigenheit der verschiedenen Eiweisskorper der Milch. *Muench. Med. Wochsehr.* 1:597
50. Schroten H, Hanisch FG, Plogmann R, Hacker J, Uhlenbruck G, et al. 1992. Inhibition of adhesion of S-fimbriated *Escherichia coli* to buccal epithelial cells by human milk fat globule membrane components: a novel aspect of the protective function of mucins in the nonimmunoglobulin fraction. *Infect. Immun.* 60:2893–99
51. Stahl B, Thurl S, Zeng J, Karas M, Hillenkamp F, et al. 1994. Oligosaccharides from human milk as revealed by matrix-assisted laser desorption/ionization mass spectrometry. *Anal. Biochem.* 223:218–26
52. Stehle T, Yan Y, Benjamin TL, Harrison SC. 1994. Structure of murine polyomavirus complexed with an oligosaccharide receptor fragment. *Nature* 369:160–63
53. Stins MF, Prasadarao NV, Ibric L, Wass CA, Luckett P, Kim KS. 1994. Binding characteristics of S fimbriated *Escherichia coli* to isolated brain microvascular endothelial cells. *Am. J. Pathol.* 145:1228–36
54. Svanborg C, Agerstam H, Aronson A, Bjerkvig R, Duringer C, et al. 2003. HAMLET kills tumor cells by an apoptosis-like mechanism—cellular, molecular, and therapeutic aspects. *Adv. Cancer Res.* 88:1–29
55. Thurl S, Henker J, Siegel M, Tovar K, Sawatzki G. 1997. Detection of four human milk groups with respect to Lewis-blood-group-dependent oligosaccharides. *Glycoconj. J.* 14:795–99
56. Tissier H. 1905. Repartition des microbes dans l'intestin du nourisson. *Ann. de l'Institut de Pasteur* 19:109
57. Virkola R, Parkkinen J, Hacker J, Korhonen TK. 1993. Sialyloligosaccharide chains of laminin as an extracellular matrix target for S fimbriae of *Escherichia coli. Infect. Immun.* 61:4480–84
58. Viverge D, Grimmonprez L, Cassanas G, Bardet L, Solere M. 1990. Discriminant carbohydrate components of human milk according to donor secretor types. *J. Pediatr. Gastroenterol. Nutr.* 11:365–70
59. Viveros-Rogel M, Soto-Ramirez L, Chaturvedi P, Newburg DS, Ruiz-Palacios GM. 2004. Inhibition of HIV-1 infection in vitro by human milk sulfated glycolipids and glycosaminoglycans. *Adv. Exp. Med. Biol.* 554:481–87
60. Wilson EO. 1980. *Sociobiology*. Cambridge, MA: Harvard Univ. Press
61. Yalom M. 1997. *A History of the Breast.* New York: Random House
62. Yolken RH, Peterson JA, Vonderfecht SL, Fouts ET, Midthun K, Newburg DS. 1992. Human milk mucin inhibits rotavirus replication and prevents experimental gastroenteritis. *J. Clin. Invest.* 90:1984–91

Annu. Rev. Nutr. 2005. 25:59–85
doi: 10.1146/annurev.nutr.24.012003.132145

First published online as a Review in Advance on May 4, 2005

NUTRITIONAL CONTROL OF GENE EXPRESSION: How Mammalian Cells Respond to Amino Acid Limitation*

M.S. Kilberg, Y.-X. Pan, and H. Chen
Department of Biochemistry and Molecular Biology, University of Florida College of Medicine, Gainesville, Florida 32610-0245; email: mkilberg@ufl.edu

V. Leung-Pineda
Department of Cell Biology and Physiology, Washington University School of Medicine, Saint Louis, Missouri 63110-1093

Key Words nutrient starvation, metabolite control, protein metabolism, transcription, mRNA stability

■ **Abstract** The amino acid response (AAR) pathway in mammalian cells is designed to detect and respond to amino acid deficiency. Limiting any essential amino acid initiates this signaling cascade, which leads to increased translation of a "master regulator," activating transcription factor (ATF) 4, and ultimately, to regulation of many steps along the pathway of DNA to RNA to protein. These regulated events include chromatin remodeling, RNA splicing, nuclear RNA export, mRNA stabilization, and translational control. Proteins that are increased in their expression as targets of the AAR pathway include membrane transporters, transcription factors from the basic region/leucine zipper (bZIP) superfamily, growth factors, and metabolic enzymes. Significant progress has been achieved in understanding the molecular mechanisms by which amino acids control the synthesis and turnover of mRNA and protein. Beyond gaining additional knowledge of these important regulatory pathways, further characterization of how these processes contribute to the pathology of various disease states represents an interesting aspect of future research in molecular nutrition.

*ABBREVIATIONS: AAR, amino acid response (pathway); AARE, amino acid response element; ARE, AU-rich elements; ASNS, asparagine synthetase; Cdk, cyclin-dependent kinase; CdkI, cyclin-dependent kinase inhibitor; C/EBP, CCAAT-enhancer binding protein; ChIP, chromatin immunoprecipitation; CHOP, C/EBP homology protein/growth arrest and DNA damage 153; EMSA, electrophoresis mobility shift analysis; mTOR, mammalian target of rapamycin; NSRE, nutrient-sensing response element; UPR, unfolded protein response.

CONTENTS

DETECTION OF AMINO ACID AVAILABILITY

Mammalian cells have two recognized pathways for monitoring and responding to amino acid availability. These two pathways change the rate of protein synthesis in opposite directions, but whether they are linked in a more direct manner is not known. The mammalian target of rapamycin (mTOR) pathway functions to confirm a sufficient level of amino acids to support protein synthesis and cell growth. Through an unknown amino acid detection mechanism, amino acid sufficiency activates the mTOR kinase cascade that ultimately results in phosphorylation of the ribosome-associated S6 kinase. Activation of the S6 kinase permits a high level of translation of mRNA species that encode ribosomal proteins. In this way, protein synthesis and cell growth rates are maintained at a rate consistent with nutrient availability. How the extracellular or cellular amino acid level is detected remains unknown, as do the exact events that exist between that detection mechanism and the activation of the mTOR kinase. A number of excellent reviews on the mTOR pathway and control of translation have been published recently (35, 50, 65, 98). The second known amino acid responsive pathway is designed to detect amino acid deficiency. Limiting the availability for any single amino acid initiates this signaling cascade, which is referred to here as the amino acid response (AAR) pathway. The substrate specificity for this pathway is not well understood, but in general, if an amino acid is "essential" to the cell, an insufficient amount of that amino acid will trigger pathway activation. In this instance, the definition of an essential amino acid must be considered in the context of a particular cell type rather than the whole organism. For example, acute lymphoblastic leukemia cells express particularly low levels of asparagine synthetase, and therefore, asparagine is an essential amino acid for this specific cell type. In fact, this cell-specific need for extracellular asparagine is the basis for the use of asparaginase as a chemotherapeutic drug for childhood acute lymphoblastic leukemia (7), and as expected, the drug-induced asparagine deprivation triggers the AAR pathway in MOLT4 leukemia cells (8).

Limiting the extracellular supply of an essential amino acid or blocking the synthesis of an otherwise nonessential one results in an increase in uncharged tRNA that binds to and activates the general control nonderepressible protein 2 (GCN2) kinase (13, 110, 130). In this manner, the GCN2 protein serves as a sensor of amino acid insufficiency. It is interesting that suppressed activity for any one of the tRNA synthetases can also trigger the AAR pathway, despite a normal cytoplasmic level of that amino acid (6). Once activated, GCN2 kinase phosphorylates the translation initiation factor eIF-2α, which leads to a decrease in global protein synthesis (64). However, selected mRNAs exhibit increased translation under these circumstances, as first demonstrated for the yeast transcription factor GCN4 (52), and more recently shown for the mammalian GCN4 counterpart, activating transcription factor 4 (ATF4) (46, 103). This translational control is modulated by short upstream open reading frames in the GCN4 (52) and ATF4 (77, 115) mRNA, which permit translation of the transcription factor primarily when translation initiation has been slowed in response to eIF-2α phosphorylation. GCN4 has been called a "master regulator" of nutrient sensing in yeast, as its elevated production following amino acid deprivation results in a change in the transcriptional rate for literally hundreds of genes (85). Although the entire mammalian genome has yet to be screened for responsiveness to ATF4, it also appears to serve as an important regulator of cell stress based on an initial array analysis (47). In support of this interpretation, genomic analysis of specific genes for which the amino acid response elements have been identified has demonstrated that ATF4 plays a key role in the transcriptional control of these genes (see below).

AMINO ACID REGULATION OF RNA SYNTHESIS AND METABOLISM

Amino acid deprivation has been demonstrated to regulate gene expression at a number of steps along the pathway of DNA to RNA to protein (Figure 1). As mentioned above, amino acid–dependent control of protein synthesis has been reviewed elsewhere. Therefore, the following is a summary of the influence that amino acid availability has at steps from DNA to RNA, as well as mRNA turnover. The published observations are described briefly to illustrate the breadth of mechanisms that cells use to regulate gene expression in response to amino acid limitation. Examples from yeast are given for those steps not yet investigated in mammalian cells.

Chromatin Structure and Transcription Factor Recruitment

Eukaryotic DNA is packaged with core histone proteins to form chromatin, with the nucleosome serving as the basic structural repeating unit. In addition, the chromatin fiber contains a large number of other proteins, such as linker histones and nonhistone proteins, to stabilize the folded nucleosomal arrays and to perform specialized functions within tightly bundled chromatin domains. Transcriptional activation of a particular gene is thought to require a transition from a compacted

D, and other members of the hnRNP family, interact with AREs and affect the stability of ARE-containing mRNA. All of the above-mentioned proteins except HuR function as destabilizers of the ARE-containing mRNA to which they bind (76). It has been shown that HuR and AUF1 can bind to common target mRNA molecules in a competitive fashion, but AUF1-bound mRNA undergoes exosome-mediated decay, whereas HuR-bound mRNA is stabilized (69). HuR is a member of the human embryonic lethal abnormal vision family of RNA-binding proteins, ubiquitously expressed in all cell types. In addition to stabilization of ARE-containing mRNA molecules, HuR also plays a role in the nuclear export of mRNA and in the control of translation (16).

Yaman et al. (128) demonstrated by in vitro RNA gel shift experiments that HuR could bind to an ARE within the 3′ UTR sequence of the CAT-1 cationic amino acid transporter mRNA. They were also the first to report that amino acid limitation causes increased HuR accumulation in the cytoplasm. Consistent with that observation, cytoplasmic HuR binding to the CAT-1 ARE was increased during amino acid deprivation, resulting in stabilization of the mRNA. Like CAT-1, the 3′ region of the ATF3 mRNA contains several AUUUA sequences. Immunoprecipitation of HuR-RNA complexes followed by real time PCR analysis showed that HuR also interacts with ATF3 mRNA in vivo and that the interaction increases following amino acid limitation of HepG2 hepatoma cells (Y.-X. Pan, H. Chen, & M.S. Kilberg, manuscript submitted). As originally shown by Yaman et al. (128) for C6 glioma cells, after amino acid limitation the total amount of HuR was increased in the HepG2 cells and it was translocated from the nucleus to the cytoplasm. Importantly, these changes in cytoplasmic accumulation of HuR paralleled the kinetics of ATF3 mRNA accumulation in vivo. Furthermore, suppression of HuR protein content using RNAi partially blocked the increase in ATF3 mRNA in histidine-deprived HepG2 cells.

Leung-Pineda et al. (72) have shown that the cyclin-dependent kinase inhibitors (CdkIs) p21 and p27 also represent an example of mRNA stabilization in response to amino acid deprivation. The progression of the cell cycle from one phase to the next is tightly controlled by three classes of proteins: cyclins, cyclin-dependent kinases (Cdks), and CdkIs. Cyclins and Cdks act as positive regulators by forming complexes with each other to cause phosphorylation of specific cell cycle–promoting substrates and thus advancement into the next phase. Individual CdkIs function as negative regulators of the cell cycle by inhibiting the action of specific cyclin-Cdk complexes.

A long-standing model of how amino acid limitation may block cell cycle progression is based on the observation that amino acid deprivation has the same effect as protein synthesis inhibition and serum starvation (83). All three treatments can lead to cell cycle arrest in G0, a resting state that the cell can enter from the G1 phase. This transition is thought to occur because of a general decrease in global protein synthesis, which leads to a decreased rate of cyclin D synthesis (105). However, more recent studies demonstrate that amino acids can act as signaling molecules, and this research has led to the hypothesis that amino acid limitation controls cell cycle progression by specifically modulating the gene expression of individual regulators of the cell cycle, independent of global effects on protein synthesis. For example, Leung-Pineda et al. (72) observed that limitation for the essential amino acid histidine leads to increased mRNA and protein expression for the CdkIs p21 and p27 in HepG2 human hepatoma cells (72). This increase in p21 and p27 expression occurs in the presence of actinomycin D, and extensive promoter analysis provided no evidence for transcriptional control of the p21 gene (72). Additional experiments showed that the increase in p21 and p27 mRNA was dependent on mRNA stabilization rather than transcription. Furthermore, as described above for ATF3, siRNA-induced blockade of HuR protein expression following amino acid deprivation prevented the increase in p21 mRNA (Y.-X. Pan & M.S. Kilberg, unpublished observations). These observations not only provide an example of amino acid–regulated mRNA stabilization, but also are consistent with the proposal by Leung-Pineda et al. (72) that through the increased expression of the CdkIs p21 and p27, cells have more specific mechanisms for amino acid–dependent control of the cell cycle than relying on a global decline in protein synthesis with its subsequent pleiotropic effects. Collectively, the CAT-1, ATF3, and p21/p27 data illustrate the critical role that mRNA destabilization and stabilization plays in the amino acid response, and it is likely that many other examples will be discovered.

TARGET GENES FOR AMINO ACID LIMITATION

Array analysis of amino acid–deprived yeast has illustrated that the spectrum of GCN4-activated genes goes well beyond amino acid transport and biosynthesis (85). Although there is not yet an array covering an entire mammalian genome, partial screening has identified a large number of ATF4 target genes (47) and similarities to yeast counterparts are clear. In addition to those described in more detail in this section, other amino acid–responsive genes include transcription factors such as CCAAT-enhancer binding protein-α (C/EBPα) (79), as well as c-jun, junB, c-myc, and c-fos (96). As mentioned above, the mRNA content for the ribosomal proteins L17 and S25 is increased (67, 68, 104), as is expression of the ER chaperone protein calreticulin (51). Cytokines and growth factors that have been confirmed to be amino acid responsive include interleukin-8 (IL-8) (14) and glucagon (93). This list is increasing steadily and it is expected to get much longer. More important than the number of genes induced by amino acid limitation, the breadth of their function illustrates the organism's need to globally modulate its gene expression profile to adapt to a changing nutritional environment. A few examples of amino acid–regulated genes are described below in more detail to illustrate the molecular mechanisms by which gene expression is controlled.

Transporter Proteins

A number of plasma membrane amino acid transport activities have been demonstrated to be responsive to amino acid availability. The two most extensively studied include neutral amino acid transport System A, mediated by the SNAT2 gene product, and cationic amino acid transport, mediated by the CAT-1 transporter. These two examples are discussed in greater detail below, but other examples include one or more members of the excitatory amino acid transporter (EAAT) family, which mediate the uptake of the anionic amino acids glutamate and aspartate. McGivan and colleagues (86, 94) have demonstrated that the transport of glutamate across the cell membrane of the kidney cell line NBL-1 increased following amino acid limitation. Glutamate transport in this cell line is thought to be mediated by the EAAT3 transporter (86, 94), but the EAAT3 protein content within the starved NBL-1 cells was not increased, a finding that suggests the increased glutamate transport activity was the result of a posttranslational mechanism on EAAT3 or that regulatory proteins or unidentified transporters contributed to this activity. Interestingly, the EAAT transporters have interacting proteins referred to as glutamate transporter-associated proteins (GTRAPs) that can modulate transport activity. For example, GTRAP3-18 binds to the C-terminal of EAAT3 and inhibits transport activity (21). Such regulatory proteins associated with specific transporters represent a relatively new area of investigation and should provide important new insight into transporter control.

Another example of amino acid–regulated transport has been demonstrated for System L transport activity mediated by the protein product LAT1, which exists as a heterodimer with the plasma membrane glycoprotein 4F2 heavy chain (116). Although not a substrate for the neutral amino acid transporter LAT1, removing arginine from the culture medium caused an activation of the transporter activity (87). It remains to be established whether this effect by arginine represents a regulatory mechanism associated with arginine itself or an indirect result of changing nitric oxide levels within the cell.

SNAT2 NEUTRAL AMINO ACID TRANSPORTER System A transport activity mediates the sodium-dependent, secondary active transport of neutral amino acids in all nucleated mammalian cells. Regulation of transport activity has been investigated extensively and is increased by a broad spectrum of hormones and growth factors as well as substrate availability and cellular growth rate (15, 62, 81, 89). Hepatic transport of alanine, in part mediated by System A activity, can be a rate-determining step for further alanine metabolism (27, 28), and thus it is hypothesized that glucagon-induced alanine delivery via System A contributes to the aberrant synthesis of glucose in diabetes (106). In addition to hormone signals, System A transport activity is increased by amino acid limitation. This activation occurs when mammalian cells are deprived of even a single amino acid that is essential for that particular cell; the amino acid may or may not be a substrate for the transporter (45). Recently, three distinct genes have been identified that encode System A transport activity, and a unified nomenclature has been proposed for these genes by Mackenzie & Erickson (78) using the term SNAT (systems N and A transporters). The genes representing System A transport activity are SNAT1 (formerly ATA1, SAT1, SA2, GlnT, NAT2), SNAT2 (formerly ATA2, SAT2, SA1), and SNAT4 (formerly ATA3, NAT3). Expression of these

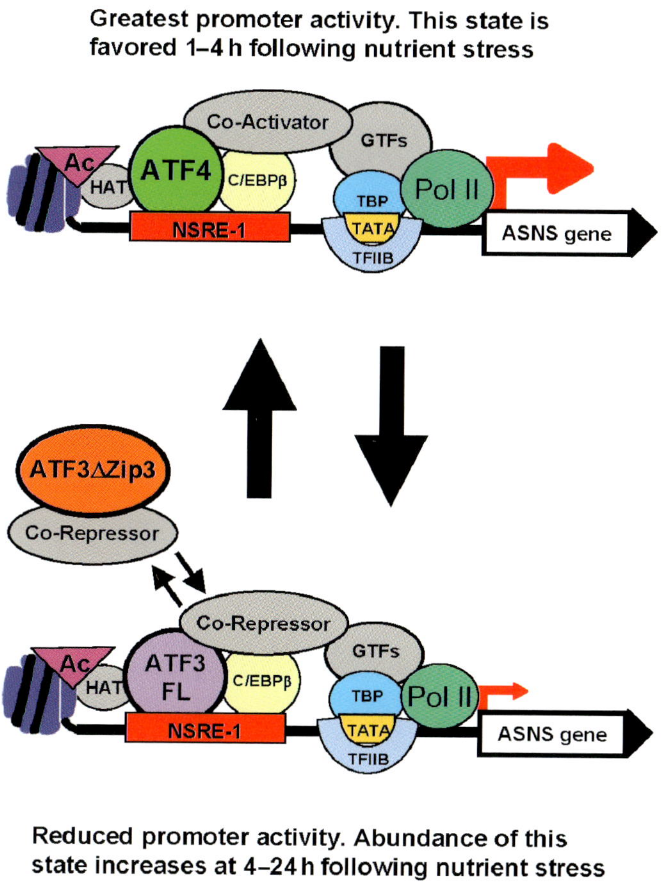

Figure 4 Working model for control of the asparagine synthetase (ASNS) gene (see text for details). Transcription factors shown in color have been localized to the ASNS promoter by chromatin immunoprecipitation analysis (24). Unidentified proteins are shown in gray.

genes is tissue specific and the functional properties are somewhat different between the three protein products. SNAT2 mRNA content is increased following amino acid deprivation (10, 38, 74), and Hyde et al. (55) have shown that there is an increase in plasma membrane SNAT2 protein following amino acid limitation of skeletal muscle cells or 3T3-L1 mouse adipocytes. The induction of System A activity (36), as well as the increase in SNAT2 mRNA (75), is largely prevented by the MAP kinase pathway inhibitor PD98059. Lopez-Fontanals et al. (75) used this sensitivity to show that the SNAT2 induction by amino acid limitation was mediated by the MAP kinase pathway, whereas transporter activation by hypertonicity was not. Two important questions about these observations remain unresolved. How is the MAP kinase pathway activated by amino acid limitation? What is the mechanism by which the kinase pathway increases SNAT2 mRNA expression?

Palii et al. (90) have established that the human, chimpanzee, mouse, and rat SNAT2 gene contains an amino acid response element (AARE) within the first intron. For the human gene, the AARE sequence is located at nucleotides +712 to +724 (Figure 3). The core sequence of the SNAT2 AARE (5′-TGATGCAAT-3′) is identical to that present in the promoter region of the human C/EBP homology protein (CHOP) gene (90). A unique feature of the SNAT2 AARE is the presence of a nearby CAAT box (Figure 3) that is not absolutely necessary for the amino acid response, but when it is mutated the response is blunted to about 60% of the maximum (90). The AARE functions as an enhancer element in that it is position and orientation independent and can convey amino acid responsiveness to a heterologous promoter. The SNAT2 intronic region near the AARE also contains a purine-rich sequence (PuR box) that contributes to maintenance of the gene's low rate of basal transcription but does not appear to play a direct role in the amino acid response (90). As shown in Figure 3, all three of these elements are completely conserved in sequence and relative intronic location across the human, chimpanzee, mouse, and rat species.

CAT-1 CATIONIC AMINO ACID TRANSPORTER The CAT-1 gene product mediates the sodium-independent transport of arginine, lysine, and, to a lesser extent, histidine and ornithine. Prior to cloning of the cDNA and gene for CAT-1, CAT-2, and CAT-3, the collective transport activity for cationic amino acids was referred to as System Ly^+ (122). Characterization of Ly^+ activity and its regulation has been described over the last three decades, and two recent reviews summarize the current knowledge regarding the transport activity and the CAT family of transporter genes (49, 116). Interestingly, the CAT-1 transporter serves as the receptor for the murine ecotropic retrovirus, and it was on the basis of this receptor function that the original mouse cDNA was cloned (63, 118). The CAT-1 transporter protein in other species does not function as a retroviral receptor because of specific amino acid differences (5), but stable expression of the murine CAT-1 protein has been used to render human cells susceptible to the murine ecotropic retrovirus (7). While investigating the viral receptor properties of the rat CAT-1 protein, Hatzoglou and colleagues determined that expression was regulated by amino acid

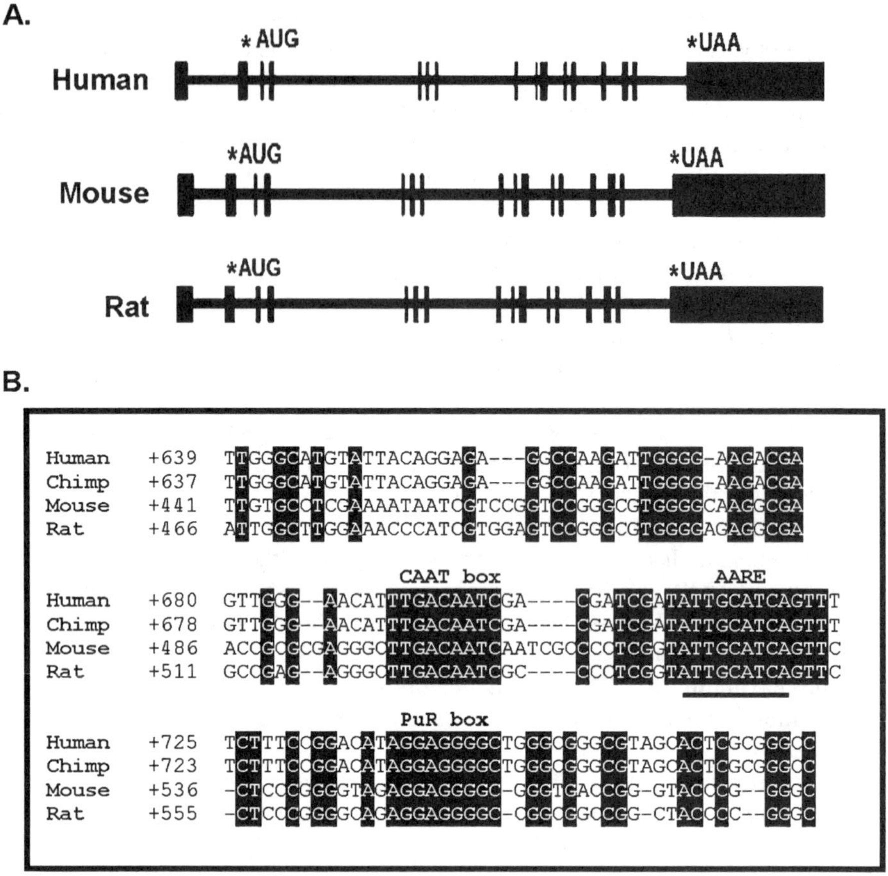

Figure 3 SNAT2 gene structure and the conserved sequences within intron 1. *Panel A* depicts the structure of the 16 exons and 15 introns within the human, chimpanzee, mouse, and rat SNAT2 genes (90). The translation start (AUG) and stop (UAA) sites are also shown. *Panel B* shows the conservation of sequence within intron 1 that contains the amino acid response element (AARE), the CAAT box, and the purine-rich element (PuR). The core sequence of the AARE that is identical to that in the C/EBP homology protein (CHOP) promoter is underlined. The numbers are the nucleotide for that particular species relative to the predicted transcription start site as +1.

availability (54). Their studies showed that removal of a single essential amino acid or all amino acids induced an increase in CAT-1 mRNA. More recently, it has been documented that expression of CAT-1 protein is increased by amino acid limitation through both transcriptional and posttranscriptional mechanisms (49). The transcriptional activation is mediated by an AARE identified within the first exon of the genomic sequence (nucleotides +45 to +53) that is identical in sequence to the nutrient-sensing response element-1 (NSRE-1) nutrient control site of the ASNS gene (125). These two genes differ in that the combination of NSRE-1/NSRE-2 sites in the ASNS gene responds to both the AAR and the unfolded protein response (UPR) stress response pathways (discussed below), whereas the CAT-1 gene lacks an NSRE-2 sequence, and control through the AARE is limited to amino acids (31). Point mutation of the CAT-1 AARE sequence abolished the amino acid–induced transcription, although the corresponding transcription factors that mediate this induction have yet to be identified.

As described above, using CAT-1 as a model, Hatzoglou and coworkers were the first to demonstrate that regulatory proteins associated with mRNA stabilization are modulated by amino acid availability (128). Those authors documented that after amino acid limitation, nuclear HuR protein was translocated to the cytoplasm and the interaction between CAT-1 and HuR protein was increased. A third form of regulation impacting CAT-1 expression arises from the presence of an internal ribosome entry sequence (IRES) in the CAT-1 mRNA, such that m^7G-cap independent translation initiation occurs, and this internal initiation is increased following amino acid deprivation (33, 34). Translation of a short uORF in the 5′ end of the CAT-1 mRNA is necessary for this amino acid–dependent translational control (32). Translation of the uORF leads to a change in mRNA structure that allows ribosome entry at the IRES, and consequently, selective translation of the CAT-1 coding sequence (127). Thus, synthesis of the CAT-1 cationic amino acid transporter is a highly regulated process that displays amino acid–dependent control at the transcriptional, mRNA stability, and translational steps of synthesis.

Transcription Factors

ACTIVATING TRANSCRIPTION FACTOR 4 The ATF family of proteins represents a subclass of the bZIP superfamily (43). Selected ATF members are known to heterodimerize within the ATF family as well as with members of another bZIP subgroup, the C/EBP family. In particular, a C/EBPβ-ATF4 complex has been detected at cAMP response elements (114) and the crystal structure of the C/EBPβ–ATF4 heterodimer has been obtained (95). As described below, the human CHOP promoter contains a C/EBP-ATF composite site (123), at which Fawcett et al. (30) observed by electrophoresis mobility shift analysis (EMSA) a transient ATF4 binding 2 hours after initiating arsenite-induced stress. The nuclear extract ATF4 binding activity was replaced at 6 hours by ATF3 binding activity that was coincident with a suppression of the gene back toward the basal rate. Bruhat et al. (17) later showed that this same C/EBP-ATF composite site functions as an AARE. Other C/EBP-ATF composite sites that function as AAREs have been reported for ASNS (107), the SNAT2 neutral amino acid transporter (90), and the CAT-1 cationic amino acid transporter (31). ATF4 has been shown to bind to the ASNS (107) and CHOP (9) sites in vitro by EMSA, and to the ASNS promoter in vivo by ChIP (24). These observations, coupled with increased translation of ATF4 following amino acid deprivation (46), are consistent with the proposed role for ATF4 as the key regulator of the AAR pathway.

following amino acid limitation requires both ATF2 phosphorylation and increased ATF4 expression (9).

Interestingly, there may be graded differences in response to depletion of a particular amino acid within a given cell type (58). Whereas the relative activation of the ASNS promoter was greater than that for CHOP when HeLa cells were deprived of leucine, cysteine, asparagine, or histidine, the activation of the CHOP promoter was nearly twice as great as that for ASNS when the cells were starved for methionine (58). Furthermore, Bruhat et al. (17) demonstrated that the relative magnitude of transcriptional activation from the CHOP AARE following depletion of leucine, methionine, or lysine was different in HeLa, Caco-2, and HepG2 hepatoma cells. How amino acid specificity relates to possible in vivo tissue-specific effects, especially at the initial detection steps in the AAR pathway, remains to be established. With regard to other factors that may influence amino acid control, Entingh et al. (26) showed that the induction of CHOP by amino acid deprivation of mouse fibroblasts required serum; they went on to document that the serum-required component was insulin-like growth factor-1 (IGF-1). Interestingly, induction of the System A amino acid transporter activity following amino acid starvation in fibroblasts is also dependent on serum (37, 61), but that is not the case in rat hepatoma cells (61).

ACTIVATING TRANSCRIPTION FACTOR 3 ATF3 is expressed at low levels in normal and quiescent cells, but can be rapidly induced in response to diverse stress signals and is likely to be involved in controlling a wide variety of cellular activities (48, 56, 91). Pan et al. (91) and Jiang et al. (56) demonstrated that the expression of ATF3 is induced in response to activation of the AAR and the UPR pathways, and the latter group showed these inductions required the eIF-2α kinases GCN2 and PERK, respectively (56). Ron and associates (47) have shown through a microarray survey that in ATF4-deficient fibroblasts, tunicamycin-induced ATF3 mRNA induction is reduced as compared with the wild type. Wek and colleagues (56) have shown that in both GCN2$^{-/-}$ and ATF4$^{-/-}$ fibroblasts, induction of ATF3 was impaired following amino acid limitation. These results illustrate the importance of ATF4 on ATF3 expression in response to a variety of stress stimuli.

The amino acid–dependent stabilization of ATF3 mRNA is briefly summarized above, but relatively little is known about the mechanisms controlling transcription of the ATF3 gene under nutritional stress conditions. The human ATF3 promoter has a consensus ATF/CRE site at nucleotides –93 to –85 (5′-TTACGTCAG-3′) and a C/EBP-ATF composite site at nucleotides –23 to –15 (5′-TGATGCAAC-3′), but there are no in vivo studies of transcription factor binding. The C/EBP-ATF element has been identified as an ATF3 binding site responsible for autoregulation of the ATF3 gene (124). The sequence of this element differs from the NSRE-1 in ASNS (5′-TGATG<u>A</u>AAC-3′) and the AARE in CHOP (3′-TGATGCAA<u>T</u>-5′) by only one nucleotide each, and ATF4 has been shown to bind this ATF3 sequence in vitro (30). However, whether this AARE-like element contributes to the increase in ATF3 mRNA following histidine deprivation is unknown.

METABOLISM AND GROWTH CONTROL

VASCULAR ENDOTHELIAL GROWTH FACTOR Vascular endothelial growth factor (VEGF) has potent angiogenic properties and is expressed as four alternative spliced variants that exert similar activity on endothelial cell proliferation and permeability. VEGF levels are higher in the serum and urine of patients with tumor or metastatic disease relative to healthy individuals (126). Abcouwer et al. (1) showed that deprivation of the amino acid glutamine caused increased VEGF mRNA expression in a retinal pigmented epithelial cell line. This induction was the result of both increased transcription and mRNA stabilization. Although glutamine deprivation induced the transcription factors NF-κB and activating protein 1 (AP-1) activities in human breast carcinoma cells, Bobrovnikova-Marjon et al. (14) showed that the induction of VEGF expression was independent of those two factors. Roybal et al. (102) reported that homocysteine or other thiol-containing compounds induced expression of VEGF and also caused transient phosphorylation of eIF2α, which, as expected, caused an increase in ATF4 protein content. Those authors showed that the VEGF induction in response to homocysteine was abolished by blockade of ATF4 function through the use of a dominant negative or in ATF4-deficient mouse embryonic fibroblasts. Collectively, these results suggest that control of expression for critical growth factors such as VEGF is sensitive to amino acid availability.

INSULIN-LIKE GROWTH FACTOR BINDING PROTEIN-1 The importance of amino acid–dependent regulation of insulin-like growth factor binding protein-1 (IGFBP-1) has been reviewed by Bruhat et al. (18), and is briefly summarized here. Protein malnutrition has been documented to decrease the circulating level of IGF-I, but to increase the level of IGFBP-1 (111). The effect on IGFBP-1 expression was demonstrated to be the result of increased mRNA content. Straus (112) showed that single amino acid limitation of hepatoma cells in culture also resulted in an increase in IGFBP-1 mRNA. Jousse et al. (57) investigated the expression of IGF-I, IGF-II, and IGFBP-1 in response to amino acid limitation in cultured cells and showed that IGFBP-1 mRNA and protein content was increased significantly, whereas the expression of the IGF-1 and IGF-II were either unaffected or slightly reduced. These observations appear to conflict with the observations of Entingh et al. (26), who reported that the activation of the CHOP gene by amino acid deprivation of fibroblasts requires the presence of IGF-1. However, those authors suggested that even a decreased level of IGF-I might still be sufficient for induction of the CHOP gene. The exact role of IGF-I in modulating the AAR pathway and the apparent cell specificity of this involvement requires further investigation. The regulation of IGFBP-1 is of particular interest because given the broad nature of its physiologic function, nutrient-dependent control of its expression is likely to impact a number of organs and cell types. An investigation of the influence of amino acid availability on the entire spectrum of hormones and cytokines has not been reported, but such a study would contribute to our understanding of the interorgan effects that protein nutrition has on cell growth and metabolism. For example, it has been demonstrated in cell culture that histidine deprivation of pancreatic cells was unique among the amino acids in causing suppression of the synthesis of glucagon (93). Relative to this observation, it will be interesting to discover how dietary amino acid availability impacts metabolic homeostasis in diabetic patients and their nutrition.

ASPARAGINE SYNTHETASE ASNS catalyzes the ATP-dependent synthesis of asparagine and glutamate from aspartate and glutamine (99). Gong et al. (40) were the first to determine that ASNS mRNA content increased in cells deprived of amino acid; subsequently, Hutson & Kilberg (53) also demonstrated increased ASNS mRNA content following total amino acid deprivation or depletion of a single essential amino acid. Guerrini et al. (42) analyzed the ASNS promoter region and determined that an AARE was present at nucleotides –70 to –64. In vivo footprinting by Barbosa-Tessmann et al. (11) revealed five protein binding sites within the ASNS proximal promoter region that contribute to nutrient control of the human ASNS gene, three GC boxes (GC-I, GC-II, and GC-III), and two novel sequences, originally labeled sites V and VI, and later renamed nutrient-sensing response element (NSRE)-1 and -2. The three GC-rich sequences are necessary to maintain the basal transcription rate and to permit maximal activation of the ASNS gene by the AAR or UPR pathways (71). Expression of either Sp1 or Sp3 in *Drosophila* SL2 cells supported basal ASNS promoter activity, but interestingly only Sp3 expression permitted the starvation-induced ASNS-driven transcription. Barbosa-Tessmann et al. (12) demonstrated that both NSRE-1 and NSRE-2 were required for activation of the human ASNS gene following activation by either the AAR or the UPR pathways. EMSA experiments revealed increased nuclear protein binding to the NSRE-1 binding site (5′-TGATGAAAC-3′, nucleotides –68 to –60) when extracts from either amino acid or glucose-deprived cells were tested (11). This broader nutrient-detecting capability is the reason that the site is referred to as an NSRE rather than solely as an AARE. Mutagenesis of the ASNS promoter confirmed the in vivo footprinting, which had suggested the presence of a second element, NSRE-2 (nucleotides –48 to –43, 5′-GTTACA-3′), positioned eleven nucleotides downstream of NSRE-1. NSRE-2 is also absolutely required for induction of the ASNS gene by both the AAR and the UPR pathway (11). The NSRE-1 and NSRE-2 sequences, as well as the 11 bp between them, are completely conserved in rat, mouse, hamster, and man. Mutagenesis studies have documented that these two elements must be aligned on the same side of the DNA helix and must be only one turn away from each other (131). It is postulated that this spatial relationship is required for protein-protein interactions that occur between the transcription factors that bind to these two sites.

In vitro binding analysis revealed ATF4 binding to the NSRE-1 sequence and that this binding activity was increased when nuclear extracts from either histidine-deprived (AAR pathway) or glucose-deprived (UPR pathway) cells were tested (107). Consistent with the translational control of ATF4, inhibition of protein synthesis blocked the starvation-dependent enhancement in ATF4-NSRE-1 complex formation. ATF4 regulation of ASNS expression in vivo was illustrated by the observation that ASNS promoter-driven transcription was induced by ATF4 overexpression (107). Subsequently, ChIP analysis documented in vivo that ATF4 binds to the ASNS promoter following amino acid deprivation (24).

Both EMSA experiments and transient expression of ATF3-FL (107, 121) and C/EBPβ (108) suggested that these bZIP transcription factors also exhibit affinity for the ASNS NSRE-1 site and that both contribute to the regulation of transcription driven by the ASNS promoter. Transient expression studies using combinations of ATF4, ATF3-FL, and C/EBPβ suggest that ATF3-FL serves as the primary antagonist to ATF4 function (24, 91). Consistent with this hypothesis, as mentioned above, Fawcett et al. (30) used nuclear extracts from arsenite-treated cells and EMSA studies to show a transient increase in ATF4 binding activity at the C/EBP-ATF composite site in the human CHOP promoter. ATF4 binding activity peaked at 2 hours after arsenite exposure, but that activity was subsequently replaced by elevated ATF3 binding activity at about 6 hours, a time at which transcription from the gene declined back toward the basal expression rate. Fawcett et al. (30) also used overexpression studies to document that elevated ATF4 activates the CHOP gene through the C/EBP-ATF composite site and that increased ATF3 production antagonizes the ATF4 function. The data of Chen et al. (24) extend the observations of Fawcett et al. (30) by showing through ChIP analysis that a similar sequence of events can be observed in vivo at the ASNS C/EBP-ATF composite site (NSRE-1).

Chen et al. (24) have proposed a working model for ASNS transcription in response to amino acid limitation (Figure 4, see color insert). Phase I encompasses the first 4 hours and phase II covers the time from 4–24 hours. During the first 30 minutes, translational control of ATF4 mRNA results in increased binding of ATF4 to the NSRE-1 site (24). A low level of C/EBPβ is constitutively bound to the ASNS promoter and this amount only increases after the transition to phase II has begun. In parallel with ATF4 binding, acetylation of histones H3 and H4 is increased, and subsequently, the general transcription factors TBP and TFIIB, as well as RNA Pol II, are recruited to the promoter. It is assumed that the ATF4 complex requires a coactivator or other bridging proteins to the general transcription machinery, which are shown as gray modules in the model (Figure 4). In phase II of amino acid deprivation, C/EBPβ binding increases at a time when the transcription rate has peaked. The synthesis and action of ATF3-FL and its alternatively spliced variant ATF3ΔZip3, also increases during this period (24), and it is believed that these three proteins act in concert to suppress, but not to completely reverse, the increased transcription. Transcription in phase II, even out to 24 hours, remains elevated relative to the status of the gene in amino acid–complete medium (24). Given that the rate of change in intracellular amino acid concentration surely varies from cell to cell and that the cells used by Chen et al. (24) were not cell cycle synchronized, it is proposed that individual cells make the transition from the "fed" state to phase I and from phase I to phase II at somewhat different rates. Therefore, it is hypothesized that what is measured as the "net" transcription rate and the "net" binding result by ChIP is actually the ratio of the number of cells in these three conditions at any single time point.

promoter binding of nutrient-responsive bZIP transcription factors as well as localized histone acetylation. *J. Biol. Chem.* 279:50829–39

25. Descombes P, Schibler U. 1991. A liver-enriched transcriptional activator protein, LAP, and a transcriptional inhibitory protein, LIP, are translated from the same mRNA. *Cell* 67:569–79
26. Entingh AJ, Law BK, Moses HL. 2001. Induction of the C/EBP homologous protein (CHOP) by amino acid deprivation requires insulin-like growth factor I, phosphatidylinositol 3-kinase, and mammalian target of rapamycin signaling. *Endocrinology* 142:221–28
27. Fafournoux P, Remesy C, Demigne C. 1983. Control of alanine metabolism in rat liver by transport processes or cellular metabolism. *Biochem. J.* 210:645–52
28. Fafournoux P, Remesy C, Demigne C. 1990. Fluxes and membrane transport of amino acids in rat liver under different protein diets. *Am. J. Physiol.* 259:E614–25
29. Fairley JA, Evans R, Hawkes NA, Roberts SG. 2002. Core promoter-dependent TFIIB conformation and a role for TFIIB conformation in transcription start site selection. *Mol. Cell Biol.* 22:6697–705
30. Fawcett TW, Martindale JL, Guyton KZ, Hai T, Holbrook NJ. 1999. Complexes containing activating transcription factor (ATF)/cAMP-responsive-element-binding protein (CREB) interact with the CCAAT/enhancer-binding protein (C/EBP)-ATF composite site to regulate *Gadd153* expression during the stress response. *Biochem. J.* 339:135–41
31. Fernandez J, Lopez AB, Wang C, Mishra R, Zhou L, et al. 2003. Transcriptional control of the arginine/lysine transporter, cat-1, by physiological stress. *J. Biol. Chem.* 278:50000–9
32. Fernandez J, Yaman I, Merrick WC, Koromilas A, Wek RC, et al. 2002. Regulation of internal ribosome entry site-mediated translation by eukaryotic initiation factor-2α phosphorylation and translation of a small upstream open reading frame. *J. Biol. Chem.* 277:2050–58
33. Fernandez J, Yaman I, Mishra R, Merrick WC, Snider MD, et al. 2001. Internal ribosome entry site-mediated translation of a mammalian mRNA is regulated by amino acid availability. *J. Biol. Chem.* 276:12285–91
34. Fernandez J, Yaman I, Sarnow P, Snider MD, Hatzoglou M. 2002. Regulation of internal ribosomal entry site-mediated translation by phosphorylation of the translation initiation factor eIF2α. *J. Biol. Chem.* 277:19198–205
35. Fingar DC, Blenis J. 2004. Target of rapamycin (TOR): an integrator of nutrient and growth factor signals and coordinator of cell growth and cell cycle progression. *Oncogene* 19:3151–71
36. Franchi-Gazzola R, Visigalli R, Bussolati O, Dall'Asta V, Gazzola GC. 1999. Adaptive increase of amino acid transport System A requires ERK1/2 activation. *J. Biol. Chem.* 274:28922–28
37. Gazzola GC, Dall'Asta V, Guidotti GG. 1981. Adaptive regulation of amino acid transport in cultured human fibroblasts. *J. Biol. Chem.* 256:3191–98
38. Gazzola RF, Sala R, Bussolati O, Visigalli R, Dall'Asta V, et al. 2001. The adaptive regulation of amino acid transport system A is associated to changes in ATA2 expression. *FEBS Lett.* 490:11–14
39. Genu V, Godecke S, Hollenberg CP, Pereira GG. 2003. The Hansenula polymorpha MOX gene presents two alternative transcription start points differentially utilized and sensitive to respiratory activity. *Eur. J. Biochem.* 270:2467–75
40. Gong SS, Guerrini L, Basilico C. 1991. Regulation of asparagine synthetase gene expression by amino acid starvation. *Mol. Cell. Biol.* 11:6059–66
41. Graveley BR. 2001. Alternative splicing: increasing diversity in the proteomic world. *Trends Genet.* 17:100–7

42. Guerrini L, Gong SS, Mangasarian K, Basilico C. 1993. *Cis-* and *trans*-acting elements involved in amino acid regulation of asparagine synthetase gene expression. *Mol. Cell. Biol.* 13:3202–12
43. Hai T, Hartman MG. 2001. The molecular biology and nomenclature of the activating transcription factor/cAMP responsive element binding family of transcription factors: activating transcription factor proteins and homeostasis. *Gene* 273:1–11
44. Hai T, Wolfgang CD, Marsee DK, Allen AE, Sivaprasad U. 1999. ATF3 and stress responses. *Gene Expr.* 7:321–35
45. Handlogten ME, Kilberg MS, Christensen HN. 1982. Incomplete correspondence between repressive and substrate action by amino acids on transport Systems A and N in monolayered rat hepatocytes. *J. Biol. Chem.* 257:345–48
46. Harding HP, Novoa I, Zhang Y, Zeng H, Wek R, et al. 2000. Regulated translation initiation controls stress-induced gene expression in mammalian cells. *Mol. Cell* 6:1099–108
47. Harding HP, Zhang Y, Zeng H, Novoa I, Lu PD, et al. 2003. An integrated stress response regulates amino acid metabolism and resistance to oxidative stress. *Mol. Cell* 11:619–33
48. Hashimoto Y, Zhang C, Kawauchi J, Imoto I, Adachi MT, et al. 2002. An alternatively spliced isoform of transcriptional repressor ATF3 and its induction by stress stimuli. *Nucleic Acids Res.* 30:2398–406
49. Hatzoglou M, Fernandez J, Yaman I, Closs EI. 2004. Regulation of cationic amino acid transport: the story of the CAT-1 transporter. *Annu. Rev. Nutr.* 24: 377–99
50. Hay N, Sonenberg N. 2004. Upstream and downstream of mTOR. *Genes Dev.* 18: 1926–45
51. Heal R, McGivan JD. 1998. Induction of calreticulin expression in response to amino acid deprivation in Chinese hamster ovary cells. *Biochem. J.* 329:389–94
52. Hinnebusch AG. 1997. Translational regulation of yeast GCN4. *J. Biol. Chem.* 272:21661–64
53. Hutson RG, Kilberg MS. 1994. Cloning of rat asparagine synthetase and specificity of the amino acid-dependent control of its mRNA content. *Biochem. J.* 303:745–50
54. Hyatt SL, Aulak KS, Malandro M, Kilberg MS, Hatzoglou M. 1997. Adaptive regulation of the cationic amino acid transporter-1 (Cat-1) in Fao cells. *J. Biol. Chem.* 272:19951–57
55. Hyde R, Christie GR, Litherland GJ, Hajduch E, Taylor PM, Hundal HS. 2001. Subcellular localization and adaptive upregulation of the System A (SAT2) amino acid transporter in skeletal-muscle cells and adipocytes. *Biochem. J.* 355:563–68
56. Jiang HY, Wek SA, McGrath BC, Lu D, Hai T, et al. 2004. Activating transcription factor 3 is integral to the eukaryotic initiation factor 2 kinase stress response. *Mol. Cell. Biol.* 24:1365–77
57. Jousse C, Bruhat A, Ferrara M, Fafournoux P. 1998. Physiological concentration of amino acids regulates insulin-like-growth-factor-binding protein 1 expression. *Biochem. J.* 334(Pt. 1):147–53
58. Jousse C, Bruhat A, Ferrara M, Fafournoux P. 2000. Evidence for multiple signaling pathways in the regulation of gene expression by amino acids in human cell lines. *J. Nutr.* 130:1555–60
59. Jousse C, Bruhat A, Harding HP, Ferrara M, Ron D, Fafournoux P. 1999. Amino acid limitation regulates CHOP expression through a specific pathway independent of the unfolded protein response. *FEBS Lett.* 448:211–16
60. Kaufman RJ. 1999. Stress signaling from the lumen of the endoplasmic reticulum: coordination of gene transcriptional and translational controls. *Gene. Dev.* 13:1211–33
61. Kilberg MS, Han HP, Barber EF, Chiles TC. 1985. Adaptive regulation of neutral amino acid transport system A in rat

H4 hepatoma cells. *J. Cell. Physiol.* 122:290–98
62. Kilberg MS, Stevens BR, Novak D. 1993. Recent advances in mammalian amino acid transport. *Annu. Rev. Nutr.* 13:137–65
63. Kim JW, Closs EI, Albritton LM, Cunningham JM. 1991. Transport of cationic amino acids by the mouse ecotropic retrovirus receptor. *Nature* 352:725–28
64. Kimball SR. 2002. Regulation of global and specific mRNA translation by amino acids. *J. Nutr.* 132:883–86
65. Kimball SR, Jefferson LS. 2004. Molecular mechanisms through which amino acids mediate signaling through the mammalian target of rapamycin. *Curr. Opin. Clin. Nutr. Metab. Care* 7:39–44
66. Lagrange T, Kapanidis AN, Tang H, Reinberg D, Ebright RH. 1998. New core promoter element in RNA polymerase II-dependent transcription: sequence-specific DNA binding by transcription factor IIB. *Genes Dev.* 12:34–44
67. Laine RO, Laipis PJ, Shay NF, Kilberg MS. 1991. Identification of an amino acid-regulated mRNA from rat liver as the mammalian equivalent of bacterial ribosomal protein L22. *J. Biol. Chem.* 266: 16969–72
68. Laine RO, Shay NF, Kilberg MS. 1994. Nuclear retention of the induced mRNA following amino acid-dependent transcriptional regulation of mammalian ribosomal proteins L17 and S25. *J. Biol. Chem.* 269:9693–97
69. Lal A, Mazan-Mamczarz K, Kawai T, Yang X, Martindale JL, Gorospe M. 2004. Concurrent versus individual binding of HuR and AUF1 to common labile target mRNAs. *EMBO J.* 23:3092–102
70. Lemon B, Tjian R. 2000. Orchestrated response: a symphony of transcription factors for gene control. *Genes Dev.* 14: 2551–69
71. Leung-Pineda V, Kilberg MS. 2002. Role of Sp1 and Sp3 in the nutrient-regulated expression of the human asparagine synthetase gene. *J. Biol. Chem.* 277: 16585–91
72. Leung-Pineda V, Pan Y, Chen H, Kilberg MS. 2004. Induction of p21 and p27 expression by amino acid deprivation of HepG2 human hepatoma cells involves mRNA stabilization. *Biochem. J.* 379:79–88
73. Lie-Venema H, Hakvoort TB, van Hemert FJ, Moorman AF, Lamers WH. 1998. Regulation of the spatiotemporal pattern of expression of the glutamine synthetase gene. *Prog. Nucleic Acid Res. Mol. Biol.* 61:243–308
74. Ling R, Bridges CC, Sugawara M, Fujita T, Leibach FH, et al. 2001. Involvement of transporter recruitment as well as gene expression in the substrate-induced adaptive regulation of amino acid transport system A. *Biochim. Biophys. Acta* 1512:15–21
75. Lopez-Fontanals M, Rodriguez-Mulero S, Casado FJ, Derijard B, Pastor-Anglada M. 2003. The osmoregulatory and the amino acid-regulated responses of System A are mediated by different signal transduction pathways. *J. Gen. Physiol.* 122:5–16
76. Lu JY, Schneider RJ. 2004. Tissue distribution of AU-rich mRNA-binding proteins involved in regulation of mRNA decay. *J. Biol. Chem.* 279:12974–79
77. Lu PD, Harding HP, Ron D. 2004. Translation reinitiation at alternative open reading frames regulates gene expression in an integrated stress response. *J. Cell Biol.* 167:27–33
78. Mackenzie B, Erickson JD. 2004. Sodium-coupled neutral amino acid (System N/A) transporters of the SLC38 gene family. *Pflugers Arch.* 447:784–95
79. Marten NW, Burke EJ, Hayden JM, Straus DS. 1994. Effect of amino acid limitation on the expession of 19 genes in rat hepatoma cells. *FASEB J.* 8:538–44
80. Marten NW, Sladek FM, Straus DS. 1996. Effect of dietary protein restriction on liver transcription factors. *Biochem. J.* 317:361–70

81. McGivan JD, Pastor-Anglada M. 1994. Regulatory and molecular aspects of mammalian amino acid transport. *Biochem. J.* 299:321–34
82. Modrek B, Lee C. 2002. A genomic view of alternative splicing. *Nat. Genet.* 30:13–19
83. Murray A, Hunt T. 1993. *The Cell Cycle: An Introduction*. New York: Freeman
84. Naar AM, Lemon BD, Tjian R. 2001. Transcriptional coactivator complexes. *Annu. Rev. Biochem.* 70:475–501
85. Natarajan K, Meyer MR, Jackson BM, Slade D, Roberts C, et al. 2001. Transcriptional profiling shows that Gcn4p is a master regulator of gene expression during amino acid starvation in yeast. *Mol. Cell Biol.* 21:4347–68
86. Nicholson B, McGivan JD. 1996. Induction of high affinity glutamate transport activity by amino acid deprivation in renal epithelial cells does not involve an increase in the amount of transporter protein. *J. Biol. Chem.* 271:12159–64
87. Padbury JF, Diah SK, McGonnigal B, Miller C, Fugere C, et al. 2004. Transcriptional regulation of the LAT-1/CD98 light chain. *Biochem. Biophys. Res. Commun.* 318:529–34
88. Pahl HL. 1999. Signal transduction from the endoplasmic reticulum to the cell nucleus. *Physiol. Rev.* 79:683–701
89. Palacín M, Estevez R, Bertran J, Zorzano A. 1998. Molecular biology of mammalian plasma membrane amino acid transporters. *Physiol. Rev.* 78:969–1054
90. Palii SS, Chen H, Kilberg MS. 2004. Transcriptional control of the human sodium-coupled neutral amino acid transporter system A gene by amino acid availability is mediated by an intronic element. *J. Biol. Chem.* 279:3463–71
91. Pan Y-X, Chen H, Siu F, Kilberg MS. 2003. Amino acid deprivation and endoplasmic reticulum stress induce expression of multiple ATF3 mRNA species which, when overexpressed in HepG2 cells, modulate transcription by the human asparagine synthetase promoter. *J. Biol. Chem.* 278:38402–12
92. Patil C, Walter P. 2001. Intracellular signaling from the endoplasmic reticulum to the nucleus: the unfolded protein response in yeast and mammals. *Curr. Opin. Cell Biol.* 13:349–55
93. Paul GL, Waegner A, Gaskins HR, Shay NF. 1998. Histidine availability alters glucagon gene expression in murine αTC6 cells. *J. Nutr.* 128:973–76
94. Plakidou-Dymock S, McGivan JD. 1993. Regulation of the glutamate transporter by amino acid deprivation and associated effects on the level of EAAC1 mRNA in the renal epithelial cell line NBL-1. *Biochem. J.* 295:749–55
95. Podust LM, Krezel AM, Kim Y. 2001. Crystal structure of the CCAAT box/enhancer-binding protein beta activating transcription factor-4 basic leucine zipper heterodimer in the absence of DNA. *J. Biol. Chem.* 276:505–13
96. Pohjanpelto P, Holtta E. 1990. Deprivation of a single amino acid induces protein synthesis-dependent increases in c-jun, c-myc, and ornithine decarboxylase mRNAs in Chinese hamster ovary cells. *Mol. Cell Biol.* 10:5814–21
97. Price BD, Calderwood SK. 1992. Gadd45 and Gadd153 messenger RNA levels are increased during hypoxia and after exposure of cells to agents which elevate the levels of the glucose-regulated proteins. *Cancer Res.* 52:3814–17
98. Proud CG. 2004. The multifaceted role of mTOR in cellular stress responses. *DNA Repair (Amst.)* 3:927–34
99. Richards NGJ, Schuster SM. 1998. Mechanistic issues in asparagine synthetase catalysis. *Adv. Enzymol.* 72:145–98
100. Ron D, Habener JF. 1992. CHOP, a novel developmentally regulated nuclear protein that dimerizes with transcription factors C/EBP and LAP and functions as a dominant-negative inhibitor of gene transcription. *Genes Dev.* 6:439–53

101. Roy B, Lee AS. 1999. The mammalian endoplasmic reticulum stress response element consists of an evolutionarily conserved tripartite structure and interacts with a novel stress-inducible complex. *Nucleic Acids Res.* 27:1437–43
102. Roybal CN, Yang S, Sun CW, Hurtado D, Vander Jagt DL, et al. 2004. Homocysteine increases the expression of vascular endothelial growth factor by a mechanism involving endoplasmic reticulum stress and transcription factor ATF4. *J. Biol. Chem.* 279:14844–52
103. Scheuner D, Song B, McEwen E, Liu C, Laybutt R, et al. 2001. Translational control is required for the unfolded protein response and in vivo glucose homeostasis. *Mol. Cell* 7:1165–76
104. Shay NF, Nick HS, Kilberg MS. 1990. Molecular cloning of an amino acid-regulated mRNA (amino acid starvation-induced) in rat hepatoma cells. *J. Biol. Chem.* 265:17844–48
105. Sherr CJ, Roberts JM. 1995. Inhibitors of mammalian G1 cyclin-dependent kinases. *Genes Dev.* 9:1149–63
106. Sips HJ, Groen AK, Tager JM. 1990. Plasma-membrane transport of alanine is rate-limiting for its metabolism in rat-liver parenchymal cells. *FEBS Lett.* 119:271–74
107. Siu F, Bain PJ, LeBlanc-Chaffin R, Chen H, Kilberg MS. 2002. ATF4 is a mediator of the nutrient-sensing response pathway that activates the human asparagine synthetase gene. *J. Biol. Chem.* 277:24120–27
108. Siu FY, Chen C, Zhong C, Kilberg MS. 2001. CCAAT/enhancer-binding protein beta (C/EBPb) is a mediator of the nutrient sensing response pathway that activates the human asparagine synthetase gene. *J. Biol. Chem.* 276:48100–7
109. Smale ST, Kadonaga JT. 2003. The RNA polymerase II core promoter. *Annu. Rev. Biochem.* 72:449–79
110. Sood R, Porter AC, Olsen DA, Cavener DR, Wek RC. 2000. A mammalian homologue of GCN2 protein kinase important for translational control by phosphorylation of eukaryotic initiation factor-2α. *Genetics* 154:787–801
111. Straus DS. 1994. Nutritional regulation of hormones and growth factors that control mammalian growth. *FASEB J.* 8:6–12
112. Straus DS, Burke EJ, Marten NW. 1993. Induction of insulin-like growth factor binding protein-1 gene expression in liver of protein-restricted rats and in rat hepatoma cells limited for a single amino acid. *Endocrinology* 132:1090–100
113. Takiguchi M. 1998. The C/EBP family of transcription factors in the liver and other organs. *Int. J. Exp. Pathol.* 79:369–91
114. Vallejo M, Ron D, Miller CP, Habener JF. 1993. C/ATF, a member of the activating transcription factor family of DNA-binding proteins, dimerizes with CAAT/enhancer-binding proteins and directs their binding to cAMP response elements. *Proc. Natl. Acad. Sci. USA* 90: 4679–83
115. Vattem KM, Wek RC. 2004. Reinitiation involving upstream ORFs regulates ATF4 mRNA translation in mammalian cells. *Proc. Natl. Acad. Sci. USA* 101:11269–74
116. Verrey F, Closs EI, Wagner CA, Palacin M, Endou H, Kanai Y. 2004. CATs and HATs: the SLC7 family of amino acid transporters. *Pflugers Arch.* 447:532–42
117. Vinson C, Myakishev M, Acharya A, Mir AA, Moll JR, Bonovich M. 2002. Classification of human B-ZIP proteins based on dimerization properties. *Mol. Cell Biol.* 22:6321–35
118. Wang H, Kavanaugh MP, North RA, Kabat D. 1991. Cell-surface receptor for ecotropic murine retroviruses is a basic amino-acid transporter. *Nature* 352:729–31
119. Wang J, Cao Y, Steiner DF. 2003. Regulation of proglucagon transcription by activated transcription factor (ATF) 3 and a novel isoform, ATF3b, through the cAMP-response element/ATF site of

the proglucagon gene promoter. *J. Biol. Chem.* 278:32899–904

120. Wang X-Z, Kuroda M, Sok J, Batchvarova N, Kimmel R, et al. 1998. Identification of novel stress-induced genes downstream of *chop. EMBO J.* 17:3619–30
121. Waye MM, Stanners CP. 1981. Role of asparaginase synthetase and asparagyl-transfer RNA synthetase in the cell-killing activity of asparaginase in Chinese hamster ovary cell mutants. *Cancer Res.* 41: 3104–6
122. White MF. 1985. The transport of cationic amino acids across the plasma membrane of mammalian cells. *Biochim. Biophys. Acta* 822:355–74
123. Wolfgang CD, Chen BP, Martindale JL, Holbrook NJ, Hai T. 1997. gadd153/Chop10, a potential target gene of the transcriptional repressor ATF3. *Mol. Cell Biol.* 17:6700–7
124. Wolfgang CD, Liang G, Okamoto Y, Allen AE, Hai T. 2000. Transcriptional autorepression of the stress-inducible gene ATF3. *J. Biol. Chem.* 275:16865–70
125. Xie Y, Davies SM, Xiang Y, Robison LL, Ross JA. 2003. Trends in leukemia incidence and survival in the United States (1973–1998). *Cancer* 97:2229–35
126. Yamamoto Y, Toi M, Kondo S, Matsumoto T, Suzuki H, et al. 1996. Concentrations of vascular endothelial growth factor in the sera of normal controls and cancer patients. *Clin. Cancer Res.* 2:821–26
127. Yaman I, Fernandez J, Liu H, Caprara M, Komar AA, et al. 2003. The zipper model of translational control. A small upstream ORF is the switch that controls structural remodeling of an mRNA leader. *Cell* 113:519–31
128. Yaman I, Fernandez J, Sarkar B, Schneider RJ, Snider MD, et al. 2002. Nutritional control of mRNA stability is mediated by a conserved AU-rich element that binds the cytoplasmic shuttling protein HuR. *J. Biol. Chem.* 277:41539–46
129. Yoshida H, Haze K, Yanagi H, Yura T, Mori K. 1998. Identification of the cis-acting endoplasmic reticulum stress response element responsible for transcriptional induction of mammalian glucose-regulated proteins. *J. Biol. Chem.* 273:33741–49
130. Zhang P, McGrath BC, Reinert J, Olsen DS, Lei L, et al. 2002. The GCN2 eIF2α kinase is required for adaptation to amino acid deprivation in mice. *Mol. Cell Biol.* 22:6681–88
131. Zhong C, Chen C, Kilberg MS. 2003. Characterization of the nutrient sensing response unit in the human asparagine synthetase promoter. *Biochem. J.* 372: 603–9
132. Zinszner H, Kuroda M, Wang XZ, Batchvarova N, Lightfoot RT, et al. 1998. CHOP is implicated in programmed cell death in response to impaired function of the endoplasmic reticulum. *Genes. Dev.* 12:982–95

potatoes, and spinach. Analysis of recent NHANES data (77), for both genders and all age groups, showed that the mean intake of vitamin A in the United States was about 600 μg RAE/day from food and that 70% to 75% of this was as preformed vitamin A (retinol).

DIGESTION OF RETINYL ESTERS

Solubilization

The digestion of REs requires catalysis by lipases, enzymes that hydrolyze water-insoluble substrates. The fundamental distinction between esterases and lipases is the involvement of a lipid-water interface in the catalytic process for the latter class of enzymes. Esterases function on water-soluble substrates and hence catalyze reactions in which the enzyme, substrate, and products are homogeneously distributed in a single (aqueous) phase. With lipases and water-insoluble substrates like REs, this is not the case. The presence of heterogeneous phases per se, and the fact that they change in composition during the course of the lipolytic reaction, makes the interpretation of enzyme kinetic data much more complicated than for homogeneous catalysis. A full discussion of lipase kinetics is beyond the scope of the present review, and the reader is referred to the excellent monograph edited by Borgstrom & Brockman (11). However, a few points of particular relevance to the study of the hydrolysis of highly apolar lipids such as REs should be made. The composition and packing of nonsubstrate molecules at the interface (the "quality" of the interface) plays a large role in the binding of the enzyme and the rates of substrate hydrolysis observed. Obviously, the availability of substrate molecules is also important. The point is that the observed kinetic "preference" for one substrate over another may reflect more its interactions with other lipids that allow it to achieve a high concentration at the interface than preferential binding to the enzyme itself. In other words, the apparent specificity of a lipolytic enzyme may reflect mostly the physical availability of the substrate at the interface. The physiological relevance of this is that the detailed composition of luminal lipids has a major impact on the digestion and absorption of dietary vitamin A.

Studies of the enzymatic hydrolysis of retinyl esters generally have been conducted under conditions in which the interfacial concentration of substrate (and other lipids or detergents) is undefined. This does not preclude making certain operational comparisons of the rates of hydrolysis of different potential substrates. It does mean, however, that it is problematic to conclude that the higher rate of hydrolysis of one ester over another tells much about the enzyme's specificity. This is especially true when one considers that even fairly well characterized substrate forms (i.e., micelles, liposomes, or monolayers of defined composition) probably do not closely resemble the physical forms adopted by REs in vivo (e.g., the complex emulsions, micelles, and vesicles in the intestinal lumen).

It is worth pointing out, too, that there is almost no detailed information on the physical forms or "phases" that REs adopt in the intestinal lumen. Much more detailed information on these issues is available for other major dietary lipids such as triglycerides, phospholipids, and cholesterol (31, 68). Nonetheless, it is clear from studies both in experimental animals and in humans that the co-ingestion of dietary fat markedly enhances the intestinal absorption of dietary vitamin A (8, 55, 74). The presence of dietary fat in the intestine can stimulate RE digestion by (*a*) stimulating pancreatic enzyme secretion, (*b*) stimulating the secretion of bile salts, which serve to form mixed micelles of lipids, and (*c*) providing products of lipid digestion (i.e., lysophospholipids, monoglycerides, and free fatty acids), which themselves can serve as components of micelles. Finally, fat ingestion promotes vitamin A absorption by providing the lipid components for intestinal chylomicron assembly, a process discussed in more detail below.

Pancreatic Enzymes

More than three decades ago Erlanson & Borgström (18) reported the partial separation of two different pancreatic RE hydrolase (REH) activities in the rat using a Sephadex G100 column. These two activities hydrolyzed different physical forms of the retinyl palmitate substrate. The early peak mainly hydrolyzed retinyl palmitate, which was dispersed in millimolar concentrations of taurodeoxycholate [a condition known to stimulate carboxylester lipase (CEL) and to inhibit pancreatic triglyceride lipase (PTL) (10)], whereas the subsequent peak was more effective in hydrolyzing dispersed retinyl palmitate in the absence of bile salt. These two different REH elution patterns were consistent with CEL and PTL, respectively.

Pancreatic carboxylester lipase catalyzes the hydrolysis of cholesteryl esters, triglycerides, and lysophospholipids. It was thought to hydrolyze retinyl esters also in the intestine. CEL knockout (KO) mice were generated to study the functions of CEL (80, 83). Though neither CEL KO nor wild-type (WT) mice absorbed nonhydrolyzable cholesteryl ether, CEL KO mice absorbed about half the amount of cholesterol provided as cholesteryl ester compared with WT mice. These data indicated that hydrolysis of cholesteryl esters is necessary prior to absorption, and that CEL plays an important role in cholesterol absorption. In contrast to the results for cholesteryl ester, CEL KO mice absorbed the same amount of retinol, when provided as RE, as did WT mice. On the other hand, neither mouse absorbed the nonhydrolyzable retinyl hexadecyl ether. These data suggested that RE hydrolysis was required for absorption and that CEL was not the responsible enzyme (at least under conditions where the amount of dietary RE was in the ug range, as used in this study). Triglyceride absorption was also comparable between CEL KO and WT mice, indicating that absence of CEL does not affect triglyceride hydrolysis. Therefore, if intestinal RE absorption is unaffected in CEL KO mice, one or more other RE hydrolytic enzymes must be present in the gut lumen or on the enterocyte surface.

Studies were then conducted to identify the non-CEL pancreatic REH activity that appeared to be present in CEL KO mice, as well as to investigate this activity in WT mice and in rats. Several lines of evidence suggest that this activity is due to PTL (79). First, the dependence of pancreatic REH on different types of bile salt was investigated in pancreatic homogenates of WT mice and rats. When assayed utilizing different bile salt conditions, cholesteryl ester hydrolase activity was detected only in the presence of trihydroxy bile salts, consistent with previous results (25, 84). Pancreatic REH activity, however, was not absolutely dependent on trihydroxy bile salts. RE hydrolysis not only was detected in the presence of trihydroxy bile salts, but also in the presence of dihydroxy bile salts and CHAPS, a bile salt analog, as well as in the absence of bile salts. The finding that REH activity was supported by dihydroxy bile salts is consistent with PTL-mediated hydrolysis. Second, when total pancreatic homogenates obtained from rats, WT mice, and CEL KO mice are used to assay REH activity, a considerable stimulation of the REH activity by colipase was observed; this indicates that PTL was at least partially contributing to the pancreatic bile salt–dependent REH activity. Third, when pancreatic homogenates from rats, WT mice, and CEL KO mice were applied to diethylaminoethanol chromatography, the majority of REH activity co-eluted with PTL activity in the unbound fraction. In contrast, a minor peak eluted with CEL activity during the KCl gradient elution in both species. This further supports the notion of PTL-mediated RE hydrolysis. Fourth, because of the possibility that multiple proteins are involved in pancreatic RE hydrolysis, the enzymatic characteristics of purified human PTL, using either triolein or retinyl palmitate as a substrate, were studied. Both REH and triglyceride hydrolase activities of the enzyme were completely dependent on the presence of colipase. In addition, identical patterns of bile salt inhibition were observed using either triolein or retinyl palmitate as a substrate. Based on these data, PTL may be the main REH activity in the intestinal lumen of both mice and rats.

Although these data strongly suggest that PTL may be a major REH in rat and mouse intestinal lumen, they do not provide final proof for this concept. In addition, other enzymes synthesized and secreted by the pancreas may also play a role in the lumenal hydrolysis of REs. For example, some triglyceride hydrolysis was observed in the absence of colipase in pancreatic homogenates from both rats and mice, which may point to the presence of other related enzyme activities, such as pancreatic lipase-related protein 2 (PLRP2). It is possible that the triglyceride hydrolase activity observed in the absence of colipase is due to endogenous colipase present in the pancreatic homogenates. Nonetheless, PLRP2 is 65% identical to PTL and hydrolyzes phospholipids and shows activity toward triglycerides in the classical PTL assay (39). At present, the percentage of PLRP2's contribution to pancreatic bile salt–dependent REH activity is not known. In addition, yet another pancreatic lipase-related protein (PLRP1) has been cloned that is 68% homologous to PTL but for which the substrate is still unknown (20). Thus, more than one enzyme may be responsible for the complete hydrolysis of REs in the intestinal lumen.

Intestinal Enzymes

In addition to pancreatic bile salt–dependent REH activities, an REH activity that is intrinsically located in the brush border membrane of the absorptive enterocytes

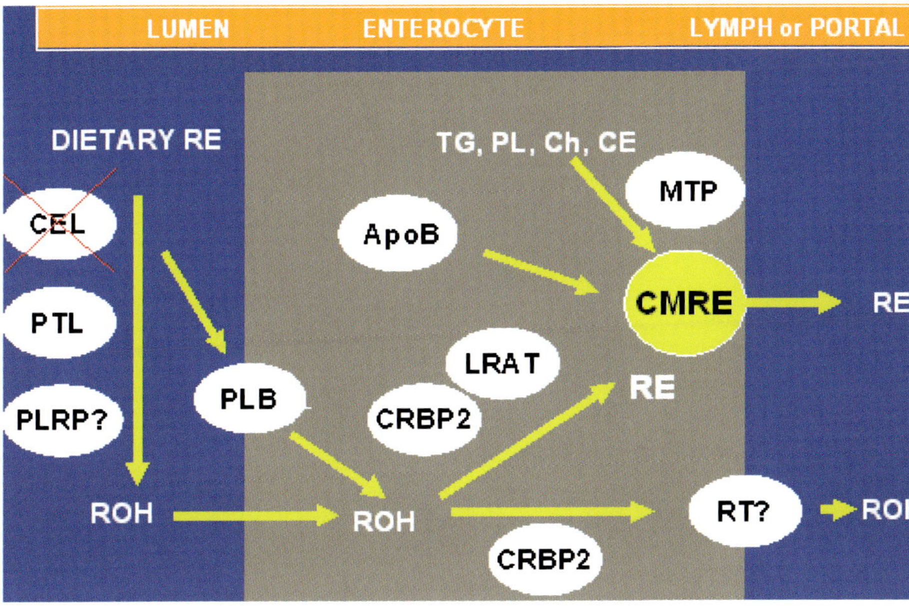

Figure 1 Overview of digestion and absorption of vitamin A. Dietary retinyl esters (REs) are hydrolyzed in the lumen by the pancreatic enzyme pancreatic triglyceride lipase (PTL) and intestinal brush border enzyme phospholipase B (PLB). Studies of the carboxylester lipase (CEL) knockout mouse suggest that CEL is not involved in dietary RE digestion. The possible roles of the pancreatic lipase-related proteins (PLRPs) 1 and 2 and other enzymes require further investigation. Unesterified retinol (ROH) is taken up by the enterocyte, perhaps facilitated by a yet unidentified retinol transporter. Once in the cell, retinol is complexed with cellular retinol-binding protein type 2 (CRBP2) and the complex serves as a substrate for reesterification of the retinol by the enzyme lecithin:retinol acyltransferase (LRAT). The REs are then incorporated into chylomicrons, intestinal lipoproteins containing other dietary lipids such as triglyceride (TG), phospholipid (PL), cholesterol (Ch) and cholesteryl esters (CEs), and apolipoprotein B (apoB). The incorporation of some of these lipids is dependent on the activity of microsomal triglyceride transfer protein (MTP). Chylomicrons containing newly absorbed retinyl esters (CMRE) are then secreted into the lymph. Unesterified retinol is also absorbed into the portal circulation and its efflux from the basolateral cell membrane may also be facilitated by retinol transporter (RT) proteins.

was shown in rat and human intestines (64, 65). It was suggested that this enzyme activity is due to an intestinal phospholipase B (63). These authors showed that rat brush border membrane isolated from rats in which the common pancreatic duct had been ligated for two days (thus prohibiting contamination of brush border membrane with any enzymes secreted by the pancreas, such as CEL or PTL) had a greatly decreased hydrolytic activity against short-chain REs (in the presence of trihydroxy bile salts) and a smaller (30%) decrease in the activity against long-chain REs (such as retinyl palmitate) as compared with sham-operated rats. Therefore, they suggested that short-chain REH was mainly due to enzymes of pancreatic origin (and could be due to CEL), whereas the majority (70%) of long-chain REH was intrinsic to the brush border. The remaining 30% of REH activity, however, could be due to PTL, as this REH activity was detected in both the presence of trihydroxy and dihydroxy bile salts. It is important to point out, however, that the relative activities observed in vitro may not reflect the relative contributions of the various enzymes in vivo. It is likely that both PTL and phospholipase B contribute to RE digestion. In order to determine their relative roles in intestinal RE digestion and absorption, it will become essential to perform RE absorption experiments in the appropriate KO mice strains and in mice deficient in more than one enzyme. The enzymes potentially involved in hydrolysis of dietary REs are outlined in Table 1 and Figure 1 (see color insert).

TABLE 1 Proteins involved in the digestion, absorption, and transport of retinol

1. Retinyl ester hydrolysis	a. Lumen	Pancreatic triglyceride lipase Pancreatic lipase-related protein 1 (?) Pancreatic lipase-related protein 2 (?) Carboxyl ester lipase (probably NOT involved)
	b. Brush border membrane	Phospholipase B
2. Retinol uptake, transfer, and efflux		
	Retinol transporters (CD36, SRB1, NPC1L1, ABCA1, etc.) (?) Cellular retinol binding protein I (?) Cellular retinol binding protein II	
3. Retinyl ester synthesis		
	Lecithin:retinol acyltransferase Acyl-CoA:retinol acyltransferase (probably NOT involved)	
4. Chylomicron assembly		
	Apolipoprotein B Microsomal triglyceride transfer protein	

INTESTINAL ABSORPTION OF VITAMIN A

Mechanisms of Cellular Uptake and Efflux of Unesterified Retinol in Enterocytes—Portal Secretion

Studies concerning the uptake of retinol by the human intestinal cell line, Caco-2, indicated that retinol at physiologic and pharmacologic concentrations was taken up by saturable carrier-mediated processes and nonsaturable diffusion-dependent processes, respectively (61). The retinol taken up by these cells was esterified, and the REs mainly contained palmitic and oleic acids (43, 61). Studies showed that retinol uptake is a rapid process with a half-life of minutes (52). This uptake was not affected by the presence of high concentrations of free fatty acids.

Recent experiments in the author's laboratory have further examined the role of transporters in retinol flux in Caco-2 cells (16). When cells were incubated with 3 μM retinol for varying times up to 24 hours, cellular retinol plateaued within 2 hours, whereas there was continuous formation of REs. Both retinol and REs secreted in basolateral medium increased linearly with time (up to 20 hours). REs were associated with chylomicrons and retinol with the nonlipoprotein fraction. After incubation with retinol concentrations of 0.5–130 μM, cellular uptake of retinol was directly proportional to initial retinol concentration. However, the kinetics of efflux of retinol into basolateral medium revealed two processes. Retinol secretion showed saturation at concentrations $<10\ \mu$M, which suggests a mediated transport out of the cell, and linearity with higher concentrations, which suggests passive diffusion. One interpretation of these data is that free retinol enters into intestinal cells by simple diffusion, whereas its secretion may require a facilitated transport at physiological doses. This notion is supported by other experiments in which glyburide, a known inhibitor of the ABCA1 transporter, caused marked inhibition of the efflux of free retinol into basolateral medium (but not cell uptake). Of course, it is also possible that cellular uptake at the apical membrane is also facilitated, but that the rapid esterification of retinol after uptake makes it difficult to demonstrate kinetically that the transport is rate limiting.

Early studies using intestinal segments also suggested that the unesterified retinol was taken up by protein-mediated facilitated diffusion and passive diffusion mechanisms at physiologic (150 nM) and pharmacological (450 nM–2700 nM) concentrations, respectively (33, 34). Other evidence for protein-mediated uptake of retinol has been presented using intestinal segments (15). However, no protein has yet been identified and characterized that might be involved in the uptake of retinol.

There is an enormous amount of current interest in the role of membrane-bound lipid transporters in the cellular uptake and efflux of fat-soluble molecules. For example, three different membrane-bound proteins—CD36, membrane-bound fatty acid–binding protein, and a fatty acid transport protein—that might be involved in fatty acid uptake have been identified (for review, see 1, 21). In the case of cholesterol, SRB1, CD36, NPC1L1, and a variety of ABC transporters have been implicated in its uptake and/or efflux from various cells (2, 13, 14, 75, 81, 82). It is possible that these or other proteins play a role in the transport of retinol across cell membranes. Defining the exact mechanisms of cellular uptake of retinol (or other lipids) is complicated by the fact that, as indicated above, multiple mechanisms (both facilitated and passive) may exist in a single cell. An additional problem is that much of the work in this area relies on the use of membrane transporter inhibitors, and there is increasing evidence that some of these compounds inhibit multiple transporter types (54). A final complication is that some of the transport inhibitors also affect the expression of transporter genes and, thus, exert effects on transporter number and function simultaneously.

The general perception that retinol is efficiently absorbed and quantitatively transported on chylomicrons may need reevaluation (for review, see 5, 6). First, it should be pointed out that the recovery of ingested retinol into lymph varies between 20% and 60% (6, 22, 35). Second, Hollander showed that approximately 60% and 30% of the absorbed retinol is secreted into lymph and portal circulation, respectively (32). Furthermore, he showed that secretion of retinol into lymph was modulated by the presence of different concentrations of taurocholate and different fatty acids (32). Third, oral supplementation of retinol into abetalipoproteinemia patients, who do not assemble and secrete chylomicrons, results in partial recovery from symptoms of retinol deficiency (40). Fourth, cell culture studies showed that free retinol or its metabolized products are transported across the cells independent of the assembly and secretion of lipoproteins (52). Thus, much of the absorbed retinol is secreted into lymph in esterified form. However, a significant amount is also secreted into portal circulation, probably as free retinol. The transport of free retinol to the portal circulation is expected to be physiologically significant in pathologic conditions that affect the secretion of chylomicrons. Thus, the transport of free retinol may be an essential back-up mechanism for the homoeostasis of vitamin A under some conditions.

Intracellular Transport by Cellular Retinol-Binding Protein (II)

After cellular uptake, free retinol is probably immediately sequestered by cellular retinol-binding proteins (CRBPs) (Table 1). Two CRBPs, CRBP(I) and CRBP(II), have been purified and characterized extensively. They have considerable sequence identity and belong to a family of fatty acid–binding proteins. Both of the proteins are highly conserved during evolution, which indicates their physiologic importance. These proteins share considerable structural, genetic, and biochemical properties. However, the cellular expression pattern of these proteins is very different. The CRBP(I), a 14.6 kDa polypeptide, is expressed in many tissues, whereas CRBP(II), a 16 kDa polypeptide, is expressed primarily in the absorptive cells of the small intestine. The CRBP(II) is one of the most abundant proteins and accounts for approximately 1% of the total soluble proteins recovered from the jejunal mucosa. The tissue distribution and abundance indicate that it must be uniquely suited for retinol absorption by the intestine (for reviews, see 45, 53, 56, 57).

In vitro studies indicate that CRBP(II) can play several functions in the trafficking of retinol. It has been speculated that it can bind to specific transporters on the brush border membrane and permit facilitated diffusion. It can serve as a reservoir to keep the concentrations of free retinoids very low and protect cells from their detergent-like properties. More important, it may present retinoids to different enzymes and direct their metabolism (56, 57).

In vivo studies showed that CRBP(II) mRNA levels are increased in the small intestine of retinoid-deficient rats (62) and rats fed with long-chain fatty acids (70). In Caco-2 cells, CRBP(II) mRNA was shown to be increased (two- to threefold) after treatment of the differentiated cells with retinoic acid. More importantly, this resulted in increased absorption and intracellular esterification of radiolabeled retinol. Furthermore, absorption and esterification was also increased after the overexpression of CRBP(II) in these cells (48). These studies indicate that changes in CRBP(II) expression results in the modulation of retinol metabolism (44, 69, 71). However, it is not known whether the increased expression of CRBP(II) results in increased secretion of REs in chylomicrons.

Recent characterization of the CRBP(II) knockout mouse has clarified that CRBP(II) plays an important, but not absolutely essential, role in the intestinal absorption of vitamin A (85). Using the methodology originally described by Dew & Ong (15), Li & coworkers showed that the saturable component of retinol uptake by jejunal segments was reduced to about half that of tissue from WT littermates (85). The CRBP(II) knockout mice, when maintained on a vitamin A–enriched diet, also had reduced (about 40%) hepatic stores of vitamin A, which suggests that the incomplete impairment of retinol processing in the intestine nonetheless affects whole-body vitamin A status.

Reesterification and Incorporation into Chylomicrons—Lymphatic Secretion

Early studies in intact rats and humans clearly demonstrated that after uptake of newly absorbed retinol, the retinol was largely reesterified with long-chain fatty acids (mostly palmitate) and secreted into the lymphatics along with other dietary lipids in chylomicrons. Caco-2 cells have been used to study mechanisms of vitamin A absorption that are difficult to study in intact animals. The differentiated Caco-2 cells were shown to express CRBP(II), ARAT, LRAT, and retinal reductase (43, 61). Studies on retinol secretion revealed that Caco-2 cells supplemented with no fatty acids secreted only free retinol. However, cells incubated with oleic acid were shown to secrete REs in addition to free retinol (43). Based on these observations, it has been suggested that lipoprotein particles secreted by these cells may contain retinol and REs (43). However, no data about the secretion of either free or esterified retinol as part of different lipoprotein particles were reported in these studies.

In the cells, the free retinol can remain associated with its cellular retinol binding proteins. However, much of the retinol is usually esterified and stored. In enterocytes, two enzymes—LRAT and ARAT—have been identified that can catalyze the esterification of free retinol in vitro (30, 49). It has been suggested, but not shown, that REs formed by LRAT and ARAT may be targeted for secretion with chylomicrons and storage, respectively (5, 6). The recent characterization of the LRAT knockout mouse has largely resolved the question of whether enzymes other than LRAT play any physiological role in retinol esterification. Given that the LRAT knockout mouse has no detectable tissue REs (3), it is unlikely that other enzymes such as ARAT are physiologically involved in retinol esterification in intestine. Obviously, this issue warrants further investigation. It is possible, and even likely, that other acyltransferases can catalyze the acyl-CoA-dependent esterification of retinol in vitro. It is also possible that other enzymes are involved in the esterification of retinol if given to animals in very large quantities.

It is generally believed that retinol is mainly secreted into the lymph as retinyl palmitate. During metabolic studies, analysis of the plasma revealed that most of the REs are present in small chylomicrons (42). Significant amounts of REs are also found in large chylomicrons, followed by smaller amounts in very-low-density lipoproteins (42). In contrast to triglycerides, cholesterol esters, and other lipids, REs are not present in other lipoproteins such as intermediate-density lipoproteins, low-density lipoproteins, or high-density lipoproteins. These studies indicate that REs are mainly present in large and small chylomicrons and behave very differently from other neutral lipids, such as triglycerides and cholesterol esters.

To understand the mechanism of secretion of RE by the intestine under the fasting and postprandial states, studies were conducted in which differentiated Caco-2 cells were supplemented with radiolabeled retinol under conditions that support (postprandial) or do not support (fasting) chylomicron secretion (52). These cells assimilated vitamin A by a very rapid uptake mechanism under both conditions. After uptake, the cells stored retinol in both esterified and unesterified forms. Under fasting conditions, the cells mainly secreted variable amounts of free retinol unassociated with lipoproteins. However, under postprandial conditions, these cells secreted significant amounts of REs, mainly with chylomicrons. The secretion of RE with chylomicrons was independent of the rate of uptake of retinol, intracellular free, and esterified retinol levels, and was dependent on the assembly and secretion of chylomicrons. The secretion of RE was correlated with the secretion of chylomicrons and not with the secretion of total apoB. Inhibition of chylomicron secretion by Pluronic L81 decreased the secretion of RE and did not result in their increased secretion with smaller lipoproteins. These data strongly suggest that RE secretion by the intestinal cells is a highly specific and regulated process that is dependent on the assembly and secretion of chylomicrons. These data also indicate that the incorporation of RE into chylomicrons is not a passive process but rather is an exquisitely orchestrated event. RE secretion does not occur at all times. It is induced when cells can assemble and secrete chylomicrons. Thus, it appears that intestinal cells may have a specific mechanism for the targeting of REs to nascent chylomicrons.

As discussed above, Caco-2 cells do not secrete REs under conditions simulating a fasting state. In recent work on the kinetics of retinol uptake by Caco2 cells, a five-day "washout" experiment was conducted in which cells were incubated with retinol for 16 hours to accumulate cellular retinol and REs, followed by incubation with retinoid-free medium (containing fatty acids and thus mimicking the "fed" state) that was changed every 24 hours (16). This resulted in the release of the free retinol but not the accumulated REs. This implies that only newly synthesized REs are incorporated into chylomicrons and that preformed REs cannot be used for chylomicron assembly. Thus, the synthesis of REs and their incorporation into chylomicrons appear to be concerted processes.

Due to the specificity of the secretion of REs, it was proposed that REs could be used as signposts to study chylomicron assembly (36, 38). Two different mechanisms have been proposed for the assembly and secretion of chylomicrons (for review, see 36–38). First, in the independent pathway, very-low-density lipoproteins and chylomicrons have been proposed to be synthesized by two independent mechanisms (72, 73). If chylomicron assembly occurs by an independent pathway that is induced during the postprandial state, REs may be used to differentiate between chylomicron and very-low-density lipoprotein assembly pathways. The second, sequential assembly mechanism suggests that the assembly of chylomicrons and very-low-density lipoproteins involves a common first event resulting in the synthesis of primordial lipoproteins. Another important event hypothesized for the assembly of chylomicrons and other lipoproteins is the formation of different-sized lipid droplets. Subsequently, the larger lipid droplets are proposed to fuse with primordial lipoproteins, resulting in the "core expansion" of primordial lipoproteins (36, 37). If this is true, REs may be incorporated at the terminal stages of lipoprotein assembly. Both of these mechanisms can be distinguished by studying the presence of REs in different intracellular lipoproteins. It is clear that RE synthesis and the incorporation and secretion of REs in chylomicrons are concerted processes.

PROSPECTIVE

The literature reviewed above suggests that the intestinal digestion and absorption of vitamin A is a highly complex process, and that a number of enzymes and other proteins participate in the process. Table 1 and Figure 1 summarize some of the proteins described in this review. Given the complexity of the process, caution is urged in attempts to define a single enzyme or protein that is the physiologically relevant one in a given step. Several of the proteins studied may be relevant, and certainly, a number will be found that are involved in the overall process. Further use of techniques such as overexpression of specific proteins or gene ablation might ultimately lead to a definition of which proteins play which roles in vitamin

A absorption. In addition, the development of highly specific inhibitors could also shed light on these issues.

ACKNOWLEDGMENTS

I thank my colleagues Susan Gebhardt and David Haytowitz of the Nutrient Data Laboratory for their analysis of the food sources of vitamin A in the diet, and Alanna Moshfegh of the Food Surveys Research Group for her analysis of the vitamin A intake of the U.S. population. I also thank the USDA and the NIH (DK44498 and HL49879) for financial support of my research, and the many students, fellows, and colleagues who have been my collaborators.

The *Annual Review of Nutrition* is online at http://nutr.annualreviews.org

LITERATURE CITED

1. Abumrad N, Harmon C, Ibrahimi A. 1998. Membrane transport of long-chain fatty acids: evidence for a facilitated process. *J. Lipid Res.* 39:2309–18
2. Altmann SW, Davis HR Jr, Zhu LJ, Yao X, Hoos LM, et al. 2004. Niemann-Pick C1 Like 1 protein is critical for intestinal cholesterol absorption. *Science* 303:1201–4
3. Batten ML, Imanishi Y, Maeda T, Tu DC, Moise AR, et al. 2004. Lecithin-retinol acyltransferase is essential for accumulation of all-trans-retinyl esters in the eye and in the liver. *J. Biol. Chem.* 279:10422–32
4. Blaner WS, Hendricks HFJ, Brouwer A, de Leeuw AM, Knook DL, et al. 1985. Retinoids, retinoid-binding proteins, and retinyl palmitate hydrolase distributions in different types of rat liver cells. *J. Lipid Res.* 26:1241–51
5. Blomhoff R, Green MH, Berg T, Norum KR. 1990. Transport and storage of vitamin A. *Science* 250:399–404
6. Blomhoff R, Green MH, Green JB, Berg T, Norum KR. 1991. Vitamin A metabolism: new perspectives on absorption, transport, and storage. *Physiol. Rev.* 71:951–90
7. Blomhoff R, Helgerud P, Rasmussen M, Berg T, Norum KR. 1982. In vivo uptake of chylomicron [^{3}H]retinyl ester by rat liver: evidence for retinol transfer from parenchymal to nonparenchymal cells. *Proc. Natl. Acad. Sci. USA* 79:7326–30
8. Blomhoff R, Holte K, Naess L, Berg T. 1984. Newly administered [^{3}H]retinol is transferred from hepatocytes to stellate cells in liver storage. *Exp. Cell Res.* 150:186–93
9. Blomhoff R, Rasmussen M, Nilsson A, Norum KR, Berg T, et al. 1985. Hepatic retinol metabolism. Distribution of retinoids, enzymes, and binding proteins in isolated rat liver cells. *J. Biol. Chem.* 260:13560–65
10. Borgström B, Erlanson C. 1973. Pancreatic lipase and co-lipase. Interactions and effects of bile salts and other detergents. *Eur. J. Biochem.* 37:60–68
11. Brockman HL. 1984. General features of lipolysis: reaction scheme, interfacial structure and experimental approaches. In *Lipases*, ed. B. Borgström, HL Brockman, pp. 3–46. Amsterdam/NY/Oxford: Elsevier
12. Burri BJ, Clifford AJ. 2004. Carotenoid and retinoid metabolism: insights from isotope studies. *Arch. Biochem. Biophys.* 430:110–19
13. Chen HC. 2001. Molecular mechanisms of sterol absorption. *J. Nutr.* 131:2603–5
14. Davis HR Jr, Zhu LJ, Hoos LM, Tetzloff G, Maguire M, et al. 2004. Niemann-Pick C1-like 1 (NPC1L1) is the intestinal

phytosterol and cholesterol transporter and a key modulator of whole-body cholesterol homeostasis. *J. Biol. Chem.* 279:33586–92

15. Dew SE, Ong DE. 1994. Specificity of the retinol transporter of the rat small intestine brush border. *Biochemistry* 33:12340–45
16. During A, Harrison EH. 2003. Kinetics of retinol uptake and secretion by Caco-2 cells: mechanistic implications. *FASEB J.* 17:A314
17. During A, Harrison EH. 2004. Intestinal absorption and metabolism of carotenoids: insights from cell culture. *Arch. Biochem. Biophys.* 430:77–88
18. Erlanson C, Borgström B. 1968. The identity of vitamin A esterase activity of rat pancreatic juice. *Biochim. Biophys. Acta* 167:629–31
19. Futterman S, Andrews JS. 1964. The composition of liver vitamin A ester and the synthesis of vitamin A ester by liver microsomes. *J. Biol. Chem.* 239:4077–80
20. Giller T, Buchwald P, Blum-Kaelin D, Hunziker W. 1992. Two novel human pancreatic lipase related proteins, hPLRP1 and hPLRP2: differences in colipase dependence and in lipase activity. *J. Biol. Chem.* 267:16509–16
21. Glatz JFC, van Nieuwenhoven FA, Luiken JJFP, Schaap FG, van der Vusse GJ. 1997. Role of membrane-associated and cytoplasmic fatty acid-binding proteins in cellular fatty acid metabolism. *Prostaglandins Leukot. Essent. Fatty Acids* 57:373–78
22. Goodman DS, Blomstrand R, Werner B, Huang HS, Shiratori T. 1966. The intestinal absorption and metabolism of vitamin A and beta-carotene in man. *J. Clin. Invest.* 45:1615–23
23. Goodwin TW. 1963. *The Biosynthesis of Vitamin A and Related Compounds*. London: Academic
24. Goodwin TW. 1971. Biosynthesis. In *Carotenoids*, ed. O Isler, pp. 577–86. Switzerland: Birkhauser
25. Harrison EH. 1998. Lipases and carboxylesterases: possible roles in the hepatic metabolism of retinol. *Annu. Rev. Nutr.* 18:259–76
26. Harrison EH, Blaner WS, Goodman DS, Ross AC. 1987. Subcellular localization of retinoids, retinoid-binding proteins, and acyl-CoA:retinol acyltransferase in rat liver. *J. Lipid Res.* 28:973–81
27. Harrison EH, Gad MZ, Ross AC. 1995. Hepatic uptake and metabolism of chylomicron retinyl esters: probable role of plasma membrane/endosomal retinyl ester hydrolases. *J. Lipid Res.* 36:1498–506
28. Harrison EH, Hussain MM. 2001. Mechanisms involved in the intestinal digestion and absorption of dietary vitamin A. *J. Nutr.* 131:1405–8
29. Hazzard WR, Bierman EL. 1976. Delayed clearance of chylomicron remnants following vitamin A–containing oral fat loads in broad-beta disease (type III hyperlipoproteinemia). *Metab. Clin. Exp.* 25:777–801
30. Helgerud P, Peterson LB, Norum KR. 1982. Acyl CoA:retinol acyltransferase in rat small intestine: its activity and some properties of the enzymatic reaction. *J. Lipid Res.* 23:609–18
31. Hernell O, Staggers JE, Carey MC. 1990. Physical-chemical behavior of dietary and biliary lipids during intestinal digestion and absorption. 2. Phase analysis and aggregation states of luminal lipids during duodenal fat digestion in healthy adult human beings. *Biochemistry* 29:2041–56
32. Hollander D. 1980. Retinol lymphatic and portal transport: influence of pH, bile, and fatty acids. *Am. J. Physiol.* 239:G210–14
33. Hollander D. 1981. Intestinal absorption of vitamins A, E, D, and K. *J. Lab. Clin. Med.* 97:449–62
34. Hollander D, Muralidhara KS. 1977. Vitamin A1 intestinal absorption in vivo: influence of luminal factors on transport. *Am. J. Physiol.* 232:E471–77
35. Huang HS, Goodman DS. 1965. Vitamin A and carotenoids. I. Intestinal absorption and metabolism of ^{14}C-labeled vitamin A alcohol and β-carotene in the rat. *J. Biol. Chem.* 240:2839–44

36. Hussain MM. 2000. A proposed model for the assembly of chylomicrons. *Atherosclerosis* 148:1–15
37. Hussain MM, Kancha RK, Zhou Z, Luchoomun J, Zu H, Bakillah A. 1996. Chylomicron assembly and catabolism: role of apolipoproteins and receptors. *Biochim. Biophys. Acta* 1300:151–70
38. Hussain MM, Kedees MH, Singh K, Athar H, Jamali NZ. 2001. Signposts in the assembly of chylomicrons. *Front. Biosci.* 6:D320–31
39. Jennens ML, Lowe ME. 1995. Rat GP-3 is a pancreatic lipase with kinetic properties that differ from colipase-dependent pancreatic lipase. *J. Lipid Res.* 36:2374–82
40. Kane JP, Havel RJ. 1995. Disorders of the biogenesis and secretion of lipoproteins containing the B apolipoproteins. In *The Metabolic and Molecular Bases of Inherited Disorders*, ed. CR Scriver, AL Beaudet, WS Sly, D Valle, pp. 1853–85. New York: McGraw-Hill
41. Lawrence CW, Crain FD, Lotspeich FJ, Krause RF. 1966. Absorption, transport, and storage of retinyl-15-^{14}C palmitate-9,10-^{3}H in the rat. *J. Lipid Res.* 7:226–29
42. Lemieux S, Fontani R, Uffelman KD, Lewis GF, Steiner G. 1998. Apolipoprotein B-48 and retinyl palmitate are not equivalent markers of postprandial intestinal lipoproteins. *J. Lipid Res.* 39:1964–71
43. Levin MS. 1993. Cellular retinol-binding proteins are determinants of retinol uptake and metabolism in stably transfected Caco-2 cells. *J. Biol. Chem.* 268:8267–76
44. Levin MS, Davis AE. 1997. Retinoic acid increases cellular retinol binding protein II mRNA and retinol uptake in the human intestinal Caco-2 cell line. *J. Nutr.* 127:13–17
45. Li E, Norris AW. 1996. Structure/function of cytoplasmic vitamin A–binding proteins. *Annu. Rev. Nutr.* 16:205–34
46. Li E, Tso P. 2003. Vitamin A uptake from foods. *Curr. Opin. Lipidol.* 14:241–47
47. Linder MC, Anderson H, Ascarelli I. 1971. Quantitative distribution of vitamin A in Kupffer cell and hepatocyte populations of rat liver. *J. Biol. Chem.* 246:5538–40
48. Lissoos TW, Davis AE, Levin MS. 1995. Vitamin A trafficking in Caco-2 cells stably transfected with cellular retinol binding proteins. *Am. J. Physiol.* 268:G224–31
49. MacDonald PN, Ong DE. 1988. Evidence for a lecithin-retinol acyltransferase activity in the rat small intestine. *J. Biol. Chem.* 263:12478–82
50. Matsuura T, Gad MZ, Harrison EH, Ross AC. 1997. Lecithin:retinol acyltransferase and retinyl ester hydrolase activities are differentially regulated by retinoids and have distinct distribution between hepatocyte and nonparenchymal cell fractions of rat liver. *J. Nutr.* 127:218–24
51. Miller M, Humphrey J, Johnson E, Marinda E, Brookmeyer R, Katz J. 2002. Why do children become vitamin A deficient? *J. Nutr.* 132(9 Suppl.)2867–80
52. Nayak N, Harrison EH, Hussain MM. 2001. Retinyl ester secretion by the intestinal cells is a specific and regulated process that is dependent on the assembly and secretion of chylomicrons. *J. Lipid Res.* 42:272–80
53. Newcomer ME, Jamison RS, Ong DE. 1998. Structure and function of retinoid-binding proteins. *Subcell. Biochem.* 30:53–80
54. Nieland TJ, Chroni A, Fitzgerald ML, Maliga Z, Zannis VI, et al. 2004. Cross-inhibition of SR-BI- and ABCA1-mediated cholesterol transport by the small molecules BLT-4 and glyburide. *J. Lipid Res.* 45:1256–65
55. Noh SK, Koo SI. 2001. Intraduodenal infusion of lysophosphatidylcholine restores the intestinal absorption of vitamins A and E in rats fed a low-zinc diet. *Exp. Biol. Med.* 226:342–48
56. Ong DE. 1985. Vitamin A–binding proteins. *Nutr. Rev.* 43:225–32
57. Ong DE. 1994. Cellular transport and metabolism of vitamin A: roles of the cellular retinoid-binding proteins. *Nutr. Rev.* 52:S24–31

Annu. Rev. Nutr. 2005. 25:105–25
doi: 10.1146/annurev.nutr.25.050304.092647

First published online as a Review in Advance on February 10, 2005

REGULATION OF VITAMIN C TRANSPORT

John X. Wilson
Department of Exercise and Nutrition Sciences, School of Public Health and Health Professions, University at Buffalo, Buffalo, New York 14214-3079; email: jxwilson@buffalo.edu

Key Words ascorbic acid, dehydroascorbic acid, transporters, ion channels, bioavailability

■ **Abstract** Ascorbic acid and dehydroascorbic acid (DHAA, oxidized vitamin C) are dietary sources of vitamin C in humans. Both nutrients are absorbed from the lumen of the intestine and renal tubules by, respectively, enterocytes and renal epithelial cells. Subsequently vitamin C circulates in the blood and enters all of the other cells of the body. Concerning flux across the plasma membrane, simple diffusion of ascorbic acid plays only a small or negligible role. More important are specific mechanisms of transport and metabolism that concentrate vitamin C intracellularly to enhance its function as an enzyme cofactor and antioxidant. The known transport mechanisms are facilitated diffusion of DHAA through glucose-sensitive and -insensitive transporters, facilitated diffusion of ascorbate through channels, exocytosis of ascorbate in secretory vesicles, and secondary active transport of ascorbate through the sodium-dependent vitamin C transporters SVCT1 and SVCT2 proteins that are encoded by the genes Slc23a1 and Slc23a2, respectively. Evidence is reviewed indicating that these transport pathways are regulated under physiological conditions and altered by aging and disease.

CONTENTS

INTRODUCTION

Most mammalian species synthesize ascorbic acid de novo from glucose in the liver, through a biosynthetic pathway involving gulono-gamma-lactone oxidase for the terminal step. But primates and guinea pigs are absolutely dependent on exogenously supplied dietary vitamin C due to inactivation of the gulono-gamma-lactone oxidase gene by mutation (33).

Ingestion of ascorbic acid or its reversibly oxidized metabolite, dehydroascorbic acid (DHAA), raises the plasma concentration of ascorbate (the predominant form of reduced vitamin C at physiological pH) in normal human subjects (40, 79). Transport systems associated with cells' plasma membranes determine the distribution of vitamin C between extracellular and intracellular fluids. Simple diffusion, facilitated diffusion, and active mechanisms may potentially contribute to the membrane transport of vitamin C.

SIMPLE DIFFUSION

Ascorbic acid is a lactone ($C_6H_8O_6$) and its hydroxyl groups at positions 2 and 3 ionize with pK values of 4.17 and 11.57. Therefore, reduced vitamin C exists predominantly as the ascorbate anion in most body fluids. Molecules that are comparably water soluble but smaller and nonionized, such as ethanol and glycerol, diffuse rapidly through nonspecific pathways in cell membranes, especially through the lipid bilayer. In contrast, ascorbate, because of its size and charge, does not readily permeate the lipid bilayer. Simple diffusion of DHAA into cells is negligible, too, because the oil:water distribution coefficient of DHAA is similar to that of an osmotic diuretic, mannitol, which is excluded from lipid bilayers (76).

Weak organic acids can enter cells by simple diffusion of their undissociated forms. Once in the cytoplasm, these acids dissociate into organic ions (e.g., propionic acid becomes propionate) and protons. To investigate if appreciable uptake of ascorbic acid might occur this way, bone-derived osteoblasts were incubated with 5 mM sodium ascorbate or sodium propionate at pH 7.3 and cytoplasmic pH was monitored to detect uptake of the organic acids (99). Sodium propionate caused rapid acidification of the cytoplasm but ascorbate had little effect, which indicates that osteoblasts do not take up appreciable amounts of undissociated ascorbic acid. Further studies showed that these cells increase their intracellular concentration of vitamin C through plasma membrane transport systems that translocate either the ascorbate anion (99) or DHAA (72). Therefore, simple diffusion across the plasma membrane at physiological pH comprises only a slow component of vitamin C accumulation and may be negligibly small in those cells that contain transport systems with high affinity for ascorbate or DHAA.

FACILITATED DIFFUSION

Specific proteins mediate the entry and exit of vitamin C in cells by facilitated diffusion or active transport. Facilitated diffusion achieves net movement only in the direction of a chemical or electrochemical gradient of the transported solute, whereas active transport can move solute against this gradient by using energy derived from cellular metabolism. The facilitated diffusion of DHAA and ascorbate is discussed in this section.

Uptake of Dehydroascorbic Acid into Cells

When ascorbate acts as an antioxidant or enzyme cofactor, it becomes oxidized to DHAA. This oxidization product evidently plays physiologically important roles because it can be used by cells to regenerate ascorbate, and directly or indirectly, it can change the redox state of many other molecules. DHAA is a dietary source of vitamin C in humans because cellular mechanisms of transport and metabolism convert DHAA to ascorbate (40, 79). It is widely understood that dietary ascorbate and DHAA possess roughly equivalent bioavailability, which is the fraction of the ingested amount that has the potential to meet the functional requirements of tissues for vitamin C. Indeed, the vitamin C content of food is commonly reported as the sum of the ascorbate and DHAA contents.

Bioavailability is determined by the rates of absorption, distribution, and metabolism within the body, and by excretion. Absorption of vitamin C from food occurs across the epithelium of the small intestine, which is comprised of polarized enterocytes. Both ascorbate and DHAA are absorbed along the entire length of the human intestine, as has been shown by measuring transport activities in luminal (brush-border) membrane vesicles (59). For both the DHAA and ascorbate transport systems, initial rates of uptake saturate with increasing external substrate concentration, reflecting high-affinity interactions that can be described by Michaelis-Menten kinetics. A transport system's affinity is reflected in the substrate concentrations required for half-maximal flux, which is the Michaelis constant, K_m. In human intestinal brush-border membranes, DHAA is taken up with lower affinity than ascorbate because the apparent K_m values are 0.8 and 0.2 mM, respectively. However, the maximal rates of uptake are similar for DHAA and ascorbate when glucose is absent.

The mechanism of DHAA uptake by luminal membranes of human jejunum has pharmacological characteristics that clearly differ from those of ascorbate uptake. Sodium-independent carriers take up DHAA by facilitated diffusion, and these are distinct from the sodium-dependent transporters of ascorbate. Glucose inhibits ascorbate uptake but not DHAA uptake, which raises the possibility that glucose derived from food may increase the bioavailability of DHAA relative to ascorbate (59). Human enterocytes contain reductases that convert DHAA to ascorbate (12). This conversion maintains the intracellular level of DHAA low and the resulting concentration gradient favors uptake of oxidized vitamin C across the enterocytes' plasma membrane. Intestinal DHAA absorption may be especially important during gastritis, since chronic gastritis decreases the concentration of ascorbate in gastric juice and yet does not cause scurvy (80). Inflammation in the gastric mucosa may accelerate oxidation of ascorbate to DHAA, but intestinal absorption of the latter may prevent gastritis patients from becoming scorbutic.

ascorbate concentration is decreased and DHAA is increased in the plasma and sciatic nerve of rats made diabetic by streptozotocin (66, 67). Moreover, because intracellular ascorbate is required for collagen synthesis by osteoblasts (29), deficient recycling of ascorbate in this bone cell type may contribute to the development of osteopenia. It is consistent with this hypothesis that feeding ascorbate to diabetic pregnant rats has been found to improve skeletal development in their offspring (9).

DHAA uptake occurs through relatively glucose-insensitive mechanisms in rat astrocytes and human erythrocytes, enterocytes, and renal epithelial cells.

DHAA is filtered from the plasma at the renal glomerular capillaries and then reabsorbed across the luminal membranes of the epithelial cells that comprise the renal proximal tubules. These cells are the principal sites where vitamin C is removed from the lumen of the renal tubule and translocated toward the blood. Studies of brush-border membrane vesicles prepared from rat renal cortex, which are representative of the luminal membranes of proximal tubule cells, have shown that ascorbate uptake occurs through sodium-ascorbate cotransport, whereas DHAA uptake occurs by a sodium-independent process (60). Neither ascorbate nor DHAA uptake is inhibited by glucose; hence, the facilitative and sodium-dependent glucose transporters present in the luminal membranes cannot be the routes of vitamin C uptake. Perhaps a previously unidentified, specific DHAA transporter exists in epithelial cells.

Uptake of DHAA (5–200 uM) by brain-derived astrocytes is inhibited only partially by a supraphysiological concentration of glucose (10 mM) (17). The remaining glucose-insensitive accumulation of intracellular ascorbate from DHAA is blocked by phloretin and cytochalasin B, which are antagonists of facilitative glucose transporters, but it is also inhibited reversibly by sulfinpyrazone. Astrocytes are an abundant cell type in the brain. These nonneuronal, glial cells regulate the composition of extracellular fluid and thus influence the environment and activity of neurons. DHAA is lethal to neurons in the absence of astrocytes (87), whereas the latter cells are capable of regenerating ascorbate without ill effect (17, 84). Brain cells produce cyclic AMP in response to neurotransmitters and ischemia and this intracellular messenger stimulates astrocytic uptake of DHAA and accumulation of ascorbate (84). Thus, astrocytes clear neurotoxic DHAA from extracellular fluid through a transport system that is not very sensitive to inhibition by glucose and that is upregulated by cyclic AMP.

It has been suggested that DHAA can be injected as a prodrug to treat cerebral ischemia (1, 38). The aim is to increase cerebral ascorbate concentration and thereby counter the oxidative stress caused by ischemia and reperfusion. Radiotracer experiments have shown that blood-borne DHAA enters the brain and is converted to ascorbate (1). Intravenous injection of DHAA improves neurologic outcome in mice subjected to experimental stroke, although it is not known if elevation of the vitamin C concentration in brain parenchyma is the cause of this improvement (38). The acute effect of DHAA on normal brain parenchymal cells may be to inhibit behavioral activation (i.e., open-field locomotion, approach of novel objects, and social interactions with other rats), since infusion of ascorbate oxidase into rat brain converts extracellular ascorbate to DHAA and leads to a rapid decline in behavioral activation; in fact, oxidation of 50% to 70% of extracellular ascorbate is associated with a near-total inhibition of all recorded behavior (75).

Within various cell types, the most important enzymes for DHAA reduction are thioredoxin, protein disulfide isomerase, and thioredoxin reductase. Additionally, 3-hydroxysteroid dehydrogenase may reduce DHAA in hepatocytes. Glucose-6-phosphate dehydrogenase (G6PD) activity provides nicotinamide adenine dinucleotide phosphate (NADPH) as a source of reducing equivalents for DHAA reduction. Using DHAA-stimulated reduction of cationic nitroxides, which is an indirect measure of the rate of DHAA reduction, Mehlhorn (62) found that DHAA reduction is slower in human erythrocytes deficient in G6PD than in normal erythrocytes. Because low-activity alleles of G6PD are common genetic polymorphisms in human populations and the resulting G6PD deficiency could impair DHAA reduction (62), it may be desirable to screen for G6PD status before administering high doses of DHAA parenterally. If the amount of DHAA administered exceeds the capacity for its reduction, then DHAA concentration may rise high enough to inhibit transporters and enzymes (27).

Ascorbate Efflux from Cells

There has been relatively little research on how vitamin C is transported out of cells. Incubation with extracellular vitamin C stimulates efflux of preloaded [^{14}C]vitamin C, as has been shown for various cells of both epithelial and nonepithelial types (26, 42, 85). This effect has been interpreted as transstimulation of ascorbate efflux by extracellular ascorbate, which is supposed to enter cells through a homeoexchange transport system. However, the existence of ascorbate homeoexchange systems has not been demonstrated conclusively and the molecular identities of the membrane proteins responsible for homeoexchange have not been determined.

Intracellular reduction of DHAA to ascorbate can lead to ascorbate efflux, as reported for erythrocytes, endothelial cells, and hepatocyte-like HepG cells (63, 93). It is not known if a single transporter exchanges extracellular DHAA for intracellular ascorbate or if different transporters mediate uptake than efflux. Nevertheless, this recycling mechanism allows the reducing equivalents derived from cell metabolism to be transferred to DHAA and carried into the extracellular fluid as ascorbate, thus becoming available to neighboring cells.

Efflux of ascorbate from enterocytes and renal tubular cells, to the blood, is essential for intestinal absorption and renal conservation of vitamin C. Because enterocytes and renal tubular cells swell markedly during transepithelial transport of nutrients such as glucose or alanine (4, 10, 58), it may be hypothesized that ascorbate diffuses from the cytoplasm to the extracellular fluid through volume-sensitive anion channels in the epithelial cells' basolateral membrane and then enters the blood plasma through discontinuities in the capillary wall. Indeed, there is functional evidence that volume-sensitive anion channels are permeant to ascorbate, although the molecular identities of these channels have not been determined (31).

Volume-sensitive pathways may mediate ascorbate efflux from nonepithelial cells, too. Adrenal chromaffin cells release vitamin C from multiple intracellular compartments to the extracellular fluid when incubated with high-potassium solutions that both depolarize and swell the cells (19), whereas depolarization of the plasma membrane by itself is not a sufficient stimulus to elicit ascorbate efflux (13). Cerebral astrocytes also rapidly release ascorbate when stimulated appropriately. Swelling of astrocytes transiently and reversibly permits large quantities of ascorbate to move from the cells to the extracellular fluid (83, 104). Based on its osmotic and pharmacological characteristics, it may be inferred that volume-sensitive anion channels in the plasma membrane mediate this efflux (83, 104). Thus, astrocytes condition the extracellular fluid for neurons by clearing DHAA and replacing ascorbate.

Glutamate uptake into brain cells triggers ascorbate efflux (74, 106). In vitro experiments have shown that astrocytes release ascorbate when exposed to glutamate (104). Astrocytes are in close contact with neuronal synapses and respond to the glutamate released there. Thus, a demand-driven component of ascorbate efflux from astrocytes may appear just in time and place to reach active neurons. A putative glutamate-ascorbate heteroexchanger has been proposed to mediate the counter movements of glutamate and ascorbate (74). However, it is more likely that glutamate uptake through sodium-glutamate cotransporters, located in astrocyte processes (end feet), causes swelling of the end feet and thereby activates a volume-sensitive efflux pathway (104). Exocytosis of ascorbate in secretory vesicles may also raise extracellular ascorbate (95). The physiological consequences may be enormous because changes in the brain's extracellular level of ascorbate play a critical role in behavioral activation. In rats that are awake, for example, ascorbate iontophoresis enhances the magnitude of glutamate-induced neuronal excitations (44). In contrast, intrastriatal infusion of ascorbate oxidase, to convert extracellular ascorbate to DHAA, causes a rapid and severe inhibition of behavior in rats (75).

Connexin proteins, which aggregate to form gap junctions and hemichannels in plasma membranes, may increase membrane permeability to ascorbate. This has been shown by reconstituting microsomes containing connexin proteins into liposomes (2). The liposomes were incubated with ascorbate for 2 minutes and ascorbate uptake was detected by measuring the reduction of cytochrome c that had been trapped in the lumen of the liposomes during their formation. Incorporation of connexin 26 into the liposomes greatly increased their apparent ascorbate uptake (2). Presumably, the connexin 26 formed gap-junction hemichannels that are bidirectional and can facilitate ascorbate efflux as well as uptake.

ACTIVE TRANSPORT

Sodium-Ascorbate Cotransport Mediates High-Affinity Absorption

Ascorbate is absorbed from the lumen of the human intestine by sodium-ascorbate cotransport in enterocytes, as has been shown by measuring transport activities in luminal (brush-border) membrane vesicles (59). This is an example of secondary active transport because it couples ascorbate uptake to the concentration gradient of sodium ion across the plasma membrane that is maintained by sodium/potassium-ATPase. It is likely because of the limited capacity of enterocytes for sodium-ascorbate cotransport that large oral doses of ascorbate are absorbed less completely than are small doses. How ascorbate is administered affects how much reaches the bloodstream and may affect the results of studies of its potential effect on health and disease. For instance, peak plasma ascorbate concentrations are higher after administration of intravenous ascorbate doses than after administration of oral doses and the difference increases with increasing dose (70). Clinical consequences arise from the limited bioavailability of oral ascorbate. For example, when oral and intravenous routes of ascorbate administration (500 mg/day for 30 days) were compared in sedentary older men, only intravenous ascorbate restored endothelial function as indicated by flow-mediated dilatation in the brachial artery (24).

Absorption sites for ascorbate are found along the entire length of the small intestine (59). In vesicles prepared from the jejunum, intravesicular (cytoplasmic) glucose inhibits ascorbate uptake. This observation does not implicate sodium-glucose cotransporters (i.e., SGLT proteins) as carriers of ascorbate because only glucose on the cytoplasmic side of the plasma membrane slows sodium-dependent ascorbate uptake (59). If trans-inhibition by glucose occurs in vivo then it may permit ingested glucose and hyperglycemia to decrease ascorbate bioavailability by slowing intestinal absorption of the vitamin. Other ingredients in foods and drugs may have comparable effects. For instance, the inhibition by salicylate of sodium-ascorbate cotransport that has been demonstrated in vitro (20) may explain the decrease in ascorbate bioavailability caused by aspirin (39).

Flavonoids, such as the dietary component quercetin, reversibly inhibit vitamin C uptake in human colon cancer cells and rat nontransformed intestinal crypt cells, as well as in Chinese hamster ovary cells and Xenopus laevis oocytes transfected with human sodium-dependent vitamin C transporter SVCT1 (52, 86). However, it has not been determined if inhibition of SVCTs and glucose transporters by quercetin, or oxidation of ascorbate by quercetin metabolites (32), causes the decrease in ascorbate bioavailability after quercetin administration in vivo (86). The high content of quercetin and other flavonoids in red grape juice may account for the observation that drinking this juice decreases absorption into blood of [^{13}C]ascorbate administered orally to human subjects (3).

Besides intestinal absorption, another important determinant of bioavailability is secondary active transport of ascorbate in the kidney. Most vitamin C circulates in the blood in the form of the ascorbate anion. The ascorbate in the blood plasma is freely filtered at the renal glomerulus, but much of it is reabsorbed in the proximal tubule. Ascorbate uptake across the luminal membranes of renal proximal tubule cells occurs through sodium-ascorbate cotransport. The amount of ascorbate lost in the urine rises when the plasma ascorbate concentration exceeds the renal threshold. Above this threshold the tubular reabsorptive capacity is overwhelmed. This phenomenon is exploited clinically when urinary acidification with ascorbate is used for treatment and prevention of urinary tract infection (14). The renal threshold for vitamin C is reported to be slightly higher in men than in women (plasma ascorbate concentrations of 86 and 71 uM, respectively), but the underlying mechanism and physiological importance of this difference are unknown (68). Unlike the sodium-dependent ascorbate transport system in the luminal membrane of human jejunum that is inhibited by cytoplasmic glucose (59), Malo & Wilson (60) observed that the initial rate of ascorbate uptake by the luminal membrane of rat proximal tubule is not retarded by glucose. A previous study found a small, low-potency inhibitory action of glucose (30% inhibition by 100 mM glucose) during relatively long uptake periods, which is attributable to sodium loading of the membrane vesicles by prolonged, maximal operation of the sodium-glucose cotransporter (91). The briefer uptake period employed by Malo & Wilson (60) did not allow glucose-coupled sodium entry to increase intracellular sodium concentration to levels that inhibit ascorbate uptake during the transport assay.

Evidently, ascorbate and DHAA uptakes are not mediated by glucose transporters in these rat kidney membranes, since they are not inhibited by glucose directly or by the SGLT blocker phlorizin (60). Nevertheless, patients with diabetic nephropathy have lower plasma ascorbate concentration and higher renal clearance of ascorbate than do control subjects (35). Since tubular atrophy and interstitial fibrosis are common in the diabetic kidney, it is likely that structural damage impairs renal tubular reabsorption of ascorbate in these patients and thus diminishes plasma ascorbate concentration (35).

Many nonepithelial cell types also are capable of high-affinity vitamin C uptake through sodium-ascorbate cotransporters, including bone osteoblasts, cerebral astrocytes, ovarian granulosa cells, and vascular smooth muscle and endothelial cells (37, 49, 100, 101, 107). The apparent K_m values for sodium-ascorbate cotransport range from 200 uM L-ascorbate in absorptive epithelia [luminal membranes of human jejunum (59) and rodent renal cortex (91)] to 20 uM L-ascorbate in nonepithelial cells [osteoblasts (21)]. Thus, the secondary active transport of ascorbate occurs with higher affinity than does facilitated transport of DHAA.

Sodium-ascorbate cotransporters are remarkably specific for L-ascorbate (20, 29, 54, 59, 99). Among the molecules that have been tested and found not to be substrates for these cotransporters are ascorbate-2-O-phosphate, DHAA, glucose, 2-deoxyglucose, xanthine, hypoxanthine, L-gulono-lactone, formate, lactate, pyruvate, gluconate, oxalate, malonate, succinate, and an assortment of nucleosides and nucleotides. The cotransporters' stereoselectivity has been demonstrated as a greater affinity for L-ascorbate over the epimer D-isoascorbate, which leads to higher intracellular ascorbate concentrations of L-ascorbate than D-isoascorbate at steady state (29). The cotransporters are absolutely dependent on sodium and translocate at least two sodium cations with each ascorbate anion, thus employing the electrochemical gradient of sodium ion across the plasma membrane to provide the energy required for concentrative uptake of ascorbate (29, 54, 59, 99, 102).

Distinct Properties of the Cotransporters SVCT1 and SVCT2

Two isoforms of sodium-ascorbate cotransporters have been cloned and named SVCT1 and SVCT2 (16, 54, 55, 73, 88, 92, 96, 97). They are encoded by the genes Slc23a1 and Slc23a2, respectively. The majority of single nucleotide polymorphisms (SNPs) in Slc23a1 are population-specific in either African Americans or Caucasians, including three of four nonsynonymous SNPs (23). Most SNPs in Slc23a2 are shared between African Americans and Caucasians, and there are no nonsynonymous SNPs in Slc23a2 (23). In humans, rats, and mice, SVCT1 and SVCT2 have extensive sequence identity with each other but do not share structural homology with other families of sodium cotransporters. Hydropathy plots of the amino acid sequences are consistent with 12 transmembrane domains. Both SVCT isoforms are glycoproteins containing *N*-linked oligosaccharides when expressed in heterologous systems such as *Xenopus* oocytes, HRPE cells, and COS-1 cells (55).

Heterologous expression of either SVCT1 or SVCT2 confers concentrative ascorbate uptake. SVCT1 has consistently been found to have a higher capacity for ascorbate than does the other isoform. It has not been determined if this greater capacity is an inherent property of the SVCT1 protein (i.e., a larger turnover number) or simply reflects a larger abundance of SVCT1 than SVCT2 in the plasma membrane of the transfected cells (55).

SVCT1 and SVCT2 are remarkably specific for L-ascorbate (54, 73, 96). Their stereoselectivity for L-ascorbate over the epimer D-isoascorbate (erythorbate) likely accounts for the low antiscorbutic activity of the latter. Most studies have found that SVCT2 has a higher affinity for L-ascorbate than does SVCT1, with SVCT2 being approximately half saturated at the low end of the normal range of plasma ascorbate concentrations (90).

Endogenous mRNA for one or both of the SVCT isoforms has been found in most organs (16, 51, 73, 92, 96, 97). Reverse transcription-polymerase chain reaction (RT-PCR) analysis showed that brain, skeletal muscle, and spleen express predominantly SVCT2, whereas liver and kidney express mainly SVCT1; indeed, quantitative RT-PCR showed that SVCT2 mRNA levels in liver and kidney are less than 5% of SVCT1 levels (51). SVCT1 is localized mostly in epithelial tissues, whereas SVCT2 has a wider distribution. On the one hand, the high capacity of SVCT1 is appropriate for epithelial cells that transport much more ascorbate than required for their own internal use. On the other hand, the affinities of both SVCT1 and SVCT2 are sufficiently high to enable cells to absorb ascorbate effectively from extracellular fluid where—in most tissues except the stomach, eye, and central nervous system—the concentration of ascorbate may approximate the 20–80 uM normally found in plasma.

Transfection of an antisense oligonucleotide of SVCT2 into cells that otherwise express this transporter endogenously suppresses their sodium-dependent uptake of ascorbate in vitro (82). Concerning manipulation of this transporter in vivo, heterozygous SVCT2 knockout (*Slc23a2+/−*) mice comprise a valuable model because they survive to adulthood, unlike the homozygous *Slc23a2−/−* mice that die shortly after birth (88). The SVCT isoforms appear to function independently of each other because SVCT1 expression and ascorbate concentrations in SVCT1-predominant organs are not affected by SVCT2 deficiency (51). Ascorbate concentrations are lower for *Slc23a2+/−* than wild-type (*Slc23a2+/+*) mice in tissues where SVCT2 is the main isoform, such as brain, spleen, and skeletal muscle (51, 88). Therefore, SVCT2 is a major determinant of ascorbate accumulation in tissues lacking SVCT1.

Selective sorting to the apical plasma membrane has been demonstrated for SVCT1 in the human colon adenocarcinoma cell line CaCo-2 (61) and the human nasal epithelial cell line CF15 (28). The evidence for the latter is that, first, cells cultured from human airway epithelia express SVCT1 and SVCT2 mRNA and are capable of sodium-dependent ascorbate uptake, and second, recombinantly expressed SVCT2-enhanced green fluorescent fusion protein is targeted exclusively to the apical membrane pole of the CF15 nasal epithelial cell line (28). Confocal imaging of hSVCT1 truncation mutants expressed in CaCo-2 cells and Madin-Darby canine kidney cells demonstrated that hSVCT1 was expressed at the apical cell surface and also resided in a heterogeneous population of intracellular organelles (89). Progressive truncation of the cytoplasmic COOH-terminal tail of hSVCT1 showed that an embedded ten-amino-acid sequence PICPVFKGFS, in amino acids 563–572, was required for targeting of hSVCT1 (89).

Elderly human subjects require more vitamin C in their diet than do young subjects to reach a desired plasma ascorbate concentration (11). Animal studies have revealed a diminished expression of SVCT1 mRNA and a decline in the capacity of cells to absorb vitamin C during aging (64). The ascorbate concentration in the liver of male rats decreases with age even though the rate of de novo ascorbate synthesis does not (64). When incubated with ascorbate, isolated hepatocytes from old as compared with young rats show decreased maximal rate of ascorbate uptake and lower steady state intracellular ascorbate concentration. Sodium-free media significantly reduces ascorbate uptake, implicating sodium-ascorbate cotransporters. Hepatic SVCT1 mRNA levels decline 45% with age, with no significant changes in SVCT2 mRNA abundance. It thus appears likely that a fall in SVCT1 expression changes hepatic ascorbate concentration. This finding may indicate a dominant role for plasma membrane transporters in the regulation of ascorbate levels, even in cells capable of synthesizing the vitamin. Moreover, the deficit in intracellular ascorbate concentration can be overcome by increasing the external supply of the vitamin, which suggests that intervention to increase plasma ascorbate concentrations might be beneficial for hepatic function in elderly subjects (64). Another potential therapeutic approach is to elevate the activity of sodium-ascorbate cotransporters.

Much research has been directed to identifying mechanisms that control the ascorbate transport in various cell types. Transport activity may be altered by changes in the affinity of substrate binding, the translocation capacity (i.e., turnover number) of each transporter protein, or the number of transporter proteins present in the plasma membrane.

Sodium-ascorbate cotransport may be regulated kinetically by changes in either the concentrations of the transported solutes or membrane potential. Ascorbate downregulates the maximal rate of sodium-ascorbate cotransport. This has been shown for absorptive epithelia by feeding excess ascorbate to guinea pigs and afterward measuring the rate of sodium-dependent uptake of vitamin C into the intestinal mucosal (41). Downregulation of SVCT1 by ascorbate may limit its usefulness for raising intracellular ascorbate concentration. Evidence for downregulation is that incubation of the human colon adenocarcinoma cell line CaCo-2 TC7 with ascorbate for 24 hours leads to decreases in SVCT1 mRNA level and ascorbate uptake rate (57). Thus, it appears that the activity of SVCT1 in enterocytes is regulated to adjust for the recent history of ascorbate absorption.

Substrate downregulation of SVCT2 activity has been induced by preincubating astrocytes and osteoblasts with ascorbate for 10 to 24 hours and subsequently determining the kinetic properties of the initial rate of [^{14}C]ascorbate uptake (22, 103). Changes in SVCT2 activity are rapid and large. The observation that SVCT2 activity varies inversely with intracellular ascorbate concentration is consistent with the hypothesis that this transporter regulates the intracellular concentration of its organic substrate. Upregulation of SVCT2 in cells depleted of ascorbate leads to more efficient absorption of extracellular ascorbate and tends to restore the intracellular concentration of the vitamin (22, 103). Therefore, in the absence of neurohormonal or paracrine signals, SVCT2 acts to maintain intracellular ascorbate concentration constant. Experiments with transgenic mice lacking Slc23a2 indicate that SVCT2 normally maintains the high ascorbate concentration found in brain (51, 88). In situ hybridization of mRNA indicated that the ependymal cells of the choroid plexus express SVCT2, where it may be involved in the transepithelial transport of ascorbate between the blood and the cerebrospinal fluid (92). Brain neurons and astrocytes also express SVCT2 (5, 15, 49, 92). However, because sodium-ascorbate cotransporters become downregulated when intracellular ascorbate concentration is high (103), they may not be suitable targets for therapeutic strategies that attempt to raise intracellular ascorbate to supraphysiological levels. Instead it has been suggested that DHAA be injected as a prodrug to increase tissue—particularly brain—ascorbate concentration (1, 38), as discussed in the "Uptake of Dehydroascorbic Acid into Cells" section of this review.

The limited capacities of SVCT isoforms and their susceptibility to downregulation by ascorbate may have influenced the many human clinical trials with oral vitamin C supplements that failed to confer antioxidant protection or clinical benefit. Optimization of the dosing regime may be critical to the success of future intervention studies using vitamin C (69). An important consequence of substrate regulation of SVCT1 and SVCT2 activities may be more efficient absorption by the intestine, conservation by the kidney, and uptake into target cells of intermittent doses than of continuously ingested doses of ascorbate. This phenomenon

The *Annual Review of Nutrition* is online at http://nutr.annualreviews.org

LITERATURE CITED

1. Agus DB, Gambhir SS, Pardridge WM, Spielholz C, Baselga J, et al. 1997. Vitamin C crosses the blood-brain barrier in the oxidized form through the glucose transporters. *J. Clin. Invest.* 100:2842–48
2. Ahmad S, Evans WH. 2002. Post-translational integration and oligomerization of connexin 26 in plasma membranes and evidence of formation of membrane pores: implications for the assembly of gap junctions. *Biochem. J.* 365:693–99
3. Bates CJ, Jones KS, Bluck LJ. 2004. Stable isotope-labelled vitamin C as a probe for vitamin C absorption by human subjects. *Br. J. Nutr.* 91:699–705
4. Beck JS, Potts DJ. 1990. Cell swelling, co-transport activation and potassium conductance in isolated perfused rabbit kidney proximal tubules. *J. Physiol.* 425:369–78
5. Berger UV, Lu XC, Liu W, Tang Z, Slusher BS, Hediger MA. 2003. Effect of middle cerebral artery occlusion on mRNA expression for the sodium-coupled vitamin C transporter SVCT2 in rat brain. *J. Neurochem.* 86:896–906
6. Blee TH, Cogbill TH, Lambert PJ. 2002. Hemorrhage associated with vitamin C deficiency in surgical patients. *Surgery* 131:408–12
7. Blom JH, Dabrowski K. 1998. Continuous or "pulse-and-withdraw" supply of ascorbic acid in the diet: a new approach to altering the bioavailability of ascorbic acid, using teleost fish as a scurvy-prone model. *Int. J. Vitam. Nutr. Res.* 68:88–93
8. Borrelli E, Roux-Lombard P, Grau GE, Girardin E, Ricou B. et al. 1996. Plasma concentrations of cytokines, their soluble receptors, and antioxidant vitamins can predict the development of multiple organ failure in patients at risk. *Crit. Care Med.* 24:392–97
9. Braddock R, Siman CM, Hamilton K, Garland HO, Sibley CP. 2002. Gamma-linoleic acid and ascorbate improves skeletal ossification in offspring of diabetic rats. *Pediatr. Res.* 51:647–52
10. Breton S, Marsolais M, Lapointe JY, Laprade R. 1996. Cell volume increases of physiologic amplitude activate basolateral K and CI conductances in the rabbit proximal convoluted tubule. *J. Am. Soc. Nephrol.* 7:2072–87
11. Brubacher D, Moser U, Jordan P. 2000. Vitamin C concentrations in plasma as a function of intake: a meta-analysis. *Int. J. Vitam. Nutr. Res.* 70:226–37
12. Buffinton GD, Doe WF. 1995. Altered ascorbic acid status in the mucosa from inflammatory bowel disease patients. *Free Radic. Res.* 22:131–43
13. Cahill PS, Wightman RM. 1995. Simultaneous amperometric measurement of ascorbate and catecholamine secretion from individual bovine adrenal medullary cells. *Anal. Chem.* 67:2599–605
14. Carlsson S, Wiklund NP, Engstrand L, Weitzberg E, Lundberg JON. 2001. Effects of pH, nitrite, and ascorbic acid on nonenzymatic nitric oxide generation and bacterial growth in urine. *Nitric Oxide* 5: 580–86
15. Castro M, Caprile T, Astuya A, Millan C, Reinicke K, et al. 2001. High-affinity sodium-vitamin C co-transporters (SVCT) expression in embryonic mouse neurons. *J. Neurochem.* 78:815–23
16. Daruwala R, Song J, Koh WS, Rumsey SC, Levine M. 1999. Cloning and functional characterization of the human sodium-dependent vitamin C transporters hSVCT1 and hSVCT2. *FEBS Lett.* 460:480–84
17. Daskalopoulos R, Korcok J, Tao L, Wilson JX. 2002. Accumulation of intracellular ascorbate from dehydroascorbic acid

by astrocytes is decreased after oxidative stress and restored by propofol. *Glia* 39:124–32
18. Demling R, Ikegami K, Picard L, Lalonde C. 1994. Administration of large doses of vitamin C does not decrease oxidant-induced lung lipid peroxidation caused by bacterial-independent acute peritonitis. *Inflammation* 18:499–510
19. Diliberto EJ, Menniti FS, Knoth J, Daniels AJ, Kizer JS, Viveros OH. 1987. Adrenomedullary chromaffin cells as a model to study the neurobiology of ascorbic acid: from monooxygenation to neuromodulation. *Ann. NY Acad. Sci.* 498:28–53
20. Dixon SJ, Kulaga A, Jaworski EM, Wilson JX. 1991. Ascorbate uptake by ROS 17/2.8 osteoblast-like cells: substrate specificity and sensitivity to transport inhibitors. *J. Bone Miner. Res.* 6:623–29
21. Dixon SJ, Wilson JX. 1992. Transforming growth factor-β stimulates ascorbate transport activity in osteoblastic cells. *Endocrinology* 130:484–89
22. Dixon SJ, Wilson JX. 1992. Adaptive regulation of ascorbate transport in osteoblastic cells. *J. Bone Miner. Res.* 7:675–81
23. Eck P, Erichsen HC, Taylor JG, Yeager M, Hughes AL, et al. 2004. Comparison of the genomic structure and variation in the two human sodium-dependent vitamin C transporters, SLC23A1 and SLC23A2. *Hum. Genet.* 115:285–94
24. Eskurza I, Monahan KD, Robinson JA, Seals DR. 2004. Effect of acute and chronic ascorbic acid on flow-mediated dilatation with sedentary and physically active human ageing. *J. Physiol.* 556:315–24
25. Fain O, Paries J, Jacquart B, Le Moel G, Kettaneh A, et al. 2003. Hypovitaminosis C in hospitalized patients. *Eur. J. Intern. Med.* 14:419–25
26. Finn FM, Johns PA. 1980. Ascorbic acid transport by isolated bovine adrenal cortical cells. *Endocrinology* 106:811–17
27. Fiorani M, De Sanctis R, Scarlatti F, Stocchi V. 1998. Substrates of hexokinase, glucose-6-phosphate dehydrogenase, and glyceraldehyde-3-phosphate dehydrogenase prevent the inhibitory response induced by ascorbic acid/iron and dehydroascorbic acid in rabbit erythrocytes. *Arch. Biochem. Biophys.* 356:159–66
28. Fischer H, Schwarzer C, Illek B. 2004. Vitamin C controls the cystic fibrosis transmembrane conductance regulator chloride channel. *Proc. Natl. Acad. Sci. USA* 101:3691–96
29. Franceschi RT, Wilson JX, Dixon SJ. 1995. Requirement for Na^+-dependent ascorbic acid transport in osteoblast function. *Am. J. Physiol.* 268:C1430–39
30. Fujita I, Hirano J, Itoh N, Nakanishi T, Tanaka K. 2001. Dexamethasone induces sodium-dependant vitamin C transporter in a mouse osteoblastic cell line MC3T3-E1. *Br. J. Nutr.* 86:145–49
31. Furst J, Gschwentner M, Ritter M, Botta G, Jakab M, et al. 2002. Molecular and functional aspects of anionic channels activated during regulatory volume decrease in mammalian cells. *Pflugers Arch.* 444:1–25
32. Galati G, Sabzevari O, Wilson JX, O'Brien PJ. 2002. Prooxidant activity and cellular effects of the phenoxyl radicals of dietary flavonoids and other polyphenolics. *Toxicology* 177:91–104
33. Ha MN, Graham FL, D'Souza CK, Muller WJ, Igdoura SA, Schellhorn HE. 2004. Functional rescue of vitamin C synthesis deficiency in human cells using adenoviral-based expression of murine l-gulono-gamma-lactone oxidase. *Genomics* 83:482–92
34. Himmelreich U, Drew KN, Serianni AS, Kuchel PW. 1998. ^{13}C NMR studies of vitamin C transport and its redox cycling in human erythrocytes. *Biochemistry* 37:7578–88
35. Hirsch IB, Atchley DH, Tsai E, Labbe RF, Chait A. 1998. Ascorbic acid clearance in

diabetic nephropathy. *J. Diabetes Complications* 12:259–63
36. Holmes ME, Mwanjewe J, Samson SE, Haist JV, Wilson JX et al. 2002. Dehydroascorbic acid uptake by coronary artery smooth muscle: effect of intracellular acidification. *Biochem. J.* 362:507–12
37. Holmes ME, Samson SE, Wilson JX, Dixon SJ, Grover AK. 2000. Ascorbate transport in pig coronary artery smooth muscle: Na^+ removal and oxidative stress increase loss of accumulated cellular ascorbate. *J. Vasc. Res.* 37:390–98
38. Huang J, Agus DB, Winfree CJ, Kiss S, Mack WJ, et al. 2001. Dehydroascorbic acid, a blood-brain barrier transportable form of vitamin C, mediates potent cerebroprotection in experimental stroke. *Proc. Natl. Acad. Sci. USA* 98:11720–24
39. Ioannides C, Stone AN, Breacker PJ, Basu TK. 1982. Impairment of absorption of ascorbic acid following ingestion of aspirin in guinea pigs. *Biochem. Pharmacol.* 31:4035–38
40. Jacob RA, Spinozzi GM, Simon VA, Kelley DS, Prior RL, et al. 2003. Consumption of cherries lowers plasma urate in healthy women. *J. Nutr.* 133:1826–29
41. Karasov WH, Darken BW, Bottum MC. 1991. Dietary regulation of intestinal ascorbate uptake in guinea pigs. *Am. J. Physiol.* 260:G108–18
42. Khatami M, Stramm LE, Rockey JH. 1986. Ascorbate transport in cultured cat retinal pigment epithelial cells. *Exp. Eye Res.* 43:607–15
43. Kim M, Otsuka M, Yu R, Kurata T, Arakawa N. 1994. The distribution of ascorbic acid and dehydroascorbic acid during tissue regeneration in wounded dorsal skin of guinea pigs. *Int. J. Vitam. Nutr. Res.* 64:56–59
44. Kiyatkin EA, Rebec GV. 1998. Heterogeneity of ventral tegmental area neurons: single-unit recording and iontophoresis in awake unrestrained rats. *Neuroscience* 85:1285–309
45. Klepper J, Wang D, Fischbarg J, Vera JC, Jarjour IT, et al. 1999. Defective glucose transport across brain tissue barriers: a newly recognized neurological syndrome. *Neurochem. Res.* 24:587–94
46. Kodaman PH, Behrman HR. 1999. Hormone-regulated and glucose-sensitive transport of dehydroascorbic acid in immature rat granulosa cells. *Endocrinology* 140:3659–65
47. Korcok J, Dixon SJ, Lo TCY, Wilson JX. 2003. Differential effects of glucose on dehydroascorbic acid transport and intracellular ascorbate accumulation in astrocytes and skeletal myocytes. *Brain Res.* 993:201–7
48. Korcok J, Wu F, Tyml K, Hammond RR, Wilson JX. 2002. Sepsis inhibits reduction of dehydroascorbic acid and accumulation of ascorbate in astroglial cultures: Intracellular ascorbate depletion increases nitric oxide synthase induction and glutamate uptake inhibition. *J. Neurochem.* 81:185–93
49. Korcok J, Yan R, Siushansian R, Dixon SJ, Wilson JX. 2000. Sodium-ascorbate cotransport controls intracellular ascorbate concentration in primary astrocyte cultures expressing the SVCT2 transporter. *Brain Res.* 881:144–51
50. Kubin A, Kaudela K, Jindra R, Alth G, Grunberger W, et al. 2003. Dehydroascorbic acid in urine as a possible indicator of surgical stress. *Ann. Nutr. Metab.* 47:1–5
51. Kuo SM, MacLean ME, McCormick K, Wilson JX. 2004. Gender and sodium-ascorbate transporters determine ascorbate concentrations in mice. *J. Nutr.* 134:2216–21
52. Kuo SM, Morehouse HF Jr, Lin CP. 1997. Effect of antiproliferative flavonoids on ascorbic acid accumulation in human colon adenocarcinoma cells. *Cancer Lett.* 116:131–37
53. Lee W, Davis KA, Rettmer RL, Labbe RF. 1988. Ascorbic acid status: biochemical and clinical considerations. *Am. J. Clin. Nutr.* 48:286–90

54. Liang WJ, Johnson D, Jarvis SM. 2001. Vitamin C transport systems of mammalian cells. *Mol. Membr. Biol.* 18:87–95
55. Liang WJ, Johnson D, Ma LS, Jarvis SM, Wei-Jun L. 2002. Regulation of the human vitamin C transporters expressed in COS-1 cells by protein kinase C. *Am. J. Physiol.* 283:C1696–704
56. Louw JA, Werbeck A, Louw ME, Kotze TJ, Cooper R, Labadarios D.1992. Blood vitamin concentrations during the acute-phase response. *Crit. Care Med.* 20:934–41
57. MacDonald L, Thumser AE, Sharp P. 2002. Decreased expression of the vitamin C transporter SVCT1 by ascorbic acid in a human intestinal epithelial cell line. *Br. J. Nutr.* 87:97–100
58. MacLeod RJ, Lembessis P, Hamilton JR. 1992. Differences in Ca^{2+}-mediation of hypotonic and Na^{+}-nutrient regulatory volume decrease in suspensions of jejunal enterocytes. *J. Membr. Biol.* 130:23–31
59. Malo C, Wilson JX. 2000. Glucose modulates vitamin C transport in adult human small intestinal brush border membrane vesicles. *J. Nutr.* 130:63–69
60. Malo C, Wilson JX. 2001. Transport of ascorbic acid and dehydroascorbic acid in rat kidney cortex. *FASEB J.* 15:A838
61. Maulen NP, Henriquez EA, Kempe S, Carcamo JG, Smid-Kotsas A, et al. 2003. Upregulation and polarized expression of the sodium-ascorbic acid transporter SVCT1 in post-confluent differentiated CaCo-2 cells. *J. Biol. Chem.* 278:9035–41
62. Mehlhorn RJ. 1991. Ascorbate- and dehydroascorbic acid–mediated reduction of free radicals in the human erythrocyte. *J. Biol. Chem.* 266:2724–31
63. Mendiratta S, Qu ZC, May JM. 1998. Erythrocyte ascorbate recycling: antioxidant effects in blood. *Free Radic. Biol. Med.* 24:789–97
64. Michels AJ, Joisher N, Hagen TM. 2003. Age-related decline of sodium-dependent ascorbic acid transport in isolated rat hepatocytes. *Arch. Biochem. Biophys.* 410: 112–20
65. Ng LL, Ngkeekwong FC, Quinn PA, Davies JE. 1998. Uptake mechanisms for ascorbate and dehydroascorbate in lymphoblasts from diabetic nephropathy and hypertensive patients. *Diabetologia* 41:435–42
66. Obrosova IG, Fathallah L, Liu E, Nourooz-Zadeh J. 2003. Early oxidative stress in the diabetic kidney: effect of DL-alpha-lipoic acid. *Free Radic. Biol. Med.* 34:186–95
67. Obrosova IG, Fathallah L, Stevens MJ. 2001. Taurine counteracts oxidative stress and nerve growth factor deficit in early experimental diabetic neuropathy. *Exp. Neurol.* 172:211–19
68. Oreopoulos DG, Lindeman RD, VanderJagt DJ, Tzamaloukas AH, Bhagavan HN, Garry PJ. 1993. Renal excretion of ascorbic acid: effect of age and sex. *J. Am. Coll. Nutr.* 12:537–42
69. Padayatty SJ, Katz A, Wang Y, Eck P, Kwon O, et al. 2003. Vitamin C as an antioxidant: evaluation of its role in disease prevention. *J. Am. Coll. Nutr.* 22:18–35
70. Padayatty SJ, Sun H, Wang Y, Riordan HD, Hewitt SM, et al. 2004. Vitamin C pharmacokinetics: implications for oral and intravenous use. *Ann. Intern. Med.* 140:533–37
71. Pandipati S, Driscoll JE, Franceschi RT. 1998. Glucocorticoid stimulation of Na^{+}-dependent ascorbic acid transport in osteoblast-like cells. *J. Cell. Physiol.* 176: 85–91
72. Qutob S, Dixon SJ, Wilson JX. 1998. Insulin stimulates vitamin C recycling and ascorbate accumulation in osteoblastic cells. *Endocrinology* 139:51–56
73. Rajan DP, Huang W, Dutta B, Devoe LD, Leibach FH, et al. 1999. Human placental sodium-dependent vitamin C transporter (SVCT2): molecular cloning and transport function. *Biochem. Biophys. Res. Commun.* 262:762–68

74. Rebec GV, Pierce RC. 1994. A vitamin as neuromodulator: Ascorbate release into the extracellular fluid of the brain regulates dopaminergic and glutamatergic transmission. *Prog. Neurobiol.* 43:537–65
75. Rebec GV, Wang Z. 2001. Behavioral activation in rats requires endogenous ascorbate release in striatum. *J. Neurosci.* 21:668–75
76. Rose RC. 1987. Solubility properties of reduced and oxidized ascorbate as determinants of membrane permeation. *Biochim. Biophys. Acta* 924:254–56
77. Rumsey SC, Daruwala R, Al-Hasani H, Zarnowski MJ, Simpson IA, Levine M. 2000. Dehydroascorbic acid transport by GLUT4 in *Xenopus* oocytes and isolated rat adipocytes. *J. Biol. Chem.* 275:28246–53
78. Rumsey SC, Kwon O, Xu GW, Burant CF, Simpson I, Levine M. 1997. Glucose transporter isoforms GLUT1 and GLUT3 transport dehydroascorbic acid. *J. Biol. Chem.* 272:18982–89
79. Sabry JH, Fisher KH, Dodds ML.1958. Human utilization of dehydroascorbic acid. *J. Nutr.* 64:457–64
80. Schorah CJ. 1992. The transport of vitamin C and effects of disease. *Proc. Nutr. Soc.* 51:189–98
81. Schorah CJ, Downing C, Piripitsi A, Gallivan L, Al-Hazaa AH, et al. 1996. Total vitamin C, ascorbic acid, and dehydroascorbic acid concentrations in plasma of critically ill patients. *Am. J. Clin. Nutr.* 63:760–65
82. Seno T, Inoue N, Matsui K, Ejiri J, Hirata KI, et al. 2004. Functional expression of sodium-dependent vitamin C transporter 2 in human endothelial cells. *J. Vasc. Res.* 41:345–51
83. Siushansian R, Dixon SJ, Wilson JX. 1996. Osmotic swelling stimulates ascorbate efflux from cerebral astrocytes. *J. Neurochem.* 66:1227–33
84. Siushansian R, Tao L, Dixon SJ, Wilson JX. 1997. Cerebral astrocytes transport ascorbic acid and dehydroascorbic acid through distinct mechanisms regulated by cyclic AMP. *J. Neurochem.* 68:2378–85
85. Socci RR, Delamere NA. 1988. Characteristics of ascorbate transport in the rabbit iris-ciliary body. *Exp. Eye Res.* 46:853–61
86. Song J, Kwon O, Chen S, Daruwala R, Eck P, et al. 2002. Flavonoid inhibition of sodium-dependent vitamin C transporter 1 (SVCT1) and glucose transporter isoform 2 (GLUT2), intestinal transporters for vitamin C and glucose. *J. Biol. Chem.* 277:2252–60
87. Song JH, Shin SH, Ross GM. 2001. Oxidative stress induced by ascorbate causes neuronal damage in an in vitro system. *Brain Res.* 895:66–72
88. Sotiriou S, Gispert S, Cheng J, Wang Y, Chen A, et al. 2002. Ascorbic-acid transporter Slc23a1 is essential for vitamin C transport into the brain and for perinatal survival. *Nat. Med.* 8:514–17
89. Subramanian VS, Marchant JS, Boulware MJ, Said HM. 2004. A carboxy-terminal region dictates the apical plasma membrane targeting of the human sodium-dependent vitamin C transporter-1 in polarized epithelia. *J. Biol. Chem.* 279: 27719–28
90. Takanaga H, Mackenzie B, Hediger MA. 2004. Sodium-dependent ascorbic acid transporter family SLC23. *Pflugers Arch.* 447:677–82
91. Toggenburger G, Hausermann M, Mutsch B, Genoni G, Kessler M, et al. 1981. Na^+-dependent, potential-sensitive L-ascorbate transport across brush border membrane vesicles from kidney cortex. *Biochim. Biophys. Acta* 646:433–43
92. Tsukaguchi H, Tokui T, Mackenzie B, Berger UV, Chen XZ, et al. 1999. A family of mammalian Na^+-dependent L-ascorbic acid transporters. *Nature* 399:70–75
93. Upston JM, Karjalainen A, Bygrave FL, Stocker R. 1999. Efflux of hepatic

ascorbate: a potential contributor to the maintenance of plasma vitamin C. *Biochem. J.* 342:49–56

94. Vera JC, Rivas CI, Zhang RH, Golde DW. 1998. Colony-stimulating factors signal for increased transport of vitamin C in human host defense cells. *Blood* 91:2536–46
95. von Zastrow M, Tritton TR, Castle JD. 1986. Exocrine secretion granules contain peptide amidation activity. *Proc. Natl. Acad. Sci. USA* 83:3297–301
96. Wang H, Dutta B, Huang W, Devoe LD, Leibach FH, et al. 1999. Human Na^+-dependent vitamin C transporter 1 (hSVCT1): primary structure, functional characteristics and evidence for a non-functional splice variant. *Biochim. Biophys. Acta* 1461:1–9
97. Wang Y, Mackenzie B, Tsukaguchi H, Weremowicz S, Morton CC, Hediger MA. 2000. Human vitamin C (L-ascorbic acid) transporter SVCT1. *Biochem. Biophys. Res. Commun.* 267:488–94
98. Wilson JX. 1989. Ascorbic acid uptake by a high-affinity sodium-dependent mechanism in cultured rat astrocytes. *J. Neurochem.* 53:1064–71
99. Wilson JX, Dixon SJ. 1989. High-affinity sodium-dependent uptake of ascorbic acid by rat osteoblasts. *J. Membr. Biol.* 111:83–91
100. Wilson JX, Dixon SJ. 1995. Ascorbate concentration in osteoblastic cells is elevated by transforming growth factor-β. *Am. J. Physiol.* 268:E565–71
101. Wilson JX, Dixon SJ, Yu J, Nees S, Tyml K. 1996. Ascorbate uptake by microvascular endothelial cells of rat skeletal muscle. *Microcirculation* 3:211–21
102. Wilson JX, Jaworski EM, Dixon SJ. 1991. Evidence for electrogenic sodium-dependent ascorbate transport in rat astroglia. *Neurochem. Res.* 16:73–78
103. Wilson JX, Jaworski EM, Kulaga A, Dixon SJ. 1990. Substrate regulation of ascorbate transport activity in astrocytes. *Neurochem. Res.* 15:1037–43
104. Wilson JX, Peters C, Sitar SM, Daoust P, Gelb AW. 2000. Glutamate stimulates ascorbate transport by astrocytes. *Brain Res.* 858:61–66
105. Wu X, Itoh N, Taniguchi T, Hirano J, Nakanishi T, Tanaka K. 2004. Stimulation of differentiation in sodium-dependent vitamin C transporter 2 overexpressing MC3T3-E1 osteoblasts. *Biochem. Biophys. Res. Commun.* 317:1159–64
106. Yusa T. 2001. Increased extracellular ascorbate release reflects glutamate re-uptake during the early stage of reperfusion after forebrain ischemia in rats. *Brain Res.* 897:104–13
107. Zreik TG, Kodaman PH, Jones EE, Olive DL, Behrman H. 1999. Identification and characterization of an ascorbic acid transporter in human granulosa-lutein cells. *Mol. Hum. Reprod.* 5:299–302

Annu. Rev. Nutr. 2005. 25:127–49
doi: 10.1146/annurev.nutr.25.050304.092713

THE VITAMIN K–DEPENDENT CARBOXYLASE

Kathleen L. Berkner
Department of Molecular Cardiology, Cleveland Clinic Lerner College of Medicine at Case Western Reserve University, Lerner Research Institute, Cleveland, Ohio 44195; email: berknek@ccf.org

Key Words VKOR, vitamin K–dependent protein, hemostasis, carboxylation, vitamin K oxidoreductase

■ **Abstract** The vitamin K–dependent (VKD) carboxylase uses the oxygenation of vitamin K to convert glutamyl residues (Glus) to carboxylated Glus (Glas) in VKD proteins, rendering them active in a broad range of physiologies that include hemostasis, apoptosis, bone development, arterial calcification, signal transduction, and growth control. The carboxylase has a high-affinity site that selectively binds VKD proteins, usually through their propeptide, and also has a second low-affinity site of VKD protein interaction. Propeptide binding increases carboxylase affinity for the Glu substrate, and the coordinated binding of the VKD propeptide and Glu substrate increases carboxylase affinity for vitamin K and activity, possibly through a mechanism of substrate-assisted catalysis. Tethering of VKD proteins to the carboxylase allows clusters of Glus to be modified to Glas by a processive mechanism that becomes disrupted during warfarin therapy. Warfarin inhibits a vitamin K oxidoreductase that generates the reduced vitamin K cofactor required for continuous carboxylation and causes decreased carboxylase catalysis and increased dissociation of partially carboxylated, inactive VKD proteins. The availability of reduced vitamin K may also control carboxylation in r-VKD protein-expressing cells, where the amounts of reduced vitamin K are sufficient for full carboxylation of low, but not high, expression levels of VKD proteins, and where carboxylation is not improved by overexpression of r-carboxylase. This review discusses these recent advances in understanding the mechanism of carboxylation. Also covered is the identification of functional carboxylase residues, a brief description of the role of VKD proteins in mammalian and lower organisms, and the potential impact of quality control components on carboxylation, which occurs in the endoplasmic reticulum during the secretion of VKD proteins.

CONTENTS

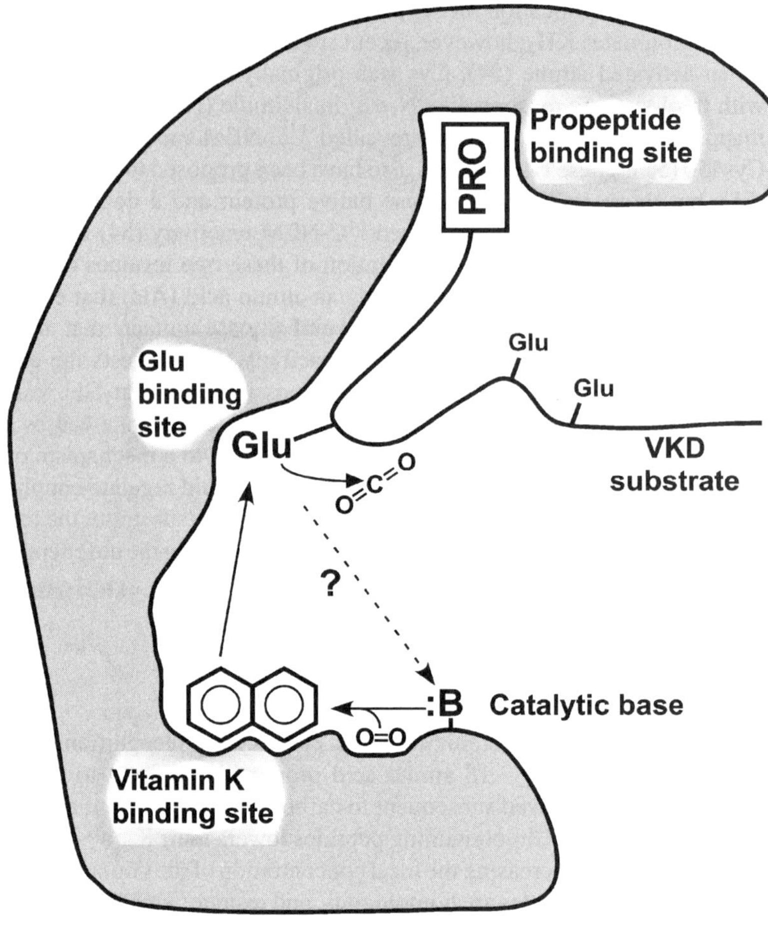

Figure 2 The carboxylase active site. The carboxylase binds vitamin K–dependent (VKD) proteins through their propeptide (PRO), a high-affinity domain in most VKD proteins that is cleaved after carboxylation. Propeptide binding increases the affinity of the carboxylase for the Glu substrate, and propeptide and Glu binding together increase the affinity of carboxylase for the vitamin K cofactor. Osteocalcin is unusual among VKD proteins in having a low-affinity propeptide and high-affinity sequence in the mature protein that binds a different site in the carboxylase (which is undefined and not indicated here). Carboxylation is initiated when the catalytic base deprotonates reduced vitamin K (described in Figure 1), and the Glu substrate may regulate carboxylation by activating the catalytic base, i.e., to increase its reactivity, as indicated by the dashed arrow. The Glu and vitamin K binding sites and catalytic base are drawn as spatially distinct entities for the purpose of illustration and almost certainly exist in a tightly coordinated complex during catalysis. Multiple Glus in the Gla domain of VKD substrates are carboxylated, which is accomplished by a processive mechanism.

by mutagenesis experiments (21). Nonetheless, the propeptides show substantial differences in carboxylase affinity when tested for their ability to compete with a truncated factor IX substrate that contains the propeptide and Gla domain (66). The osteocalcin propeptide shows the lowest affinity ($K_i > 500\ \mu M$), consistent with the divergence of two of the three highly conserved propeptide residues (at positions –10 and –6). However, even VKD propeptides that have all three of the conserved residues show up to a 100-fold difference in carboxylase affinity, with the factor X propeptide showing the highest and prothrombin and protein C propeptides the lowest affinities [K_i's of 3 nM or ~200 nM, respectively (66)]. Thus, other propeptide residues are also important to VKD protein-carboxylase interaction, and residues -18, -17, -15, and -9 have been functionally implicated (21).

Interestingly, the carboxylase has high affinity for mature osteocalcin, i.e., osteocalcin that does not contain the propeptide. Thus, the K_m for mature osteocalcin (~2 μM) is ~100- to 1000-fold lower than small Glu-containing peptides lacking the propeptide domain (26) and at least 70-fold lower than the factor IX Gla domain (68). Competition experiments indicate that mature osteocalcin does not bind the carboxylase through its propeptide binding site (26) nor is the high affinity simply due to osteocalcin Glu residue interaction with the carboxylase Glu binding site (27). Thus, the carboxylase has at least two sites for mediating high-affinity binding of VKD proteins: the propeptide binding site (Figure 2) that confers tight interaction with most of the VKD proteins and a second site that has not yet been identified that mediates high-affinity binding to mature osteocalcin.

Substrate binding causes allosteric changes that regulate carboxylation. Thus, free propeptide stimulates carboxylase activity on noncovalently attached Glu-containing substrates through a decrease in their K_m (14, 28). In addition, substrates in which the propeptide and Glu-containing sequences are covalently attached increase the affinity of the carboxylase for the vitamin K cofactor (63). Covalent attachment introduces a conformational constraint because the carboxylase Glu- and propeptide-binding sites are physically linked by the substrate (Figure 2), and this linkage may cause a structural change in the carboxylase that increases vitamin K binding. Alternatively, covalent attachment may generate a specific VKD structure that activates the carboxylase at a site distinct from Glu or propeptide binding, leading to increased vitamin K affinity. Regardless of the mechanism, the consequence of VKD protein binding regulating vitamin K affinity is increased efficiency of vitamin K utilization, which is important because the availability of vitamin K appears to control carboxylation in vivo (discussed below). Mutations in the carboxylase that decrease its affinity for the Glu or propeptide domain of VKD proteins might then be predicted to affect vitamin K binding, which is in fact the case: Patients with such mutations (described in more detail below) show at least partial correction for carboxylase function when administered supraphysiological doses of vitamin K (11, 64).

The vitamin K cofactor required by the carboxylase is the reduced form, KH_2 (Figure 1), which is generated largely by recycling of the vitamin K epoxide product (KO, Figure 1*C*). Recycling is accomplished by the combined actions of VKOR

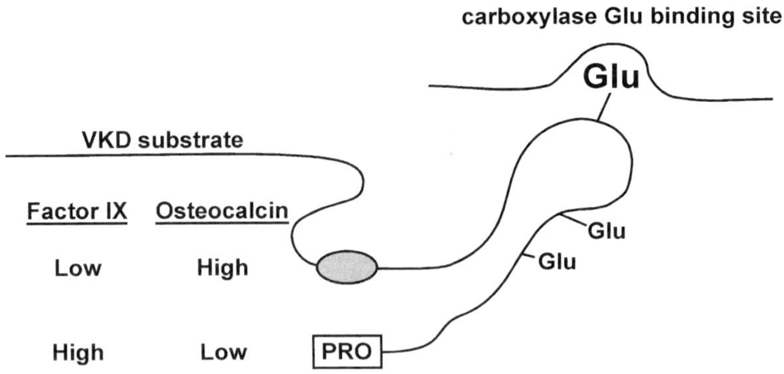

Figure 4 Two sites of vitamin K–dependent (VKD) protein-carboxylase interaction. Most VKD proteins (e.g., factor IX) have a high-affinity propeptide (PRO) and a second sequence (the shaded oval) of unknown identity that mediates low-affinity binding to the carboxylase. Osteocalcin has a low-affinity propeptide and a high-affinity domain of unknown identity. Whether the high-affinity osteocalcin and low-affinity factor IX sequences bind the same carboxylase site is also unknown. Two sites of VKD protein-carboxylase interaction can facilitate efficient carboxylation by juxtaposing the Gla domain near the carboxylase active site and can explain why carboxylation is restricted to the Gla domain.

i.e., the propeptide binding site, varies widely for different VKD proteins. However, the second site of VKD protein-carboxylase interaction could significantly impact the overall affinity, especially if there are differences in affinity at this second site.

Both partially carboxylated intermediates and fully carboxylated VKD product have the propeptide that mediates carboxylase interaction, raising the question of whether there is some change at the end of the reaction that effects preferential release of the fully carboxylated product. One change that marks when carboxylation is finished is the loss of Glu binding, and propeptide binding has been shown to be weaker in the absence of Glu substrate (47), which indicates that the effect of propeptide on Glu binding (discussed above) is reciprocated. However, loss of Glu binding is probably not the only factor that facilitates release because carboxylase isolated from r-carboxylase, factor IX–expressing cells remains associated with fully carboxylated factor IX (23), which indicates a dissociation rate far too slow to reconcile with normal in vivo turnover. This study also suggested that r-carboxylase overexpression titrates out a factor (e.g., excess VKD protein or a quality control component) that facilitates carboxylated VKD protein release.

DISRUPTION OF PROCESSIVITY

Carboxylase processivity is disrupted when vitamin K is limiting, for example during therapy with warfarin, which inhibits VKOR to cause a decreased rate of catalysis and premature dissociation of partially carboxylated VKD proteins

(Figure 3). The importance of the relative rates of catalysis versus dissociation to processivity was dramatically revealed by the phenotype of hemophiliacs who show an unusual sensitivity to warfarin (15, 45, 65). These patients exhibited normal hemostasis until they underwent warfarin therapy, which caused a selective decrease in factor IX activity, i.e., to ~1% of normal levels, which was well below the activities of other hemostatic VKD proteins (~30%–40%). Sequence analysis identified two independent mutations in the factor IX propeptide at either position –9 or at the highly conserved –10 position, and functional analysis showed substantial decreases in the affinity of these factor IX mutants for the carboxylase (15, 65). The weakened affinity of the mutant propeptides, then, caused an increased rate of dissociation that only became significant when the rate of catalysis was slowed by warfarin treatment.

Interestingly, the carboxylase affinity of the factor IX propeptide with the mutation at the –9 position is almost identical to that of the propeptides for protein C and prothrombin (66), yet neither of these VKD proteins shows a selective decrease in activity during warfarin anticoagulation (11, 38, 64). Thus, protein C and prothrombin, like factor X, are reduced to the 30%–40% activity level despite the fact that the carboxylase affinity for the factor X propeptide is about 100-fold higher than for that of the protein C and prothrombin propeptides (66). If the propeptide alone determines the rate of dissociation of VKD proteins from the carboxylase, then protein C and prothrombin would be predicted to behave like the factor IX mutant, i.e., showing a selectively larger decrease during warfarin therapy. The similarity in response of prothrombin, protein C, and factor X to warfarin therefore suggests that while there may be differences in carboxylase interaction and processivity among individual VKD proteins, they may not be as vast as suggested by the differences in propeptide affinities. Modulation of carboxylase interaction and processivity could be due to intrinsic effects, e.g., from the second site of VKD protein-carboxylase interaction, or extrinsic effects, i.e., from quality control components (discussed below).

The factor IX propeptide mutants were well carboxylated when vitamin K was available (i.e., in the absence of warfarin), which indicates that normally the rate of catalysis is so much faster than dissociation that processive carboxylation is not disrupted even by weakened affinity. This observation is of interest with respect to a separate study that analyzed a prothrombin mutant in which the Gla domain was deleted and the propeptide was fused to an unrelated Glu-rich portion of the molecule (22). Expression of this mutant in cultured cells produced a secreted protein that was multiply carboxylated. Thus, so long as vitamin K in the cultured cells supports a high rate of catalysis, propeptide tethering confers a rate of dissociation sufficiently slow to result in multiple carboxylations, even of an irrelevant sequence that may not have a second site of VKD protein-carboxylase interaction. It would be of interest to see whether the mutant prothrombin shows decreased processivity compared with normal prothrombin when tested at low vitamin K concentrations, where low rates of catalysis can reveal differences in the efficiency of carboxylation.

QUALITY CONTROL AND CARBOXYLATION

A full understanding of VKD protein carboxylation must consider how the secretory process affects carboxylation. One example is whether VKD proteins compete for carboxylase binding: Thus, multiple VKD proteins are expressed in some tissues [e.g., osteocalcin, Gas 6, protein S and matrix Gla protein in bone, and seven hemostatic VKD proteins in liver (7)] and these proteins may not bind equivalently to the carboxylase if there are large differences in affinities. However, as discussed above, the association of VKD proteins and carboxylase almost certainly is mediated by chaperones (Figure 3), and the increase in local concentration of VKD proteins and carboxylase due to the chaperones could override the differences in VKD protein affinities. Cargo receptors also have the potential to influence carboxylation by translocating VKD proteins to a different compartment, the Golgi, where the VKD proteins no longer have the opportunity to bind carboxylase. Consequently, under normal conditions, i.e., when reduced vitamin K is available to confer a high rate of catalysis, there may not be competition between VKD proteins. In contrast, during warfarin therapy the decreased rate of catalysis results in the accumulation of a precursor pool (because carboxylase turnover is slower but VKD protein synthesis still occurs) that disrupts the normal process. Precursor pool buildup may disrupt carboxylation directly, through competition between VKD proteins for the carboxylase, or indirectly, by saturating quality control components necessary for facilitating carboxylation. Studies in warfarin-treated tissue and cultured cells show a higher proportion of factor X than prothrombin complexed to carboxylase (18, 69), but it is unknown whether this result is due to differences in competition between prothrombin and factor X for initial binding to the carboxylase and/or to differences in the dissociation of prothrombin and factor X and/or to differences in quality control regulation. Thus, the multiple mechanisms involved in VKD protein carboxylation complicate interpretation of in vivo studies. Interpretation is even more difficult when the analysis is performed on secreted VKD proteins, e.g., those present in blood or secreted from cultured cells, because of an additional component of quality control: Undercarboxylated and uncarboxylated VKD proteins are preferentially degraded (i.e., versus fully carboxylated protein) by the proteasome pathway (76, 84). Consequently, this filtering can generate a secreted VKD protein subpopulation different from the original carboxylation product population. In summary, then, secreted VKD proteins represent the endpoint of a complex process that must be considered when extrapolating in vitro results to what actually occurs in vivo.

CELL LINES AS MODEL SYSTEMS FOR ANALYZING CARBOXYLATION

Many of the r-VKD proteins have been expressed in mammalian cells, where inefficient carboxylation often occurs. Thus, fully carboxylated VKD proteins are secreted when expression levels are low but uncarboxylated and undercarboxylated forms are observed when the levels are high. Individual VKD proteins do not all respond the same; for example, secreted factor X is a mixture of uncarboxylated and fully carboxylated, but not partially carboxylated, protein, whereas secreted factor IX comprises all of these forms (5, 33). Variation among individual VKD proteins could be due to differences in their affinities for the carboxylase and/or how they are processed by quality control mechanisms (e.g., the efficiency of degradation of undercarboxylated forms by the proteosome pathway may not be the same for all VKD proteins). Overexpression of r-carboxylase does not improve the efficiency of VKD protein carboxylation even though the recombinant carboxylase is functional, i.e., showing an increase in activity proportional to the amount of overexpressed protein (23, 52). Inefficient carboxylation has confounded the functional analysis of r-VKD proteins, and has been a major impediment in producing large amounts of therapeutic VKD proteins for applications like treatment of hemophilia and sepsis.

Intracellular analyses of cell lines that express r-factor IX and either endogenous or r-carboxylase suggest that the reason r-carboxylase does not improve carboxylation efficiency is because it saturates the supply of reduced vitamin K. Thus, r-carboxylase overexpression results in a proportional increase in the number of intracellular factor IX-carboxylase complexes but not in the total rate of factor IX carboxylation (23). Pulse-chase analysis indicates that there is a threshold amount of reduced vitamin K sufficient for rapid catalysis of factor IX-carboxylase complexes in cells expressing endogenous carboxylase but not in cells overexpressing r-carboxylase (23). r-Carboxylase overexpression may saturate VKOR capacity in supplying reduced vitamin K (Figure 3), and studies that test the ability of r-VKOR to improve carboxylation will be of interest.

Although vitamin K availability can explain why r-carboxylase does not improve carboxylation, it cannot explain why high-level VKD protein expression causes the secretion of undercarboxylated protein. Thus, stably transfected clones isolated from the same progenitor cell line that express either high or low levels of an r-VKD protein have the same amount of endogenous carboxylase and reduced vitamin K, and therefore the rate of carboxylation of VKD protein-carboxylase complexes should be the same in both cell lines. The secretion of undercarboxylated protein must therefore be due to an increase in the rate of dissociation rather than a decrease in the rate of catalysis, which indicates that high-level VKD protein expression somehow perturbs the VKD protein-carboxylase complex. High-level expression leads to a large VKD precursor pool (Figure 3) that may perturb the complex by saturating the normal process of carboxylation facilitated by quality control components.

The events resulting from high-level expression are similar to those caused by warfarin, which also results in a large precursor pool (discussed above) and the secretion of undercarboxylated protein [shown for prothrombin (40)]. These similarities raise the question of whether the increased dissociation of partially carboxylated VKD proteins during warfarin therapy is actually due to two different effects: (*a*) a slow catalytic rate that increases the probability of dissociation and (*b*) a large precursor pool that disrupts the complexes through an unknown mechanism. In reconsidering the factor IX mutants that show selective decreases in activity during warfarin therapy (discussed above), then, the preferential dissociation of the mutants may be due not only to a decrease in the rate of catalysis but also to precursor pool buildup that increases dissociation, with the mutants being more susceptible because of their weakened affinity for the carboxylase.

IS CARBOXYLATION EFFICIENCY THE SAME IN ALL TISSUES?

Vitamin K availability and consequent effect on the rate of catalysis impacts the efficiency of processive carboxylation, but whether this efficiency is the same in all tissues is unknown. Vitamin K is a family of forms comprising phylloquinone and menaquinones (Figure 1*B*), which share a common 2-methyl 1,4-naphthoquinone nucleus and differ by the polyisoprenoid at the 3-position (the "R" in Figure 1*A*). The main source of phylloquinone is green, leafy vegetables, whereas menaquinones, in the American diet, are obtained primarily from animal products. Phylloquinone and menaquinones show differences in tissue distribution and in lability (reviewed in 7, 9), which could impact their intracellular concentrations, and the functional contribution of these forms to in vivo carboxylation is not well understood. The quality of the diet therefore has the potential to vary the form and concentration of vitamin K in different tissues, which may impact the efficiency of processive carboxylation. This efficiency has important physiological consequences since full carboxylation is required for activity, as shown by the extensive characterization of hemostatic VKD proteins.

The carboxylation status in the general population has been assessed for only a subset of VKD proteins, i.e., hemostatic VKD proteins and osteocalcin. The hemostatic proteins are well carboxylated, and their main site of synthesis is liver, which is well vascularized to receive dietary vitamin K absorbed from the gut into blood. Whether dietary vitamin K is as equally available to other tissues is unknown. Undercarboxylated osteocalcin is frequently observed in the general population (8), which indicates that incomplete carboxylation occurs in bone where osteocalcin is synthesized. The extent of undercarboxylation is unknown because the analysis is indirect, i.e., on blood samples rather than bone tissue. Osteocalcin undercarboxylation could be due to decreased processivity that results from inefficient vitamin K delivery to bone and a consequent slow rate of catalysis, or could be due to a less processive mechanism because of the unique way osteocalcin interacts with the carboxylase (Figure 4). Evaluating other VKD proteins will clearly be of interest, given the number of additional physiologies also impacted by vitamin K.

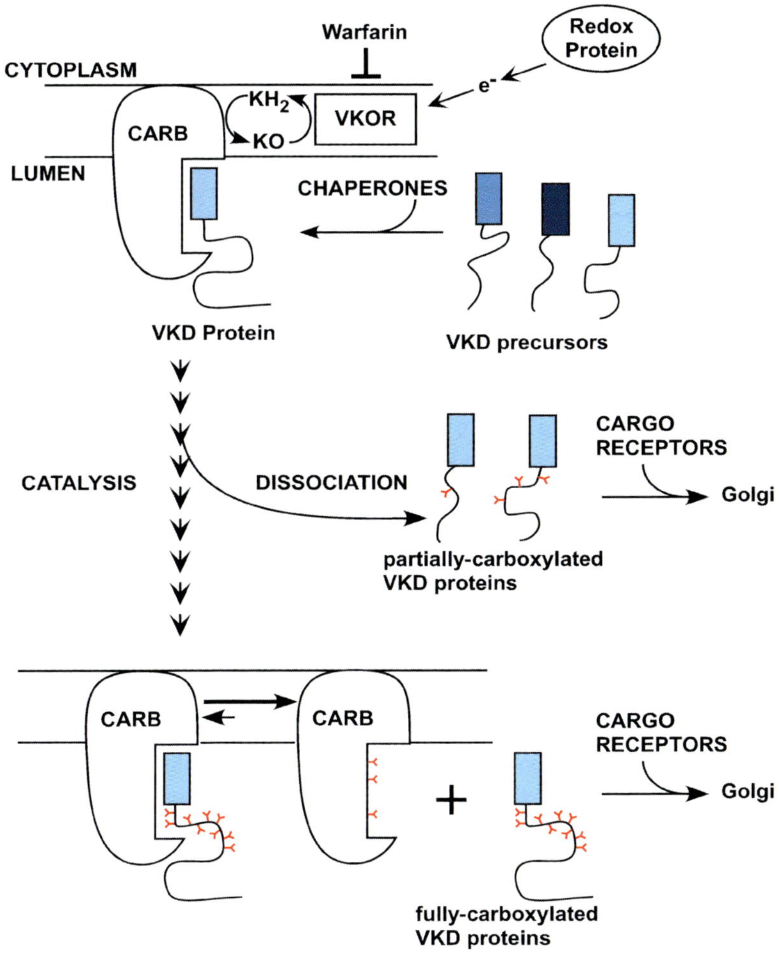

Figure 3 Vitamin K–dependent (VKD) protein carboxylation in the endoplasmic reticulum. VKD proteins contain propeptides with different affinities (indicated by the blue shading) for the carboxylase (CARB), and binding results in the conversion of multiple Glus to Glas (the red "Y's"; a VKD protein undergoing nine modifications is shown as an example). The carboxylase is also carboxylated, subsequent to the carboxylation of the VKD substrate. Each Glu to Gla conversion requires one reduced vitamin K (KH_2), which is recycled from the epoxide (KO) product of carboxylation by a vitamin K oxidoreductase (VKOR) and a redox protein of unknown identity. KH_2 availability supports a high rate of catalysis and low rate of dissociation that results in processive carboxylation, and warfarin disrupts normal carboxylation by blocking the supply of KH_2. Quality control components that affect carboxylation are chaperones, which mediate VKD protein-carboxylase assembly, and cargo receptors, which transport fully and partially carboxylated VKD proteins out of the endoplasmic reticulum. The quality control components specific to carboxylation have not yet been identified.

STRUCTURE-FUNCTION ANALYSIS OF THE CARBOXYLASE

Identifying functional residues in the carboxylase has been difficult because it is an integral membrane enzyme without an available crystal structure or homology to other proteins that might provide clues to function. The general approaches used to identify functional carboxylase residues have included mutagenesis, biochemical mapping, interspecies homology comparison, and analysis of naturally occurring variants. The natural mutations are very rare: Only three have been reported so far, which is not surprising since carboxylation is required for a broad range of functions. The mutations are autosomal recessive and cause a combined defect in VKD hemostatic protein functions (11, 58, 64). The first carboxylase mutant identified, L394R (11), resides within a region (amino acids 374–418) that is evolutionarily highly conserved (2, 3, 16, 35, 78). L394R is impaired in both Glu and propeptide interaction (44), which is likely due to their reciprocal effects on carboxylase binding (discussed above) and which demonstrates the difficulties in designating residues as part of the Glu- or propeptide-binding site. Mutagenesis of neighboring residues revealed a mutant, Y395A, with normal propeptide but defective Glu binding (43), supporting the identification of this region as part of the Glu-binding site (Figure 5, see color insert). L394R and Y395A show small decreases in vitamin K affinity (43), consistent with the observed effect of VKD protein binding on vitamin K affinity discussed above, and high concentrations of vitamin K partially correct hemostasis in the patients with the L394R mutation (11).

A second natural variant, W501S (64), appears to be important to propeptide interaction, as this mutant is associated with decreased propeptide binding but normal carboxylation of a small Glu substrate lacking the propeptide (62). W501 resides within a region (amino acids 495–518) that, interestingly, shares homology with VKD propeptides, and this similarity led to an initial proposal that this region is an autoregulatory domain that restricts carboxylation to propeptide-containing substrates (49). However, mutational analysis of W501S (62), and of mutants substituted at neighboring residues (36), suggests that this region may instead be the propeptide binding site (Figure 5). Like L394R, the W501S mutant shows a decrease in vitamin K affinity (62), and hemostasis can be partially corrected in patients by vitamin K supplementation (64). W501 is located in one of the two regions cross-linked by propeptide in vitro (83, 85; Figure 5) and is near R513, which also has been proposed to have a role in propeptide binding (71). R513 was identified by scanning mutagenesis, which also implicated the charged residue clusters R234/H235 and R406/H408 as important for propeptide interaction.

Other mutants that implicate functionally important residues are R485P, a third naturally occurring variant, which has not yet been characterized (58), K218A, which appears to be completely inactive (61), and C99A and C450A, which show decreases in activity that are propeptide dependent (54). Other relevant regions include the N-terminus (i.e., amino acids 1–218; Figure 5), which has been functionally implicated by covalent modification with a suicide substrate (29), and the site of low-affinity VKD protein-carboxylase interaction (discussed above), which includes residues C343 and Y345 (50) and may also include R359 and H360 (61, 71). Sequences not yet identified include the catalytic base, the high-affinity osteocalcin binding site, and the vitamin K–binding domain.

One additional unknown is the membrane topology of the carboxylase. A key question regarding topology is how the carboxylase active site accesses both hydrophobic vitamin K and hydrophilic VKD proteins (that contain a basic propeptide and acidic Gla domain). The carboxylase sequence predicts seven hydrophobic regions (Figure 5), five of which act as signal anchor sequences in an in vitro assay (74), and the assumption that the hydrophobic regions are transmembrane in nature has led to a model in which the carboxylase resembles a seven-transmembrane receptor (Figure 6*A*, see color insert). However, hydrophobic sequences can also form a different type of structural motif, observed in a new class of integral membrane enzymes whose crystal structures have recently been determined (reviewed in 10). These hydrophobic sequences run parallel to the lipid bilayer and insert into only one leaflet of the membrane (i.e., they are monotopic), thereby forming a tight interface between the membrane and aqueous environment (Figure 6*B*, see color insert). A commonality of these enzymes, which are all structurally unrelated, is that they utilize hydrophobic substrates. Thus, the monotopic domains form an entrance that allows the hydrophobic substrates to move from the phospholipid bilayer into the active site, located in the cytoplasm or ER lumen. With the carboxylase, then, some of the hydrophobic sequences may form an entryway that allows vitamin K in the membrane to access the lumenal active site. At present, it is not possible to extrapolate broad generalities from this new class of enzymes to the carboxylase: Only a handful of crystal structures are known and they reveal significant diversity (e.g., some have both monotopic and transmembrane sequences while others are only monotopic). Their characterization demonstrates the uncertainty in predicting membrane topology; for example, the cytochrome P450 sequence predicts a transmembrane domain (shown in Figure 6*B*) (80) that is not supported by nuclear magnetic resonance analysis (10). The carboxylase must have at least one transmembrane sequence because it has a lumenal active site (13) but no leader sequence (82); however, the complexities described here indicate a need for further studies to define the actual topology. Given this limited understanding, designating residues as lumenal or cytoplasmic simply on the basis of the proposed topological structure (Figure 6*A*), as recently done (37), is premature.

NONMAMMALIAN CARBOXYLASES

The *Conus* carboxylase, like the mammalian ortholog, has epoxidase and carboxylase activities that are dependent upon vitamin K (2, 16). *Conus* VKD substrates have the same organization as that of mammals, i.e., with a propeptide adjacent to the Glus undergoing carboxylation. However, there are differences: Carboxylation and subsequent propeptide cleavage in *Conus* results in small (10–20 amino acid) peptides that are not homologous to the larger mammalian VKD Gla domains (~40 amino acids) and that contain fewer Glas (2–5 in *Conus* versus up to 13 for the mammalian VKD proteins). The mammalian and *Conus* propeptides are not homologous, which likely reflects the fact that while the mammalian propeptide is restricted to carboxylated proteins, the *Conus* propeptide is also present in peptides that are not carboxylated. Thus, the *Conus* propeptide has an additional function unrelated to carboxylation, which is proposed to be directing the proper disulfide bond formation and folding of these highly disulfide-bonded and conformationally constrained peptides (81). In *Conus* peptides that are carboxylated, the propeptide is also a carboxylase recognition signal: The propeptide increases carboxylase affinity for the Glu substrate (1, 12), although the effect is much smaller than observed in the mammalian system (i.e., ~10-fold versus 1000-fold affinity increases). The specific residues in the *Conus* propeptide that mediate carboxylase binding have been difficult to identify. Early studies suggested the importance of hydrophobic residues (12) that were later ruled out, and basic residues have been proposed both to be (25) and to not be (1) important to carboxylase recognition. The *Conus* carboxylase can modify a mammalian propeptide-containing Glu substrate (16): Carboxylation is observed with *Conus* carboxylase isolated from *Spodoptera frugiperda* cells (16) but not from tissue (67), and the difference is probably due to the presence of interfering VKD substrates in the tissue.

Drosophila VKD proteins have not been isolated nor have orthologs been revealed by homology searches with mammalian proteins, and so the role of carboxylation in this organism is unknown. Carboxylase activity that depends on vitamin K has been demonstrated for the *Drosophila* carboxylase on small Glu-containing substrates (35, 78), and this ortholog contains the conserved sequences thought to be part of the Glu binding site (Figure 5) in mammalian carboxylases. Thus, the conversion of Glus to Glas is a likely function for the *Drosophila* carboxylase.

In contrast to *Conus* and *Drosophila*, bacterial orthologs of the carboxylase are divergent in the Glu binding region. As discussed above, these orthologs are thought to have been acquired by horizontal transfer of metazoan sequences, which may not have included transfer of VKD substrates. One intriguing possibility, then, is that the bacterial orthologs have adapted the ability to generate the strong vitamin K base (Figure 1) for some other metabolic use. Determining whether these orthologs even have epoxidase activity, then, will clearly be of interest.

FUTURE PERSPECTIVES

The carboxylase field is in an exciting phase, with recent significant advances having been made toward understanding the mechanism of carboxylation but with multiple areas yet to explore. Important goals include determining how processive carboxylation is accomplished, defining the carboxylase active site, and obtaining structural information. Determining how VKOR supplies reduced vitamin K to the carboxylase and how quality control components affect carboxylation also will be critical to understanding the overall process. Finally, the function of the carboxylase in invertebrates and bacteria should be an interesting area of discovery.

ACKNOWLEDGMENTS

The author thanks Drs. Kurt Runge, Mark Rishavy, and John Suttie for their helpful comments on the review. This work is supported by NIH55666.

The *Annual Review of Nutrition* is online at http://nutr.annualreviews.org

LITERATURE CITED

1. Bandyopadhyay PK, Colledge CJ, Walker CS, Zhou LM, Hillyard DR, Olivera BM. 1998. Conantokin-G precursor and its role in gamma-carboxylation by a vitamin K-dependent carboxylase from a *Conus* snail. *J. Biol. Chem.* 273:5447–50
2. Bandyopadhyay PK, Garrett JE, Shetty RP, Keate T, Walker CS, Olivera BM. 2002. gamma-Glutamyl carboxylation: an extracellular posttranslational modification that antedates the divergence of molluscs, arthropods, and chordates. *Proc. Natl. Acad. Sci. USA* 99:1264–69
3. Begley GS, Furie BC, Czerwiec E, Taylor KL, Furie GL, et al. 2000. A conserved motif within the vitamin K-dependent carboxylase gene is widely distributed across animal phyla. *J. Biol. Chem.* 275:36245–49
4. Benton ME, Price PA, Suttie JW. 1995. Multi-site-specificity of the vitamin K-dependent carboxylase: in vitro carboxylation of des-gamma-carboxylated bone Gla protein and Des-gamma-carboxylated pro bone Gla protein. *Biochemistry* 34:9541–51
5. Berkner KL. 1993. Expression of recombinant vitamin K-dependent proteins in mammalian cells: factors IX and VII. *Methods Enzymol.* 222:450–77
6. Berkner KL, Pudota BN. 1998. Vitamin K-dependent carboxylation of the carboxylase. *Proc. Natl. Acad. Sci. USA* 95:466–71
7. Berkner KL, Runge KW. 2004. The physiology of vitamin K nutriture and vitamin K-dependent protein function in atherosclerosis. *J. Thromb. Haemost.* 2:2118–32
8. Binkley NC, Krueger DC, Engelke JA, Foley AL, Suttie JW. 2000. Vitamin K supplementation reduces serum concentrations of under-γ-carboxylated osteocalcin in healthy young and elderly adults. *Am. J. Clin. Nutr.* 72:1523–28
9. Booth SL, Suttie JW. 1998. Dietary intake and adequacy of vitamin K. *J. Nutr.* 128:785–88
10. Bracey MH, Cravatt BF, Stevens RC. 2004. Structural commonalities among integral membrane enzymes. *FEBS Lett.* 567:159–65
11. Brenner B, Sanchez-Vega B, Wu SM, Lanir N, Stafford DW, Solera J. 1998. A missense mutation in gamma-glutamyl carboxylase gene causes combined deficiency of all vitamin K-dependent blood coagulation factors. *Blood* 92:4554–59
12. Bush KA, Stenflo J, Roth DA, Czerwiec E, Harrist A, et al. 1999. Hydrophobic amino acids define the carboxylation recognition site in the precursor of the gamma-carboxyglutamic-acid-containing conotoxin epsilon-TxIX from the marine cone snail *Conus* textile. *Biochemistry* 38:14660–66
13. Carlisle TL, Suttie JW. 1980. Vitamin K dependent carboxylase: subcellular

location of the carboxylase and enzymes involved in vitamin K metabolism in rat liver. *Biochemistry* 19:1161–67
14. Cheung A, Engelke JA, Sanders C, Suttie JW. 1989. Vitamin K-dependent carboxylase: influence of the "propeptide" region on enzyme activity. *Arch. Biochem. Biophys.* 274:574–81
15. Chu K, Wu SM, Stanley T, Stafford DW, High KA. 1996. A mutation in the propeptide of factor IX leads to warfarin sensitivity by a novel mechanism. *J. Clin. Invest.* 98:1619–25
16. Czerwiec E, Begley GS, Bronstein M, Stenflo J, Taylor K, et al. 2002. Expression and characterization of recombinant vitamin K-dependent gamma-glutamyl carboxylase from an invertebrate, *Conus* textile. *Eur. J. Biochem.* 269:6162–72
17. Dam H. 1935. The antihaemorrhagic vitamin of the chick. Occurrence and chemical nature. *Nature (Lond.)* 135:652–53
18. DeMetz M, Vermeer C, Soute BAM, Van Scharrenburg GJM, Slotboom AJ, Hemker HC. 1981. Partial purification of bovine liver vitamin K-dependent carboxylase by immunospecific adsorption onto antifactor X. *FEBS Lett.* 123:215–18
19. Dowd P, Hershline R, Ham SW, Naganathan S. 1995. Vitamin K and energy transduction: a base strength amplification mechanism. *Science* 269:1684–91
20. Fraser JD, Price PA. 1988. Lung, heart, and kidney express high levels of mRNA for the vitamin K-dependent matrix Gla protein. Implications for the possible functions of matrix Gla protein and for the tissue distribution of the gamma-carboxylase. *J. Biol. Chem.* 263:11033–36
21. Furie B, Bouchard BA, Furie BC. 1999. Vitamin K-dependent biosynthesis of gamma-carboxyglutamic acid. *Blood* 93:1798–808
22. Furie BC, Ratcliffe JV, Tward J, Jorgensen MJ, Blaszkowsky LS, et al. 1997. The gamma-carboxylation recognition site is sufficient to direct vitamin K-dependent carboxylation on an adjacent glutamate-rich region of thrombin in a propeptide-thrombin chimera. *J. Biol. Chem.* 272:28258–62
23. Hallgren KW, Hommema EL, McNally BA, Berkner KL. 2002. Carboxylase overexpression impairs factor IX secretion: implications for the release of vitamin K-dependent proteins. *Biochemistry* 41:15045–55
24. Hammond C, Helenius A. 1995. Quality control in the secretory pathway. *Curr. Opin. Cell. Biol.* 7:523–29
25. Hansson K, Ma X, Eliasson L, Czerwiec E, Furie B, et al. 2004. The first gamma-carboxyglutamic acid-containing contryphan. A selective L-type calcium ion channel blocker isolated from the venom of *Conus marmoreus*. *J. Biol. Chem.* 279:32453–63
26. Houben RJ, Jin D, Stafford DW, Proost P, Ebberink RH, et al. 1999. Osteocalcin binds tightly to the gamma-glutamylcarboxylase at a site distinct from that of the other known vitamin K-dependent proteins. *Biochem. J.* 341:265–69
27. Houben RJ, Rijkers DT, Stanley TB, Acher F, Azerad R, et al. 2002. Characteristics and composition of the vitamin K-dependent gamma-glutamyl carboxylase-binding domain on osteocalcin. *Biochem. J.* 364:323–28
28. Knobloch JE, Suttie JW. 1987. Vitamin K-dependent carboxylase. Control of enzyme activity by the "propeptide" region of factor X. *J. Biol. Chem.* 262:15334–37
29. Kuliopulos A, Nelson NP, Yamada M, Walsh CT, Furie B, et al. 1994. Localization of the affinity peptide-substrate inactivator site on recombinant vitamin K-dependent carboxylase. *J. Biol. Chem.* 269:21364–70
30. Kulman JD, Harris JE, Haldeman BA, Davie EW. 1997. Primary structure and tissue distribution of two novel proline-rich gamma-carboxyglutamic acid

proteins. *Proc. Natl. Acad. Sci. USA* 94:9058–62
31. Kulman JD, Harris JE, Xie L, Davie EW. 2001. Identification of two novel transmembrane gamma–carboxyglutamic acid proteins expressed broadly in fetal and adult tissues. *Proc. Natl. Acad. Sci. USA* 98:1370–75
32. Kuo WL, Stafford DW, Cruces J, Gray J, Solera J. 1995. Chromosomal localization of the gamma-glutamyl carboxylase gene at 2p12. *Genomics* 25:746–48
33. Larson PJ, Camire RM, Wong D, Fasano NC, Monroe DM, et al. 1998. Structure/function analyses of recombinant variants of human factor Xa: Factor Xa incorporation into prothrombinase on the thrombin-activated platelet surface is not mimicked by synthetic phospholipid vesicles. *Biochemistry* 37:5029–38
34. Li T, Chang CY, Jin DY, Lin PJ, Khvorova A, Stafford DW. 2004. Identification of the gene for vitamin K epoxide reductase. *Nature* 427:541–44
35. Li T, Yang CT, Jin D, Stafford DW. 2000. Identification of a *Drosophila* vitamin K-dependent gamma-glutamyl carboxylase. *J. Biol. Chem.* 275:18291–96
36. Lin PJ, Jin DY, Tie JK, Presnell SR, Straight DL, Stafford DW. 2002. The putative vitamin K-dependent gamma-glutamyl carboxylase internal propeptide appears to be the propeptide binding site. *J. Biol. Chem.* 277:28584–91
37. Lin PJ, Straight DL, Stafford DW. 2004. Binding of the factor IX gamma-carboxyglutamic acid domain to the vitamin K-dependent gamma-glutamyl carboxylase active site induces an allosteric effect that may ensure processive carboxylation and regulate the release of carboxylated product. *J. Biol. Chem.* 279:6560–66
38. Lind SE, Callas PW, Golden EA, Joyner KA Jr, Ortel TL. 1997. Plasma levels of factors II, VII and X and their relationship to the international normalized ratio during chronic warfarin therapy. *Blood Coagul. Fibrinolysis* 8:48–53
39. Liu Y, Nelson AN, Lipsky JJ. 1996. Vitamin K-dependent carboxylase: mRNA distribution and effects of vitamin K-deficiency and warfarin treatment. *Biochem. Biophys. Res. Commun.* 224: 549–54
40. Malhotra OP. 1987. Purification and characterization of dicoumarol-induced prothrombins. Evidence of 5-Gla variant with two (or more) polypeptide chains. *Thromb. Res.* 47:485–92
41. Manfioletti G, Brancolini C, Avanzi G, Schneider C. 1993. The protein encoded by a growth arrest-specific gene (gas6) is a new member of the vitamin K-dependent proteins related to protein S, a negative coregulator in the blood coagulation cascade. *Mol. Cell. Biol.* 13:4976–85
42. Morris DP, Stevens RD, Wright DJ, Stafford DW. 1995. Processive post-translational modification. Vitamin K-dependent carboxylation of a peptide substrate. *J. Biol. Chem.* 270:30491–98
43. Mutucumarana VP, Acher F, Straight DL, Jin DY, Stafford DW. 2003. A conserved region of human vitamin K-dependent carboxylase between residues 393 and 404 is important for its interaction with the glutamate substrate. *J. Biol. Chem.* 278:46488–93
44. Mutucumarana VP, Stafford DW, Stanley TB, Jin DY, Solera J, et al. 2000. Expression and characterization of the naturally occurring mutation L394R in human gamma-glutamyl carboxylase. *J. Biol. Chem.* 275:32572–77
45. Oldenburg J, Quenzel EM, Harbrecht U, Fregin A, Kress W, et al. 1997. Missense mutations at ALA-10 in the factor IX propeptide: an insignificant variant in normal life but a decisive cause of bleeding during oral anticoagulant therapy. *Br. J. Haematol.* 98:240–44
46. Pan LC, Price PA. 1985. The propeptide of rat bone gamma-carboxyglutamic acid protein shares homology with other

vitamin K-dependent protein precursors. *Proc. Natl. Acad. Sci. USA* 82:6109–13
47. Presnell SR, Tripathy A, Lentz BR, Jin DY, Stafford DW. 2001. A novel fluorescence assay to study propeptide interaction with gamma-glutamyl carboxylase. *Biochemistry* 40:11723–33
48. Price PA, Fraser JD, Metz VG. 1987. Molecular cloning of matrix Gla protein: implications for substrate recognition by the vitamin K-dependent gamma-carboxylase. *Proc. Natl. Acad. Sci. USA* 84:8335–39
49. Price PA, Williamson MK. 1993. Substrate recognition by the vitamin K-dependent gamma-glutamyl carboxylase: identification of a sequence homology between the carboxylase and the carboxylase recognition site in the substrate. *Protein Sci.* 2:1987–88
50. Pudota BN, Hommema EL, Hallgren KW, McNally BA, Lee S, Berkner KL. 2001. Identification of sequences within the γ-carboxylase that represent a novel contact site with vitamin K-dependent proteins and that are required for activity. *J. Biol. Chem.* 276:46878–86
51. Pudota BN, Miyagi M, Hallgren KW, West KA, Crabb JW, et al. 2000. Identification of the vitamin K-dependent carboxylase active site: Cys-99 and Cys-450 are required for both epoxidation and carboxylation. *Proc. Natl. Acad. Sci. USA* 97:13033–38
52. Rehemtulla A, Roth DA, Wasley LC, Kuliopulos A, Walsh CT, et al. 1993. In vitro and in vivo functional characterization of bovine vitamin K-dependent gamma-carboxylase expressed in Chinese hamster ovary cells. *Proc. Natl. Acad. Sci. USA* 90:4611–15
53. Rezende SM, Simmonds RE, Lane DA. 2003. Coagulation, inflammation, and apoptosis: different roles for protein S and the protein S-C4b binding protein complex. *Blood* 103:1192–201
54. Rishavy MA, Pudota BN, Hallgren KW, Qian W, Yakubenko AV, et al. 2004. A new model for vitamin K-dependent carboxylation: The catalytic base that deprotonates vitamin K hydroquinone is not Cys but an activated amine. *Proc. Natl. Acad. Sci. USA* 101:13732–37
55. Romero EE, Marvi U, Niman ZE, Roth DA. 2003. The vitamin K-dependent gamma-glutamyl carboxylase gene contains a TATA-less promoter with a novel upstream regulatory element. *Blood* 102:1333–39
56. Romero EE, Velazquez-Estades LJ, Deo R, Schapiro B, Roth DA. 1998. Cloning of rat vitamin K-dependent gamma-glutamyl carboxylase and developmentally regulated gene expression in postimplantation embryos. *Exp. Cell Res.* 243: 334–46
57. Rost S, Fregin A, Ivaskevicius V, Conzelmann E, Hortnagel K, et al. 2004. Mutations in VKORC1 cause warfarin resistance and multiple coagulation factor deficiency type 2. *Nature* 427:537–41
58. Rost S, Fregin A, Koch D, Compes M, Muller CR, Oldenburg J. 2004. Compound heterozygous mutations in the gamma-glutamyl carboxylase gene cause combined deficiency of all vitamin K-dependent blood coagulation factors. *Br. J. Haematol.* 126:546–49
59. Roth DA, Rehemtulla A, Kaufman RJ, Walsh CT, Furie B, Furie BC. 1993. Expression of bovine vitamin K-dependent carboxylase activity in baculovirus-infected insect cells. *Proc. Natl. Acad. Sci. USA* 90:8372–76
60. Schultz J. 2004. HTTM, a horizontally transferred transmembrane domain. *Trends Biochem. Sci.* 29:4–7
61. Shimizu A, Sugiura I, Matsushita T, Kojima T, Hirai M, Saito H. 1998. Identification of the five hydrophilic residues (Lys-217, Lys-218, Arg-359, His-360, and Arg-513) essential for the structure and activity of vitamin K-dependent carboxylase. *Biochem. Biophys. Res. Commun.* 251:22–26

62. Soute BA, Jin DY, Spronk HM, Mutucumarana VP, Lin PJ, et al. 2004. Characteristics of recombinant W501S mutated human gamma-glutamyl carboxylase. *J. Thromb. Haemost.* 2:597–604
63. Soute BA, Ulrich MM, Watson AD, Maddison JE, Ebberink RH, Vermeer C. 1992. Congenital deficiency of all vitamin K-dependent blood coagulation factors due to a defective vitamin K-dependent carboxylase in Devon Rex cats. *Thromb. Haemost.* 68:521–25
64. Spronk HM, Farah RA, Buchanan GR, Vermeer C, Soute BA. 2000. Novel mutation in the gamma-glutamyl carboxylase gene resulting in congenital combined deficiency of all vitamin K-dependent blood coagulation factors. *Blood* 96:3650–52
65. Stanley TB, Humphries J, High KA, Stafford DW. 1999. Amino acids responsible for reduced affinities of vitamin K-dependent propeptides for the carboxylase. *Biochemistry* 38:15681–87
66. Stanley TB, Jin DY, Lin PJ, Stafford DW. 1999. The propeptides of the vitamin K-dependent proteins possess different affinities for the vitamin K-dependent carboxylase. *J. Biol. Chem.* 274:16940–44
67. Stanley TB, Stafford DW, Olivera BM, Bandyopadhyay PK. 1997. Identification of a vitamin K-dependent carboxylase in the venom duct of a *Conus* snail. *FEBS Lett.* 407:85–88
68. Stanley TB, Wu SM, Houben RJ, Mutucumarana VP, Stafford DW. 1998. Role of the propeptide and gamma-glutamic acid domain of factor IX for in vitro carboxylation by the vitamin K-dependent carboxylase. *Biochemistry* 37:13262–68
69. Stanton C, Ross P, Hutson S, Wallin R. 1995. Evidence for competition between vitamin K-dependent clotting factors for intracellular processing by the vitamin K-dependent gamma-carboxylase. *Thromb. Res.* 80:63–73
70. Stenina O, Pudota BN, McNally BA, Hommema EL, Berkner KL. 2001. Tethered processivity of the vitamin K-dependent carboxylase: Factor IX is efficiently modified in a mechanism which distinguishes Gla's from Glu's and which accounts for comprehensive carboxylation in vivo. *Biochemistry* 40:10301–9
71. Sugiura I, Furie B, Walsh CT, Furie BC. 1996. Profactor IX propeptide and glutamate substrate binding sites on the vitamin K-dependent carboxylase identified by site-directed mutagenesis. *J. Biol. Chem.* 271:17837–44
72. Sugiura I, Furie B, Walsh CT, Furie BC. 1997. Propeptide and glutamate-containing substrates bound to the vitamin K-dependent carboxylase convert its vitamin K epoxidase function from an inactive to an active state. *Proc. Natl. Acad. Sci. USA* 94:9069–74
73. Suttie JW. 1985. Vitamin K-dependent carboxylase. *Annu. Rev. Biochem.* 54: 459–77
74. Tie J, Wu SM, Jin D, Nicchitta CV, Stafford DW. 2000. A topological study of the human gamma-glutamyl carboxylase. *Blood* 96:973–78
75. Tie JK, Mutucumarana VP, Straight DL, Carrick KL, Pope RM, Stafford DW. 2003. Determination of disulfide bond assignment of human vitamin K-dependent gamma-glutamyl carboxylase by matrix-assisted laser desorption/ionization time-of-flight mass spectrometry. *J. Biol. Chem.* 278:45468–75
76. Tokunaga F, Wakabayashi S, Koide T. 1995. Warfarin causes the degradation of protein C precursor in the endoplasmic reticulum. *Biochemistry* 34:1163–70
77. Venter JC, Remington K, Heidelberg JF, Halpern AL, Rusch D, et al. 2004. Environmental genome shotgun sequencing of the Sargasso Sea. *Science* 304:66–74
78. Walker CS, Shetty RP, Clark KA, Kazuko SG, Letsou A, et al. 2001. On a potential global role for vitamin K-dependent gamma-carboxylation in animal systems: evidence for a gamma-glutamyl

carboxylase in *Drosophila*. *J. Biol. Chem.* 276:7769–74

79. Webb JH, Blom AM, Dahlbäck B. 2002. Vitamin K-dependent protein S localizing complement regulator C4b-binding protein to the surface of apoptotic cells. *J. Immunol.* 169:2580–86
80. Williams PA, Cosme J, Sridhar V, Johnson EF, McRee DE. 2000. Mammalian microsomal cytochrome P450 monooxygenase: structural adaptations for membrane binding and functional diversity. *Mol. Cell* 5:121–31
81. Woodward SR, Cruz LJ, Olivera BM, Hillyard DR. 1990. Constant and hypervariable regions in conotoxin propeptides. *EMBO J.* 9:1015–20
82. Wu SM, Cheung WF, Frazier D, Stafford DW. 1991. Cloning and expression of the cDNA for human gamma-glutamyl carboxylase. *Science* 254:1634–36
83. Wu SM, Mutucumarana VP, Geromanos S, Stafford DW. 1997. The propeptide binding site of the bovine γ-glutamyl carboxylase. *J. Biol. Chem.* 272:11718–22
84. Wu W, Bancroft JD, Suttie JW. 1997. Structural features of the kringle domain determine the intracellular degradation of under-γ-carboxylated prothrombin: studies of chimeric rat/human prothrombin. *Proc. Natl. Acad. Sci. USA* 94:13654–60
85. Yamada M, Kuliopulos A, Nelson NP, Roth DA, Furie B, et al. 1995. Localization of the factor IX propeptide binding site on recombinant vitamin K-dependent carboxylase using benzoylphenylalanine photoaffinity peptide inactivators. *Biochemistry* 34:481–89

Annu. Rev. Nutr. 2005. 25:151–74
doi: 10.1146/annurev.nutr.24.012003.132446

VITAMIN E, OXIDATIVE STRESS, AND INFLAMMATION

U. Singh, S. Devaraj, and I. Jialal
Laboratory for Atherosclerosis and Metabolic Research, University of California Davis Medical Center, Sacramento, California 95817;
email: ishwarlal.jialal@ucdmc.ucdavis.edu, sridevi.devaraj@ucdmc.ucdavis.edu, usingh@ucdavis.edu

Key Words α-tocopherol, oxidation, antioxidant, CRP, atherosclerosis

■ **Abstract** Cardiovascular disease (CVD) is the leading cause of morbidity and mortality in the Western world. Its incidence has also been increasing lately in developing countries. Several lines of evidence support a role for oxidative stress and inflammation in atherogenesis. Oxidation of lipoproteins is a hallmark in atherosclerosis. Oxidized low-density lipoprotein induces inflammation as it induces adhesion and influx of monocytes and influences cytokine release by monocytes. A number of proinflammatory cytokines such as interleukin-1β (IL-1β), IL-6, and tumor necrosis factor-α (TNF-α) modulate monocyte adhesion to endothelium. C-reactive protein (CRP), a prototypic marker of inflammation, is a risk marker for CVD and it could contribute to atherosclerosis. Hence, dietary micronutrients having anti-inflammatory and antioxidant properties may have a potential beneficial effect with regard to cardiovascular disease. Vitamin E is a potent antioxidant with anti-inflammatory properties. Several lines of evidence suggest that among different forms of vitamin E, α-tocopherol (AT) has potential beneficial effects with regard to cardiovascular disease. AT supplementation in human subjects and animal models has been shown to decrease lipid peroxidation, superoxide (O_2^-) production by impairing the assembly of nicotinamide adenine dinucleotide phosphate (reduced form) oxidase as well as by decreasing the expression of scavenger receptors (SR-A and CD36), particularly important in the formation of foam cells. AT therapy, especially at high doses, has been shown to decrease the release of proinflammatory cytokines, the chemokine IL-8 and plasminogen activator inhibitor-1 (PAI-1) levels as well as decrease adhesion of monocytes to endothelium. In addition, AT has been shown to decrease CRP levels, in patients with CVD and in those with risk factors for CVD. The mechanisms that account for nonantioxidant effects of AT include the inhibition of protein kinase C, 5-lipoxygenase, tyrosine–kinase as well as cyclooxygenase-2. Based on its antioxidant and anti-inflammatory activities, AT (at the appropriate dose and form) could have beneficial effects on cardiovascular disease in a high-risk population.

CONTENTS

INTRODUCTION

Atherosclerosis is the leading cause of mortality in the Western world. Oxidative stress and inflammation are important in the pathogenesis of atherogenesis. Epidemiological studies suggest an association between increased antioxidant intake, especially vitamin E, and reduced morbidity and mortality from coronary artery disease. The focus in this review is on α-tocopherol (AT), the major and most bioavailable form of vitamin E.

Oxidative Stress and Atherosclerosis

Clinical and epidemiological studies show that increased levels of low-density lipoprotein (LDL) cholesterol promote premature atherosclerosis. According to the oxidative modification hypothesis, the most plausible and biologically relevant modification of LDL is oxidation (Figure 1). In the early phase, mild oxidation of LDL results in the formation of minimally modified LDL (MM-LDL) in the subendothelial space. MM-LDL stimulates production of monocyte chemotactic protein-1 (MCP-1) that promotes monocyte chemotaxis. These molecular events result in monocyte binding to the endothelium and its subsequent migration into the subendothelial space, where MM-LDL also stimulates production of monocyte colony stimulating factor (M-CSF). M-CSF promotes the differentiation and proliferation of monocytes into macrophages. The initial interest in a role for lipid oxidation in the development of atherosclerotic lesions was in its ability to modify LDL sufficiently to promote its uptake by macrophages. The extensively modified LDL (oxidized LDL, or ox-LDL) is not recognized by the LDL receptor but is taken up avidly by the scavenger receptor pathway in macrophages, leading to appreciable cholesterol ester accumulation and foam cell formation (131).

Ox-LDL has several biological consequences (52, 56, 107, 134); it is proinflammatory, it causes inhibition of endothelial nitric oxide synthase (eNOS), it promotes vasoconstriction and monocyte adhesion, it stimulates cytokines such

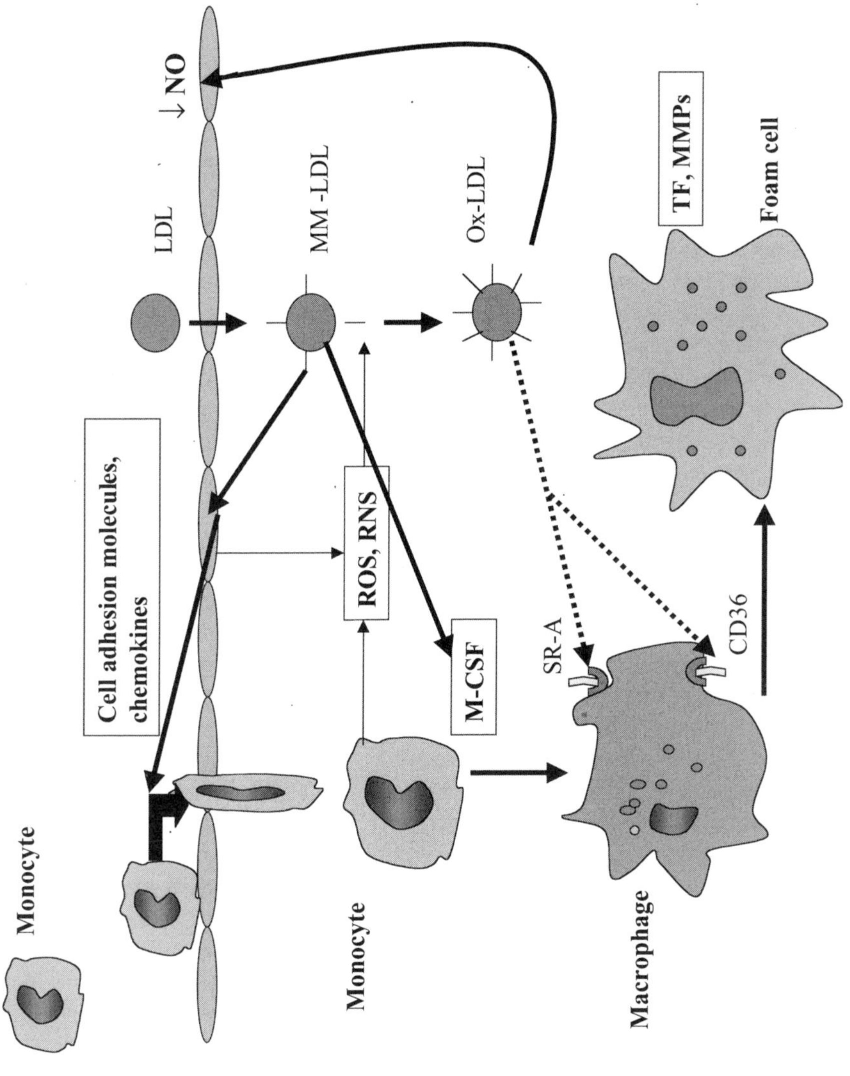

Figure 1 A schema depicting the role of oxidized LDL in atherosclerosis.

as IL-1, and it increases platelet aggregation. Ox-LDL also has been shown to upregulate vascular endothelial growth factor (VEGF) expression in macrophages as well as endothelial cells (ECs) through activation of peroxisome proliferator-activated receptor-γ (PPAR-γ) (44). Ox-LDL-derived products are cytotoxic and can induce apoptosis. Ox-LDL can adversely affect coagulation by stimulating tissue factor (TF) and plasminogen activator inhibitor-1 (PAI-1) synthesis (47). Another atherogenic property of ox-LDL is its immunogenicity and its ability to promote retention of macrophages in the arterial wall by inhibiting macrophage motility (47). Several factors may influence the susceptibility of LDL to oxidation, including its site and composition and the presence of endogenous antioxidant compounds (e.g., AT).

The more direct evidence for the role of oxidative stress in atherosclerosis comes from studies with apoE−/− mice that spontaneously develop atherosclerosis similar to that found in humans. F_2-isoprostanes, prostaglandin-like products of the free radical–catalyzed peroxidation of arachidonic acid and an established biomarker of in vivo lipid peroxidation (18, 84, 92), have been found to localize in foam cells in atherosclerotic lesions of humans as well as of animals and are significantly increased in the tissue, plasma, and urine of apoE knockout mice (38, 88). In addition to serving as biomarkers of in vivo oxidative stress, F_2-isoprostanes, including 8-epiPGF$_{2\alpha}$, exert (patho)physiological effects such as vasoconstriction (92). Both reactive oxygen species [superoxide anion (O_2^-), hydroxyl radical ($OH^\cdot$), and hydrogen peroxide (H_2O_2)] and reactive nitrogen species [nitric oxide (NO) and peroxynitrite ($ONOO^\cdot$)] have been implicated in atherogenesis (107). Although the phagocytic NAD(P)H oxidase is the major source of reactive oxygen species (ROS) in the circulatory system, vascular ECs, smooth muscle cells (SMCs), and fibroblasts also express functional leukocyte-type NAD(P)H oxidases (54). Five major components comprise the endothelial NAD(P)H oxidase: gp91^{phox} (and/or its homologues) and p22^{phox} in the membrane, and p47^{phox}, p67^{phox}, and Rac in the cytosol, and it has been suggested to be the major source of ROS in these cells (107). p47^{phox} in ECs has been shown to play an essential role in activation of NAD(P)H oxidase and in the production of O_2^- (107). Nitric oxide is released from ECs and has many beneficial effects against atherosclerosis through inhibition of platelet aggregation, SMC proliferation, leukocyte recruitment, and stimulation of vasodilation. Excess O_2^- reacts with $NO^\cdot$ to form $ONOO^\cdot$ within the vessel, leading to vascular dysfunction. The decreased bioactivity of NO in the vascular wall provides evidence that the generation of $ONOO^\cdot$ may be involved in the development of atherosclerosis (107). Furthermore, treatment of hypercholesterolemic rabbits with liposomal or polyethylene glycol-conjugated superoxide dismutase, but not with native superoxide dismutase, improves vascular responses (78). This confirms a role for oxidative stress in vascular dysfunction (73).

Inflammation and Atherosclerosis

Much evidence supports a pivotal role for inflammation in all phases of atherosclerosis, from the initiation of the fatty streak to the culmination in acute coronary syndromes (plaque rupture) (68, 93). Various noxious insults, including hypertension, diabetes, smoking, dyslipidemia, and hyperhomocysteinemia, can result in EC dysfunction. Major cellular participants in atherosclerosis include monocytes, macrophages, activated vascular endothelium, T lymphocytes, platelets, and SMCs.

Monocytes and macrophages are critical cells present at all stages of atherogenesis and, when stimulated, can produce biologically active mediators that have a profound influence on the progression of atherosclerosis (Figure 1). Monocytes promote the peroxidation of lipids such as LDL through the generation of ROS. Monocytes and macrophages secrete several proinflammatory, proatherogenic cytokines, such as IL-1β, TNF-α, and IL-6, which have been shown to be present in the atherosclerotic lesions and are known to augment monocyte-endothelial adhesion. IL-1β has been shown to stimulate procoagulant activity, promote cholesterol esterification in macrophages, and stimulate SMC proliferation via platelet-derived growth factor (PDGF). Supportive evidence for the central role played by IL-1 in the development of atherosclerosis has been recently documented by Kirii et al. (60), who demonstrated the decreased severity of atherosclerosis in apoE−/− mice deficient for IL-1β. TNF-α has been shown to promote monocyte adhesion to endothelium and contribute to the necrotic core by promoting apoptosis of macrophages and SMCs (50). Activated macrophages also release matrix metalloproteinases (MMPs) that cause a rent in the endothelium and tissue factor that promotes thrombus formation.

Atherosclerosis is associated with endothelial dysfunction, and these changes induce adhesion and transendothelial migration of monocytes (50). Both IL-1β and TNF-α stimulate expression of adhesion molecules, such as vascular cell adhesion molecule-1 (VCAM-1), intercellular cell adhesion molecule-1 (ICAM-1), and E-selectin. Chemotaxis and entry of monocytes into the subendothelial space is promoted by monocyte chemoattractant protein-1 (MCP-1), interleukin-8 (IL-8), and fractalkine. Several studies have shown a strong association between levels of soluble CAMs (which are shed from activated cells such as ECs) and coronary as well as carotid atherosclerosis (100).

Many stimuli (e.g., angiotensin II and PDGF) are released in response to inflammation, growth, and chemotactic factors from neighboring ECs, monocytes, macrophages, and platelets. These induce SMC migration and subsequent proliferation, thereby resulting in the formation of the fibrous cap (50). The earliest event following plaque fissure is the adhesion and aggregation of platelets leading to thrombus formation. Increased platelet aggregation contributes to acute coronary syndrome such as myocardial infarction. Specific subtypes of T lymphocytes also mediate the inflammatory response of atherosclerosis at every stage. Thus, there is a complex interaction of a wide variety of cells, and their activation leads to release of hydrolytic enzymes, cytokines, chemokines, and growth factors that can result in further injury.

Several large population studies have indicated that biomarkers of inflammation predict an increased risk for CVD (50, 68, 93). The prototypic marker of inflammation is C-reactive protein (CRP), a member of the pentraxin family

(48, 50). Its synthesis in the liver is triggered by various proinflammatory cytokines derived from numerous sources, including monocytes, macrophages, and adipose tissue. The proinflammatory response includes an increased secretion of IL-1β and TNF-α, which then results in the release of the principal messenger cytokine, IL-6 from macrophages. IL-6, after engagement of its receptor on the liver, results in the secretion and release of CRP. Recent evidence points to the role of vascular cells, such as ECs (125) and SMCs (135), in the production of CRP. CRP mRNA and protein have been shown to be expressed in the cells of the lesion in an order of magnitude higher than that observed in plasma (61, 135).

Numerous prospective studies from populations throughout the world have shown that elevated levels of CRP confer a greater risk of CVD (for a recent review, see Reference 50). In addition to being a risk marker, a large body of evidence points to a proatherogenic role of CRP in vascular SMCs, monocyte-macrophages, and ECs. In monocytes, CRP induces the production of inflammatory cytokines and TF expression as well as promotes uptake of ox-LDL. CRP upregulates endothelin-1, PAI-1, and chemokines such as MCP-1 and IL-8, as well as increases expression of CAMs. CRP downregulates synthesis and bioactivity of eNOS (50) and decreases another potent vasodilator and inhibitor of platelet aggregation, prostacyclin (PGI_2) release from aortic ECs via increased ONOO formation, resulting in nitration of PGI_2 synthase, which renders the enzyme inactive (123). In addition to the numerous reported proatherogenic properties of CRP in in vitro studies, there is direct evidence for a proatherosclerotic and prothrombotic effect of CRP in vivo. The exposure to CRP (200 ug/ml) resulted in an increase in SMC migration and proliferation, collagen and elastin content, and AT_1-R expression, as well as an increase in neointimal formation in a rat carotid angioplasty model (128). CRP also has been shown to promote arterial thrombosis following femoral injury in transgenic mice that express the human CRP gene (15). Further, human CRP Tg mice in apoE−/− background also have been shown to have increased CRP levels and a modest increase in aortic atherosclerosis in male mice only (83). Inflammation (as manifested by an increase in CRP) is not only increased in CVD but also in diseases with increased cardiovascular risk, e.g., end-stage renal disease (ESRD) (42), metabolic syndrome (91), and diabetes (87).

Vitamin E

CHEMICAL FORM AND ABSORPTION The term "vitamin E" covers eight different forms of the vitamin that are produced by plants alone and have similar chromanol structures: trimethyl (α-), dimethyl (β- or γ-) and monomethyl (δ-) tocopherol, and the corresponding tocotrienols (T3) (116). T3 have an unsaturated side chain, whereas tocopherols contain a saturated phytyl tail with three chiral centers that naturally occur in the *RRR* configuration (110). Commercially available vitamin E consists of either a mixture of naturally occurring tocopherols and tocotrienols; *RRR*-AT (formerly called *d*-AT); synthetic AT (*all rac*-AT, formerly called *dl*-AT), which consists of the eight possible stereoisomers in equal amounts; or their esters. The ester form prevents the oxidation of vitamin E and prolongs its shelf life. Except for individuals with malabsorption syndromes, these esters are readily hydrolyzed in the gut and are absorbed in the unesterified form (116). The natural vitamin E sources are vegetable oils: Safflower seed oil contains almost exclusively AT (59.3 mg/1 g oil), soy oil is rich in γ-, δ-, and AT (62.4, 20.4, 11.0 mg/1 g of oil, respectively), and palm oil contains T3 (17.2 mg/1 g of oil) in addition to AT (18.3 mg/1 g oil) (79).

The bioavailability of the different forms of vitamin E is highly differential. For example, although the amount of γ-tocopherol in the diet is higher than that of AT, the plasma γ-tocopherol concentration is only 10% of that of AT, which is the most abundant form in plasma (36). Once ingested, all forms of vitamin E are taken up by intestinal cells and released into the circulation in chylomicrons. The vitamins reach the liver via chylomicron remnants. In the liver, a specific protein, α-tocopherol transfer protein (α-TTP), selectively targets RRR-AT for incorporation into very-low-density lipoprotein. Other forms are much less well retained and are excreted via the bile, the urine (as carboxyethyl hydroxychromans), or unknown routes. Relative affinities of tocopherol analogs for α-TTP, calculated from the degree of competition for the α form, are as follows: α-tocopherol, 100%; β-tocopherol, 38%; γ-tocopherol, 9%; δ-tocopherol, 2% (5). The significance of α-TTP and AT is evident from a recent report showing increased basal oxidative stress and inflammatory status in α-TTP-null mice (Ttpa−/−) (97) as well as increased severity of atherosclerotic lesions in these mice in apoE−/− background (113).

In vitro studies demonstrate superior antioxidant properties of AT in the prevention of LDL lipid peroxidation due to its lipid solubility and preferential incorporation into lipoproteins (115). Overall, AT is the principal and most potent lipid-soluble antioxidant in plasma and LDL. AT is present in LDL particle in quantities (5–9 molecules/LDL particle) that can be easily modified by dietary intake or oral supplementation (46). Several lines of evidence support a relationship between low AT levels and the development of atherosclerosis (for a review, see Reference 56). Hence, dietary micronutrients, especially with anti-inflammatory and antioxidant properties (e.g., AT) have potential beneficial effects with regard to cardiovascular disease.

Animal Studies

Animal studies generate useful, and often otherwise unattainable, information on the content of arterial lipids, antioxidants, and lipid oxidation in vivo. Verlangieri & Buxh (127) reported 35% inhibition of atherosclerotic lesion formation in cholesterol-fed macaques with AT supplementation as assessed by carotid Doppler studies over a three-year period. Reduced restenosis after angioplasty in rabbits with established experimental atherosclerosis was seen following AT supplementation (66). Dietary AT led to a hypocholesterolemic and antioxidative response in rabbits (98, 130) as well as to less aortic intimal thickening in chickens

(102). Furthermore, 2000 IU/kg chow of AT supplementation significantly reduced isoprostanes generation and aortic lesion without affecting plasma cholesterol levels in apoE−/− mice. The effect of AT (400 mg/kg atherogenic diet) has been shown not only in reducing aortic lesions in 4- to 10-week-old apoE−/− mice, when fatty streaks are absent or very sparse (86), but also after the establishment of the initial aortic lesion (85), which suggests that this vitamin has a protective effect during the establishment of fatty streaks as well.

Furthermore, in addition to some in vitro studies showing the influence of AT supplementation on the production of MCP-1 (132), there also exists in vivo evidence for the increased expression of MCP-1 in aortic lesions of apoE−/− mice (86). Thus, one of the favorable effects of AT is changing the expression of some important chemotactic molecules such as MCP-1; this suggests the efficacy of vitamin E in reducing fatty streak formation by reducing cell migration to the lesion site (85).

α-Tocopherol Supplementation in Humans

Several groups have also shown that AT supplementation decreases LDL oxidation initiated by copper in vitro (52, 90) or by cells in culture (103). Esterbauer et al. (32) have shown that increasing LDL AT in vitro can prolong the lag phase of oxidation. Human studies have demonstrated that AT supplementation can reduce the susceptibility of LDL to oxidation (21, 53). The minimum dose of AT required to obtain a beneficial effect on LDL was found to be 400 IU/d (21, 32, 51).

In human subjects, AT supplementation (100–600 mg/d for two weeks) has been shown to lower urinary F_2-isoprostanes by 34%–36% in hypercholesterolemic subjects and in diabetic individuals (16, 17). Our group has shown that supplementation of healthy adults with 400 IU/d *RRR*-AT for eight weeks resulted in lower levels of urinary F_2-isoprostanes (70). However, other studies (129) have suggested there is a pro-oxidant effect of vitamin E (400 IU *dl*-AT acetate) in cigarette smokers consuming a high (20%) polyunsaturated fat (PUFA) diet. Although the supplementation of vitamin E prolonged mean LDL oxidation lag time, it paradoxically increased F_2-isoprostanes as well as $PGF_{2\alpha}$. These data suggest that vitamin E may function as a pro-oxidant in cigarette smokers consuming a high-PUFA diet that is far in excess of the normal American diet. In another study carried out by same group (96), the PUFA diet consumption for three weeks increased the mean HDL2 lag time ~1.8-fold with no change in oxidation rate. Supplementation of vitamin E (800 IU/d for three weeks as *dl*-AT acetate) further increased the HDL2 lag time ~1.3-fold and decreased the HDL2 oxidation rate ~1.3-fold. Hence, vitamin E supplementation reduces the oxidation susceptibility of HDL2, which suggests that vitamin E could influence HDL function in vivo (2). The timing of antioxidant intake has been suggested to be a variable factor on postprandial (e.g., a McDonald's Big Mac meal) markers of inflammation and fibrinolysis (12). The measurement of CRP, IL-6, PAI-1, malondialdehyde, and total radical antioxidant parameter four hours before and after the test meal revealed that there was a significant rise in CRP and PAI-1 after the test supper compared with no meal. Either presupper or prebreakfast vitamins E (800 IU *RRR*-AT) and C (1 g ascorbic acid) significantly prevented the meal-induced rise in CRP, although presupper vitamins were more effective. In contrast, only prebreakfast vitamins significantly prevented the meal-induced rise in PAI-1. However, no significant meal-related changes were found in the concentrations of IL-6, malondialdehyde, or total radical antioxidant parameter.

The supplementation of *all-rac* AT (600 IU/d for four weeks) in diabetic patients and smokers decreased oxidative stress (measured as plasma thiobarbituric acid-reacting substances and lag time of oxidation) in both groups; however, supplementation decreased inflammatory status (as reflected by circulating levels of IL-1, TNF, and IL-1 RA in whole blood) in smokers but not in diabetic patients (75). A subsequent study by Heitzer et al. (40) showed that the long-term supplementation of vitamin E (544 IU/d as *dl*-AT acetate for four months) improved endothelium-dependent relaxation in forearm vessels as well as significantly decreased autoantibodies to ox-LDL in hypercholesterolemic smokers but not in patients with either hypercholesterolemia or chronic smoking. These findings suggested that the beneficial effect of vitamin E might be confined to subjects with increased exposure to oxidized LDL. In this regard, Hodis et al. (43) reported that AT supplementation reduces LDL oxidation without affecting atherosclerosis in healthy individuals. Recently, AT supplementation (400 IU/d of *RRR*-AT acetate for six months) in smokers with acute coronary syndrome (characterized by sustained inflammatory upregulation in terms of the release of proinflammatory cytokines and elevated levels of CRP) has been shown to decrease CRP without affecting other inflammatory biomarkers such as IL-6 or sCAMs (81). Importantly, this was the first report showing an association of AT with a reduction in inflammatory markers in patients with acute coronary syndromes. This finding warrants a larger clinical trial assessing the impact of *RRR*-AT on outcome in this patient population with a sustained elevation in inflammatory markers and a high short-term clinical event rate. The anti-inflammatory activity (measured as decrease in CRP) and antioxidant function (in terms of lag time in oxidation of LDL) has also been reported by Upritchard et al. (118) in patients with diabetes after supplementation of *RRR*-AT (800 IU/d for six weeks).

Interestingly, Van Tits et al. (121), in a clinical trial of *RRR*-AT administration (600 IU/d for six weeks) in primary hypertriglyceridemic ($n = 12$) and normolipidemic subjects ($n = 8$), measured the release of cytokines (TNFα, IL-1β) and the chemokine (IL-8) from peripheral blood mononuclear cells before and after intervention. Following AT supplementation, in vitro cytokine production and IL-8 in response to LPS decreased significantly in both groups. Thus, it is suggested that AT may influence the inflammatory response of immune cells infiltrating subendothelial spaces and hence AT's therapeutic implications become relevant in chronic inflammatory processes such as atherogenesis. This study confirms in vitro reports in the literature that AT inhibited PMA-induced IL-1β expression in human monocyte leukemic cell line THP-1 (1).

In another small clinical trial of patients with ESRD undergoing hemodialysis, oxidative stress (plasma concentrations of vitamin E metabolites, F_2 isoprostanes) as well as inflammatory biomarkers (TNF-α, IL-6, and CRP) was assessed in blood samples obtained from a group of patients (n = 11). Assessments were made before and after dialysis at two occasions prior to, and at one and two months of, daily vitamin E supplementation (400 IU *RRR*-AT) (101). AT supplementation significantly increased plasma AT and decreased γ-tocopherol concentrations. Circulating vitamin E metabolites increased up to tenfold in ESRD patients without affecting plasma IL-6, CRP, TNF, and free F_2-isoprostanes concentration. These findings suggest a complex interrelationship between inflammation and oxidative stress that is not mitigated by short-term vitamin E supplementation. In support of this study, Islam et al. (45) also failed to show any significant effect on any of the parameters studied (autoantibodies to ox-LDL, Mo-EC adhesion, sICAM, and VCAM) by supplementation of *all-rac* AT (800 IU/d for 12 weeks), however, results showed significant enrichment with AT in LDL and increased lag phase of oxidation in chronic renal failure patients.

We have tested the effect of *RRR*-AT supplementation on monocyte function and inflammatory markers. Our group (26, 27) has shown that supplementation with 1200 IU/d AT in normal volunteers (n = 21) as well as in type 2 diabetic patients (T2DM) with and without macrovascular disease (n = 25/group) significantly influenced monocyte function by decreasing lipid oxidation (release of O_2^- and H_2O_2), decreasing release of the proatherogenic cytokine IL-1β, and decreasing monocyte-EC adhesion, clearly documenting that supplementation with *RRR*-AT is anti-inflammatory. In a subsequent report, we documented increased IL-6 release from monocytes and increased serum CRP levels in these diabetic patients (25). Both high-sensitivity CRP and monocyte IL-6 were significantly decreased with AT therapy. This finding was confirmed by another group (118). They showed that *RRR*-AT supplementation (800 IU/d, n = 13) in T2DM compared with placebo (n = 12) for a duration of four weeks resulted in a significant decrease in plasma CRP. AT therapy also decreased serum P-selectin and PAI-1 levels in T2DM patients (22). These findings were suggested to be relevant to strategies aimed at reducing risk of CVD in patients with diabetes.

Furthermore, as discussed above, one of the earliest events in atherosclerosis is endothelial dysfunction. Much of the data obtained from animal studies show that AT supplementation (1000 IU/kg diet of *RRR*-AT) preserved endothelium-dependent vasorelaxation in cholesterol-fed rabbits by a mechanism independent of its antioxidant effect (57, 106). Vascular incorporation of AT has been shown to prevent endothelial dysfunction due to oxidized LDL by inhibiting protein kinase C (PKC) stimulation (59). However, in humans, the data on AT and endothelial dysfunction are conflicting. In hypercholesterolemic subjects, *RRR*-AT (1000 IU for four weeks) significantly increased acetylcholine-mediated vasodilation expressed as changes in absolute forearm blood flow, forearm vascular resistance, or forearm blood flow ratios (39). However, Elliott et al. (30) failed to show any improvement in endothelial function after three months of therapy with vitamin E

(800 IU/d of *RRR*-AT). Another study by Simons et al. (99) also failed to show any improvement in endothelial function in older persons receiving vitamin E (1000 IU/d of *RRR*-AT compared with placebo). In patients with chronic spastic angina, treatment with vitamin E (AT acetate as 300 mg/d compared with placebo) significantly restored flow-dependent vasodilation, and this improvement was associated with the decreases in plasma thiobarbituric acid-reacting substances levels and anginal attacks (76). Also, in hypercholesterolemic smokers, Heitzer et al. (40) showed that vitamin E significantly augmented endothelium-dependent relaxation. AT supplementation (1600 IU/d *RRR*-AT) in T2DM patients also has been shown to improve endothelial function (37). In addition, Paolisso et al. (82) have shown in 40 T2DM patients that supplementation with AT (600 mg/d of *all-rac* AT for eight weeks) was associated with a significant improvement in brachial artery reactivity compared with placebo, along with an improvement in oxidative stress indices. Kinlay et al. (59) reported a positive correlation between measurement of plasma AT and preservation of endothelium-dependent vasomotor function in patients with coronary atherosclerosis.

Furthermore, arterial compliance or elasticity is a potential index of arterial function that has been shown to be dependent upon endothelial function (67, 89). Short-term AT supplementation (400 IU/d for four and eight weeks) recently has been reported to improve arterial compliance in middle-aged men and women (77). Beckman et al. (6) recently showed that administration of vitamin C (1000 mg) and vitamin E (800 IU AT) daily compared to placebo for six months significantly increased endothelium-dependent vasodilation in type 1 but not in T2DM subjects. A trial by Engler et al. (31) examined the effect of supplementation of antioxidant vitamins C (500 mg/d) and E (400 IU/d) for six weeks and the National Cholesterol Education Program Step II diet for six months on endothelium-dependent flow-mediated dilation of the brachial artery in 15 children with familial hypercholesterolemia or the phenotype of familial combined hyperlipidemia. Antioxidant vitamin therapy significantly improved flow-mediated dilation of the brachial artery compared with baseline. Furthermore, Ulker et al. (117) recently reported the efficacy of supplementing vitamin E along with C in reversing endothelial dysfunction via regulation of eNOS and nicotinamide adenine dinucleotide phosphate (reduced form) (NADPH) oxidase activities. Recently, an open-label pilot interventional study (95) using 800 IU of vitamin E was undertaken in eight stable outpatients with nondiabetic chronic kidney disease and six healthy controls, with the objective of measuring plasma asymmetrical dimethylarginine levels at baseline and after eight weeks of treatment. After treatment with vitamin E, plasma asymmetrical dimethylarginine significantly decreased in six of eight patients, a finding that implies increased NO availability (95). Thus, although the results from studies on EC dysfunction with AT are equivocal, it appears that the combination of vitamins E and C is more effective in ameliorating EC dysfunction.

In addition, very recently (74) vitamin E (AT acetate 400 mg/d for one month) has been shown to improve fibrinolytic activity (measured as PAI-1 activity) as well as decrease oxidative stress (thioredoxin levels) in patients with coronary spastic angina as compared with baseline levels, whereas placebo had no effect on these variables. PAI activity as well as thioredoxin levels were significantly high in patients with coronary spastic angina as compared with control subjects ($n = 17$) at day 0.

The antioxidant and anti-inflammatory activity of vitamin E was also explored to improve the biocompatibility of materials such as cellulosic membranes for hemodialysis (9). This group of authors enrolled two group of patients on regular hemodialysis [one group had cellulosic dialyzers whereas the other group had vitamin E–modified dialyzers (CLE)] without clinical atherosclerotic cardiovascular disease, and compared plasma levels of autoantibodies for ox-LDL, von Willebrand factor, and thromomodulin as markers of endothelial damage. In the CLE group, ox-LDL-Ab and von Willebrand factor, but not thrombomodulin levels, decreased significantly and vitamin E increased up to two fold, which indicates efficacy of CLE versus cellulosic in lowering the indices of damage to LDL and ECs.

A recent clinical trial by Micheletta et al. (72) enrolled 16 patients who were candidates for carotid endartectomy and 32 age- and sex-matched controls. Patients were randomly allocated to standard treatment with or without AT (*all-rac*-AT as 450 mg/d for six weeks). At the end of treatment, the different variables (plasma levels of 7-beta-hydroxycholesterol, 7-ketocholesterol, cholesterol, and vitamin E) were measured in plasma and plaques. Patients who were given vitamin E supplementation showed a significant increase of plasma vitamin E with concomitant decrease of 7-beta-hydroxycholesterol. However, no treatment effect was observed in oxysterol or vitamin E content of plaques. This study formed the basis for facilitation of vitamin E transport within atherosclerotic plaque representing an important target for treatment of early-stage atherosclerotic progression. However, this study has been contradicted and brought into question in a recently published editorial (62)—based on previously documented reports (108, 119)—that states vitamin E is not deficient in human atherosclerotic plaques.

Finally, a re-evaluation report on the relative potency of synthetic and natural AT based on experimental and clinical observations concluded that both of these are not equivalent in any dosage ratio (7). The relative bioavailability of *all-rac*-AT and *RRR*-AT varies between tissues as well as with dose, time after dosing, and duration of dosing, which suggests that a fixed dosage ratio of *all-rac*- and *RRR*-AT cannot produce a fixed ratio of effects on all processes after all dosages. In this regard, it is important to mention that most of the reported anti-inflammatory effects of AT have been due to *RRR*-AT, probably because of its higher bioavailability and decreased degradation as compared to *all-rac*-AT. In this regard, we have shown that both 400 IU (55) and 800 IU (122) of *all-rac*-AT, containing the eight isomers, failed to have any significant anti-inflammatory effects in normal subjects.

Molecular and Cellular Effects of α-Tocopherol

Advances have been made in understanding the molecular effects of AT beyond that of preventing LDL oxidation. The understanding of various regulatory, nonoxidative responses to AT by crucial cells involved in the pathogenesis of atherosclerosis is very important. Such responses include inhibition of SMC proliferation, preservation of endothelial function, inhibition of monocyte-endothelial adhesion, inhibition of monocyte ROS and cytokine release, and inhibition of platelet adhesion and aggregation (3). These cellular responses to AT are associated with transcriptional and post-transcriptional events. Activation of diacylglycerol (DAG) kinase and protein phosphatase 2A, and the inhibition of PKC, COX, lipoxygenase, tyrosine kinase phosphorylation, and cytokine release by AT are all examples of post-transcriptional regulation.

α-Tocopherol and Endothelial Cells

AT enrichment of monocytes or ECs decreases adhesion of monocytes to human ECs in vitro and depends on the expression of various adhesion molecules (14, 34) that correlated with a decrease in cell-surface expression of E-selectin, ICAM-1, and VCAM-1. Martin et al. (71) further showed that in vitro enrichment of human aortic ECs with AT significantly inhibited LDL-induced adhesion of monocytes to EC in a dose-dependent manner with a concomitant reduction in levels of ICAM. Recently, Fan et al. (33) reported the inhibition of ox-LDL mediated ICAM-1 expression in human umbilical vein ECs by different forms of tocopherols. The mixed tocopherols (α and γ) were more potent than AT or γ-tocopherol alone. The inhibitory effect of tocopherols was not seen on recombinant human CRP-mediated adhesion of monocytes to endothelium.

Data from our laboratory have shown that pretreatment of monocytic cells with AT resulted in a decrease in monocyte-EC adhesion mediated by decreased expression of CD11b and VLA-4, via inhibition of NF-kB activity (for a review, see Reference 56). AT acetate and succinate also have been shown to inhibit TNF-α-induced NF-kB activation in vitro (109). Thus, AT has been shown to have beneficial effects in inhibiting monocyte-endothelial adhesion when incubated with either EC or monocytes; it is very likely that following supplementation it partitions into both monocytes and EC and its ability to reduce monocyte-EC adhesion is greater.

Van Aalst et al. (120) recently reported that AT but not probucol or BHT resulted in preservation of EC migration in the presence of ox-LDL. The lack of effect of other antioxidants suggested that the effect of AT is via nonantioxidant action and is probably the result of membrane stabilizing properties. Exploration of the latter revealed that pretreatment with AT inhibited the increase in membrane fluidity of ECs incubated in the presence of physiologically relevant monocyte/macrophage-oxidized LDL. This action of AT might prove to be of clinical significance for improving the healing of endothelial injury.

In recent pioneering work, Dhanasekaran et al. (29) explored the strategy of supplementation of ECs with mitochondrial targeted antioxidants and reported their better efficacy for inhibition of peroxide-induced mitochondrial iron uptake, oxidative damage, and apoptosis. The mitochondria-targeted drugs mitoquinone and mitovitamin E are a new class of antioxidants containing the triphenylphosphonium cation moiety that facilitates drug accumulation in mitochondria. Pretreatment of bovine aortic ECs with mitoquinone (1 μM) and mitovitamin E (1 μM), but not untargeted antioxidants (e.g., vitamin E), significantly abrogated H_2O_2 and lipid peroxide–induced 2′,7′-dichlorofluorescein fluorescence and protein oxidation.

α-Tocopherol and Platelets

AT inhibits aggregation of platelets both in vitro and in vivo and delays intra-arterial thrombus formation (94). Higashi & Kikuchi (41) were the first to demonstrate the inhibitory effect of AT on platelet aggregation in vitro. Steiner (105) has shown that AT in doses of 200 IU/d decreases platelet adhesion. In hypercholesterolemic subjects, two weeks of supplementation with AT (600 mg/d) reduced elevated plasma concentrations of the platelet-derived adhesion molecule P-selectin by 40% (19). Furthermore, Steiner (104) has shown that at doses of 1200 IU/d, AT produced only a mild inhibition of collagen-induced platelet aggregation, whereas platelet adhesion to collagen was markedly inhibited in its presence. In another study (111), platelet adhesion was significantly reduced in 100 patients with transient ischemic attacks who were given 400 IU/d of AT. A double-blind, randomized, placebo-controlled study was performed on 40 healthy volunteers (20–50 years of age) supplemented daily with vitamin E [*dl*-AT acetate (300 mg/d)], vitamin C (250 mg), or β-carotene (15 mg) for eight weeks (11). Platelet function was significantly decreased by vitamin E as revealed by the decreased platelet aggregation in response to ADP and arachidonic acid, the increased sensitivity to inhibition by prostaglandin E_1 (PGE_1), the decreased plasma α-thromboglobulin concentration, and the decreased ATP secretion. Freedman et al. (35) have shown that supplementation with 400 IU of *RRR*-AT inhibits platelet aggregation through a PKC-dependent mechanism. In another published study, Mabile et al. (69) showed that *RRR*-AT uptake by platelets is optimal at 75 IU/d, and this correlates with the maximal influence on platelet aggregation and platelet responsiveness to inhibition by PGE_1. Increased supplemental levels (200, 400 IU/d) failed to exert greater effects. Thus, the majority of studies support an antiplatelet effect of AT.

α-Tocopherol and Monocytes/Macrophages

It has been shown that AT decreases monocyte $O_2^{\cdot}$ release and monocyte-mediated lipid oxidation (23), and this appears to be via inhibition of PKC. Furthermore, results from an in vitro study (10) revealed that AT inhibits $O_2^{\cdot}$ production by monocytes by impairing the assembly of NADPH oxidase, the enzyme responsible for generating the respiratory burst. AT inhibits $p47^{phox}$ translocation to the membrane and also impairs phosphorylation of $p47^{phox}$. This study also suggests that inhibition of PKC activity is not due directly to the antioxidant capacity of AT but requires AT integration into the cell membrane where it can interact directly with PKC. In addition, data showed that under hyperglycemic conditions, using antisense to PKCα and PKCβ, AT inhibits the increased $O_2^{\cdot}$ released from monocytes via inhibition of p47^{phox} phosphorylation through inhibition of α-isoform of PKC (126).

With regard to cytokine release, we (24) have shown that AT inhibits IL-1 release from activated human monocytes by inhibiting 5-lipoxygenase at post-transcriptional levels. Also, as discussed above, we have shown that AT enrichment of monocytes inhibits subsequent adhesion to human endothelium via inhibition of counterreceptors CD11b and VLA-4 on monocytes and inhibition of the transcription factor NF-kB (56). Furthermore, using siRNA technology, we recently showed that the increased IL-6 release from monocytes under hyperglycemia is mediated via upregulation of both PKCα and PKCβ, through p38 MAPK and NFκB, resulting in increased mRNA and protein for IL-6. We also showed that cells enriched with AT, which inhibits both PKCα and PKCβ, released significantly decreased amounts of IL-6 under hyperglycemia (28). In addition, AT has been demonstrated to downregulate scavenger receptor activity and CD36 receptor expression in human blood–derived macrophages in vitro, whereas γ-tocopherol showed only a weak suppression of scavenger receptor activity, scavenger receptor class A expression, and AP-1 activity (114). Very recently, we reported that inhibition of CD36 expression in human monocyte–derived macrophages is via inhibition of tyrosine kinase phosphorylation (124). An age-associated increase in PGE_2 synthesis and COX-2 activity in murine macrophages has been shown to be reversed by AT treatment (133). There was no effect on COX mRNA and protein levels, which indicates a post-translational regulation of COX by AT.

α-Tocopherol and Smooth Muscle Cells

The antiproliferative effects of AT have been well demonstrated in rat aortic SMC stimulated with PDGF (4, 8, 13), and the effect has not been related to its antioxidant effect (112). These studies collectively suggest that AT inhibits SMC proliferation in vivo and thus retards narrowing of the artery lumen. The role of AT in cellular signaling, especially in relation to PKC, has been delineated by Azzi et al. (5). It has been shown that this effect is not related to antioxidant effects of AT because only *RRR*-AT, and not β-tocopherol, binds to a receptor resulting in activation of AP-1, leading to the dephosphorylation of PKC, even though both have similar antioxidant activity. Thus, *RRR*-AT appears to act as a sensor of the oxidation status of the cell and as a transducer capable of informing cells of the oxidation status. Compelling data suggests that antioxidant activity alone cannot mediate PKC inhibition (56). Direct inhibition of PKC by AT does not appear likely because several studies showed no effect on DAG or on calcium-stimulated PKCα and PKC β-2 activity (63, 65). An indirect mechanism for AT inhibition of PKC seems more likely, and data to support this come from SMCs (4), where PKCβ-2 is activated by hyperglycemia and AT inhibits this effect by decreasing cellular DAG levels through stimulation of DAG kinase activity. In addition, it has been demonstrated that okadaic acid prevents the antiproliferative effect of AT in SMC proliferation, a finding that clearly indicates PKC phosphorylation and/or protein phosphatase activity is involved. Evidence for AT inhibition of SMC proliferation is mostly in vitro, and there are few data available in vivo. De Maio et al. (20) reported that supplementation with AT (1200 IU/d for four months) resulted in a trend to decreased restenosis in coronary artery after angioplasty. The ability of AT to reduce restenosis after angioplasty was further tested in a rabbit model in which angioplasty was performed on established atherosclerotic lesions (66). Ox-LDL stimulated DNA synthesis in rabbit vascular SMCs, and AT was found to inhibit this effect. These findings support the hypothesis that oxidized lipids can stimulate hyperplasia, and AT can limit this effect by inhibiting either oxidation or the proliferative effects of oxidants on cells. Recently, the effect of a mixture of AT phosphate and *dl*-AT PO_4 was shown to inhibit the proliferation of rat aortic SMCs at doses lower than the dose of AT alone (80). The higher potency of the former has been attributed to better uptake of this molecule and its intracellular hydrolysis.

Intervention Studies

Although AT has several beneficial effects on oxidation and on different cells that participate in atherogenesis, the results of randomized clinical trials have been equivocal (see References 49 and 64 for recent reviews).

CONCLUSION

Vitamin E, especially AT, exhibits antioxidant as well as anti-inflammatory activity and inhibits several biological events involved in atherogenesis (as summarized in Table 1). Although the studies carried out with cell culture and animal models suggest that AT has promising antiatherosclerotic effects, the results of its supplementation in humans are somewhat controversial, possibly because of inadequate

TABLE 1 Effect of α-tocopherol on biomarkers of oxidative stress and inflammation/thrombosis in atherosclerosis

Oxidative stress	Inflammation/thrombosis
↓ LDL oxidative susceptibility	↓ hs-CRP
↓ Autoantibodies to ox-LDL	↓ Pro-inflammatory cytokines (IL-1 & 6, TNF)
↓ Urinary isoprostanes	↓ Monocyte adhesion to endothelium
↓ ROS (O_2^-) production in monocytes	↓ Soluble cell adhesion molecules
	↓ PAI-1
	↓ PGE_2 synthesis
	↓ Platelet aggregation

Abbreviations: hs-CRP, high sensitivity C-reactive protein; LDL, low-density lipoprotein; ox-LDL, oxidative low-density lipoprotein; PAI-1, plasminogen activator inhibitor-1; PGE_2, prostaglandin E_2; ROS, reactive oxygen species; TNF, tumor necrosis factor; IL, interleukin.

selection of subjects (by gender, vitamin E status, etc.) or of the dose, timing of intake, and chemical form of tocopherol. Despite some of these limitations, it appears that *RRR*-AT demonstrates a multifaceted effect on vascular homeostasis.

ACKNOWLEDGMENTS

This work was supported by National Institutes of Health Grants NIH K24 AT00596 and RO1 AT00005.

The *Annual Review of Nutrition* is online at http://nutr.annualreviews.org

LITERATURE CITED

1. Akeson AL, Woods CW, Mosher LB, Thomas CE, Jackson RL. 1991. Inhibition of IL-1 beta expression in THP-1 cells by probucol and tocopherol. *Atherosclerosis* 86:261–70
2. Arrol S, Mackness MI, Durrington PN. 2000. Vitamin E supplementation increases the resistance of both LDL and HDL to oxidation and increases cholesteryl ester transfer activity. *Atherosclerosis* 150:129–34
3. Azzi A. 2004. The role of alpha-tocopherol in preventing disease. *Eur. J. Nutr.* 43(Suppl. 1):I18–25
4. Azzi A, Breyer I, Feher M, Ricciarelli R, Stocker A, et al. 2001. Nonantioxidant functions of alpha-tocopherol in smooth muscle cells. *J. Nutr.* 131:378S–81S
5. Azzi A, Ricciarelli R, Zingg JM. 2002. Non-antioxidant molecular functions of alpha-tocopherol (vitamin E). *FEBS Lett.* 519:8–10
6. Beckman JA, Goldfine AB, Gordon MB, Garrett LA, Keaney JF Jr, Creager MA. 2003. Oral antioxidant therapy improves endothelial function in Type 1 but not Type 2 diabetes mellitus. *Am. J. Physiol. Heart Circ. Physiol.* 285:H2392–98
7. Blatt DH, Pryor WA, Mata JE, Rodriguez-Proteau R. 2004. Re-evaluation of the relative potency of synthetic and natural alpha-tocopherol: experimental and clinical observations. *J. Nutr. Biochem.* 15:380–95
8. Boscoboinik D, Szewczyk A, Hensey C, Azzi A. 1991. Inhibition of cell proliferation by α-tocopherol, role of PKC. *J. Biol. Chem.* 266:6188–94
9. Bufano G, Usberti M, Mandolfo S, Malberti F, Piroddi M, Galli F. 2004. Von Willebrand factor and autoantibodies against oxidized LDL in hemodialysis patients treated with vitamin E–modified dialyzers. *Int. J. Artif. Organs* 27:214–21
10. Cachia O, Benna JE, Pedruzzi E, Descomps B, Gougerot-Pocidalo MA, Leger CL. 1998. α-Tocopherol inhibits the respiratory burst in human monocytes: attenuation of p47 (phox) membrane translocation and phosphorylation. *J. Biol. Chem.* 273:32801–5
11. Calzada C, Bruckdorfer K, Rice Evans C. 1997. The influence of antioxidant nutrients on platelet function in healthy volunteers. *Atherosclerosis* 128:97–105
12. Carroll MF, Schade DS. 2003. Timing of antioxidant vitamin ingestion alters postprandial proatherogenic serum markers. *Circulation* 108:24–31
13. Chatelain E, Boscoboinik DO, Bartoli GM, Kagan VE, Gey FK, et al. 1993. Inhibition of smooth muscle cell proliferation and protein kinase C activity by tocopherols and tocotrienols. *Biochim. Biophys. Acta* 1176:83–89
14. Cominacini L, Garbin U, Pasini AF, Davoli A, Campagnola M, et al. 1997. Antioxidants inhibit the expression of

intercellular cell adhesion molecule-1 and vascular cell adhesion molecule-1 induced by oxidized LDL on human umbilical vein endothelial cells. *Free Radic. Biol. Med.* 22:117–27
15. Danenberg HD, Szalai AJ, Swaminathan RV, Peng L, Chen Z, et al. 2003. Increased thrombosis after arterial injury in human C-reactive protein-transgenic mice. *Circulation* 108:512–15
16. Davi G, Alessandrini P, Mezzetti A, Minotti G, Bucciarelli T, et al. 1997. In vivo formation of 8-epi-prostaglandin-F_2 is increased in hypercholesterolemia. *Arterioscler. Thromb. Vasc. Biol.* 17:3230–35
17. Davi G, Ciabattoni G, Consoli A, Mezzetti A, Falco A, et al. 1999. In vivo formation of 8-epi-PGF_2- and platelet activation in diabetes mellitus: effect of improved metabolic control and vitamin E supplementation. *Circulation* 99:224–29
18. Davi G, Falco A, Patrono C. 2004. Determinants of F2-isoprostane biosynthesis and inhibition in man. *Chem. Phys. Lipids* 128:149–63
19. Davi G, Romano M, Mezzetti A, Procopio A, Iacobelli S, ct al. 1998. Increased levels of soluble P-selectin in hypercholesterolemic patients. *Circulation* 97:953–57
20. DeMaio SJ, King SB III, Lembo NJ, Roubin GS, Hearn JA, et al. 1992. Vitamin E supplementation, plasma lipids, and incidence of restenosis after percutaneous transluminal coronary angioplasty (TCA). *J. Am. Coll. Nutr.* 11:68–73
21. Devaraj S, Adams-Huet B, Fuller CJ, Jialal I. 1997. Dose-response comparison of RRR-AT and all-rac-tocopherol on LDL oxidation. *Arterioscler. Thromb. Vasc. Biol.* 17:2273–79
22. Devaraj S, Chan AV Jr, Jialal I. 2002. Alpha-tocopherol supplementation decreases plasminogen activator inhibitor-1 and P-selectin levels in type 2 diabetic patients. *Diabetes Care* 25:524–29
23. Devaraj S, Jialal I. 1998. The effects of α-tocopherol on critical cells in atherogenesis. *Curr. Opin. Lipidol.* 9:1115–17
24. Devaraj S, Jialal I. 1999. Alpha-tocopherol decreases interleukin-1 beta release from activated human monocytes by inhibition of 5-lipoxygenase. *Arterioscler. Thromb. Vasc. Biol.* 19:1125–33
25. Devaraj S, Jialal I. 2000. Alpha-tocopherol supplementation decreases serum C-reactive protein and monocyte interleukin-6 levels in normal volunteers and type 2 diabetic patients. *Free Radic. Biol. Med.* 29:790–92
26. Devaraj S, Jialal I. 2000. Low-density lipoprotein postsecretory modification, monocyte function, and circulating adhesion molecules in type 2 diabetic patients with and without macrovascular complications: the effect of alpha-tocopherol supplementation. *Circulation* 102:191–96
27. Devaraj S, Li D, Jialal I. 1996. The effects of alpha-tocopherol supplementation on monocyte function. Decreased lipid oxidation, interleukin 1 beta secretion, and monocyte adhesion to endothelium. *J. Clin. Invest.* 98:756–63
28. Devaraj S, Venugopal SK, Singh U, Jialal I. 2005. Hyperglycemia induces monocytic IL-6 via induction of PK-C alpha and beta. *Diabetes* 54:85–91
29. Dhanasekaran A, Kotamraju S, Kalivendi SV, Matsunaga T, Shang T, et al. 2004. Supplementation of endothelial cells with mitochondria-targeted antioxidants inhibit peroxide-induced mitochondrial iron uptake, oxidative damage and apoptosis. *J. Biol. Chem.* 279:37575–87
30. Elliott TG, Barth JD, Mancini GB. 1995. Effects of vitamin E on endothelial function in men after myocardial infarction. *Am. J. Cardiol.* 76:1188–90
31. Engler MM, Engler MB, Malloy MJ, Chiu EY, Schloetter MC, et al. 2003. Antioxidant vitamins C and E improve endothelial function in children with

hyperlipidemia: Endothelial Assessment of Risk from Lipids in Youth (EARLY) Trial. *Circulation* 108:1059–63

32. Esterbauer H, Dieber-Rothcneder M, Striegl G, Waeg G. 1991. Role of vitamin E in preventing the oxidation of low-density lipoprotein. *Am. J. Clin. Nutr.* 53(Suppl. 1):314S–21S
33. Fan Y, Liu ML, Qi YY, Ren ZW. 2004. Effect of different isoforms of tocopherols on expression of intercellular adhesion molecule-1 in human umbilical vein endothelial cells. *Beijing Da Xue Xue Bao* 36:70–74
34. Faruqui R, De La Motte C, Dicorleto P. 1994. α-Tocopherol inhibits agonist-induced monocyte cell adherence to cultured human endothelial cells. *J. Clin. Invest.* 94:592–600
35. Freedman JE, Farhat JH, Loscalzo J, Keaney JF Jr. 1996. α-Tocopherol inhibits aggregation of human platelets by a protein kinase C–dependent mechanism. *Circulation* 94:2434–40
36. Friedrich MJ. 2004. To "E" or not to "E," vitamin E's role in health and disease is the question. *JAMA* 292:671–73
37. Gazis A, White DJ, Page SR, Cockcroft JR. 1999. Effect of oral vitamin E (alpha-tocopherol) supplementation on vascular endothelial function in type 2 diabetes mellitus. *Diabet. Med.* 16:304–11
38. Gniwotta C, Morrow JD, Roberts LJ II, Kuhn H. 1997. Prostaglandin F_2-like compounds, F_2 isoprostanes, are present in increased amounts in human atherosclerotic lesions. *Arterioscler. Thromb. Vasc. Biol.* 17:3236–41
39. Green D, O'Driscoll G, Rankin JM, Maiorana AJ, Taylor RR. 1998. Beneficial effect of vitamin E administration on nitric oxide function in subjects with hypercholesterolaemia. *Clin. Sci. (Lond.)* 95:361–67
40. Heitzer T, Yla Herttuala S, Wild E, Luoma J, Drexler H. 1999. Effect of vitamin E on endothelial vasodilator function in patients with hypercholesterolemia, chronic smoking or both. *J. Am. Coll. Cardiol.* 33:499–505
41. Higashi O, Kikuchi Y. 1974. Effects of vitamin E on the aggregation and lipid peroxidation of platelets exposed to hydrogen peroxide. *Tohoku J. Exp. Med.* 112:271–78
42. Himmelfarb J, Kane J, McMonagle E, Zaltas E, Bobzin S, et al. 2003. Alpha and gamma tocopherol metabolism in healthy subjects and patients with end-stage renal disease. *Kidney Int.* 64:978–91
43. Hodis HN, Mack WJ, LaBree L, Mahrer PR, Sevanian A, et al. 2002. Alpha-tocopherol supplementation in healthy individuals reduces low-density lipoprotein oxidation but not atherosclerosis. *Circulation* 106:1453–59
44. Inoue M, Itoh H, Tanaka T, Chun TH, Doi K, et al. 2001. Oxidized LDL regulates vascular endothelial growth factor expression in human macrophages and endothelial cells through activation of peroxisome proliferator-activated receptor-gamma. *Arterioscler. Thromb. Vasc. Biol.* 21:560–66
45. Islam KN, O'Byrne D, Devaraj S, Palmer B, Grundy SM, Jialal I. 2000. Alpha-tocopherol supplementation decreases the oxidative susceptibility of LDL in renal failure patients on dialysis therapy. *Atherosclerosis* 150:217–24
46. Jessup W, Kritharides L, Stocker R. 2004. Lipid oxidation in atherogenesis: an overview. *Biochem. Soc. Trans.* 32:134–38
47. Jialal I. 1998. Evolving lipoprotein risk factors: lipoprotein(a) and oxidized low-density lipoprotein. *Clin. Chem.* 44:1827–32
48. Jialal I, Devaraj S. 2001. Inflammation and atherosclerosis: the value of the high-sensitivity C-reactive protein assay as a risk marker. *Am. J. Clin. Pathol.* 116(Suppl.):S108–15
49. Jialal I, Devaraj S. 2003. Antioxidants and atherosclerosis: Don't throw out the baby

with the bath water. *Circulation* 107:926–28
50. Jialal I, Devaraj S, Venugopal. 2004. C-reactive protein: risk marker or mediator in atherothrombosis? *Hypertension* 44:1–6
51. Jialal I, Fuller C, Huet B. 1995. The effect of AT supplementation on LDL oxidation: a dose-response study. *Arterioscler. Thromb. Vasc. Biol.* 15:190–98
52. Jialal I, Grundy SM. 1992. Effect of dietary supplementation with α-tocopherol on the oxidative modification of low-density lipoprotein. *J. Lipid Res.* 33:899–906
53. Jialal I, Grundy SM. 1992. Influence of antioxidant vitamins on LDL oxidation. *Ann. N.Y. Acad. Sci.* 669:237–48
54. Jones SA, O'Donnell VB, Wood JD, Broughton JP, Hughes EJ, et al. 1996. Expression of phagocytic NADPH oxidase components in human endothelial cells. *Am. J. Phys.* 271:H1626–34
55. Kaul N, Devaraj S, Grundy SM, Jialal I. 2001. Failure to demonstrate a major anti-inflammatory effect with alpha tocopherol supplementation (400 IU/day) in normal subjects. *Am. J. Cardiol.* 87:1320–23
56. Kaul N, Devaraj S, Jialal I. 2001. Alpha-tocopherol and atherosclerosis. *Exp. Biol. Med.* (Maywood) 226:5–12
57. Keaney JF Jr, Gaziano JM, Xu A, Frei B, Curran-Celentano J, et al. 1994. Low-dose α-tocopherol improves and high-dose α-tocopherol worsens endothelial vasodilator function in cholesterol-fed rabbits. *Clin. Invest.* 93:844–51
58. Keaney JF Jr, Guo Y, Cunningham D, Shwaery GT, Xu A, Vita JA. 1996. Vascular incorporation of α-tocopherol prevents endothelial dysfunction due to oxidized LDL by inhibiting protein kinase C stimulation. *J. Clin. Invest.* 98:386–94
59. Kinlay S, Fang JC, Hikita H, Ho I, Delagrange DM, et al. 1999. Plasma alpha-tocopherol and coronary endothelium-dependent vasodilator function. *Circulation* 100:219–21
60. Kirii H, Niwa T, Yamada Y, Wada H, Saito K, et al. 2003. Lack of interleukin-1ß decreases the severity of atherosclerosis in apoE-deficient mice. *Arterioscler. Thromb. Vasc. Biol.* 23:656–60
61. Kobayashi S, Inoue N, Ohashi Y, Terashima M, Matsui K, et al. 2003. Interaction of oxidative stress and inflammatory response in coronary plaque instability: important role of C-reactive protein. *Arterioscler. Thromb. Vasc. Biol.* 23:1398–404
62. Kontush A, Chapman MJ, Stocker R. 2004. Vitamin E is not deficient in human atherosclerotic plaques. *Arterioscler. Thromb. Vasc. Biol.* 24:e139–40
63. Koya D, Haneda M, Kikkawa R, King GL. 1998. α- and δ-Tocopherol treatment prevents glomerular dysfunctions in diabetic rats through inhibition of protein-kinase C–diacylglycerol pathway. *Biofactors* 7:69–76
64. Kris-Etherton PM, Lichtenstein AH, Howard BV, Steinberg D, Witztum JL. 2004. Nutrition Committee of the American Heart Association Council on Nutrition, Physical Activity, and Metabolism. Antioxidant vitamin supplements and cardiovascular disease. *Circulation* 110:637–40
65. Kunisaki M, Bursell SE, Umeda F, Nawata H, King GL. 1994. Normalization of DAG-PKC activation by vitamin E in aorta of diabetic rats and cultured rat SMC exposed to elevated glucose levels. *Diabetes* 42:1372–77
66. Lafont AM, Chai YC, Cornhill JF, Whitlow PL, Howe PH, et al. 1995. Effect of α-tocopherol on restenosis after angioplasty in a model of experimental atherosclerosis. *J. Clin. Invest.* 95:1018–25
67. Laursen JB, Boesgaard S, Trautner S, Rubin I, Poulsen HE, Aldershvile J. 2001. Endothelium-dependent vasorelaxation in inhibited by in vivo depletion of vascular thiol levels: role of endothelial nitric oxide synthase. *Free Radic. Res.* 35:387–94

68. Libby P. 2002. Inflammation in atherosclerosis. *Nature* 420:868–74
69. Mabile L, Bruckdorfer K, Rice Evans C. 1999. Moderate supplementation with natural alpha-tocopherol decreases platelet aggregation and low-density lipoprotein oxidation. *Atherosclerosis* 147:177–85
70. Marangon K, Devaraj S, Jialal I. 1999. The effect of α-lipoate and α-tocopherol on plasma, whole body, and LDL oxidation. *Free Radic. Biol. Med.* 27:1114–21
71. Martin A, Foxall T, Blumberg JB, Meydani M. 1997. AT inhibits LDL-induced adhesion of monocytes to human aortic endothelial cells *in vitro*. *Arterioscler. Thromb. Vasc. Biol.* 17:429–36
72. Micheletta F, Natoli S, Misuraca M, Sbarigia E, Diczfalusy U, Iuliano L. 2004. Vitamin E supplementation in patients with carotid atherosclerosis: reversal of altered oxidative stress status in plasma but not in plaque. *Arterioscler. Thromb. Vasc. Biol.* 24:136–40
73. Miller FJ Jr, Gutterman DD, Rios CD, Heistad DD, Davidson BL. 1998. Superoxide production in vascular smooth muscle contributes to oxidative stress and impaired relaxation in atherosclerosis. *Circ. Res.* 82:1298–305
74. Miyamoto S, Kawano H, Takazoe K, Soejima H, Sakamoto T, et al. 2004. Vitamin E improves fibrinolytic activity in patients with coronary spastic angina. *Thromb. Res.* 113:345–51
75. Mol MJ, de Rijke YB, Demacker PN, Stalenhoef AF. 1997. Plasma levels of lipid and cholesterol oxidation products and cytokines in diabetes mellitus and cigarette smoking: effects of vitamin E treatment. *Atherosclerosis* 129:169–76
76. Motoyama T, Kawano H, Kugiyama K, Hirashima O, Ohgushi M, et al. 1998. Vitamin E administration improves impairment of endothelium-dependent vasodilation in patients with coronary spastic angina. *J. Am. Coll. Cardiol.* 32:1672–79
77. Mottrram P, Shige H, Nestel P. 1999. Vitamin E improves arterial compliance in middle-aged men and women. *Atherosclerosis* 145:399–404
78. Mugge A, Elwell JH, Peterson TE, Hofmeyer TG, Heistad DD, Harrison DG. 1991. Chronic treatment with PEG-SOD partially restores endothelial-dependent vascular relaxation in cholesterol-fed rabbits. *Circ. Res.* 69:1293–300
79. Munteanu A, Zingg JM, Azzi A. 2004. Anti-atherosclerotic effects of vitamin E—myth or reality? *J. Cell. Mol. Med.* 8:59–76
80. Munteanu A, Zingg JM, Ogru E, Libinaki R, Gianello R, et al. 2004. Modulation of cell proliferation and gene expression by alpha-tocopheryl phosphates: relevance to atherosclerosis and inflammation. *Biochem. Biophys. Res. Commun.* 318:311–16
81. Murphy RT, Foley JB, Tome MT, Mulvihill NT, Murphy A, et al. 2004. Vitamin E modulation of C-reactive protein in smokers with acute coronary syndromes. *Free Radic. Biol. Med.* 36:959–65
82. Paolisso G, Tagliamonte MR, Barbieri M, Zito GA, Gambardella A, et al. 2000. Chronic vitamin E administration improves brachial reactivity and increases intracellular magnesium concentration in type II diabetic patients. *J. Clin. Endocrinol. Metab.* 85:109–15
83. Paul A, Ko KW, Li L, Yechoor V, McCrory MA, et al. 2004. C-reactive protein accelerates the progression of atherosclerosis in apolipoprotein E–deficient mice. *Circulation* 109:647–55
84. Patrano C, Fitzgerald G. 1997. Isoprostanes: potential markers of oxidant stress in atherothrombotic disease. *Arterioscler. Thromb. Vasc. Biol.* 17:2309–15
85. Peluzio MC, Homem AP, Cesar GC, Azevedo GS, Amorim R, et al. 2001. Influences of alpha-tocopherol on cholesterol metabolism and fatty streak development in apolipoprotein E–deficient mice fed an atherogenic diet. *Braz. J. Med. Biol. Res.* 34:1539–45

86. Peluzio MC, Miguel E Jr, Drumond TC, Cesar GC, Santiago HC, et al. 2003. Monocyte chemoattractant protein-1 involvement in the alpha-tocopherol-induced reduction of atherosclerotic lesions in apolipoprotein E knockout mice. *Br. J. Nutr.* 90:3–11
87. Pickup JC. 2004. Inflammation and activated innate immunity in the pathogenesis of type 2 diabetes. *Diabetes Care* 27:813–23
88. Pratico D, Juliano L, Mauriello A, Spagnoli L, Lawson JA, et al. 1998. Localization of distinct F_2-isoprostanes in human atherosclerotic lesions. *J. Clin. Invest.* 100:915–24
89. Ramsey MW, Goodfellow J, Jones CJ, Luddington LA, Lewis MJ, Henderson AH. 1995. Endothelial control of arterial distensibility is impaired in chronic heart failure. *Circulation* 92:3212–19
90. Reaven P, Witztum J. 1993. Comparison of supplementation with RRR-α-tocopherol and all-rac-tocopherol in humans. *Arterioscler. Thromb. Vasc. Biol.* 13:601–8
91. Ridker PM. 2003. Clinical application of C-reactive protein for cardiovascular disease detection and prevention. *Circulation* 168:363–69
92. Roberts LJ 2nd, Morrow JD. 2002. Products of the isoprostane pathway: unique bioactive compounds and markers of lipid peroxidation. *Cell. Mol. Life Sci.* 59:808–20
93. Ross R. 1999. Atherosclerosis: an inflammatory disease. *N. Engl. J. Med.* 340:115–26
94. Saldeen T, Li D, Mehta JL. 1999. Differential effects of alpha- and gamma-tocopherol on low-density lipoprotein oxidation, superoxide activity, platelet aggregation and arterial thrombogenesis. *J. Am. Coll. Cardiol.* 34:1208–15
95. Saran R, Novak JE, Desai A, Abdulhayoglu E, Warren JS, et al. 2003. Impact of vitamin E on plasma asymmetric dimethylarginine (ADMA) in chronic kidney disease (CKD): a pilot study. *Nephrol. Dial. Transplant.* 18:2415–20
96. Schnell JW, Anderson RA, Stegner JE, Schindler SP, Weinberg RB. 2001. Effects of a high polyunsaturated fat diet and vitamin E supplementation on high-density lipoprotein oxidation in humans. *Atherosclerosis* 159:459–66
97. Schock BC, Van der Vliet A, Corbacho AM, Leonard SW, Finkelstein E, et al. 2004. Enhanced inflammatory responses in alpha-tocopherol transfer protein null mice. *Arch. Biochem. Biophys.* 423:162–69
98. Schwenke DC, Rudel LL, Sorci-Thomas MG, Thomas MJ. 2002. Alpha-tocopherol protects against diet-induced atherosclerosis in New Zealand white rabbits. *J. Lipid Res.* 43:1927–38
99. Simons LA, von Konigsmark M, Simons J, Stocker R, Celermajer DS. 1999. Vitamin E ingestion does not improve arterial endothelial dysfunction in older adults. *Atherosclerosis* 143:193–99
100. Singh U, Jialal I. 2004. Anti-inflammatory effects of alpha-tocopherol. *Ann. N.Y. Acad. Sci.* 1031:195–203
101. Smith KS, Lee CL, Ridlington JW, Leonard SW, Devaraj S, Traber MG. 2003. Vitamin E supplementation increases circulating vitamin E metabolites tenfold in end-stage renal disease patients. *Lipids* 38:813–19
102. Smith T, Kummerow F. 1989. Effect of dietary vitamin E on plasma lipids and atherogenesis in restricted ovulator chicken. *Atherosclerosis* 75:105–9
103. Steinbrecher U. 1984. Modification of low-density lipoprotein by endothelial cells involves lipid peroxidation and degradation of low-density lipoprotein phospholipids. *Proc. Natl. Acad. Sci. USA* 81:3883–87
104. Steiner M. 1983. Effect of alpha-tocopherol administration on platelet function in man. *Thromb. Haemost.* 49:73–77
105. Steiner M. 1991. Influence of vitamin E on

platelet function in humans. *J. Am. Coll. Nutr.* 10:466–73
106. Stewart-Lee AL, Forster LA, Nourooz-Zadeh J, Ferns GA, Anggard EE. 1994. Vitamin E protects against impairment of endothelium-mediated relaxations in cholesterol-fed rabbits. *Arterioscler. Thromb. Vasc. Biol.* 14:494–99
107. Stocker R, Keaney JF Jr. 2004. Role of oxidative modifications in atherosclerosis. *Physiol. Rev.* 84:1381–478
108. Suarna C, Dean RT, May J, Stocker R. 1995. Human atherosclerotic plaque contains both oxidized lipids and relatively large amounts of alpha-tocopherol and ascorbate. *Arterioscler. Thromb. Vasc. Biol.* 15:1616–24
109. Suzuki YJ, Packer L. 1993. Inhibition of NF-κB DNA binding activity by AT succinate. *Biochem. Mol. Biol. Int.* 31:693–700
110. Suzuki YJ, Tsuchiya M, Wassall SR, Choo YM, Govil G, et al. 1993. Structural and dynamic properties of AT and T3: implication to the molecular mechanism of their antioxidant potency. *Biochemistry* 32:10692–99
111. Takamatsu S, Takamatsu M, Satoh K. 1995. Effects on health of dietary supplementation with 100 mg α- and δ-tocopheryl acetate, daily for 6 years. *J. Int. Med. Res.* 23:342–57
112. Tasinato A, Boscoboinik D, Bartoli GM, Maroni P, Azzi A. 1995. d-α-Tocopherol inhibition of vascular smooth muscle cell proliferation occurs at physiological concentrations, correlates with protein kinase C inhibition, and is independent of its antioxidant properties. *Proc. Natl. Acad. Sci.* USA 92:12190–94
113. Terasawa Y, Ladha Z, Leonard SW, Morrow JD, Newland D, et al. 2000. Increased atherosclerosis in hyperlipidemic mice deficient in alpha-tocopherol transfer protein and vitamin E. *Proc. Natl. Acad. Sci. USA* 97:13830–34
114. Teupser D, Thiery J, Seidel D. 1999. AT downregulates SR activity in macrophages. *Atherosclerosis* 144:109–15
115. Thomas SR, Stocker R. 2000. Molecular action of vitamin E in lipoprotein oxidation: implications for atherosclerosis. *Free Radic. Biol. Med.* 28(12):1795–805
116. Traber MG, Arai H. 1999. Molecular mechanism of vitamin E transport. *Annu. Rev. Nutr.* 19:343–55
117. Ulker S, McKeown PP, Bayraktutan U. 2003. Vitamins reverse endothelial dysfunction through regulation of eNOS and NAD(P)H oxidase activities. *Hypertension* 41:534–39
118. Upritchard JE, Sutherland WHE, Mann JI. 2000. Effect of supplementation with tomato juice, vitamin E, and vitamin C on LDL oxidation and products of inflammatory activity in type 2 diabetes. *Diabetes Care* 23:733–38
119. Upston JM, Terentis AC, Morris K, Keaney Jr JF, Stocker R. 2002. Oxidized lipid accumulates in the presence of alpha-tocopherol in atherosclerosis. *Biochem. J.* 363:753–60
120. van Aalst JA, Burmeister W, Fox PL, Graham LM. 2004. α-Tocopherol preserves endothelial cell migration in the presence of cell-oxidized low-density lipoprotein by inhibiting changes in cell membrane fluidity. *J. Vasc. Surg.* 39:229–37
121. Van Tits LJ, Demacker PN, de Graaf J, Hak-Lemmers HL, Stalenhoef AF. 2000. α-Tocopherol supplementation decreases production of superoxide and cytokines by leukocytes ex vivo in both normolipidemic and hypertriglyceridemic individuals. *Am. J. Clin. Nutr.* 71:458–64
122. Vega-Lopez S, Kaul N, Devaraj S, Cai RY, German B, Jialal I. 2004. Supplementation with ω3 polyunsaturated fatty acids and all-rac AT alone and in combination failed to exert an anti-inflammatory effect in human volunteers. *Metabolism* 53:236–40
123. Venugopal SK, Devaraj S, Jialal I. 2003. CRP decreases prostacyclin release from

human aortic endothelial cells. *Circulation* 108:1676–78

124. Venugopal SK, Devaraj S, Jialal I. 2004. RRR-AT decreases the expression of the major SR, CD36, in human macrophages via inhibition of tyrosine kinase (Tyk2). *Atherosclerosis* 175:213–20
125. Venugopal SK, Devaraj S, Jialal I. 2005. Macrophage conditioned medium induces the expression of CRP in human aortic endothelial cells: potential for paracrine/autocrine effects. *Am J. Pathol.* 166:1265–71
126. Venugopal SK, Devaraj S, Yang T, Jialal I. 2002. AT decreases superoxide anion release in human monocytes under hyperglycemic conditions via inhibition of PKC-α. *Diabetes* 51:3049–54
127. Verlangieri A, Buxh M. 1992. Effects of AT supplementation on experimentally induced primate atherosclerosis. *J. Am. Coll. Nutr.* 11:131–38
128. Wang CH, Li SH, Weisel RD, Fedak PW, Dumont AS, et al. 2003. C-reactive protein upregulates angiotensin type 1 receptors in vascular smooth muscle. *Circulation* 107:1783–90
129. Weinberg RB, VanderWerken BS, Anderson RA, Stegner JE, Thomas MJ. 2001. Pro-oxidant effect of vitamin E in cigarette smokers consuming a high polyunsaturated fat diet. *Arterioscler. Thromb. Vasc. Biol.* 21:1029–33
130. Williams RJ, Motteram JM, Sharp CH, Gallagher PJ. 1992. Dietary vitamin E and attenuation of early lesion development in modified Watanabe rabbits. *Atherosclerosis* 94:153–59
131. Witzum J, Steinberg D. 1991. Role of oxidized low-density lipoprotein in atherogenesis. *J. Clin. Invest.* 88:1785–92
132. Wu D, Koga T, Martin KR, Meydani M. 1999. Effect of vitamin E on human aortic endothelial cell production of chemokines and adhesion to monocytes. *Atherosclerosis* 147:297–307
133. Wu D, Mura C, Beharka AA, Han SN, Paulson KE, et al. 1998. Age-associated increase in PGE2 synthesis and COX activity in murine macrophages is reversed by vitamin E. *Am. J. Physiol.* 275:C661–68
134. Yang T, Devaraj S, Jialal I. 2001. Oxidative stress and atherosclerosis. *J. Clin. Ligand Assay* 24:13–24
135. Yasojima K, Schwab C, McGeer EG, McGeer PL. 2001. Generation of CRP and complement components in atherosclerotic plaques. *Am. J. Pathol.* 158:1039–51

Annu. Rev. Nutr. 2005. 25:175–96
doi: 10.1146/annurev.nutr.25.121304.131724

UPTAKE, LOCALIZATION, AND NONCARBOXYLASE ROLES OF BIOTIN*

Janos Zempleni
Department of Nutrition and Health Sciences and Departments of Biochemistry and Animal Science, University of Nebraska at Lincoln, Nebraska 68583-0806; email: Jzempleni2@unl.edu

Key Words biotin, cell signaling, gene expression, histones, transport

■ **Abstract** Evidence is emerging that biotin participates in processes other than classical carboxylation reactions. Specifically, novel roles for biotin in cell signaling, gene expression, and chromatin structure have been identified in recent years. Human cells accumulate biotin by using both the sodium-dependent multivitamin transporter and monocarboxylate transporter 1. These transporters and other biotin-binding proteins partition biotin to compartments involved in biotin signaling: cytoplasm, mitochondria, and nuclei. The activity of cell signals such as biotinyl-AMP, Sp1 and Sp3, nuclear factor (NF)-κB, and receptor tyrosine kinases depends on biotin supply. Consistent with a role for biotin and its catabolites in modulating these cell signals, greater than 2000 biotin-dependent genes have been identified in various human tissues. Many biotin-dependent gene products play roles in signal transduction and localize to the cell nucleus, consistent with a role for biotin in cell signaling. Posttranscriptional events related to ribosomal activity and protein folding may further contribute to effects of biotin on gene expression. Finally, research has shown that biotinidase and holocarboxylase synthetase mediate covalent binding of biotin to histones (DNA-binding proteins), affecting chromatin structure; at least seven biotinylation sites have been identified in human histones. Biotinylation of histones appears to play a role in cell proliferation, gene silencing, and the cellular response to DNA repair. Roles for biotin in cell signaling and chromatin structure are consistent with the notion that biotin has a unique significance in cell biology.

CONTENTS

---

*ABBREVIATIONS: CNS, central nervous system; ER, endoplasmic reticulum; HCS, holocarboxylase synthetase; K_m, Michaelis-Menten constant; MCT, monocarboxylate transporter; PBMC, peripheral blood mononuclear cells; SMVT, sodium-dependent multivitamin transporter; UPR, unfolded protein response.

INTRODUCTION

Soon after the discovery of biotin by Boas (12) and Kogl & Tonnis (75), biochemical functions of the vitamin were unveiled. It was demonstrated that biotin serves as a covalently bound coenzyme for the following carboxylases in eukaryotes: acetyl-CoA carboxylase, pyruvate carboxylase, propionyl-CoA carboxylase, and 3-methylcrotonyl-CoA carboxylase (74, 144). For acetyl-CoA carboxylase, a cytosolic (denoted acetyl-CoA carboxylase α) and a mitochondrial (denoted acetyl-CoA carboxylase β) form have been identified; the distinct functions of these isoforms in fatty acid metabolism have been reviewed (73). Acetyl-CoA carboxylase β may also play a role in biotin storage (120). Additional biotin-dependent carboxylases have been identified in prokaryotes (7, 49, 74, 144). Binding of biotin to carboxylases in eukaryotic cells is mediated by holocarboxylase synthetase (HCS); biotinyl-AMP occurs as an intermediate (44). Recycling of covalently bound biotin from breakdown products of carboxylases is mediated by biotinidase (142).

In the late 1960s and early 1970s, evidence began to emerge that biotin affects gene expression in mammals (45, 46). These pioneering studies can be considered the starting point for many of the exciting developments that the field of biotin research has witnessed in the recent past. Beginning with an improved understanding of cellular biotin uptake and localization, it became evident very quickly that biotin plays essential roles in cell signaling and chromatin structure. These recent advances in cellular uptake and localization, and the noncarboxylase roles of biotin, are reviewed in this chapter.

CELLULAR UPTAKE AND DISTRIBUTION

Mechanisms of biotin uptake into mammalian cells have been reviewed in detail in recent volumes in the *Annual Reviews* series (90, 116). The reader is referred to these reviews for a detailed account of biotin transporters. Here we provide a brief update on biotin transporters located in the plasma membrane. Factors that determine the intracellular distribution of biotin are also discussed as they relate to newly discovered noncarboxylase roles of the vitamin.

Biotin Transporters in the Plasma Membrane

Early investigations of biotin transport in mammals provided evidence for the existence of a biotin carrier in plasma membranes (17, 18, 35). These studies suggested that uptake of biotin is a sodium-dependent process that requires metabolic energy. The Michaelis-Menten constant (K_m) of the biotin transporter in mouse fibroblasts 3T3-L1 and mouse jejunum is 22 and 3.7 μmol/L, respectively (35, 117). At high extracellular concentrations of biotin ([biotin] $\gg K_m$), passive diffusion of biotin into cells gains importance and exceeds carrier-mediated influx (18, 35). Both carrier-mediated uptake and passive diffusion account for the very efficient uptake of biotin observed in mammals. Oral doses of biotin that exceed the normal dietary intake by about 600 times are absorbed completely (150).

The biotin transporter in mammalian cells has broad substrate specificity and carries biotin, pantothenic acid, and lipoic acid (103) with similar affinity (105). Consequently, this transporter was named the sodium-dependent multivitamin transporter (SMVT) (105). The SMVT has been detected in numerous cell lines from various species (103–105, 116). Four variants of SMVT transcripts have been identified in rats (28). The role of SMVT in biotin transport was confirmed by cloning a cDNA coding for rat SMVT, and expressing functional transporter in human-derived HeLa cells (105). Likewise, rabbit intestinal SMVT was functionally expressed in human retinal pigment epithelium (104).

The intestinal biotin uptake is regulated by protein kinase C and Ca^{2+}/calmodulin-mediated pathways (115). Activation of protein kinase C inhibits biotin uptake, whereas inhibition of protein kinase C stimulates biotin uptake by Caco-2 cells. This effect of protein kinase C is mediated by alterations in the activity or abundance of biotin transporters, as opposed to alterations in transporter affinity for substrate. SMVT contains two putative protein kinase C phosphorylation sites (28, 104, 115), but it is unknown whether these sites are involved in the regulation of biotin uptake by protein kinase C.

The 5′-regulatory regions of *SMVT* genes in rats and humans have been cloned and characterized (29, 48). The rat and human *SMVT* genes contain three and two distinct promoters, respectively. Both promoter sequences in the human gene are TATA-less, CAAT-less, contain highly GC-rich sites, and have multiple putative regulatory *cis*-elements, e.g., AP-1, AP-2, C/EBP, SP1, NF1, and GATA (48). The minimal region required for basal activity of the human SMVT promoter is encoded by a sequence between −5846 and −5313 for promoter 1 and between −4417 and −4244 for promoter 2 relative to the translation initiation codon. The three promoters in the rat SMVT gene contain *cis*-elements similar to the elements observed in the human promoters, but the rat 5′-regulatory region also contains two TATA-like elements (29).

Notwithstanding the important role of SMVT in biotin uptake, the following lines of evidence suggest that transporters other than SMVT also mediate biotin uptake in some human tissues. First, the K_m for biotin uptake into human peripheral blood mononuclear cells (PBMC) is about 1000 times smaller than the K_m for biotin transport by SMVT (57, 149, 152). Second, both lipoic acid and pantothenic acid are substrates for SMVT but do not compete with biotin for uptake into PBMC (149, 152). Third, an inborn error in biotin transport does not affect transport of pantothenic acid in PBMC (87). Fourth, human lymphoid (Jurkat) cells respond to biotin deficiency with increased rates of biotin uptake without increasing the expression of SMVT (85).

Eventually evidence was provided that biotin uptake into human lymphoid cells is mediated by monocarboxylate transporter 1 (MCT1) in addition to SMVT (42). Notwithstanding the ubiquitous expression of MCT1 in human tissues (61), it remains to be demonstrated whether MCT1 plays a role in biotin uptake in tissues other than lymphoid cells (42). MCT1 belongs to the family of monocarboxylate transporters. Nine MCT-related sequences have so far been identified in mammals, each having a distinct tissue distribution (61). It is unknown if MCTs other than MCT1 play a role in biotin uptake.

Biotin Homeostasis in the Central Nervous System

Disturbances in biotin homeostasis in the central nervous system (CNS) cause encephalopathies (41, 95). Factors leading to biotin imbalances in CNS include deficiencies of biotinidase, HCS (41), and perhaps biotin transporters (87, 95). Afflicted patients typically respond to the administration of large doses of biotin with maintaining normal neurological function (41, 95).

Moderate dietary biotin deficiency is typically not associated with neurological symptoms. This is consistent with the hypothesis that under conditions of moderate biotin deficiency the CNS maintains normal concentrations of biotin at the expense of other tissues. Indeed, research has shown that biotin deficiency causes a >90% decrease of biotinylated carboxylases in rat liver, whereas brain carboxylases remain unchanged (96). Apparently, biotin deficiency decreases expression of SMVT in rat liver while maintaining normal expression of SMVT in brain (96).

Biotin Uptake into Cellular Organelles

Biotin is distributed unequally across cellular compartments (100). If [^{14}C]biotin is administered intravenously to rats, the vast majority of biotin in liver localizes to mitochondria and cytoplasm, whereas only a small fraction localizes to microsomes (100). The relative enrichment of biotin in mitochondria and cytoplasm is consistent with the role of biotin as a coenzyme for carboxylases in these compartments. A quantitatively small but qualitatively important fraction of biotin localizes to the cell nucleus, i.e., about 0.7% of total biotin in human PBMC can be recovered from the nuclear fraction (128). The relative abundance of nuclear biotin increases to about 1% of total biotin in response to proliferation, consistent with a role for nuclear biotin-binding proteins (histones) in cell proliferation as described in the "Biological Functions of Histone Biotinylation" section.

What are the mechanisms driving the cellular partitioning of biotin? Theoretically, both transport by MCT1 (42) and binding to carboxylases (73, 74, 144) might mediate the sequestration of biotin in mitochondria. MCT1 is known to transport biotin (42) and has been detected in mitochondrial membranes (22, 61). After entry into mitochondria, biotin is trapped by covalent binding to acetyl-CoA carboxylase β, pyruvate carboxylase, propionyl-CoA carboxylase, and 3-methylcrotonyl-CoA carboxylase (74, 144). Studies of biotin turnover in human PBMC suggested that the half-life of biotin during the slow phase of elimination (half-life $= 21.9 \pm 13.6$ h) coincides with the breakdown of biotinylated carboxylases (151). Similar findings were made for biotin and holo-pyruvate carboxylase in the mouse preadipocyte cell line 3T3-L1 (54). Depletion and repletion studies of biotin-dependent carboxylases in rat liver are consistent with a role for mitochondrial acetyl-CoA carboxylase β in biotin storage (120).

Binding of biotin to proteins in cytoplasm and nucleus is likely to mediate the sequestration of biotin in these compartments. In cytoplasm, acetyl-CoA carboxylase α is the primary biotin-binding protein (147). In the cell nucleus, histones are the primary biotin-binding proteins (128).

CELL SIGNALING

Gene Expression

Pioneering studies by Dakshinamurti and coworkers (43, 45, 46) provided evidence that biotin affects gene expression in addition to its classical role as a coenzyme for carboxylases. Specifically, these studies revealed that biotin deficiency in rats causes a 40% to 45% reduction of liver glucokinase activity, and that normal enzyme activity can be restored by biotin administration (45). Administration of biotin increases the amount of mRNA coding for glucokinase in rat liver (30, 126) and in cultured beta cells (14). These observations broke the ground for current investigations at the interface of biotin, cell signaling, gene expression, and human health.

DNA microarray studies have substantially expanded the number of genes known to be affected by biotin. Most of these studies were conducted using human PBMC and hepatocarcinoma (HepG2) cells. As of today, researchers have identified greater than 2000 human genes that depend on biotin for expression (109, 139, 140). Apparently, biotin-dependent genes are not randomly distributed in the human genome but are arranged in clusters. For example, supplementation of healthy adults with 8.8 μmol/d of biotin for 21 days was associated with increased and decreased expression of 139 and 131 genes, respectively, in PBMC compared with before biotin supplementation (140). The following clusters of biotin-responsive genes were identified in this study. First, if genes were clustered by biological function, biotin-dependent genes were overrepresented among genes associated with cell signaling. For example, at least 28% of biotin-responsive genes play roles in signal transduction, and 16% of products from biotin-responsive genes localize to the cell nucleus. Second, if genes were clustered by chromosomal location,

54% of biotin-responsive genes clustered on chromosomes 1, 2, 3, 11, 12, and 19, whereas no biotin-responsive genes were found on chromosomes 10, 16, 18, 21, and heterosomes. This suggests that position effects play a role in biotin-dependent gene expression.

In another study, human HepG2 cells were cultured in media containing deficient, physiological, and pharmacological concentrations of biotin or the catabolite bisnorbiotin (109). Approximately 1800 biotin-dependent genes were identified. A large number of biotin-dependent genes could be assigned to one of the following clusters based on molecular function: DNA-binding proteins, RNA-binding proteins, genes that play roles in translational activity, nucleotide-binding proteins, and proteins with transferase activity. Gene clusters associated with DNA-binding proteins, RNA-binding proteins, and nucleotide-binding proteins are consistent with a role of biotin in cell signaling and chromatin structure as described below.

The mechanisms that mediate the occurrence of biotin-dependent gene clusters are currently unknown. Both common regulatory elements in biotin-dependent genes and biotin-dependent remodeling of chromatin appear to play a role in this process. The following cell signals and transcription factors mediate effects of biotin on gene expression: (*a*) biotinyl-AMP and cGMP (125); (*b*) nuclear factor (NF)-κB (112); (*c*) Sp1 and Sp3 (59); and (*d*) receptor tyrosine kinases. These signaling pathways are reviewed in the following sections; biotin-dependent remodeling of chromatin is discussed further in the "Chromatin Structure" section.

Biotinyl-AMP

Biotinyl-AMP is an intermediate in the synthesis of biotin-dependent holocarboxylases, catalyzed by HCS (147). In mammalian cells, HCS is localized in cytosol, mitochondria, and nucleus (27, 33, 94). Solorzano-Vargas et al. (125) proposed that biotinyl-AMP plays an essential role in regulating gene expression. According to this model, biotinyl-AMP activates soluble guanylate cyclase by a yet unknown mechanism; activation of guanylate cyclase increases the synthesis of cGMP (125). cGMP stimulates protein kinase G, leading to phosphorylation and activation of proteins that enhance the transcription of genes encoding HCS and some carboxylases. Transcriptional activation of these genes is impaired by both biotin deficiency and decreased activity of HCS; the latter can be observed in an inborn error of metabolism known as multiple carboxylase deficiency (131, 142). Consistent with the model described above, addition of biotin to biotin-deficient culture medium increased the activity of guanylate cyclase in both HeLa cells and fibroblasts (122). It remains to be determined whether activation of guanylate cyclase by biotinyl-AMP also plays a role in regulating the expression of genes other than holocarboxylase synthetase and carboxylases. Circumstantial evidence has shown that activation of guanylate cyclase by biotin supplementation is associated with increased activity of RNA polymerase II in HeLa cells and fibroblasts (122). These effects were observed at a concentration of 10 nmol/L biotin (122), which can be readily achieved in healthy adults by biotin supplementation (148).

Biotinyl-AMP-dependent cell signaling is also known from microorganisms. In *Escherichia coli* and other enteric bacteria, biotinyl-AMP [complexed with BirA (biotin-protein ligase), the microbial homolog of HCS] affects gene expression. The biotinyl-AMP/BirA complex binds to promoter regions in the biotin operon, a cluster of genes mediating biotin biosynthesis; binding of biotinyl-AMP/BirA represses the transcription of these genes (40). This feedback loop prevents excessive biosynthesis of biotin.

Nuclear Factor-κB

The transcription factor NF-κB regulates processes such as prevention of cell death, immune function, and embryonic development (81). Five members of the mammalian NF-κB/Rel family of transcription factors have been identified: c-Rel, NF-κB1 (p50/p105), NF-κB2 (p52/p100), RelA (p65), and RelB (4). Transcriptional activation of genes by NF-κB proceeds along the following mechanistic sequence. In unstimulated cells, heterodimers and homodimers of proteins from the NF-κB family reside in the cytoplasm (4). These inactive dimers are associated with the following monomers of inhibitors of NF-κB: IκBα or IκBβ (4). Binding to IκB retains NF-κB in the cytoplasm by masking the nuclear localization sequences (4). Stimulation of IκB kinases by bacteria, cytokines, mitogens, oxidative stress, growth factors, and hormones triggers phosphorylation of IκBs, which are then degraded in proteasome-dependent pathways (81). The liberated NF-κB dimers translocate to the cell nucleus, where they bind to response elements in regulatory regions of genes, triggering gene expression.

Research has shown that biotin affects cell signaling by NF-κB (112). In these studies, human-derived lymphoma (Jurkat) cells were cultured in biotin-deficient and biotin-supplemented media for five weeks; cells were stimulated with phytohemagglutinin and phorbol-12-myristate-13-acetate to induce nuclear translocation of NF-κB. The following observations are consistent with the hypothesis that biotin supply affects NF-κB signaling: (*a*) the nuclear abundance of p50 and p65 is greater in biotin-deficient cells compared with biotin-supplemented cells; (*b*) the DNA-binding activity of NF-κB is greater in biotin-deficient cells compared with biotin-supplemented cells; (*c*) the transcriptional activity of NF-κB-dependent reporter genes is greater in biotin-deficient cells compared with biotin-supplemented cells; and (*d*) the activity of IκBα kinases is greater in biotin-deficient cells compared with biotin-supplemented cells, consistent with increased rates of IκBα degradation and nuclear translocation of NF-κB.

Many cancer cells activate NF-κB in response to treatment with antineoplastic drugs (13, 47, 138), mediating expression of antiapoptotic genes such as *Bfl-1/A1* (6, 52, 66, 81). The products of these genes enhance survival of cancer cells (70, 137, 138), causing resistance to chemotherapy. Research has shown that biotin deficiency enhances the nuclear translocation of NF-κB in Jurkat cells treated with antineoplastic agents such as taxol, doxorubicin, and vinblastine (60). This is associated with increased expression of Bfl-1/A1 and a decreased rate of death in cells treated with doxorubicin and vinblastine. It is uncertain whether biotin status of cancer patients affects the resistance to chemotherapy in vivo. Notwithstanding this uncertainty, effects of biotin on NF-κB activity and cell survival are of potential relevance for health care professionals, given the high prevalence of nutrient deficiencies in cancer patients and during chemotherapy (71, 123, 124).

Sp1 and Sp3

Sp1 and Sp3 belong to the Sp/Krüppel-like factor (KLF) family of transcription factors, which contains at least 20 distinct proteins in mammals (11). Some members of this family are widespread or ubiquitously expressed, whereas other members are highly restricted in their tissue distribution (11). Sp/KLF transcription factors have overlapping DNA-binding specificities and bind to GC-rich sequences (e.g., GC boxes, CACCC boxes) located in regulatory regions of numerous genes; these sequences are collectively referred to as Sp1 sites. Competition among family members for binding to regulatory sequences in DNA plays an important role in the regulation of gene expression (11). Sp/KLF transcription factors differ in their transcriptional activity, with some being activating and some being repressive, establishing a very complex network of regulation. For example, Sp3 may repress Sp1-dependent activation of genes encoding dihydrofolate reductase and α1(II) procollagen by competing with Sp1 for binding to Sp1 sites (10, 55).

The nuclear abundance of Sp1 and Sp3 depends on biotin status in Jurkat cells; the DNA-binding activity of Sp1 and Sp3 is up to 149% greater in biotin-supplemented cells compared with biotin-deficient cells (59). The increased DNA-binding activity in biotin-supplemented cells is mediated by increased expression of genes coding for Sp1 and Sp3. In contrast, posttranslational phosphorylation of Sp1 and Sp3 [a modification known to affect DNA-binding activity (2, 80, 93, 114)] does not depend on biotin (59). Preliminary evidence suggests that Sp1 and Sp3 might be directly modified by covalent binding of biotin (J. Zempleni, unpublished observation). The increased nuclear abundance of Sp1 and Sp3 in biotin-supplemented cells is associated with increased transcriptional activity of Sp1/Sp3-dependent reporter-gene constructs compared with biotin-deficient controls (59).

Effects of biotin on the nuclear abundance of Sp1 and Sp3 are physiologically important. First, the increased nuclear abundance of Sp1 and Sp3 in biotin-supplemented lymphoid cells is associated with increased expression of the *cytochrome P450 1B1* gene (108). The 5′-flanking region of the human *cytochrome P450 1B1* gene contains 11 Sp1 sites (132, 135, 141). Cytochrome P450 1B1 hydroxylates xenobiotics and estrogens ("metabolic activation"), creating electrophilic mutagens that may cause single-stranded breaks in DNA and 8-hydroxylation of guanine bases in DNA (64, 82). Indeed, biotin supplementation is associated with increased frequency of DNA strand breaks in lymphoid cells (108).

Second, biotin supplementation is associated with decreased transcription of the *sarco/endoplasmic reticulum ATPase3* (*SERCA3*) gene (58), the expression of which is controlled by 25 Sp1 sites in its 5′-flanking region (50). Given that Sp3 may act as transcriptional repressor, it has been proposed that effects of biotin on SERCA3 expression are mediated by the increased nuclear abundance of Sp3 in biotin-supplemented cells (58). Decreased expression of SERCA3 reduces the sequestration of calcium in the endoplasmic reticulum (ER) (83). This impairs activities of calcium-dependent proteins such as calnexin (8, 63), BiP (84), and protein disulfide isomerase (84), which play essential roles in the folding of secretory proteins. Accumulation of unfolded proteins in the ER triggers a process named the unfolded protein response (UPR) (121). Hallmarks of UPR include a low global translational activity, a specific increase in the expression of chaperones and other stress-related proteins, a decreased rate of cell proliferation, and an increase in apoptotic activity (20, 25, 97, 106, 121, 146). The following lines of evidence suggest that low expression of SERCA3 in biotin-supplemented cells impairs protein folding in the ER, triggering UPR (58): (*a*) sequestration of calcium in the ER decreased by 30% in response to biotin supplementation; (*b*) secretion of interleukin-2 into the extracellular space decreased by 75% in response to biotin supplementation; and (*c*) the abundance of stress-related proteins such as UBE1, GADD153, XBP1, and phosphorylated eIF2α increased in response to biotin supplementation.

Receptor Tyrosine Kinase Signaling

Receptor tyrosine kinases span the membranes of mammalian cells (65). Various ligands have affinity for the ligand-binding site located in the extracellular domain of receptor tyrosine kinases; ligands include platelet-derived growth factor, insulin, thrombin, and various other compounds. Binding of ligands causes dimerization of receptors and activation of the tyrosine kinase domain located in the cytoplasmic region; this is associated with autophosphorylation of the C-terminus of the receptor. Phosphorylated receptor has affinity for GRB2 (and perhaps its homolog SAM68) and SOS. Binding of the G protein SOS to the phosphorylated receptor tyrosine kinase triggers a substitution of GTP for GDP in the serine/threonine kinase Ras, leading to its catalytic activation. Phosphorylated Ras mediates phosphorylation and, hence, activation of the serine/threonine kinase RAF1. RAF1 phosphorylates MAP kinase kinases (MAPKK or MEK). Phosphorylated MEK catalyze phosphorylation and, hence, activation of mitogen-activated protein kinases (MAPK) such as ERK1 and ERK2. Phosphorylated ERK mediate phosphorylation of the transcription factors Fos and Jun, which bind to AP1 sites in regulatory regions of genes, causing transcriptional activation.

Research has shown that biotin deficiency activates signaling by receptor tyrosine kinases. In these studies, human hepatocarcinoma (HepG2) cells were cultured in media containing deficient, physiological, or pharmacological concentrations of biotin for 10 days (107). Proteins in cell extracts were quantified using high-throughput immunoblots. Biotin deficiency was associated with increased abundance of GRB2, SAM68, and RAF1; the abundance of the Ras-interacting protein

AF6 decreased to nondetectable levels in response to biotin deficiency, enhancing the activity of Ras. Activation of receptor tyrosine kinase pathways was associated with nuclear translocation of AP1-binding proteins Jun and Fos, and transcriptional activation of AP1-dependent reporter genes in biotin-deficient HepG2 cells. The physiological significance of this finding is uncertain. AP1 sites render genes responsive to stimulation with phorbol esters (77); the 5′-flanking region of the human *SMVT* gene also contains AP1 sites (48). Theoretically, activation of receptor tyrosine kinase signaling in biotin-deficient cells may contribute to increasing SMVT-mediated biotin uptake.

Biotin Catabolites

McCormick and coworkers have described the two major pathways of biotin catabolism in a series of seminal papers (89). In the first pathway, biotin is catabolized by β-oxidation of the valeric acid side chain, generating compounds such as bisnorbiotin and tetranorbiotin. In the second pathway, the sulfur in the thiophane portion of the biotin molecule is oxidized, generating compounds such as biotin-*d*, l-sulfoxides and biotin sulfone. Combinations of both β-oxidation and sulfur oxidation also occur to generate compounds such as tetranorbiotin-l-sulfoxide. Biotin catabolites are quantitatively important in mammalian body fluids and cells; the total concentration of biotin catabolites approximately equals the concentration of intact biotin (91, 92).

Evidence emerged that biotin catabolites may play roles in cell signaling. In Jurkat cells, biotin deficiency is associated with decreased expression of the genes encoding interleukin-2 and interleukin-2 receptor gamma (110). Supplementation of biotin-deficient culture medium with the synthetic biotin derivatives diaminobiotin and desthiobiotin restored expression of interleukin-2 and interleukin-2 receptor gamma to control levels (110). Supplementation of culture media with diaminobiotin and desthiobiotin did not affect the abundance of holocarboxylases and activities of propionyl-CoA carboxylase. Hence, effects of biotin analogs on gene expression are not mediated by carboxylase-dependent pathways. Modulation of gene expression by biotin analogs extends to naturally occurring biotin catabolites. For example, supplementation of culture medium with bisnorbiotin altered the expression of 618 genes in HepG2 cells (109).

The mechanisms by which biotin catabolites affect gene expression are uncertain. Note that HCS cannot convert biotin analogs such as desthiobiotin to AMP esters (134); in addition, biotin analogs such as biocytin (biotin-ε-lysine), desthiobiotin, diaminobiotin, and iminobiotin do not inhibit the enzymatic conversion of biotin to biotinyl-AMP, suggesting that these analogs do not compete with biotin for binding to HCS (134). Thus, effects of biotin catabolites on gene expression cannot be explained by the biotinyl-AMP model. Future studies are likely to reveal the mechanism by which biotin catabolites modify gene expression, including the possibility that catabolites may have a biotin-sparing effect in human cells. Notwithstanding the uncertainties described above, effects of biotin catabolites on gene expression are of important consideration for nutritionists. Given that biotin catabolites account for at least 50% of total biotinyl compounds in mammalian tissues (and, hence, foodstuffs) (91), previous studies may have underestimated the true food content and dietary intake of bioactive biotinyl compounds.

Posttranscriptional Events

Effects of biotin on gene expression and cell signaling are not limited to the transcriptional level but also include posttranscriptional events. The earliest studies pointing to a role for biotin in posttranscriptional events date back to the late 1980s (38). These studies provided evidence that the expression of the asialoglycoprotein receptor is reduced in biotin-deficient HepG2 cells, whereas total cellular protein content and mRNA coding for the asialoglycoprotein receptor are comparable to those of control cells; addition of biotin or biocytin to culture media restored receptor expression (38). Analogous studies of propionyl-CoA carboxylase in rat hepatocytes suggested that biotin might also affect the expression of this carboxylase at a posttranscriptional step (111). The mechanisms leading to these effects of biotin are largely unknown. Theoretically, the formation of translation initiation complexes may depend on biotin. Consistent with this notion, the expression of ribosomal subunits LP2, L27a, L38, S11, and S19 and translation initiation factor eIF5A increases in response to biotin deficiency in HepG2 cells (109). In contrast, expression of the ribosomal subunits L37a, S5, and S21 increases in response to biotin supplementation.

HISTONES

Chromatin Structure

Chromatin in the mammalian cell nucleus is composed primarily of DNA and DNA-binding proteins, i.e., histones and nonhistone proteins. Histones play a predominant role in the folding of DNA into chromatin (143). Five major classes of histones have been identified in mammals: H1, H2A, H2B, H3, and H4. Histones are small proteins (11 to 22 kDa) consisting of a globular domain and a more flexible amino terminus (histone "tail"). Lysine and arginine residues combined account for >20% of all amino acid residues in histones, leading to a positive net charge of these proteins at physiological pH (143).

DNA and histones form repetitive nucleoprotein units, the nucleosomes (143). Each nucleosome ("nucleosomal core particle") consists of 146 base pairs of DNA wrapped around an octamer of core histones (one H3-H3-H4-H4 tetramer and two H2A-H2B dimers). The binding of DNA to histones is of electrostatic nature, and is mediated by the association of negatively charged phosphate groups of DNA with positively charged ε-amino groups (lysine moieties) and guanidino groups (arginine moieties) of histones. The DNA located between nucleosomal core particles is associated with histone H1.

The amino terminal tail of histones protrudes from the nucleosomal surface; covalent modifications of this tail affect the structure of chromatin and form the basis for gene regulation (21, 56, 69, 88, 101, 133), mitotic and meiotic chromosome condensation (34), and DNA repair (1, 9, 16, 51, 72, 145). Histone tails are modified by covalent acetylation (3, 62, 79), methylation (143), phosphorylation (143), ubiquitination (143), poly (ADP-ribosylation) (15, 16, 26), and biotinylation (see below) of ϵ-amino groups (lysine), guanidino groups (arginine), carboxyl groups (glutamate), and hydroxyl groups (serine). Multiple signaling pathways converge on histones to mediate covalent modifications of specific amino acid residues (31, 78). Site-specific modifications of histones have distinct functions; for example, dimethylation of lysine-4 in histone H3 is associated with transcriptional activation of surrounding DNA (53, 69). Modifications of histone tails ("histone code") considerably extend the information potential of the DNA code and gene regulation (69, 129, 136). Modifications of histone tails may affect binding of chromatin-associated proteins, triggering cascades of downstream histone modifications. For example, methylation of arginine-3 in histone H4 recruits the histone acetyl transferase Esa1 to yeast chromatin, leading to acetylation of lysine-5 in histone H4 (69). Histone modifications can influence each other in synergistic or antagonistic ways, mediating gene regulation. For example, phosphorylation of serine-10 inhibits methylation of lysine-9 in histone H3, but it is coupled with acetylation of lysine-9 and lysine-14 during mitogenic stimulation in mammalian cells (69). Covalent modifications of histones can be reversed by a large variety of enzymatic processes (69).

Enzymatic Biotinylation and Debiotinylation of Histones

Histones are modified by covalent attachment of the vitamin biotin. Hymes et al. (67, 68, 113) have proposed a reaction mechanism by which cleavage of biocytin (biotin-ε-lysine) by biotinidase leads to the formation of a biotinyl-thioester intermediate (cysteine-bound biotin) at or near the active site of biotinidase. In a next step, the biotinyl moiety is transferred from the thioester to the ε-amino group of lysine in histones. Biocytin is generated in the breakdown of biotin-dependent carboxylases, which contain biotin linked to the ε-amino group of a lysine moiety (102, 142).

Biotinidase belongs to the nitrilase superfamily of enzymes, which consists of 12 families of amidases, N-acyltransferases, and nitrilases (19). Some members of the nitrilase superfamily (vanins-1, -2, and -3) share significant sequence similarities with biotinidase (86); it is unknown whether vanins use histones as acceptor molecules in transferase reactions. Biotinidase is ubiquitous in mammalian cells and 26% of the cellular biotinidase activity is located in the nuclear fraction (102). Human biotinidase has been characterized at the gene level (36, 37). The 5′-flanking region of exon 1 contains a CCAAT element, three initiator sequences, an octamer sequence, three methylation consensus sites, two GC boxes, and one HNF-5 site, but has no TATA element (37). The 62-amino acid region that harbors the active site of biotinidase is highly conserved among various mammals and *Drosophila* (130).

Subsequent to the elucidation of the biotinidase-mediated mechanism of histone biotinylation in vitro (67, 68), biotinylated histones H1, H2A, H2B, H3, and H4 were detected in human PBMC in vivo (128). Biotinylated histones were also detected in human lymphoma cells (85), small cell lung cancer cells (119), choriocarcinoma cells (39), and chicken erythrocytes (98). These studies also suggested that biotinidase may not be the only enzyme mediating histone biotinylation. For example, evidence showed that biotinylation of histones increases in response to cell proliferation, whereas biotinidase activity was similar in nuclei from proliferating cells and quiescent controls (128). Finally, Gravel and coworkers (94) identified HCS as another enzyme that may catalyze biotinylation of histones.

Mechanisms mediating debiotinylation of histones are largely unknown. Recent studies suggested that biotinidase might catalyze both biotinylation and debiotinylation of histones (5). Variables such as the microenvironment in chromatin and posttranslational modifications and alternate splicing of biotinidase might determine whether biotinidase acts as biotinyl histone transferase or histone debiotinylase. This assumption is based on the following lines of reasoning. First, the availability of substrate might favor either biotinylation or debiotinylation of histones. For example, locally high concentrations of biocytin might increase the rate of histone biotinylation in confined regions of chromatin. Note that the pH is unlikely to affect the biotinylation equilibrium, given that the pH optimum is similar (pH 8) for both the biotinylating activity (67) and the debiotinylating activity of biotinidase (5). Second, proteins may interact with biotinidase at the chromatin level, favoring either biotinylation or debiotinylation of histones. Third, three alternatively spliced variants of biotinidase have been identified (127). Theoretically, these variants may have unique functions in histone metabolism. Fourth, some variants of biotinidase are modified posttranslationally by glycosylation (36, 127), potentially affecting enzymatic activity.

Identification of Biotinylation Sites

Biotinylation sites in human histones were identified by using synthetic peptides (23, 24). Briefly, this approach is based on the following analytical sequence: (*a*) short peptides (<20 amino acids in length) are synthesized chemically; the amino acid sequences in these peptides are based on the sequence in a given region of a given histone; (*b*) peptides are incubated with biotinidase or HCS to conduct enzymatic biotinylation; (*c*) peptides are resolved by electrophoresis; and (*d*) biotin in peptides is probed using streptavidin peroxidase. Amino acid substitutions (e.g., lysine-to-alanine substitutions) and modifications (e.g., acetylation of lysines) in synthetic peptides can be used to corroborate identification of biotinylation sites and to investigate the cross-talk between biotinylation and other known modifications of histones, respectively (24). Using this approach, the following biotinylation sites have been identified in human histones: K9 and K13 in histone H2A (J. Zempleni, unpublished observation), K4, K9, and K18 in histone H3 (118), and K8 and K12 in histone H4 (24). Acetylation and phosphorylation of lysine and serine residues, respectively, decrease biotinylation of adjacent lysine residues (24, 118). In contrast, dimethylation of arginine residues enhances biotinylation of adjacent lysine residues (118). This is consistent with studies suggesting that histones in livers from biotin-deficient rats showed unusual patterns of phosphorylation, methylation, and acetylation compared with biotin-sufficient controls (99).

Biological Functions of Histone Biotinylation

Biotinylation of histones is a relatively new field of research; evidence of biological roles for biotinylation of histones is scarce. However, biotinylation of histones appears to participate in the following biological processes.

First, evidence showed that biotinylation of histones increases in response to cell proliferation in human PBMC (128). Biotinylation of histones increases early in the cell cycle (G1 phase) and remains increased during later phases (S, G2, and M phase) compared with quiescent controls; the increase is greater than fourfold. Fibroblasts from patients with HCS deficiency are severely deficient in histone biotinylation (94). It remains to be determined whether this is associated with decreased proliferation rates. Note that these studies were conducted before specific biotinylation sites in histones were identified and before biotinylation site-specific antibodies became available. Thus, these studies did not allow pinpointing changes in specific biotinylation sites; rather, the global biotinylation of histones was quantified by using streptavidin or radiolabeled biotin.

Second, studies in chicken erythrocytes have provided circumstantial evidence that biotinylated histones are enriched in transcriptionally silent chromatin (98).

Third, biotinylation of histones might play a role in the cellular response to DNA damage (76, 98). If formation of thymine dimers is caused by exposure of lymphoid cells to UV light, the global biotinylation of histones increases (98). If double-stranded DNA breaks are caused by exposure of lymphoid and choriocarcinoma cells to etoposide, biotinylation of K12 in histone H4 shows a rapid and transient decrease (76). This is consistent with a role for histone biotinylation in signaling DNA damage. These studies suggest that distinct kinds of DNA damage cause unique changes in histone biotinylation. Currently, it is unknown whether biotinylation of histones is a mechanism leading to DNA repair or apoptosis.

Biotin Supply

Effects of biotin supply on biotinylation of histones have been investigated in various human-derived cell lines (39, 85, 119). In these studies, cell lines were cultured in media containing deficient, physiological, and pharmacological concentrations of biotin for several weeks. Biotin concentrations in culture media had only a moderate impact on biotinylation of histones; in contrast, biotinylation of carboxylases correlated strongly with biotin concentrations in culture media (39, 85, 119). The reader should note that even small changes in biotinylation of histones might be physiologically meaningful, given that these changes might affect other modifications of histones such as acetylation and methylation.

CONCLUSIONS AND OUTLOOK

In recent years, the groundwork has been laid to characterize roles for biotin in gene expression, cell signaling, and chromatin structure. Numerous clusters of biotin-dependent genes and signaling pathways have been identified. Biotin-dependent signaling pathways regulate the expression of genes that have important biological functions, e.g., in apoptosis and cell survival. Importantly, biotin-dependent cell signals converge at the level of chromatin: At least seven lysine residues in human histones are targets for biotinylation by biotinidase and HCS. Biotinylation of histones appears to be associated with cell proliferation, gene silencing, and the cellular response to DNA damage. Likely, more biotinylation sites in histones await identification. We anticipate that roles of biotin in cell signaling and chromatin structure will lead to the discovery of numerous novel roles for biotin in cell biology and human health, e.g., prevention of tumor initiation. Finally, one can expect to discover new biotinylated proteins in eukaryotic cells. Consistent with this assumption, we have identified novel biotinylation motifs in human proteins, including important signaling molecules (J. Zempleni, unpublished observation). Identification of new biotinylated proteins is likely to add substantially to the importance of biotin in cell biology.

ACKNOWLEDGMENTS

This work was supported by NIH grants DK 60447 and DK 063945, and by NSF EPSCoR grant EPS-0346476. This chapter is a contribution of the University of Nebraska Agricultural Research Division, Lincoln, Nebraska.

The *Annual Review of Nutrition* is online at http://nutr.annualreviews.org

LITERATURE CITED

1. Althaus F. 1992. Poly ADP-ribosylation: a histone shuttle mechanism in DNA excision repair. *J. Cell Sci.* 102:663–70
2. Armstrong SA, Barry DA, Leggett RW, Mueller CR. 1997. Casein kinase II–mediated phosphorylation of the C terminus of Sp1 decreases its DNA binding activity. *J. Biol. Chem.* 272:13489–95
3. Ausio J, van Holde KE. 1986. Histone hyperacetylation: its effect on nucleosome conformation and stability. *Biochemistry* 25:1421–28
4. Baldwin AS. 1996. The NF-κB and IκB proteins: new discoveries and insights. *Annu. Rev. Immunol.* 14:649–81
5. Ballard TD, Wolff J, Griffin JB, Stanley JS, van Calcar S, Zempleni J. 2002. Biotinidase catalyzes debiotinylation of histones. *Eur. J. Nutr.* 41:78–84
6. Barkett M, Gilmore TD. 1999. Control of apoptosis by Rel/NF-κB transcription factors. *Oncogene* 18:6910–24
7. Berg M, Dimroth P. 1998. The biotin protein MadF of the malonate decarboxylase

from *Malonomonas rubra*. *Arch. Microbiol.* 170:464–68
8. Bergeron JJM, Brenner MB, Thomas DY, Williams DB. 1994. Calnexin: a membrane-bound chaperone of the endoplasmic reticulum. *Trends Biochem. Sci.* 19:124–28
9. Bird AW, Yu DY, Pray-Grant MG, Qiu Q, Harmon KE, et al. 2002. Acetylation of histone H4 by Esa1 is required for DNA double-strand break repair. *Nature* 419:411–15
10. Birnbaum MJ, van Wijnen AJ, Odgren PR, Last TJ, Suske G, et al. 1995. Sp1 trans-activation of cell cycle regulated promoters is selectively repressed by Sp3. *Biochemistry* 34:16503–8
11. Black A, Black JD, Azizkhan-Clifford J. 2001. Sp1 and Krüppel-like factor family of transcription factors in cell growth regulation and cancer. *J. Cell. Physiol.* 188: 143–60
12. Boas MA. 1927. The effect of desiccation upon the nutritive properties of egg-white. *Biochem. J.* 21:712–24
13. Boland MP, Foster SJ, O'Neill LAJ. 1997. Daunorubicin activates NFκB and induces κB-dependent gene expression in HL-60 promyelocytic and Jurkat T lymphoma cells. *J. Biol. Chem.* 272:12952–60
14. Borboni P, Magnaterra R, Rabini RA, Staffolani R, Porzio O, et al. 1996. Effect of biotin on glucokinase activity, mRNA expression and insulin release in cultured beta-cells. *Acta Diabetol.* 33:154–58
15. Boulikas T. 1988. At least 60 ADP-ribosylated variant histones are present in nuclei from dimethylsulfate-treated and untreated cells. *EMBO J.* 7:57–67
16. Boulikas T, Bastin B, Boulikas P, Dupuis G. 1990. Increase in histone poly (ADP-ribosylation) in mitogen-activated lymphoid cells. *Exp. Cell Res.* 187:77–84
17. Bowers-Komro DM, McCormick DB. 1985. Biotin uptake by isolated rat liver hepatocytes. In *Biotin*, ed. K Dakshinamurti, HN Bhagavan, pp. 350–58. New York: NY Acad. Sci.
18. Bowman BB, Selhub J, Rosenberg IH. 1986. Intestinal absorption of biotin in the rat. *J. Nutr.* 116:1266–71
19. Brenner C. 2002. Catalysis in the nitrilase superfamily. *Curr. Opin. Struct. Biol.* 12:775–82
20. Brewer JW, Diehl JA. 2000. PERK mediates cell-cycle exit during the mammalian unfolded protein response. *Proc. Natl. Acad. Sci. USA* 97:12625–30
21. Brownell JE, Zhou J, Ranalli T, Kobayashi R, Edmondson DG, et al. 1996. *Tetrahymena* histone acetyltransferase A: a homolog to yeast Gcn5p linking histone acetylation to gene activation. *Cell* 84:843–51
22. Butz CE, McClelland GB, Brooks GA. 2004. MCT1 confirmed in rat striated muscle mitochondria. *J. Appl. Physiol.* 97: 1059–66
23. Camporeale G, Chew YC, Kueh A, Sarath G, Zempleni J. 2005. Use of synthetic peptides for identifying biotinylation sites in human histones. In *Avidin-Biotin Technology in the Life Sciences*, ed. RJ McMahon. Totowa, NJ: Humana. In press
24. Camporeale G, Shubert EE, Sarath G, Cerny R, Zempleni J. 2004. K8 and K12 are biotinylated in human histone H4. *Eur. J. Biochem.* 271:2257–63
25. Caspersen C, Pedersen PS, Treiman M. 2000. The sarco/endoplasmic reticulum calcium-ATPase 2b is an endoplasmic reticulum stress-inducible protein. *J. Biol. Chem.* 275:22363–72
26. Chambon P, Weill JD, Doly J, Strosser MT, Mandel P. 1966. On the formation of a novel adenylic compound by enzymatic extracts of liver nuclei. *Biochem. Biophys. Res. Commun.* 25:638–43
27. Chang HI, Cohen ND. 1983. Regulation and intracellular localization of the biotin holocarboxylase synthetase of 3T3-L1 Cells. *Arch. Biochem. Biophys.* 225:237–47

28. Chatterjee NS, Kumar CK, Ortiz A, Rubin SA, Said HM. 1999. Molecular mechanism of the intestinal biotin transport process. *Am. J. Physiol.* 277:C605–13
29. Chatterjee NS, Rubin SA, Said HM. 2001. Molecular characterization of the 5′ regulatory region of rat sodium-dependent multivitamin transporter gene. *Am. J. Physiol. Cell Physiol.* 280:C548–55
30. Chauhan J, Dakshinamurti K. 1991. Transcriptional regulation of the glucokinase gene by biotin in starved rats. *J. Biol. Chem.* 266:10035–8
31. Cheung P, Allis CD, Sassone-Corsi P. 2000. Signaling to chromatin through histone modifications. *Cell* 103:263–71
32. Deleted in proof
33. Chiba Y, Suzuki Y, Aoki Y, Ishida Y, Narisawa K. 1994. Purification and properties of bovine liver holocarboxylase synthetase. *Arch. Biochem. Biophys.* 313:8–14
34. Clayton AL, Mahadevan LC. 2003. MAP kinase-mediated phosphoacetylation of histone H3 and inducible gene regulation. *FEBS Lett.* 546:51–58
35. Cohen ND, Thomas M. 1982. Biotin transport into fully differentiated 3T3-L1 cells. *Biochem. Biophys. Res. Commun.* 108:1508–16
36. Cole H, Reynolds TR, Lockyer JM, Buck GA, Denson T, et al. 1994. Human serum biotinidase cDNA cloning, sequence, and characterization. *J. Biol. Chem.* 269:6566–70
37. Cole KH, Reynolds TR, Meyers GA, Pomponio RJ, Buck GA, Wolf B. 1998. Structure of the human biotinidase gene. *Mamm. Genome* 9:327–30
38. Collins JC, Paietta E, Green R, Morell AG, Stockert RJ. 1988. Biotin-dependent expression of the asialoglycoprotein receptor in HepG2. *J. Biol. Chem.* 263: 11280–83
39. Crisp SERH, Camporeale G, White BR, Toombs CF, Griffin JB, et al. 2004. Biotin supply affects rates of cell proliferation, biotinylation of carboxylases and histones, and expression of the gene encoding the sodium-dependent multivitamin transporter in JAr choriocarcinoma cells. *Eur. J. Nutr.* 43:23–31
40. Cronan JE Jr. 1989. The *E. coli* bio operon: transcriptional repression by an essential protein modification enzyme. *Cell* 58:427–29
41. Dabbagh O, Brismar J, Gascon GG, Ozand PT. 1994. The clinical spectrum of biotin-treatable encephalopathies in Saudi Arabia. *Brain Dev.* 16(Suppl.):72–80
42. Daberkow RL, White BR, Cederberg RA, Griffin JB, Zempleni J. 2003. Monocarboxylate transporter 1 mediates biotin uptake in human peripheral blood mononuclear cells. *J. Nutr.* 133:2703–6
43. Dakshinamurti K. 2003. Regulation of gene expression by biotin, vitamin B6 and vitamin C. In *Molecular Nutrition*, eds. J Zempleni, H Daniel, pp. 151–65. Oxfordshire: CAB Int.
44. Dakshinamurti K, Chauhan J. 1994. Biotin-binding proteins. In *Vitamin Receptors: Vitamins as Ligands in Cell Communication*, ed. K Dakshinamurti, pp. 200–49. Cambridge, UK: Cambridge Univ. Press
45. Dakshinamurti K, Cheah-Tan C. 1968. Liver glucokinase of the biotin-deficient rat. *Can. J. Biochem.* 46:75–80
46. Dakshinamurti K, Litvak S. 1970. Biotin and protein synthesis in rat liver. *J. Biol. Chem.* 245:5600–5
47. Das KC, White CW. 1997. Activation of NF-κB by antineoplastic agents. *J. Biol. Chem.* 272:14914–20
48. Dey S, Subramanian VS, Chatterjee NS, Rubin SA, Said HM. 2002. Characterization of the 5′ regulatory region of the human sodium-dependent multivitamin transporter, hSMVT. *Biochim. Biophys. Acta* 1574:187–92
49. Dimroth P. 1985. Biotin-dependent decarboxylases as energy transducing system. In *Biotin*, ed. K Dakshinamurti, HN Bhagavan, pp. 72–85. New York: NY Acad. Sci.

50. Dode L, Greef CD, Mountian I, Attard M, Town MM, et al. 1998. Structure of the human sarco-endoplasmic reticulum Ca^{2+}-ATPase 3 gene. *J. Biol. Chem.* 273:13982–94
51. Durkacz BW, Omidiji O, Gray DA, Shall S. 1980. (ADP-ribose)$_n$ participates in DNA excision repair. *Nature* 283:593–96
52. Edelstein LC, Lagos L, Simmons M, Tirumalai H, Gélinas C. 2003. NF-κB-dependent assembly of an enhanceosome-like complex on the promoter region of apoptosis inhibitor Bfl-1/A1. *Mol. Cell. Biol.* 23:2749–61
53. Fischle W, Wang Y, Allis CD. 2003. Histone and chromatin cross-talk. *Curr. Opin. Cell Biol.* 15:172–83
54. Freytag SO, Utter MF. 1983. Regulation of the synthesis and degradation of pyruvate carboxylase in 3T3-L1 cells. *J. Biol. Chem.* 258:6307–12
55. Ghayor G, Chadjichristos C, Herrouin J-F, Ala-Kokko L, Suske G, et al. 2001. Sp3 represses the Sp1-mediated transactivation of the human COL2A1 gene in primary and de-differentiated chondrocytes. *J. Biol. Chem.* 276:36881–95
56. Gorovsky MA. 1973. Macro- and micronuclei of *Tetrahymena pyriformis*: a model system for studying the structure of eukaryotic nuclei. *J. Protozool.* 20:19–25
57. Grafe F, Wohlrab W, Neubert RH, Brandsch M. 2003. Transport of biotin in human keratinocytes. *J. Invest. Dermatol.* 120:428–33
58. Griffin JB, Rodriguez-Melendez R, Dode L, Wuytack F, Zempleni J. 2004. Biotin supplementation decreases the expression of the *SERCA3* gene in Jurkat cells, triggering unfolded protein response. Manuscript submitted
59. Griffin JB, Rodriguez-Melendez R, Zempleni J. 2003. The nuclear abundance of transcription factors Sp1 and Sp3 depends on biotin in Jurkat cells. *J. Nutr.* 133:3409–15
60. Griffin JB, Zempleni J. 2005. Biotin deficiency stimulates survival pathways in human lymphoma cells exposed to antineoplastic drugs. *J. Nutr. Biochem.* 16:96–103
61. Halestrap AP, Price NT. 1999. The proton-linked monocarboxylate transporter (MCT) family: structure, function and regulation. *Biochem. J.* 343:281–99
62. Hebbes TR, Thorne AW, Crane-Robinson C. 1988. A direct link between core histone acetylation and transcriptionally active chromatin. *EMBO J.* 7:1395–402
63. Hebert DN, Foellmer B, Helenius A. 1995. Glucose trimming and reglycosylation determine glycoprotein association with calnexin in the endoplasmic reticulum. *Cell* 81:425–33
64. Henderson BE, Ross RK, Pike MC. 1991. Toward the primary prevention of cancer. *Science* 254:1131–38
65. Hesketh R. 1997. *The Oncogene and Tumour Suppressor Gene FactsBook*. London: Academic. 549 pp.
66. Holmes-McNary MQ, Baldwin AS Jr, Zeisel SH. 2001. Opposing regulation of choline deficiency-induced apoptosis by p53 and nuclear factor κB. *J. Biol. Chem.* 276:41197–204
67. Hymes J, Fleischhauer K, Wolf B. 1995. Biotinylation of histones by human serum biotinidase: assessment of biotinyl-transferase activity in sera from normal individuals and children with biotinidase deficiency. *Biochem. Mol. Med.* 56:76–83
68. Hymes J, Wolf B. 1999. Human biotinidase isn't just for recycling biotin. *J. Nutr.* 129:485S–89
69. Jenuwein T, Allis CD. 2001. Translating the histone code. *Science* 293:1074–80
70. Jeremias I, Kupatt C, Baumann B, Herr I, Wirth T, Debatin KM. 1998. Inhibition of nuclear factor κB activation attenuates apoptosis resistance in lymphoid cells. *Blood* 91:4624–31
71. Jonas CR, Puckett AB, Jones DP, Griffith DP, Szeszycki EE, et al. 2000. Plasma antioxidant status after high-dose

chemotherapy: a randomized trial of parenteral nutrition in bone marrow transplantation patients. *Am. J. Clin. Nutr.* 72: 181–89
72. Juarez-Salinas H, Sims JL, Jacobson MK. 1979. Poly(ADP-ribose) levels in carcinogen-treated cells. *Nature* 282:740–41
73. Kim K-H, McCormick DB, Bier DM, Goodridge AG. 1997. Regulation of mammalian acetyl-coenzyme A carboxylase. *Annu. Rev. Nutr.* 17:77–99
74. Knowles JR. 1989. The mechanism of biotin-dependent enzymes. *Annu. Rev. Biochem.* 58:195–221
75. Kogl F, Tonnis B. 1932. Uber das Bios–Problem. Darstellung von krystallisiertem Biotin aus Eigelb. *Z. Physiol. Chem.* 242: 43–73
76. Kothapalli N, Zempleni J. 2004. Double strand breaks of DNA decrease biotinylation of lysine-12 in histone H4 in JAr cells. *FASEB J.* 18:A103–4
77. Latchman DS. 1998. *Eukaryotic Transcription Factors.* San Diego, CA: Academic
78. Laudet V, Gronemeyer H. 2002. *The Nuclear Receptor Facts Book.* San Diego, CA: Academic
79. Lee DY, Hayes JJ, Pruss D, Wolffe AP. 1993. A positive role for histone acetylation in transcription factor access to nucleosomal DNA. *Cell* 72:73–84
80. Leggett RW, Armstrong SA, Barry D, Mueller CR. 1995. Sp1 is phosphorylated and its DNA binding activity down-regulated upon terminal differentiation of the liver. *J. Biol. Chem.* 270:25879–84
81. Li X, Stark GR. 2002. NFκB-dependent signaling pathways. *Exp. Hematol.* 30: 285–96
82. Liehr JG, Ricci MJ. 1996. 4-Hydroxylation of estrogens as marker of human mammary tumors. *Proc. Natl. Acad. Sci. USA* 93:3294–96
83. Lytton J, Westlin M, Burk SE, Shull GE, MacLennan DH. 1992. Functional comparisons between isoforms of the sarcoplasmic or endoplasmic reticulum family of calcium pumps. *J. Biol. Chem.* 267: 14483–89
84. Macher DRJ, Koch GLE. 1988. Identification of a set of calcium-binding proteins in reticuloplasm, the luminal content of the endoplasmic reticulum. *J. Cell Sci.* 91:61–70
85. Manthey KC, Griffin JB, Zempleni J. 2002. Biotin supply affects expression of biotin transporters, biotinylation of carboxylases, and metabolism of interleukin-2 in Jurkat cells. *J. Nutr.* 132:887–92
86. Maras B, Barra D, Dupre S, Pitari G. 1999. Is pantetheinase the actual identity of mouse and human vanin-1 proteins. *FEBS Lett.* 461:149–52
87. Mardach R, Zempleni J, Wolf B, Cannon MJ, Jennings ML, et al. 2002. Biotin dependency due to a defect in biotin transport. *J. Clin. Invest.* 109:1617–23
88. Mathis DJ, Oudet P, Waslyk B, Chambon P. 1978. Effect of histone acetylation on structure and in vitro transcription of chromatin. *Nucleic Acids Res.* 5:3523–47
89. McCormick DB, Wright LD. 1971. The metabolism of biotin and analogues. In *Metabolism of Vitamins and Trace Elements*, ed. M Florkin, EH Stotz, pp. 81–110. Amsterdam: Elsevier
90. McMahon RJ. 2002. Biotin in metabolism and molecular biology. *Annu. Rev. Nutr.* 22:221–39
91. Mock DM, Lankford GL, Cazin J Jr. 1993. Biotin and biotin analogs in human urine: biotin accounts for only half of the total. *J. Nutr.* 123:1844–51
92. Mock DM, Lankford GL, Mock NI. 1995. Biotin accounts for only half of the total avidin-binding substances in human serum. *J. Nutr.* 125:941–46
93. Mortensen ER, Marks PA, Shiotani A, Merchant JL. 1997. Epidermal growth factor and okadaic acid stimulate Sp1 proteolysis. *J. Biol. Chem.* 272:16540–47
94. Narang MA, Dumas R, Ayer LM, Gravel RA. 2004. Reduced histone biotinylation

in multiple carboxylase deficiency patients: a nuclear role for holocarboxylase synthetase. *Hum. Mol. Genet.* 13:15–23

95. Ozand PT, Gascon GG, Essa MA, Joshi S, Jishi EA, et al. 1998. Biotin-responsive basal ganglia disease: a novel entity. *Brain* 121(Pt. 7):1267–79
96. Pacheco-Alvarez D, Solorzano-Vargas RS, Gravel RA, Cervantes-Roldan R, Velazquez A, Leon-Del-Rio A. 2004. Paradoxical regulation of biotin utilization in brain and liver and implications for inherited multiple carboxylase deficiencies. *J. Biol. Chem.* 279:52312–18
97. Pahl HL. 1999. Signal transduction from the endoplasmic reticulum to the cell nucleus. *Physiol. Rev.* 79:683–700
98. Peters DM, Griffin JB, Stanley JS, Beck MM, Zempleni J. 2002. Exposure to UV light causes increased biotinylation of histones in Jurkat cells. *Am. J. Physiol. Cell Physiol.* 283:C878–84
99. Petrelli F, Coderoni S, Moretti P, Paparelli M. 1978. Effect of biotin on phosphorylation, acetylation, methylation of rat liver histones. *Mol. Biol. Rep.* 4:87–92
100. Petrelli F, Moretti P, Paparelli M. 1979. Intracellular distribution of biotin-14C COOH in rat liver. *Mol. Biol. Rep.* 4:247–52
101. Pham A-D, Sauer F. 2000. Ubiquitin-activating/conjugating activity of $TAF_{II}250$, a mediator of activation of gene expression in *Drosophila*. *Science* 289:2357–60
102. Pispa J. 1965. Animal biotinidase. *Ann. Med. Exp. Biol. Fenn.* 43:4–39
103. Prasad PD, Ramamoorthy S, Leibach FH, Ganapathy V. 1997. Characterization of a sodium-dependent vitamin transporter mediating the uptake of pantothenate, biotin and lipoate in human placental choriocarcinoma cells. *Placenta* 18:527–33
104. Prasad PD, Wang H, Huang W, Fei Y-J, Leibach FH, et al. 1999. Molecular and functional characterization of the intestinal Na^+-dependent multivitamin transporter. *Arch. Biochem. Biophys.* 366:95–106
105. Prasad PD, Wang H, Kekuda R, Fujita T, Fei Y-J, et al. 1998. Cloning and functional expression of a cDNA encoding a mammalian sodium-dependent vitamin transporter mediating the uptake of pantothenate, biotin, and lipoate. *J. Biol. Chem.* 273:7501–6
106. Rao RV, Peel A, Logviniva A, Rio GD, Hermel E, et al. 2002. Coupling endoplasmic reticulum stress to the cell death program: role of the ER chaperone GRP78. *FEBS Lett.* 514:122–28
107. Rodriguez-Melendez R, Griffin JB, Sarath G, Zempleni J. 2005. High-throughput immunoblotting identifies biotin-dependent signaling proteins in HepG2 hepatocarcinoma cells. Manuscript submitted
108. Rodriguez-Melendez R, Griffin JB, Zempleni J. 2004. Biotin supplementation increases expression of the cytochrome P450 1B1 gene in Jurkat cells, increasing the occurrence of single-stranded DNA breaks. *J. Nutr.* 134:2222–28
109. Rodriguez-Melendez R, Griffin JB, Zempleni J. 2005. The expression of genes encoding ribosomal subunits and eukaryotic translation initiation factor 5A depends on biotin and bisnorbiotin in HepG2 cells. Manuscript submitted
110. Rodriguez-Melendez R, Lewis B, McMahon RJ, Zempleni J. 2003. Diaminobiotin and desthiobiotin have biotin-like activities in Jurkat cells. *J. Nutr.* 133:1259–64
111. Rodriguez-Melendez R, Perez-Andrade ME, Diaz A, Deolarte A, Camacho-Arroyo I, et al. 1999. Differential effects of biotin deficiency and replenishment on rat liver pyruvate and propionyl-CoA carboxylases and on their mRNAs. *Mol. Genet. Metabol.* 66:16–23
112. Rodriguez-Melendez R, Schwab LD, Zempleni J. 2004. Jurkat cells respond to biotin deficiency with increased nuclear translocation of NF-κB, mediating cell survival. *Int. J. Vitam. Nutr. Res.* 74:209–16

113. Rodriguez-Melendez R, Zempleni J. 2003. Regulation of gene expression by biotin. *J. Nutr. Biochem.* 14:680–90
114. Rohlff C, Ahmad S, Borellini F, Lei J, Glazer RI. 1997. Modulation of transcription factor Sp1 by cAMP-dependent protein kinase. *J. Biol. Chem.* 272:21137–41
115. Said HM. 1999. Cellular uptake of biotin: mechanisms and regulation. *J. Nutr.* 129:490S–93
116. Said HM. 2004. Recent advances in carrier-mediated intestinal absorption of water-soluble vitamins. *Annu. Rev. Physiol.* 66:419–46
117. Said HM, Redha R. 1987. A carrier-mediated system for transport of biotin in rat intestine in vitro. *Am. J. Physiol.* 252:G52–55
118. Sarath G, Kobza K, Rueckert B, Camporeale G, Zempleni J, Haas E. 2004. Biotinylation of human histone H3 and interactions with biotinidase. *FASEB J.* 18:A103
119. Scheerger SB, Zempleni J. 2003. Expression of oncogenes depends on biotin in human small cell lung cancer cells NCI-H69. *Int. J. Vitam. Nutr. Res.* 73:461–67
120. Shriver BJ, Roman-Shriver C, Allred JB. 1993. Depletion and repletion of biotinyl enzymes in liver of biotin-deficient rats: evidence of a biotin storage system. *J. Nutr.* 123:1140–49
121. Sidrauski C, Brickner JH, Walter P. 2002. The unfolded protein response. In *Protein Targeting, Transport & Translocation*, ed. RE Dalbey, GV Heijne, pp. 151–79. San Diego, CA: Academic
122. Singh IN, Dakshinamurti K. 1988. Stimulation of guanylate cyclase and RNA polymerase II activities in HeLa cells and fibroblasts by biotin. *Mol. Cell. Biochem.* 79:47–56
123. Slaviero KA, Read JA, Clarke SJ, Rivory LP. 2003. Baseline nutritional assessment in advanced cancer patients receiving palliative chemotherapy. *Nutr. Cancer* 46:148–57
124. Sloan GM, Maher M, Brennan MF. 1981. Nutritional effects of surgery, radiation therapy, and adjuvant chemotherapy for soft tissue sarcomas. *Am. J. Clin. Nutr.* 34:1094–102
125. Solorzano-Vargas RS, Pacheco-Alvarez D, Leon-Del-Rio A. 2002. Holocarboxylase synthetase is an obligate participant in biotin-mediated regulation of its own expression and of biotin-dependent carboxylases mRNA levels in human cells. *Proc. Natl. Acad. Sci. USA* 99:5325–30
126. Spence JT, Koudelka AP. 1984. Effects of biotin upon the intracellular level of cGMP and the activity of glucokinase in cultured rat hepatocytes. *J. Biol. Chem.* 259:6393–96
127. Stanley CM, Hymes J, Wolf B. 2004. Identification of alternatively spliced human biotinidase mRNAs and putative localization of endogenous biotinidase. *Mol. Genet. Metab.* 81:300–12
128. Stanley JS, Griffin JB, Zempleni J. 2001. Biotinylation of histones in human cells: effects of cell proliferation. *Eur. J. Biochem.* 268:5424–29
129. Strahl BD, Allis CD. 2000. The language of covalent histone modifications. *Nature* 403:41–45
130. Swango KL, Wolf B. 2001. Conservation of biotinidase in mammals and identification of the putative biotinidase gene in *Drosophila melanogaster*. *Mol. Genet. Metabol.* 74:492–99
131. Sweetman L. 1981. Two forms of biotin-responsive multiple carboxylase deficiency. *J. Inherit. Metab. Dis.* 4:53–54
132. Tang YM, Wo Y-YP, Stewart J, Hawkins AL, Griffin CA, et al. 1996. Isolation and characterization of the human cytochrome P450 *CYP1B1* gene. *J. Biol. Chem.* 271:28324–30
133. Taunton J, Hassig CA, Schreiber SL. 1996. A mammalian histone deacetylase related to a yeast transcriptional regulator Rpd3. *Science* 272:408–11
134. Tissot G, Pepin R, Job D, Douce R, Alban C. 1998. Purification and properties of the chloroplastic form of biotin holocarboxylase synthetase from Arabidopsis thaliana

overexpressed in Escherichia coli. *Eur. J. Biochem.* 258:586–96
135. Tsuchiya Y, Nakajima M, Yokoi Y. 2003. Critical enhancer region to which AhR/ARNT and Sp1 bind in the human *CYP1B1* gene. *J. Biochem.* 133:583–92
136. Turner BM. 2000. Histone acetylation and epigenetic code. *Bioessays* 22:836–45
137. Wang C-Y, Guttridge DC, Mayo MW, Baldwin AS. 1999. NF-κB induces expression of the Bcl-2 homologue A1/Bfl-1 to preferentially suppress chemotherapy-induced apoptosis. *Mol. Cell. Biol.* 19: 5923–29
138. Wang C-Y, Mayo MW, Baldwin AS. 1996. TNF- and cancer therapy-induced apoptosis: potentiation by inhibition of NF-κB. *Science* 274:784–87
139. Wiedmann S, Eudy JD, Zempleni J. 2003. Biotin supplementation causes increased expression of genes encoding interferon-γ, interleukin-1β, and 3-methylcrotonyl-CoA carboxylase, and causes decreased expression of the gene encoding interleukin-4 in human peripheral blood mononuclear cells. *J. Nutr.* 133:716–19
140. Wiedmann S, Rodriguez-Melendez R, Ortega-Cuellar D, Zempleni J. 2004. Clusters of biotin-responsive genes in human peripheral blood mononuclear cells. *J. Nutr. Biochem.* 15:433–39
141. Wo Y-YP, Stewart J, Greenlee WF. 1997. Functional analysis of the promoter for the human *CYP1B1* gene. *J. Biol. Chem.* 272:26702–7
142. Wolf B, Heard GS. 1991. Biotinidase deficiency. In *Advances in Pediatrics*, ed. L Barness, F Oski, pp. 1–21. Chicago: Medical Book Publ.
143. Wolffe A. 1998. *Chromatin*. San Diego, CA: Academic
144. Wood HG, Barden RE. 1977. Biotin enzymes. *Annu. Rev. Biochem.* 46:385–413
145. Yoon YS, Kim JW, Kang KW, Kim YS, Choi KH, Joe CO. 1996. Poly(ADP-ribosyl)ation of histone H1 correlates with internucleosomal DNA fragmentation during apoptosis. *J. Biol. Chem.* 271: 9129–34
146. Yoshida H, Matsui T, Yamamoto A, Okada T, Mori K. 2001. XBP1 mRNA is induced by ATF6 and spliced by IRE1 in response to ER stress to produce a highly active transcription factor. *Cell* 107:881–91
147. Zempleni J. 2001. Biotin. In *Present Knowledge in Nutrition*, ed. BA Bowman, RM Russell, pp. 241–52. Washington, DC: ILSI Press
148. Zempleni J, Helm RM, Mock DM. 2001. In vivo biotin supplementation at a pharmacologic dose decreases proliferation rates of human peripheral blood mononuclear cells and cytokine release. *J. Nutr.* 131:1479–84
149. Zempleni J, Mock DM. 1998. Uptake and metabolism of biotin by human peripheral blood mononuclear cells. *Am. J. Physiol. Cell Physiol.* 275:C382–88
150. Zempleni J, Mock DM. 1999. Bioavailability of biotin given orally to humans in pharmacologic doses. *Am. J. Clin. Nutr.* 69:504–8
151. Zempleni J, Mock DM. 1999. The efflux of biotin from human peripheral blood mononuclear cells. *J. Nutr. Biochem.* 10: 105–9
152. Zempleni J, Mock DM. 1999. Human peripheral blood mononuclear cells: Inhibition of biotin transport by reversible competition with pantothenic acid is quantitatively minor. *J. Nutr. Biochem.* 10: 427–32

Annu. Rev. Nutr. 2005. 25:197–214
doi: 10.1146/annurev.nutr.25.050304.092642

First published online as a Review in Advance on February 11, 2005

REGULATION OF PHOSPHORUS HOMEOSTASIS BY THE TYPE IIa Na/PHOSPHATE COTRANSPORTER

Harriet S. Tenenhouse
Departments of Pediatrics and Human Genetics, McGill University, Montreal Children's Hospital Research Institute, Montreal, Quebec, H3Z 2Z3 Canada; email: harriet.tenenhouse@mcgill.ca

Key Words kidney, hypophosphatemia, Npt2a, FGF-23, PHEX, genetic disease

■ **Abstract** The type IIa Na/phosphate (Pi) cotransporter (Npt2a) is expressed in the brush border membrane (BBM) of renal proximal tubular cells where the bulk of filtered Pi is reabsorbed. Disruption of the *Npt2a* gene in mice elicits hypophosphatemia, renal Pi wasting, and an 80% decrease in renal BBM Na/Pi cotransport, and led to the demonstration that Npt2a is the target for hormonal and dietary regulation of renal Pi reabsorption. Regulation is achieved by changes in BBM abundance of Npt2a protein and requires the interaction of Npt2a with various scaffolding and regulatory proteins. Molecular studies in patients with renal Pi wasting resulted in the identification of novel regulators of Pi homeostasis: fibroblast growth factor-23 (FGF-23) and a phosphate-regulating gene with homologies to endopeptidases on the X chromosome (PHEX). In mouse models, increased FGF-23 production or loss of Phex function causes hypophosphatemia and decreased renal Pi reabsorption, secondary to decreased BBM Npt2a protein abundance. Thus, Npt2a plays a major role in the maintenance of Pi homeostasis in both health and disease.

CONTENTS

0199-9885/05/0714-0197$20.00

INTRODUCTION

Inorganic phosphate (Pi) is fundamental to cellular function and skeletal mineralization. Pi is sufficiently abundant in the normal diet and Pi deficiency is unlikely to develop except under conditions of extreme starvation or as a consequence of administration of a class of therapeutic agents known as Pi binders. Normal Pi intake in the adult human is in the range of 800 to 1600 mg/day. Approximately 65% to 75% of ingested Pi is absorbed in the small intestine, regardless of the level of Pi intake, and hormonal regulation of this process plays only a minor role in normal Pi homeostasis. Absorbed Pi is eliminated or reabsorbed by the kidney, incorporated into organic forms in proliferating cells, and/or deposited as a component of bone mineral (hydroxyapatite). Bone deposition accounts for a much larger percentage of retained Pi during the growth period. However, even in the growing organism only a small percentage of dietary Pi is retained. Most of the absorbed Pi is excreted in the urine. This means that Pi homeostasis and plasma Pi concentration depend primarily on renal mechanisms that regulate tubular Pi transport. In addition, during times of severe dietary Pi deprivation, the Pi contained in bone provides the only source of Pi for the metabolic needs of the organism.

Pi accounts for approximately 1% of body weight (50). Approximately 85% of body Pi is in the skeleton and teeth, 15% in soft tissue, and the remainder (<1%) in extracellular fluid. Pi exists in the plasma in two forms: an organic form, consisting principally of phospholipids and phosphate esters, and an inorganic form (44). Of the total plasma Pi concentration, approximately 29% is in the inorganic form, and only this form of Pi is routinely measured in clinical settings. Of this, 10% to 15% is protein bound and the remainder, which is freely filtered by the renal glomerulus, exists either as "free" Pi ions or as Pi ions complexed with Na, Ca, or Mg. In principle, four forms of inorganic Pi are present in biological solutions: H_3PO_4, $H_2PO_4^-$, HPO_4^{2-}, PO_4^{3-}. However, only HPO_4^{2-} and $H_2PO_4^-$ are present at significant concentrations at physiological pH. The ratio of divalent to monovalent forms can be determined by the Henderson-Hasselbalch equation, $pH = pKa + \log (HPO_4^{2-}/H_2PO_4^-)$. The dissociation constant, pKa, for Pi is 6.8. Thus, at pH 7.4, the ratio of divalent to monovalent Pi anions is essentially 4:1.

In measuring plasma Pi and relating this value to a clinical situation, it is necessary to take into account the diurnal variation in plasma Pi concentration, with a nadir occurring at 9:30 to 10:00 AM and a peak at 4:00 AM (43). The change in Pi concentration from nadir to peak may be as much as 1 mg/dl, which represents a 25% to 35% change in plasma concentration. Plasma Pi concentration also varies as a function of age, with levels highest in the first three months of life in humans. Mice and rats have higher normal plasma Pi values than humans. This difference correlates with differences in basal metabolic rate, which is higher in both rodent species than in humans.

RENAL PHOSPHATE REABSORPTION

The kidney is a major regulator of Pi homeostasis by virtue of its ability to increase or decrease its Pi reabsorptive capacity to accommodate Pi need. Thus, considerable effort has been devoted to the study of Pi transport in the kidney (for reviews, see 12, 46–48, 65, 69).

Physiology and Tubular Localization

The proximal tubule is the major site of Pi reabsorption, with 60% to 80% of the filtered load reclaimed in the proximal convoluted tubule, 15% to 20% in the proximal straight tubule, and a small but variable portion (<10%) in more distal segments of the nephron.

Clearance studies in humans and experimental animals show that when the filtered load of Pi is progressively increased, Pi reabsorption increases until a maximum tubular reabsorptive rate for Pi, or TmP, is reached, after which urinary Pi excretion increases in proportion to the filtered load. The measurement of TmP varies among individuals and within the same individual, due in part to variation in glomerular filtration rate (GFR). Thus, the ratio, TmP/GFR, or maximum tubular reabsorption of Pi per unit of GFR, is the most reliable estimate of the overall tubular Pi reabsorptive capacity (8).

Cellular Aspects

Transepithelial Pi transport across the renal proximal tubular cell is essentially unidirectional and involves uptake across the apical brush border membrane (BBM), translocation across the cell, and efflux at the basolateral membrane. Pi uptake at the apical cell surface is the rate-limiting step in the overall Pi reabsorptive process and the major site of its regulation. It is mediated by Na^+-dependent Pi transporters that depend on the basolateral membrane-associated Na^+/K^+-ATPase to maintain the Na^+-gradient (outside > inside). Na/Pi cotransport is electrogenic and sensitive to changes in pH, with 10- to 20-fold increases documented when the pH is raised from 6 to 8.5. Little is known about the translocation of Pi across the cell or the mechanisms involved in the efflux of Pi at the basolateral cell surface.

Molecular Identification of Na/Phosphate Cotransporters

cDNAs encoding Na/Pi cotransporters, designated type I (Npt1, SLC17A1) and type IIa (Npt2a, SLC34A1; formerly type II, Npt2), were identified in mammalian kidney and share only 20% identity (42, 75). Renal expression of Npt1 and Npt2a is restricted to the proximal tubule where the bulk of filtered Pi is reabsorbed. Although both Npt1 and Npt2a mediate high-affinity Na/Pi cotransport, Npt1, which mediates the flux of Cl and organic anions as well as Pi (9), is not an important player in proximal tubular Pi flux. Npt2a-mediated transport is specific for Pi, is electrogenic, and has a pH profile that bears close resemblance to the pH dependence of Na/Pi cotransport across the renal BBM.

A Na/Pi cotransporter with homology to Npt2a, designated Npt2c, was also identified in mammalian kidney (51, 58). Npt2c is approximately one order of magnitude less abundant than Npt2a at the mRNA level and is expressed exclusively in the BBM of proximal tubular cells (51, 58). The relative abundance of Npt2c protein is significantly higher in kidneys of 22-day-old rats than in those of 60-day-old rats, which suggests that Npt2c is a growth-related renal Na/Pi cotransporter (58).

Two additional Na/Pi cotransporters, designated type III, have been detected in mammalian kidney and account for <1% of renal Na/Pi cotransporter mRNAs. Both are cell-surface viral receptors [gibbon ape leukemia virus (Glvr-1, Pit-1, SLC20A1) and murine amphotropic virus (Ram-1, Pit-2, SLC20A2)] that mediate high-affinity, electrogenic Na-dependent Pi transport (12, 30). Glvr-1 and Ram-1 are widely expressed in mammalian tissues and may serve as "housekeeping" Na/Pi cotransporters. Their precise membrane localization in kidney is not known.

Structure-Function Studies of Npt2a

There is considerable information on the structure of Npt2a (Figure 1). The analytical approaches used to arrive at this structure are summarized as follows: (*a*) hydrophobicity predictions (42); (*b*) antibody accessibility combined with epitope insertion (38); (*c*) cysteine insertion and accessibility of permeant and impermeant sulfhydryl reagents (36, 37); and (*d*) glycosylation (20). These studies demonstrated several important features of Npt2a (Figure 1). The transporter has a large extracellular loop that separates it into two domains (20, 42). There is intramolecular homology within the ICL-1 and ECL-3 domains (36) and both the NH_2- and COOH-termini are oriented intracellularly (38; Figure 1).

The studies described above also addressed the functional significance of specific domains of Npt2a (Figure 1). Cysteine-insertion studies suggested that ICL-1 and ECL-3 comprise an important part of a "permeation pore" that participates in both "cotransport" and "Na^+ leak" function (36, 37). Chimera construction—based on different transport properties of Npt2a and NPT2b, which is not expressed in kidney (22, 42)—suggested the involvement of three amino acid residues in determining the pH dependence of Npt2a, namely, increased transport at higher pH

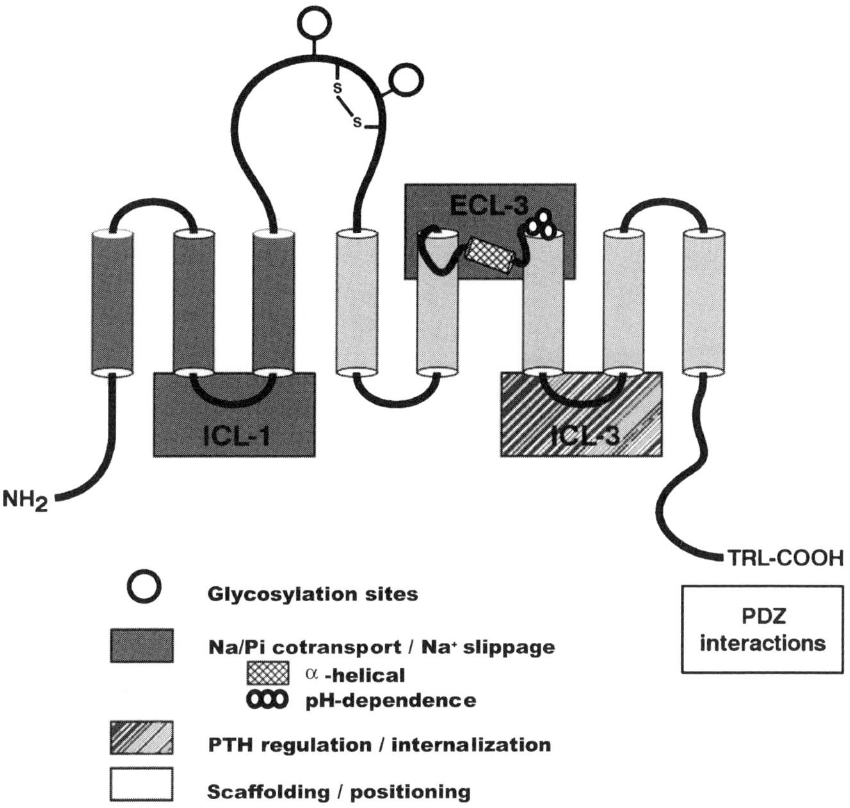

Figure 1 Structure-function relationship of the renal NPT2a Na/Pi cotransporter. See text for details. Reprinted with permission from Reference 69. PDZ, postsynaptic density-95/discs-large/zona occludens-1; PTH, parathyroid hormone.

(13, 14). The chimera approach also suggested the importance of two basic amino acid residues in ICL-3 for parathyroid hormone (PTH)-dependent internalization (28) (see "Parathyroid Hormone" section below). Deletion studies documented that the COOH-terminus contains recognition sequences that play an important role in Npt2a trafficking in response to factors that stimulate or inhibit renal Pi transport (29).

Both the NH_2- and COOH-terminal portions of Npt2a are required for transport activity. However, cleavage of the Npt2a protein backbone, between the two glycosylation sites in the large extracellular loop, does not interfere with transport function (15, 34). It is assumed that under this condition a disulfide bridge within this large extracellular loop stabilizes the transporter (Figure 1). Although Npt2a appears to be part of a multimeric complex (see below), one transporter unit is sufficient to mediate Na/Pi cotransport (35).

REGULATION OF Npt2a AND MOLECULAR MECHANISMS

Regulation of renal Pi reabsorption is achieved primarily by alterations in the abundance of Npt2a protein in the BBM of proximal tubular cells and occurs largely in the absence of changes in Npt2a mRNA (for review, see 47). Variation in apical Npt2a protein amount is accomplished by either membrane insertion or retrieval/lysosomal degradation of the transporter. Although membrane trafficking of Npt2a is a key element in the regulation of renal Pi handling, little is known about the molecular signals that confer specificity to this process, i.e., why other transporters are not inserted into or retrieved from the membrane along with Npt2a. Scaffolding proteins such as PDZK1 (NaPi-Cap1, diphor-1) and NHERF-1 have been shown to interact with Npt2a (16, 17) and play a key role in the maintenance of Npt2a polarity and the formation of regulatory complexes necessary for Npt2a trafficking in response to factors that stimulate or inhibit renal Pi transport (7, 21).

Dietary Phosphate Intake

Dietary Pi intake is a key determinant of renal Pi handling. Both acute and chronic Pi deprivation induce increases in BBM Na/Pi cotransport V_{max} and Npt2a protein abundance but not in Npt2a mRNA (53). The response to Pi deprivation is mediated by microtubule-dependent recruitment of existing Npt2a protein to the apical membrane (41). In contrast, exposure to high dietary Pi intake leads to the internalization of cell surface Npt2a protein into the endosomal compartment by a microtubule-independent mechanism (41). Internalized Npt2a protein is then delivered to the lysosome, by a microtubule-dependent process, for degradation (53).

Parathyroid Hormone

PTH acts directly on proximal tubular cells and inhibits both apical and basolateral Na/Pi cotransport by mechanisms that involve the internalization of cell surface Npt2a protein (31) and its subsequent lysosomal degradation (54). PTH binding to receptors on the basolateral membrane activates protein kinase A (PKA) and/or protein kinase C (PKC) signaling pathways, whereas PTH binding to apical receptors activates PKC (73). The PKA and PKC signaling pathways converge on the extracellular signal-regulated kinase/mitogen-activated protein kinase (ERK/MAPK) pathway to internalize Npt2a protein (3). Although the downstream targets for ERK/MAPK-mediated phosphorylation remain unknown, changes in the phosphorylation state of Npt2a are not associated with its PTH-induced internalization (25). Rather, regulation of Na/Pi cotransport by PTH may be achieved by the phosphorylation of proteins that associate with Npt2a.

AKAP79, an A kinase anchoring protein (33), and RAP, a receptor-associated protein (2), participate in the PTH-mediated retrieval of Npt2a from the plasma membrane of proximal tubular cells. In opossum kidney (OK) cells, AKAP79 associates with Npt2a and the regulatory and catalytic subunits of PKA, and this process is necessary for PKA-dependent inhibition of Na/Pi cotransport (33). In RAP-deficient mice, PTH-induced internalization of Npt2a is significantly delayed (2).

Other Hormonal and Novel Regulators

Other hormones also contribute to the regulation of proximal tubular Pi transport. Growth hormone, insulin-like growth factor-I, insulin, 1,25-dihydroxyvitamin D_3 [1,25$(OH)_2$D], thyroid hormone, and stanniocalcin all stimulate Pi reabsorption, whereas PTH-related peptide, calcitonin, atrial natriuretic factor, epidermal growth factor, transforming growth factor-α, and glucocorticoids inhibit Pi reclamation (for review, see 47). Although there is some evidence that the actions of 1,25$(OH)_2$D, thyroid hormone, and dexamethasone may occur via alterations in *Npt2a* gene transcription, hormonal regulation of renal Pi reabsorption is accomplished for the most part by changes in Npt2a protein abundance without corresponding changes in Npt2a mRNA.

Fibroblast growth factor (FGF)-23 is a novel secreted peptide that regulates renal Pi handling. It is produced by tumors from patients with oncogenic hypophosphatemic osteomalacia (OHO, or tumor-induced osteomalacia) (61), and mutations in the corresponding gene were identified in patients with autosomal dominant hypophosphatemic rickets (ADHR) (1) (see "Disorders of FGF-23 Production and Processing" section below). Administration of FGF-23 to mice elicits significant decreases in serum Pi, renal Pi reabsorption (61), and renal BBM Npt2a protein abundance (59). The hypophosphatemic effect of FGF-23 is independent of PTH (59) and robust in transgenic mice expressing the human *FGF23* gene (39). Targeted disruption of the *Fgf23* gene in mice leads to increases in serum Pi, TmP/GFR, and renal BBM Npt2a protein abundance (60). Thus, FGF-23 is an important regulator of Pi homeostasis.

Secreted frizzled protein-4 (sFRP-4), like FGF-23, is highly expressed in OHO tumors and, when infused in rats, induces an increase in urinary Pi excretion and hypophosphatemia (6). sFRP-4 also inhibits Na/Pi cotransport in OK cell cultures (6).

DISRUPTION OF THE *Npt2a* GENE IN MICE

Given that Npt2a mediates Na/Pi cotransport that is regulated by dietary Pi and PTH, major regulators of renal Pi handling, and is abundantly expressed in the nephron segment where the bulk of filtered Pi is reabsorbed, it was of interest to define its precise contribution to the overall maintenance of Pi homeostasis. To accomplish this goal and determine the impact of Npt2a on skeletal mineralization, the *Npt2a* gene was cloned and characterized (19), and inactivated in mice by targeted mutagenesis (4).

Effect of *Npt2a* Gene Disruption on Clinical and Biochemical Phenotype

Mice homozygous for the disrupted *Npt2a* gene (*Npt2a*$^{-/-}$) are viable, fertile, and do not display any gross physical or behavioral abnormalities. The mutants exhibit increased urinary Pi excretion, an ~80% decrease in renal BBM Na/Pi cotransport, and hypophosphatemia (4). Npt2c is upregulated in *Npt2a*$^{-/-}$ mice and likely accounts for residual renal BBM Na/Pi cotransport in the mutants (64).

Npt2a$^{-/-}$ Mice Fail to Respond to Major Regulators of Renal Pi Transport

PTH had no effect on serum Pi concentration, fractional Pi excretion, and BBM Na/Pi cotransport in *Npt2a*$^{-/-}$ mice, whereas the expected changes in these parameters were elicited in wild-type littermates (78). PTH did elicit a significant increase in urine cAMP in *Npt2a*$^{-/-}$ mice, which indicates that the absence of the PTH response could not be attributed to generalized PTH resistance (78). Moreover, appropriate PTH responses were elicited in Pi-depleted wild-type mice, a finding which suggests that Pi deficiency per se was not responsible for PTH resistance in the mutants (78). *Npt2a*$^{-/-}$ mice also failed to exhibit an adaptive increase in BBM Na/Pi cotransport in response to Pi restriction and to show an age-related decrease in BBM Na/Pi cotransport (23). These findings provide compelling evidence that Npt2a is the target for regulation of renal Pi reabsorption by PTH and dietary Pi and is responsible for the ontogenic pattern of renal Pi handling.

Npt2a Heterozygotes

We reported that urine Pi/creatinine and fractional Pi excretion are modestly increased in mice heterozygous for the disrupted *Npt2a* gene (*Npt2a*$^{+/-}$), relative to wild-type littermates (4). However, these differences were not apparent in mice backcrossed to C57Bl/6J mice for nine generations (Table 1). *Npt2a*$^{+/-}$ mice exhibit a 50% decrease in renal *Npt2a* mRNA abundance, relative to wild-type littermates, whereas both renal BBM Npt2a protein abundance and Na/Pi cotransport are normal in heterozygotes (Table 1), as reported previously (4). These findings indicate that *Npt2a*$^{+/-}$ mice exhibit appropriate adaptive upregulation of Npt2a protein in response to the loss of one *Npt2a* allele. In light of these results, the effects of Pi deprivation were compared in wild-type and *Npt2a*$^{+/-}$ mice. A low-Pi diet elicits significant decreases in serum Pi, urine Pi/creatinine, and fractional Pi excretion, and significant increases in BBM Na/Pi cotransport and Npt2a protein abundance in both groups of mice (Table 1). However, the adaptive BBM responses to Pi restriction are blunted in heterozygotes relative to wild-type littermates (Table 1), consistent with the loss of one *Npt2a* allele. Npt2a mRNA is not increased by Pi deprivation in either wild-type or *Npt2a*$^{+/-}$ mice, confirming that post-transcriptional mechanisms mediate the adaptive response.

TABLE 1 Effect of one copy of the disrupted *Npt2a* gene and dietary Pi intake on serum and urine Pi and renal Na/Pi cotransport and *Npt2a* gene expression

	Wild-type mice		***Npt2a***$^{+/-}$ **mice**	
Genotype diet	**1% Pi**	**0.02% Pi**	**1% Pi**	**0.02% Pi**
Serum Pi (mM)	2.5 ± 1.3	1.3 ± 0.2[a]	2.6 ± 0.3	1.4 ± 0.3[a]
Urine Pi/Cr	34 ± 7	0.5 ± 0.2[a]	36 ± 4	0.7 ± 0.7[a]
FEI-Pi	15 ± 3	0.4 ± 0.2[a]	15 ± 4	0.5 ± 0.2[a]
Npt2a mRNA (%)	100 ± 13	76 ± 23	47 ± 5[b]	59 ± 8
Npt2a protein (%)	100 ± 16	1727 ± 226[a]	108 ± 17	808 ± 76[a,b]
Na/Pi cotransport (%)	100 ± 6	412 ± 36[a]	102 ± 19	274 ± 43[a,b]

Wild-type (+/+) and *Npt2a*$^{+/-}$ (+/−) mice (70 ± 10 days of age, n = 5–8 mice/group) were fed diets containing 1% and 0.02% Pi for five days and serum, urine, and renal parameters determined as described in text (4).

[a]Effect of diet.

[b]Effect of genotype, $p < 0.05$.

Abbreviations: Pi, inorganic phosphate; Cr, creatinine; FEI, fractional excretion index; NPT2a, type IIa Na/phosphate cotransporter.

CALCIUM HOMEOSTASIS IN *Npt2a*$^{-/-}$ MICE

The serum concentration of 1,25(OH)$_2$D and the serum and urine concentrations of Ca are significantly increased in *Npt2a*$^{-/-}$ mice when compared with wild-type littermates (4). To define the mechanisms responsible for these increases, the effects of *Npt2a* gene ablation on intestinal Ca absorption and renal vitamin D metabolism were examined.

Intestinal Calcium Hyperabsorption

The observation that hypercalcemia and hypercalciuria are corrected in *Npt2a*$^{-/-}$ mice after an overnight fast suggested that dietary Ca intake is necessary for these abnormalities to manifest (63). Subsequent studies revealed that both absorption of ^{45}Ca by isolated duodenal loops and ^{45}Ca appearance in the plasma are increased in *Npt2a*$^{-/-}$ mice relative to wild-type littermates (63). In addition, the increase in duodenal Ca absorption in *Npt2a*$^{-/-}$ mice is associated with significant increases in the duodenal expression of ECaC1 (TRPV5) and ECaC2 (TRPV6), thereby implicating both epithelial Ca channels in mediating the intestinal response (63).

Upregulation of Renal 1,25-Dihydroxyvitamin D Synthesis

The elevated serum concentration of 1,25(OH)$_2$D in *Npt2a*$^{-/-}$ mice suggested that the mutants can increase their renal synthesis of the vitamin D hormone in response to endogenous hypophosphatemia (4). This notion was confirmed by the demonstration of increased activity and mRNA abundance of renal mitochondrial

1α-hydroxylase, the enzyme responsible for the biosynthesis of 1,25$(OH)_2$D (68). In addition, the mutants exhibit a decrease in the mRNA abundance of renal 24-hydroxylase (68), the enzyme responsible for catabolism of 1,25$(OH)_2$D to its final inactivation product. Furthermore, *Npt2a*$^{-/-}$ mice mounted a further increase in renal 1α-hydroxylase activity and mRNA and serum 1,25$(OH)_2$D concentration in response to dietary Pi restriction (68). Therefore, contrary to a previously held notion, normal renal Na/Pi cotransport is not necessary for the regulation of renal 1,25$(OH)_2$D production by Pi.

Thus, hypophosphatemia, secondary to targeted disruption of the *Npt2a* gene, serves as a trigger for increased renal synthesis and decreased renal catabolism of 1,25$(OH)_2$D. This results in increased serum 1,25$(OH)_2$D levels, intestinal Ca hyperabsorption, increased intestinal expression of ECaC1 and ECaC2, and the development of hypercalcemia and hypercalciuria in the mutant strain. Reduced serum PTH levels, secondary to increased serum 1,25$(OH)_2$D, also contribute to hypercalciuria in *Npt2a*$^{-/-}$ mice (4).

Renal Calcification

Because hypercalciuria is a risk factor for the development of nephrocalcinosis, kidneys from wild-type and knockout mice were examined for renal calcification (11). Von Kossa staining of renal sections and microcomputed tomography of intact kidneys revealed mineral deposits, composed of Ca and Pi, in kidneys of *Npt2a*$^{-/-}$ mice but not in wild-type littermates (11) or in *Npt2a* heterozygotes (unpublished findings). Pi supplementation or 1α-hydroxylase gene ablation reduced urine Ca/creatinine and renal calcification in *Npt2a*$^{-/-}$ mice (67). Furthermore, both treatments were associated with significant decreases in serum 1,25$(OH)_2$D levels, attesting to a key role of the vitamin D hormone in the development of nephrocalcinosis in *Npt2a*$^{-/-}$ mice (67).

Npt2a IN BONE

Npt2a Expression and Protein Interactions in the Osteoclast

Npt2a mRNA and protein were detected in osteoclasts, the cells mediating bone resorption (18, 32), but not in osteoblasts, the cells responsible for bone formation. Furthermore, Npt2a in mouse osteoclasts interacts with NHERF-1, a PDZ protein that is essential for Npt2a trafficking in kidney (see "Regulation of Npt2a and Molecular Mechanisms" section above), and colocalizes with NHERF-1 and actin at the osteoclast plasma membrane (32). These findings suggest that similar mechanisms are involved in Npt2a membrane sorting and regulation in both tissues.

Skeletal Phenotype in *Npt2a*$^{-/-}$ Mice

Npt2a gene disruption is associated with age-dependent skeletal abnormalities (4). At weaning, *Npt2a*$^{-/-}$ mice exhibit retarded secondary ossification, increased

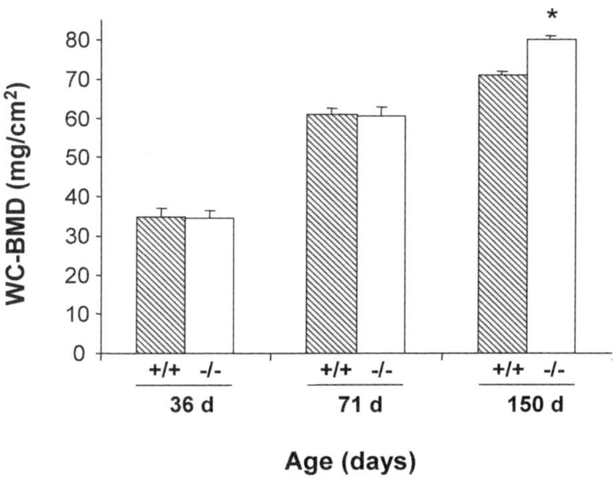

Figure 2 Effect of the *Npt2a* gene knockout on longitudinal bone mineral density. Bone mineral density was determined in vivo on both femora in wild-type (+/+) and *Npt2a*$^{-/-}$ mice at 36, 71, and 150 days of age. Weight-corrected bone mineral density (WC-BMD) was calculated by regression residuals as described by Orwoll et al. (52). Means ± SD for each 10–12 mice per group are shown. *$P < 0.05$.

trabecular thickness, and a reduction in osteoclast number (4, 18). With increasing age, the decrease in osteoclast number is less pronounced and indices of bone formation are increased in the mutants, relative to wild-type littermates (18). These studies provide evidence for osteoclast dysfunction and osteoblast adaptation in Npt2a-deficient mice, and demonstrate that both the osteoclast and the proximal tubule must be considered in the role of Npt2a on Pi homeostasis.

Based on the above findings (18, 32), we hypothesized that bone resorption is compromised and bone mineral density increased in the mutants. A longitudinal study revealed that bone mineral density is significantly increased in 150-day-old *Npt2a*$^{-/-}$ mice when compared with age-matched wild-type mice (Figure 2, unpublished data, H.S. Tenenhouse). Further work is necessary to establish whether loss of Npt2a function protects the skeleton from age-related bone loss.

Npt2a IN PHOSPHATE-DEFICIENCY DISORDERS

Disorders of FGF-23 Production and Processing

One acquired (OHO) and two Mendelian [ADHR and X-linked hypophosphatemia (XLH)] hypophosphatemic bone disorders are characterized by hypophosphatemia, decreased renal Pi reabsorption, normal-to-low serum $1,25(OH)_2D$ concentrations that are inappropriate for the degree of hypophosphatemia, and rickets and osteomalacia (66). Based on these similarities and the studies described below, it has been hypothesized that defects in a common metabolic pathway involving FGF-23 can explain the underlying basis for renal Pi wasting in all three disorders.

Excision of tumors from OHO patients corrects the clinical and biochemical abnormalities, which indicates that factors secreted by the tumor are responsible for the phenotypic features that characterize this disorder (for review, see 57). Molecular analysis of OHO tumors led to the demonstration of abundant expression of FGF-23 (61) (see "Other Hormonal and Novel Regulators" section above). In addition, serum FGF-23 concentrations are markedly elevated in OHO patients (27). These findings support the hypothesis that renal Pi wasting in OHO can be attributed to excess tumor production of FGF-23 and is likely associated with decreased renal BBM NPT2a abundance, as reported in mice (39).

Missense mutations in the *FGF23* gene were identified in patients with ADHR (1). The mutations involve two Arg residues that reside in a consensus proprotein convertase cleavage site, RHTR (ArgHisThrArg), and prevent the processing of the secreted, 227 amino acid FGF-23 peptide to its 155 amino acid N-terminal and 72 amino acid C-terminal fragments (76). The mutant FGF-23 peptide retains full phosphaturic activity, whereas neither the N- nor C-terminal fragments derived from the wild-type peptide exhibit phosphaturic activity (62). Because the arg mutations stabilize the full-length FGF-23 peptide, it is likely that in ADHR the mutant peptide is responsible for Pi wasting by decreasing the BBM abundance of NPT2a protein. Serum concentrations of FGF-23 have not yet been reported in ADHR patients.

XLH is caused by mutations in *PHEX*, a Pi-regulating gene with homology to endopeptidases on the X-chromosome (24), which is expressed in bones and teeth but not in kidney (56). In *Hyp* mice, which harbor a large 3′ deletion in the *Phex* gene (5), renal Pi wasting has been attributed to a 50% decrease in renal BBM Na/Pi cotransport and Npt2a protein abundance (70). Furthermore, parabiosis (45) and renal transplantation (49) studies in *Hyp* mice demonstrated that a circulating factor(s) is responsible for hypophosphatemia and decreased renal Pi reabsorption in the mutants. In this regard, it is of interest that serum FGF-23 levels are more than tenfold higher in *Hyp* mice (77) and significantly elevated in XLH patients (27), relative to normal counterparts. However, the mechanisms whereby loss of Phex/PHEX function leads to FGF-23 accumulation are unknown. Both decreases in FGF-23 degradation (10) and increases in FGF-23 synthesis (40) have been proposed.

Hereditary Hypophosphatemic Rickets with Hypercalciuria

Hereditary hypophosphatemic rickets with hypercalciuria (HHRH) is a Pi wasting disorder first described in a large Bedouin kindred (66, 71, 72). Although the biochemical features of HHRH patients closely resemble those of $Npt2a^{-/-}$ mice and clinical studies suggest that HHRH is a primary renal Pi wasting disorder (71), putative disease-causing mutations in the *NPT2a* gene were not identified in patients with this disorder (26). Furthermore, two single-nucleotide polymorphisms in the *NPT2a* gene failed to segregate with HHRH in the Bedouin kindred (26). These studies excluded *NPT2a* as a candidate gene and suggested that another Na/Pi cotransporter or a regulator thereof is responsible for HHRH.

Heterozygous *Npt2a* Mutations

Heterozygous missense mutations in the *NPT2a* gene were identified in two individuals with renal Pi wasting and hypophosphatemia, associated with either urolithiasis or osteoporosis (55). Although it was suggested that each amino acid substitution was sufficient for the expression of the respective phenotypic abnormalities (55), functional studies of the mutant *NPT2a* cDNAs in Xenopus oocytes failed to provide evidence for altered kinetics or dominant negative effects (74). The latter findings and the demonstration that BBM Na/Pi cotransport and Npt2a protein abundance are normal in mice heterozygous for the disrupted *Npt2a* gene (Table 1) (4) indicate that the heterozygous mutations in *NPT2a* cannot account for renal Pi wasting and hypophosphatemia in the patients studied (55).

SUMMARY AND CONCLUSIONS

Npt2a resides in the BBM of renal proximal tubular cells and plays a crucial role in the maintenance of Pi homeostasis. Npt2a is a target for regulation by PTH and dietary Pi, which elicit changes in Npt2a protein abundance in the BBM and require the interaction of Npt2a with a variety of scaffolding and regulatory proteins essential for its membrane insertion, retrieval, and degradation. Targeted disruption of the *Npt2a* gene in mice underscored the importance of Npt2a in the regulation of renal Pi reabsorption and maintenance of Pi balance, and suggested a role for Npt2a in osteoclast function. Two novel Pi regulating genes, *FGF23* and *PHEX*, which are mutated in patients with Mendelian Pi wasting disorders, have been identified and studies in mouse models demonstrated that increased circulating levels of FGF-23 or loss of Phex function induces hypophosphatemia by decreasing the renal BBM abundance of Npt2a protein. Future studies are necessary to uncover additional renal Na/Pi cotransporters, and regulators thereof, and to define the precise mechanisms whereby FGF-23 and PHEX regulate renal Pi handling.

ACKNOWLEDGMENTS

Work in the author's laboratory was supported by grants from the Canadian Institutes of Health Research. Thanks to Dr. Y. Sabbagh for critical review of the manuscript.

The *Annual Review of Nutrition* is online at http://nutr.annualreviews.org

LITERATURE CITED

1. ADHR Consortium. 2000. Autosomal dominant hypophosphataemic rickets is associated with mutations in FGF23. *Nat. Genet.* 26:345–48
2. Bacic D, Capuano P, Gisler SM, Pribanic S, Christensen EI, et al. 2003. Impaired PTH-induced endocytotic down-regulation of the renal type IIa Na(+)/P(i)-cotransporter in RAP-deficient mice with reduced megalin expression. *Pflugers Arch.* 446:475–84
3. Bacic D, Schulz N, Biber J, Kaissling B, Murer H, Wagner CA. 2003. Involvement of the MAPK-kinase pathway in the PTH-mediated regulation of the proximal tubule type IIa Na(+)/P(i) cotransporter in mouse kidney. *Pflugers Arch.* 446:52–60
4. Beck L, Karaplis AC, Amizuka N, Hewson AS, Ozawa H, Tenenhouse HS. 1998. Targeted inactivation of *Npt2* in mice leads to severe renal phosphate wasting, hypercalciuria and skeletal abnormalities. *Proc. Natl. Acad. Sci. USA* 95:5372–77
5. Beck L, Soumounou Y, Martel J, Krishnamurthy G, Gauthier C, et al. 1997. *Pex/PEX* tissue distribution and evidence for a deletion in the 3′ region of the *Pex* gene in X-linked hypophosphatemic mice. *J. Clin. Invest.* 99:1200–9
6. Berndt T, Craig TA, Bowe AE, Vassiliadis J, Reczek D, et al. 2003. Secreted frizzled-related protein 4 is a potent tumor-derived phosphaturic agent. *J. Clin. Invest.* 112:785–94
7. Biber J. 2001. Emerging roles of transporter-PDZ complexes in renal proximal tubular reabsorption. *Pflugers Arch.* 443:3–5
8. Bijvoet O. 1976. The importance of the kidney in phosphate homeostasis. In *Phosphate Metabolism, Kidney and Bone*, ed. L Avioli, P Bordier, H Fleisch, S Massry, E Slatopolsky. Paris: Armour-Montagu
9. Busch AE, Schuster A, Waldegger S, Wagner CA, Zempel G, et al. 1996. Expression of a renal type I sodium/phosphate transporter (NaPi-1) induces a conductance in *Xenopus* oocytes permeable for organic and inorganic anions. *Proc. Natl. Acad. Sci. USA* 93:5347–51
10. Campos M, Couture C, Hirata IY, Juliano MA, Loisel TP, et al. 2003. Human recombinant PHEX has a strict S1′ specificity for acidic residues and cleaves peptides derived from FGF-23 and MEPE. *Biochem. J.* 373:271–79
11. Chau H, El-Maadawy S, McKee MD, Tenenhouse HS. 2003. Renal calcification in mice homozygous for the disrupted type IIa Na/Pi cotransporter gene *Npt2*. *J. Bone Miner. Res.* 18:644–57
12. Collins JF, Bai L, Ghishan FK. 2004. The SLC20 family of proteins: dual functions as sodium-phosphate cotransporters and viral receptors. *Pflugers Arch.* 447(5):647–52
13. de la Horra C, Hernando N, Forster I, Biber J, Murer H. 2001. Amino acids involved in sodium interaction of murine type II Na(+)-P(i) cotransporters expressed in *Xenopus* oocytes. *J. Physiol.* 531:383–91
14. de la Horra C, Hernando N, Lambert G, Forster I, Biber J, Murer H. 2000. Molecular determinants of pH sensitivity of the type IIa Na/P(i) cotransporter. *J. Biol. Chem.* 275:6284–7
15. Ehnes C, Forster IC, Kohler K, Biber J, Murer H. 2002. Functional studies on a split type II Na/Pi-cotransporter. *J. Membr. Biol.* 188:227–36
16. Gisler SM, Madjdpour C, Bacic D, Pribanic S, Taylor SS, et al. 2003. PDZK1: II. An anchoring site for the PKA-binding protein D-AKAP2 in renal proximal tubular cells. *Kidney Int.* 64:1746–54
17. Gisler SM, Stagljar I, Traebert M, Bacic D, Biber J, Murer H. 2001. Interaction of the type IIa Na/Pi cotransporter with

PDZ proteins. *J. Biol. Chem.* 276:9206–13
18. Gupta A, Tenenhouse HS, Hoag HM, Wang D, Khadeer MA, et al. 2001. Identification of the type II Na^+-Pi cotransporter (Npt2) in the osteoclast and the skeletal phenotype of $Npt2^{-/-}$ mice. *Bone* 29:467–76
19. Hartmann CM, Hewson AS, Kos CH, Hilfiker H, Soumoumou Y, et al. 1996. Structure of murine and human renal type II Na^+-phosphate cotransporter genes (*Npt2* and NPT2). *Proc. Natl. Acad. Sci. USA* 93:7409–14
20. Hayes G, Busch A, Lotscher M, Waldegger S, Lang F, et al. 1994. Role of *N*-linked glycosylation in rat renal Na/Pi-cotransport. *J. Biol. Chem.* 269:24143–49
21. Hernando N, Wagner CA, Gisler SM, Biber J, Murer H. 2004. PDZ proteins and proximal ion transport. *Curr. Opin. Nephrol. Hypertens.* 13:569–74
22. Hilfiker H, Hattenhauer O, Traebert M, Forster I, Murer H, Biber J. 1998. Characterization of a murine type II sodium-phosphate cotransporter expressed in mammalian small intestine. *Proc. Natl. Acad. Sci. USA* 95:14564–69
23. Hoag HM, Martel J, Gauthier C, Tenenhouse HS. 1999. Effects of *Npt2* gene ablation and low-phosphate diet on renal Na/phosphate cotransport and cotransporter gene expression. *J. Clin. Invest.* 104:679–86
24. HYP Consortium. 1995. A gene (PEX) with homologies to endopeptidases is mutated in patients with X-linked hypophosphatemic rickets. *Nat. Genet.* 11:130–36
25. Jankowski M, Hilfiker H, Biber J, Murer H. 2001. The opossum kidney cell type IIa Na/P(i) cotransporter is a phosphoprotein. *Kidney Blood Press. Res.* 24:1–4
26. Jones AO, Tzenova J, Frappier D, Crumley M, Roslin NM, et al. 2001. Hereditary hypophosphatemic rickets with hypercalciuria is not caused by mutations in the Na/Pi cotransporter *NPT2* gene. *J. Am. Soc. Nephrol.* 12:507–14
27. Jonsson KB, Zahradnik R, Larsson T, White KE, Sugimoto T, et al. 2002. Fibroblast growth factor 23 in oncogenic osteomalacia and X-linked hypophosphatemia. *N. Engl. J. Med.* 348:1656–63
28. Karim-Jimenez Z, Hernando N, Biber J, Murer H. 2000. A dibasic motif involved in parathyroid hormone-induced down-regulation of the type IIa NaPi cotransporter. *Proc. Natl. Acad. Sci. USA* 97:12896–901
29. Karim-Jimenez Z, Hernando N, Biber J, Murer H. 2001. Molecular determinants for apical expression of the renal type IIa Na+/Pi-cotransporter. *Pflugers Arch.* 442:782–90
30. Kavanaugh MP, Miller DG, Zhang W, Law W, Kozak SL, et al. 1994. Cell-surface receptors for gibbon ape leukemia virus and amphotropic murine retrovirus are inducible sodium-phosphate symporters. *Proc. Natl. Acad. Sci. USA* 91: 7071–75
31. Kempson SA, Lotscher M, Kaissling B, Biber J, Murer H, Levi M. 1995. Parathyroid hormone action on phosphate transporter mRNA and protein in rat renal proximal tubules. *Am. J. Physiol.* 268:F784–91
32. Khadeer MA, Tang Z, Tenenhouse HS, Eiden MV, Murer H, et al. 2003. Na+-dependent phosphate transporters in the murine osteoclast: cellular distribution and protein interactions. *Am. J. Physiol. Cell Physiol.* 284:1633–44
33. Khundmiri SJ, Rane MJ, Lederer ED. 2003. Parathyroid hormone regulation of type II sodium-phosphate cotransporters is dependent on an A kinase anchoring protein. *J. Biol. Chem.* 278:10134–41
34. Kohl B, Wagner CA, Huelseweh B, Busch AE, Werner A. 1998. The Na+-phosphate cotransport system (NaPi-II) with a cleaved protein backbone: implications on function and membrane insertion. *J. Physiol.* 508:341–50
35. Kohler K, Forster IC, Lambert G, Biber J, Murer H. 2000. The functional unit of the renal type IIa Na+/Pi cotransporter is a monomer. *J. Biol. Chem.* 275:26113–20

36. Kohler K, Forster IC, Stange G, Biber J, Murer H. 2002. Identification of functionally important sites in the first intracellular loop of the NaPi-IIa cotransporter. *Am. J. Physiol.* 282:F687–96
37. Lambert G, Forster IC, Stange G, Kohler K, Biber J, Murer H. 2001. Cysteine mutagenesis reveals novel structure-function features within the predicted third extracellular loop of the type IIa Na(+)/P(i) cotransporter. *J. Gen. Physiol.* 117:533–46
38. Lambert G, Traebert M, Hernando N, Biber J, Murer H. 1999. Studies on the topology of the renal type II NaPi-cotransporter. *Pflugers Arch.* 437:972–78
39. Larsson T, Marsell R, Schipani E, Ohlsson C, Ljunggren O, et al. 2004. Transgenic mice expressing fibroblast growth factor 23 under the control of the alpha1(I) collagen promoter exhibit growth retardation, osteomalacia, and disturbed phosphate homeostasis. *Endocrinology* 145:3087–94
40. Liu S, Guo R, Simpson LG, Xiao ZS, Burnham CE, Quarles LD. 2003. Regulation of fibroblastic growth factor 23 expression but not degradation by PHEX. *J. Biol. Chem.* 278:37419–26
41. Lotscher M, Kaissling B, Biber J, Murer H, Levi M. 1997. Role of microtubules in the rapid regulation of renal phosphate transport in response to acute alterations in dietary phosphate content. *J. Clin. Invest.* 99:1302–12
42. Magagnin S, Werner A, Markovich D, Sorribas V, Stange G, et al. 1993. Expression cloning of human and rat renal cortex Na/Pi cotransport. *Proc. Natl. Acad. Sci. USA* 90:5979–83
43. Markowitz M, Rotkin L, Rosen JF. 1981. Circadian rhythms of blood minerals in humans. *Science* 213:672–74
44. Marshall RW. 1976. Plasma fractions. In *Calcium, Phosphate and Magnesium Metabolism*, ed. BEC Nordin, pp. 162–85. New York: Churchill Livingstone
45. Meyer RA Jr, Tenenhouse HS, Meyer MH, Klugerman AH. 1989. The renal phosphate transport defect in normal mice parabiosed to X-linked hypophosphatemic mice persists after parathyroidectomy. *J. Bone Miner. Res.* 4:523–32
46. Murer H, Forster I, Biber J. 2004. The sodium phosphate cotransporter family SLC34. *Pflugers Arch.* 447(5):763–67
47. Murer H, Hernando N, Forster I, Biber J. 2000. Proximal tubular phosphate reabsorption: molecular mechanisms. *Physiol. Rev.* 80:1373–409
48. Murer H, Hernando N, Forster I, Biber J. 2003. Regulation of Na/Pi transporter in the proximal tubule. *Annu. Rev. Physiol.* 65:531–42
49. Nesbitt T, Coffman TM, Griffiths R, Drezner MK. 1992. Cross-transplantation of kidneys in normal and *Hyp* mice: evidence that the *Hyp* phenotype is unrelated to an intrinsic renal defect. *J. Clin. Invest.* 89:1453–59
50. Nordin BEC. 1976. Nutritional considerations. In *Calcium, Phosphate and Magnesium Metabolism*, ed. BEC Nordin, pp. 1–35. New York: Churchill Livingstone
51. Ohkido I, Segawa H, Yanagida R, Nakamura M, Miyamoto K. 2003. Cloning, gene structure and dietary regulation of the type-IIc Na/Pi cotransporter in the mouse kidney. *Pflugers Arch.* 446:106–15
52. Orwoll ES, Belknap JK, Klein RF. 2001. Gender specificity in the genetic determinants of peak bone mass. *J. Bone Miner. Res.* 16:1962–71
53. Pfister MF, Hilfiker H, Forgo J, Lederer E, Biber J, Murer H. 1998. Cellular mechanisms involved in the acute adaptation of OK cell Na/Pi-cotransport to high- or low-Pi medium. *Pflugers Arch.* 435:713–19
54. Pfister MK, Ruf I, Stange G, Ziegler U, Lederer E, Biber J. 1998. Parathyroid hormone leads to the lysosomal degradation of the renal type II Na/Pi cotransporter. *Proc. Natl. Acad. Sci. USA* 95:1909–14
55. Prie D, Huart V, Bakouh N, Planelles G, Dellis O, et al. 2002. Nephrolithiasis and osteoporosis associated with hypophosphatemia caused by mutations in the type

IIa sodium-phosphate cotransporter. *N. Engl. J. Med.* 347:983–91
56. Ruchon AF, Tenenhouse HS, Marcinkiewicz M, Siegfried G, Aubin JE, et al. 2000. Developmental expression and tissue distribution of Phex protein: effect of the Hyp mutation and relationship to bone markers. *J. Bone Miner. Res.* 15:1440–50
57. Schiavi SC, Kumar R. 2004. The phosphatonin pathway: new insights in phosphate homeostasis. *Kidney Int.* 65:1–14
58. Segawa H, Kaneko I, Takahashi A, Kuwahata M, Ito M, et al. 2002. Growth-related renal type II Na/Pi cotransporter. *J. Biol. Chem.* 277:19665–72
59. Shimada T, Hasegawa H, Yamazaki Y, Muto T, Hino R, et al. 2004. FGF-23 is a potent regulator of vitamin D metabolism and phosphate homeostasis. *J. Bone Miner. Res.* 19:429–35
60. Shimada T, Kakitani M, Yamazaki Y, Hasegawa H, Takeuchi Y, et al. 2004. Targeted ablation of Fgf23 demonstrates an essential physiological role of FGF23 in phosphate and vitamin D metabolism. *J. Clin. Invest.* 113:561–68
61. Shimada T, Mizutani S, Muto T, Yoneya T, Hino R, et al. 2001. Cloning and characterization of FGF23 as a causative factor of tumor-induced osteomalacia. *Proc. Natl. Acad. Sci. USA* 98:6500–5
62. Shimada T, Muto T, Urakawa I, Yoneya T, Yamazaki Y, et al. 2002. Mutant FGF-23 responsible for autosomal dominant hypophosphatemic rickets is resistant to proteolytic cleavage and causes hypophosphatemia in vivo. *Endocrinology* 143:3179–82
63. Tenenhouse HS, Gauthier C, Martel J, Hoenderop JGJ, Hartog A, et al. 2002. Na/Pi cotransporter (*Npt2*) gene disruption increases duodenal calcium absorption and expression of epithelial calcium channel 1 and 2. *Pflugers Arch.* 444:670–76
64. Tenenhouse HS, Martel J, Gauthier C, Segawa H, Miyamoto K. 2003. Differential effects of *Npt2a* gene ablation and the X-linked *Hyp* mutation on renal expression of type IIc Na/Pi cotransporter. *Am. J. Physiol.* 285:F1271–78
65. Tenenhouse HS. 1999. Recent advances in epithelial sodium-coupled phosphate transport. *Curr. Opin. Nephrol. Hypertens.* 8:407–14
66. Tenenhouse HS, Econs MJ. 2001. Mendelian hypophosphatemias. In *The Metabolic and Molecular Bases of Inherited Disease*, ed. CR Scriver, AL Beaudet, WS Sly, D Valle, pp. 5039–67. New York: McGraw-Hill
67. Tenenhouse HS, Gauthier C, Chau H, St Arnaud R. 2004. 1a-Hydroxylase gene ablation and Pi supplementation inhibit renal calcification in mice homozygous for the disrupted Na/Pi cotransporter gene *Npt2a*. *Am. J. Physiol. Renal Physiol.* 286:F675–81
68. Tenenhouse HS, Martel J, Gauthier C, Zhang MYH, Portale AA. 2001. Renal expression of the sodium/phosphate cotransporter gene, *Npt2*, is not required for regulation of renal 1a-hydroxylase by phosphate. *Endocrinology* 142:1124–29
69. Tenenhouse HS, Murer H. 2003. Disorders of renal tubular phosphate transport. *J. Am. Soc. Nephrol.* 14:240–47
70. Tenenhouse HS, Werner A, Biber J, Ma S, Martel J, et al. 1994. Renal Na^+-phosphate cotransport in murine X-linked hypophosphatemic rickets: molecular characterization. *J. Clin. Invest.* 93:671–76
71. Tieder M, Modai D, Samuel R, Arie R, Halabe A, et al. 1985. Hereditary hypophosphatemic rickets with hypercalciuria. *N. Engl. J. Med.* 312:611–17
72. Tieder M, Modai D, Shaked U, Samuel R, Arie R, et al. 1987. "Idiopathic" hypercalciuria and hereditary hypophosphatemic rickets. *N. Engl. J. Med.* 316:125–29
73. Traebert M, Volkl H, Biber J, Murer H, Kaissling B. 2000. Luminal and contraluminal action of 1–34 and 3–34 PTH peptides on renal type IIa Na-P-i

cotransporter. *Am. J. Physiol.* 278:F792–98
74. Virkki LV, Forster IC, Hernando N, Biber J, Murer H. 2003. Functional characterization of two naturally occurring mutations in the human sodium-phosphate cotransporter type IIa. *J. Bone Miner. Res.* 18:2135–41
75. Werner A, Moore ML, Mantei N, Biber J, Semenza G, Murer H. 1991. Cloning and expression of cDNA for a Na/Pi cotransport system of kidney cortex. *Proc. Natl. Acad. Sci. USA* 88:9608–12
76. White KE, Carn G, Lorenz-Depiereux B, Benet-Pages A, Strom TM, Econs MJ. 2001. Autosomal-dominant hypophosphatemic rickets (ADHR) mutations stabilize FGF-23. *Kidney Int.* 60:2079–86
77. Yamazaki Y, Shimada T, Imai R, Hino R, Aono Y, et al. 2003. Elevated circulatory and expression level of fibroblast growth factor (FGF)-23 in hypophosphatemic mice. *Bone* 32:S88 (Abstr.)
78. Zhao N, Tenenhouse HS. 2000. Npt2 gene disruption confers resistance to the inhibitory action of PTH on renal Na-phosphate cotransport. *Endocrinology* 141:2159–65

Annu. Rev. Nutr. 2005. 25:215–35
doi: 10.1146/annurev.nutr.24.012003.132120

First published online as a Review in Advance on February 18, 2005

SELENOPROTEIN P: An Extracellular Protein with Unique Physical Characteristics and a Role in Selenium Homeostasis

Raymond F. Burk and Kristina E. Hill
Division of Gastroenterology, Department of Medicine and Center in Molecular Toxicology, Vanderbilt University School of Medicine, Nashville, Tennessee 37232; email: raymond.burk@vanderbilt.edu, kristina.hill@vanderbilt.edu

Key Words selenoprotein, isoforms, selenenylsulfide bonds, selenium transport, multiple selenocysteine residues

■ **Abstract** Selenoprotein P is an abundant extracellular glycoprotein that is rich in selenocysteine. It has two domains with respect to selenium content. The *N*-terminal domain of the rat protein contains one selenocysteine residue in a UxxC redox motif. This domain also has a pH-sensitive heparin-binding site and two histidine-rich amino acid stretches. The smaller *C*-terminal domain contains nine selenocysteine and ten cysteine residues. Four isoforms of selenoprotein P are present in rat plasma. They share the same *N* terminus and amino acid sequence. One isoform is full length and the three others terminate at the positions of the second, third, and seventh selenocysteine residues. Selenoprotein P turns over rapidly in rat plasma with the consequence that approximately 25% of the amount of whole-body selenium passes through it each day. Evidence supports functions of the protein in selenium homeostasis and oxidant defense. Selenoprotein P knockout mice have very low selenium concentrations in the brain, the testis, and the fetus, with severe pathophysiological consequences in each tissue. In addition, those mice waste moderate amounts of selenium in the urine. Selenoprotein P binds to endothelial cells in the rat, and plasma levels of the protein correlate with prevention of diquat-induced lipid peroxidation and hepatic endothelial cell injury. The mechanisms of these apparent functions remain speculative and much work on the mechanism of selenoprotein P function lies ahead. Measurement of selenoprotein P in human plasma has shown that it is depressed by selenium deficiency and by cirrhosis. Selenium supplementation of selenium-deficient human subjects showed that glutathione peroxidase activity was optimized before selenoprotein P concentration was optimized, indicating that plasma selenoprotein P is the better index of human selenium nutritional status.

CONTENTS

INTRODUCTION

The beneficial effects of selenium as a micronutrient were first recognized in the 1950s. It was 1973, however, before the first animal selenoprotein, glutathione peroxidase, was identified in rat liver (62). With that discovery, the known biological effects of selenium appeared to be explained (40).

Research on selenium continued, however, and another selenium-containing protein was identified in 1977, this time in blood plasma (31). That protein was further characterized (9) and shown in 1982 to contain its selenium as selenocysteine (57). Because no function could be attributed to it, the letter P was used in its name in reference to its location. Thus, selenoprotein P was the second animal selenoprotein to be identified. Its discovery fostered efforts to find additional selenoproteins and to determine how selenoproteins are produced.

An elegant series of studies by Böck and his collaborators in the late 1980s characterized selenoprotein synthesis in prokaryotes (6). Building on the prokaryotic results, other workers have provided many of the details of eukaryotic selenoprotein synthesis. A description of the process is beyond the scope of this review (see 24, 47, 50), but the open reading frame of the selenoprotein mRNA contains a UGA at the position of each selenocysteine residue in the protein, and its 3′ untranslated region contains a stem loop structure with conserved features. Thus, the DNA of a selenoprotein has identifiable features.

Twelve selenoproteins had been identified by conventional means before genomic databases became available (12). Those proteins included four glutathione peroxidases, three iodothyronine deiodinases, and a thioredoxin reductase.

By the late 1990s, it had become obvious that selenoproteins have a wide variety of metabolic roles.

Efforts were made to search available databases for additional selenoproteins. Early efforts sought stem loop structures and identified more selenoproteins (46, 48). They also demonstrated that some enzymes are selenoproteins in one species but contain cysteine in place of selenocysteine in another species.

The availability of databases of complete genomes made it possible to search for all the selenoproteins. Recently a strategy that requires candidate genes to be present in both murine and human genomes has identified 25 selenoprotein genes in the human genome and 24 in the mouse genome (44). This genome-wide search has probably identified virtually all the genes that code for selenoproteins through conventional selenoprotein mRNAs. It is possible, though, that selenoproteins with forms of selenium other than selenocysteine will be found as they have been in prokaryotes (30).

Although 25 selenoprotein genes are present in the human genome, alternative splicing and other strategies to produce more than 1 protein per gene will raise the number of selenoproteins to more than 25. A few of the selenoproteins have been extensively characterized, but little beyond the genomic data is known about many of them (44). Biochemical and physiological characterization will be required for each.

As the second animal selenoprotein identified, selenoprotein P has been the subject of a number of studies over the past 20 years. It is an abundant protein that has several striking properties not present in other selenoproteins and it appears to play a major role in whole-body selenium metabolism. In this review, we discuss the genetic and physical characteristics of selenoprotein P as well as its metabolism and physiological properties. Our aims are to draw attention to unusual and unexplained properties of this complex protein that may serve as clues to its biological activity and to provide suggestions of how it contributes to selenium homeostasis.

GENE

Structure

Selenoprotein P genomic sequences have been reported in DNA from the mouse (71) and the human being (82). Each gene contains five exons with the coding sequence being restricted to exons 2–5. The first in-frame TGA (coding for selenocysteine) is in the second exon. The other nine in-frame TGAs and the two selenocysteine insertion sequence (SECIS) elements are in the fifth exon. The mouse gene is 10.3 kb in size and the human gene is 12 kb. Because their exons are the same size, this implies a difference in the size of some introns between the two species.

No evidence has been found for multiple copies of the mouse or human genes. However, two selenoprotein P genes are implied by the presence of two cDNAs in the zebrafish-expressed sequence tag database (45). One cDNA implies a protein of 367 amino acids that contains 17 selenocysteine residues and has two SECIS elements in its 3′ untranslated region. The second cDNA implies a protein of 265 amino acids that contains only one selenocysteine residue and one SECIS element. The shorter implied protein has similarity with the *N*-terminal region of the longer one and with the *N* terminus (and shorter isoforms) of rat selenoprotein P (see "Isoforms" section below and Figure 1, color insert). Thus, selenoprotein P genes encode proteins containing from 1 to 17 selenocysteine residues.

Selenoprotein P appears to be expressed only in vertebrates. It was not found in the genomes of *Caenorhabditis elegans* or *Drosophila melanogaster* (44).

Regulation

Nuclear run-on experiments were carried out in rat liver to assess the effect of selenium deficiency on selenoprotein P gene transcription (11). No effect was found. Thus, transcription of the selenoprotein P gene in liver is not sensitive to the selenium status of the animal.

The promoters of the human and mouse selenoprotein P genes have been sequenced (23, 71). They contain binding sites for numerous transcription factors, including tissue-specific ones that presumably account for the extreme variation in expression among tissues.

Transfection experiments with the human promoter region using a luciferase reporter gene showed inhibition of expression by tumor necrosis factor-alpha (TNFα), interferon γ, and interleukin 1β. This suggests that production of selenoprotein P would be inhibited in an acute phase response. Transforming growth factor-beta (TGFβ) also inhibits expression through Smad 3 and 4 (56). However, effects of cytokines and growth factors have not been evaluated in vivo.

The spatial and temporal expression of the two selenoprotein P mRNAs in zebrafish has been assessed during embryogenesis (74). The shorter isoform was expressed primarily in the liver and the longer one primarily in the brain, kidney, and intestine. This shows a differential regulation of these genes, which indicates that the functions of the short and long isoforms are different.

PROTEIN STRUCTURE

Not enough is known about the structure of selenoprotein P to allow construction of three-dimensional representations. Similarities with other proteins have not been reported and efforts to produce crystals of it for X-ray crystallography have not yet been successful (K.E. Hill, unpublished observations). Mass spectrometry and other techniques have revealed a number of characteristics of rat selenoprotein P, however, and they are shown in Figure 1 and discussed in this section.

Primary Structure

The highly unusual nature of this protein became obvious as soon as it was subjected to analysis. As purified, rat selenoprotein P had multiple selenocysteine residues per polypeptide (61) compared with a single selenium per polypeptide in glutathione peroxidase (28).

Once the selenoprotein P cDNA had been cloned from a rat liver library, an implied amino acid sequence of 366 residues (Figure 1) and a preceding 19-amino-acid signal peptide were revealed (33). The implied mature protein contained 10 selenocysteine and 17 cysteine residues. A further unusual feature of the amino acid sequence was the presence of two histidine-rich regions. One was 14 residues long (residues 185–198) and contained eight histidine and two lysine residues; the other was 10 residues long (residues 225–234) and contained eight histidine and two lysine residues. These histidine-rich regions are likely to be involved in binding other molecules (see below).

Based on its selenium content, the protein was recognized to have two domains. The first and larger one extends from the *N* terminus through the residue just before the second selenocysteine (residues 1–244). It contains one selenocysteine and seven cysteine residues as well as the two histidine-rich sequences. The smaller domain extends from the second selenocysteine to the *C* terminus (residues 245–366). It contains nine selenocysteine and ten cysteine residues. Thus, 90% of the selenocysteines and 59% of the cysteines are concentrated in this shorter stretch of residues. The selenium-rich *C*-terminal domain has some features that suggest it might be on the inside of the molecule. Chemical modification of basic amino acid residues in the native protein did not label residues distal to the lysine at residue 261 (41), and limited trypsin proteolysis occurred after residue 264 but not more distally (R.F. Burk, unpublished observation). This lack of reactivity of the *C*-terminal domain suggests that it is shielded in the native protein.

Selenoprotein P sequences from mammalian species have overall identities in the 70%–80% range, although some of them have unique features. The seven sequential proline-histidine repeats in the bovine sequence beginning at residue 196 are an example of this (63).

Isoforms

Selenoprotein P isoforms were recognized to occur in plasma after the immunoaffinity-purified protein preparation was observed to bind to heparin at pH 7 but not at pH 8.5 (21). Application of a pH gradient to the heparin column eluted several selenoprotein P peaks of different masses. Conventional peptide sequencing and mass spectrometry were used to characterize those isoforms of rat selenoprotein P (39, 53).

In addition to the full-length selenoprotein P, three shorter isoforms were identified that shared the same *N* terminus but had *C* termini at the positions of the second, third, and seventh UGAs (53). The shorter isoforms were given the names Se-P_1, Se-P_2, and Se-P_6, while the full-length isoform was named Se-P_{10}. The subscript indicates the number of selenium atoms in the isoform. These three shorter isoforms appeared to arise from the same mRNA as the full-length protein because they shared the same sequence. Moreover, only one selenoprotein P mRNA is known. Therefore, it was postulated that three of the in-frame UGAs code alternatively for insertion of selenocysteine or for termination of translation. It is not known whether cells are programmed as to which isoform(s) they produce or whether they are able to switch among isoforms according to need.

Because the isoforms terminate precisely at UGAs, it seems unlikely that they are produced from the full-length protein by proteolysis. For that to occur, a protease that cleaves at selenocysteine residues would be needed, and no such enzyme is known. Another possible mechanism of isoform production would be inefficiency of UGA translation as selenocysteine. Such an occurrence would be predicted to take place at all UGAs, however, and not just at specific ones. Moreover, it would be expected that products of premature termination would be eliminated by the quality-control mechanism of the endoplasmic reticulum. Thus, this appears to be the first demonstration of alternative use of the UGA codon to produce different isoforms of a protein.

The presence of genes in the zebrafish that code for proteins analogous to Se-P_1 and Se-P_{10} suggests that the organism needs both the shorter and the longer forms of selenoprotein P. It can be speculated that higher vertebrates have developed a mechanism for producing shorter and longer forms from one gene to accomplish what the zebrafish does with two genes.

Glycosylation

The average mass of Se-P_{10} was estimated to be 50,474 by matrix-assisted laser desorption time-of-flight (MALDI-TOF) mass spectrometry (53). Yet, its predicted peptide weight was only 41,096 (33). This large discrepancy indicated that the protein contained post-translational modifications. Purified selenoprotein P took stains for carbohydrate and treatment of it with glycosidases increased its migration on sodium dodecyl sulfate polyacrylamide gel electrophoresis (SDS-PAGE) (61). This indicated that at least part of the modification was carbohydrate.

Se-P_{10} was analyzed for glycosylation using mass spectrometry (52a). Peptides from protease digests of Se-P_{10} had carbohydrate attached. Figure 1 shows the three occupied *N*-glycosylation sites and the one *O*-glycosylation site. All sites displayed microheterogeneity but, on average, they accounted for 9330 mass units. Addition of this value to the predicted peptide weight yields 50,426, which is close to the measured mass of Se-P_{10}. Thus, additional small modifications cannot be ruled out, but carbohydrate appears to account for the nonpeptide mass of Se-P_{10}. Similar calculations were made for the shorter isoforms, based on the carbohydrate present in Se-P_{10}, and similar results were obtained for them.

Disulfide and Selenenylsulfide Linkages

Se-P_1 was analyzed by mass spectrometry for disulfide linkages (52a). The selenocysteine at residue 40 and the cysteine at residue 43 formed a selenenylsulfide bond (Figure 1) that has characteristics of a redox center (see "Enzyme Activity" section

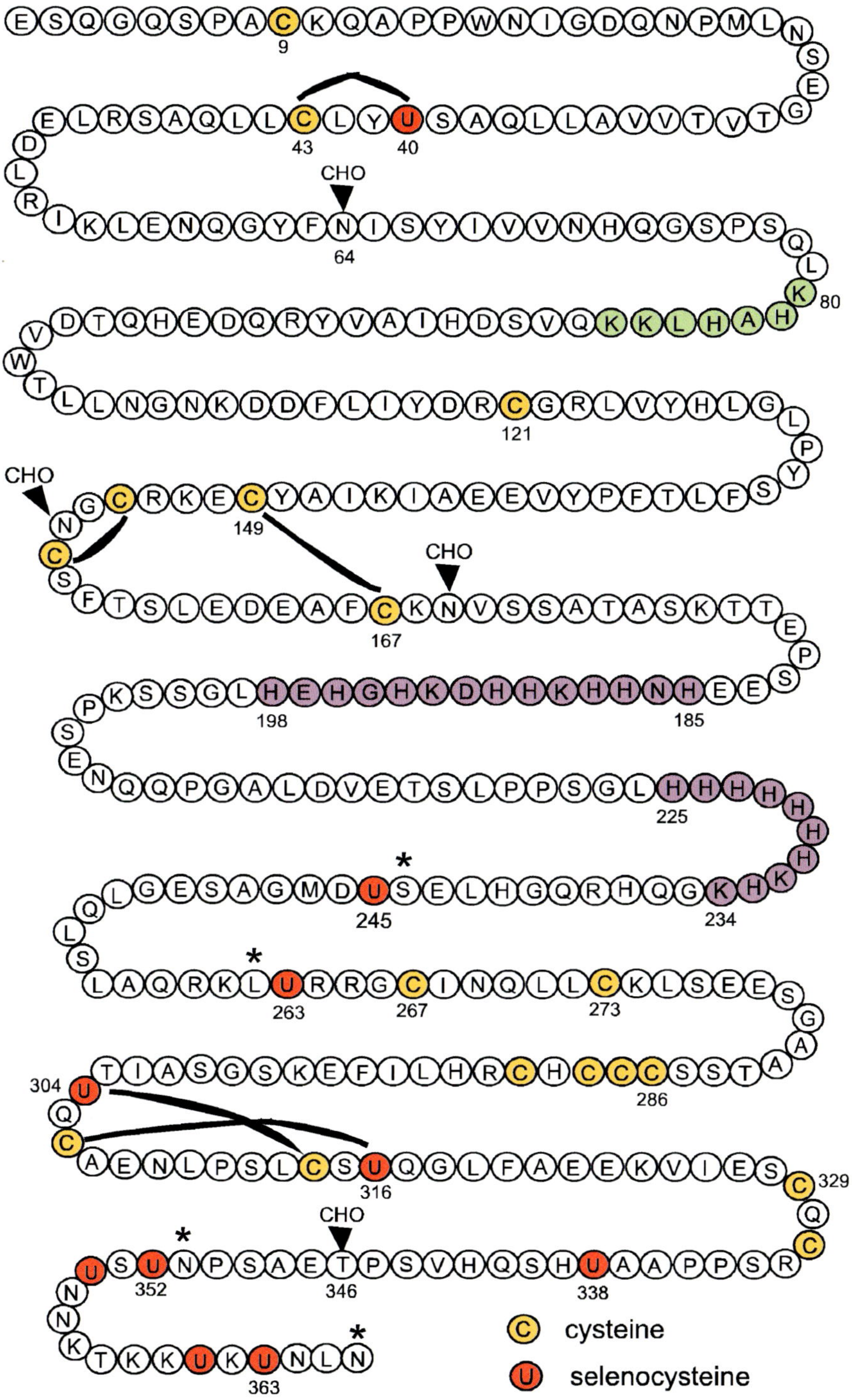

See legend on next page

Figure 1 Rat selenoprotein P. The amino acid sequence of the mature protein is presented. Asterisks denote the *C*-terminal residues of the four isoforms. CHO indicates the three occupied *N*-glycosylation sites (at residues 64, 155, and 169) and the *O*-glycosylation site (at residue 346). The heparin-binding site is shown in green and the two histidine-rich sequences are shown in purple. Selenenylsulfide and disulfide bridges are represented by dark lines that connect amino acid residues.

below). Two disulfide linkages were found between cysteine residues 149–167 and 153–156. Thus, the *N*-terminal domain has two disulfide bonds that appear to be structural and a potential redox site that contains selenocysteine.

A fragment made up of residues 298–324 was isolated from a trypsin digest of Se-P_{10} (51). Mass spectrometric analysis revealed that the fragment contained two selenenylsulfide linkages (Figure 1) (52b). This is the only structural information available on the *C*-terminal domain of selenoprotein P.

BIOCHEMICAL PROPERTIES

The study of biochemical properties of selenoproteins is often difficult because most of them, including selenoprotein P, cannot be expressed in bacteria. Thus, only the amounts of selenoprotein P that can be purified are available for study and site-directed mutagenesis cannot be employed. Initial success in expression of recombinant rat selenoprotein P in a human cell line has been reported (76). Further development of this technique will allow more extensive characterization of this protein. However, the studies reported to date have used only selenoprotein P purified from plasma.

Enzyme Activity

In general, selenoproteins serve as enzymes that catalyze redox reactions. Examples are the glutathione peroxidases, in which the selenium atom accepts electrons from GSH and transfers them to a hydroperoxide, and the thioredoxin reductases, in which the selenium atom is paired with a sulfur atom (in a cysteine residue) and this redox pair transfers electrons from the enzyme to thioredoxin (84). The primary structure of selenoprotein P (Figure 1) contains many potential redox centers in the form of cysteine and selenocysteine residues. One of them, at residues 40–43, has the classic CxxC sequence (29), with the first C being a U, or selenocysteine.

Early efforts to detect glutathione peroxidase activity of selenoprotein P were unsuccessful (81). However, Takahashi's group was able to demonstrate that their human selenoprotein P preparation weakly catalyzed the oxidation of GSH by a phosphatidylcholine hydroperoxide (64). It thus functioned as a phospholipid hydroperoxide glutathione peroxidase. Thiols such as dithiothreitol substituted effectively for GSH, but neither H_2O_2 nor small organic hydroperoxides could serve as substrates. This indicated that the peroxidase activity of selenoprotein P was highly selective, but it appeared to be suitable for acting on membrane hydroperoxides.

Further experiments revealed that an *N*-terminal fragment containing the UxxC sequence was responsible for the peroxidase activity (65). Moreover, thioredoxin was approximately 500-fold more effective as the reducing substrate than GSH (73). These findings point toward the UxxC of selenoprotein P being an enzyme active site. The nature of its endogenous substrates is uncertain, however.

Heparin Binding

A number of extracellular proteins have heparin-binding properties that allow them to bind to specific structures and thereby focus their biological activities (22). Selenoprotein P is a heparin-binding protein (2, 31). Its heparin-binding properties are highly unusual, however, because they are pH sensitive within the physiological pH range (21). Thus, rat selenoprotein P binds to heparin at pH 7.0 and becomes unbound as the pH is raised toward 8.5. This pH sensitivity was exploited to separate selenoprotein P isoforms from one another (see "Isoforms" section above). It also implies that the heparin-binding site of the protein is not typical.

Heparin binding depends on positive charge, and the basic amino acids arginine and lysine, with pK_as of >9, are almost always the constituents of heparin-binding sites. Histidine, with a pK_a in the range of 6.5–7.0, becomes positively charged as pH nears 7. In theory, it could be a factor in heparin binding at low pH. Selenoprotein P has two histidine-rich sequences (residues 185–198 and 225–234; see Figure 1) that are candidates for being heparin-binding sites.

A heparin-binding site has been identified on rat selenoprotein P using conventional chemical modification methods (41). The site was not one of the two histidine-rich sequences but was localized to residues 80–95 (Figure 1). Six positively charged residues, three lysines and three histidines, reside within that sequence. Part of the sequence, LKHAHL, is arranged in a typical heparin-binding motif xBBxBx, where B is a basic residue, and x is any other one (22). Thus, the heparin-binding site is typical in consisting of basic amino acids in a recognized motif, but it is atypical in containing histidine residues as some of the basic residues. These histidine residues are probably responsible for the pH sensitivity of heparin binding because they would become protonated only as pH fell toward 7.

The histidine-rich sequences might contribute to heparin binding under some circumstances. Peptides derived from them met some, but not all, of the criteria of heparin-binding sites (41). A separate study that used surface plasmon resonance to evaluate heparin binding of human selenoprotein P indicated that high-affinity and low-affinity binding sites were present (3). Because in vivo binding sites are heparan sulfate proteoglycans, and not heparin itself, the actual binding behavior of selenoprotein P in the organism is likely to be different from that observed in vitro. The in vivo binding should be pH sensitive, however. This allows the speculation that selenoprotein P will bind in areas of inflammation that typically have low pH. It would likely bind only to host cells in those areas because bacteria do not have heparan sulfate proteoglycans.

Mercury Binding

Interactions of selenium and mercury have been reported in a substantial literature dating back 30 years. Selenium has generally been shown to protect against the toxicity of mercury while paradoxically increasing tissue mercury concentrations.

In some instances selenium accumulated along with the mercury (8, 43); in others only mercury accumulated (10). These disparate results indicate that different mechanisms underlie each of them.

In 1997, Suzuki and colleagues reported that selenoprotein P bound a mercury-selenium complex following administration of high doses of mercuric chloride and selenite to rats (83). Our group had observed this binding much earlier in association with mutual detoxification of the elements but had not been able to identify the protein that bound the elements (8).

Suzuki reproduced the binding in vitro by adding selenite and mercuric chloride to plasma containing added GSH (83). That work indicated that reaction of selenite with GSH produced selenide, which, in turn, reacted with mercuric ion to produce a polymer that contained mercury and selenium in equimolar amounts. That this polymer bound only to selenoprotein P in plasma indicates how unusual that protein is. Competition experiments suggested that the binding was to the histidine-rich regions (72).

Although the chemistry of this binding is fascinating, there is little evidence that the phenomenon has relevance under physiological conditions. Administration of mercuric chloride alone did not result in its binding to selenoprotein P. Thus for selenoprotein P to sequester mercury, simultaneous doses of selenite and mercuric chloride would have to be administered. Such a situation is unlikely to occur outside the laboratory.

Because of its high histidine and cysteine content, selenoprotein P would appear to be suited to bind heavy metals. Evidence that it does so under conditions that are physiologically relevant is not yet available.

PHYSIOLOGICAL PROPERTIES

Expression, Turnover, and Localization

Selenoprotein P is present in extracellular fluids (11) and bound to endothelial cells (14). It is also present in milk (69). No evidence has been presented that intracellular pools of it exist, aside from those associated with its synthesis and degradation. The relative amounts of bound and free selenoprotein P have not been determined, but its concentration in plasma is high—30 mg protein per liter in the rat (61) and 5–6 mg protein per liter in the human being (67, 78). Using these figures and the amounts of selenium removed from plasma by immunoprecipitation of selenoprotein P, values of 5–6 selenium atoms per molecule of selenoprotein P are calculated. This indicates that some circulating selenoprotein P molecules contain fewer than 10 selenium atoms. Potential explanations of this are that significant amounts of the shorter isoforms are circulating or that some of the Se-P_{10} in plasma has lost selenium atoms. Although both of these are possible (39, 51), the presence of isoforms in rat plasma has been documented and so is at least part of the explanation. Methods to quantitate isoforms have not been developed, so the amounts of each of them in the plasma are not known.

Although the liver appears to be the source of 75% of plasma selenoprotein P (20), virtually all tissues express its mRNA and therefore presumably secrete it. In addition to liver, tissues with high concentrations of the mRNA are kidney and heart (11). Lesser concentrations have been detected in lung, brain, skeletal muscle, and testis. Expression of the protein by a tissue implies that it is secreted into the interstitial space of that tissue. This distinguishes selenoprotein P from proteins such as albumin that are produced solely in the liver. Proteins secreted only by the liver have limited access to the interstitial space of extrahepatic tissues. Based on its localization, a primary function of selenoprotein P in the interstitial space can be expected.

Several studies have assessed the fate of the selenium that is incorporated into selenoprotein P (15, 16, 18, 57). Absorbed selenium is removed from portal vein blood by the liver (42). Some of it is then released into the blood in the form of selenoprotein P. How selenoprotein P is degraded is not known, but the fate of its selenium has been examined in the rat. Selenoprotein P selenium has a plasma half-life of 3–4 hours and appears in peripheral tissues with a preference for testis and brain (18). Moreover, brain up-regulates its mechanism for acquiring selenium from selenoprotein P in selenium deficiency. This implies that testis and brain have receptors for selenoprotein P and that function of the putative brain receptor is regulated by the selenium status of the animal. Such a mechanism would explain how the brain conserves selenium in selenium deficiency.

Based on selenoprotein P plasma concentration and estimated turnover rate (18), 38 μg of it is synthesized per hour in a selenium-replete rat weighing 250 grams. As an indication of the magnitude of this process, this figure is just over 1% of the albumin synthesis rate (27). Moreover, it corresponds to secretion into the plasma of 440 ng of selenium per hour or just over 1% of the whole-body selenium content. This means that approximately 25% of the amount of whole-body selenium circulates through the plasma as selenoprotein P in a day. Thus, it seems likely that the functioning of selenoprotein P leads to its degradation.

Feeding a selenium-deficient diet to an animal produces selenium deficiency. The effect of selenium deficiency on rat selenoprotein P concentration has been assessed (80). Under deficient conditions, plasma glutathione peroxidase activity decreased to approximately 1% of its activity under selenium-replete conditions; selenoprotein P, however, fell only to 5%–10%. This shows that, even under severely deficient conditions, a considerable amount of the available selenium in the animal is used to synthesize selenoprotein P.

Whole-Body Selenium Metabolism

The liver is the central organ of selenium metabolism. Most ingested selenium enters specific selenium metabolism pathways there after uptake from portal vein blood or removal from selenomethionine via the transsulfuration pathway (26). This "new" selenium is used for synthesis of selenoproteins or is released as metabolites that are excreted in the urine. The selenoproteins that are synthesized by the liver include selenoenzymes that support liver function and selenoprotein P that is exported to the blood.

Insights into the role of selenoprotein P in whole-body selenium metabolism have been gained by study of mice with deletion of the selenoprotein P gene (*Sepp*). Deletion of selenoprotein P resulted in sharp decreases in brain and testis selenium concentrations, increase or no change in liver selenium concentration, and modest decreases in selenium concentrations in kidney and other tissues (37, 68). Increased urinary excretion of ingested selenium was also noted (17). These findings suggest that the $Sepp^{-/-}$ liver directs the selenium that would have been used to synthesize selenoprotein P into the production of urinary metabolites. This results in a loss of selenium from the body and a modest decrease of selenium in most tissues. The large decreases in brain and testis selenium indicate that selenoprotein P has a more direct role in supply of selenium to those tissues.

Clinical phenotypes are associated with the low concentrations of brain and testis selenium. $Sepp^{-/-}$ mice fed normal or low-selenium diets developed spasticity and progressed to paralysis and death within a few weeks of weaning (38). Feeding a high-selenium diet from weaning prevented this sequence of events. Institution of a high-selenium diet after the spasticity had appeared prevented progression of the condition but did not reverse the abnormalities that had already developed (38). These observations indicate that low selenium concentrations in the brains of mice lacking selenoprotein P led to irreversible neurological injury. They support the hypothesis that selenoprotein P supplies the brain with selenium. It is clear, however, that other forms of selenium can be taken up by the brain because feeding a high-selenium diet prevents the development of spasticity (38).

Male $Sepp^{-/-}$ mice have such low fertility that they cannot be used for breeding purposes (37, 68). Moreover, feeding a high-selenium diet does not correct the infertility (58a). The morphology of their sperm resembles that of selenium-deficient mice. There is a 180° kink at the junction of the midpiece and the principal piece. Female $Sepp^{-/-}$ mice are fertile if they are fed a high-selenium diet (35) or are given selenium in the drinking water (69).

These studies in $Sepp^{-/-}$ mice imply that selenoprotein P is essential for adequate selenium supply to the brain, testis, and fetus. Moreover, the evidence that uptake of selenium from selenoprotein P by brain increases in selenium deficiency (see above; Reference 18) is compatible with receptor-mediated uptake of the protein. Thus, a second protein, a selenoprotein P receptor, might be involved in selenium supply to these tissues. Mutations in selenoprotein P or its putative receptor could impair selenium delivery and play a role in diseases affecting these tissues.

Selenoprotein P is secreted by cells and therefore has been suggested to play a role in regulating cell selenium content. However, $Sepp^{-/-}$ mice fed a high-selenium diet did not accumulate more selenium in tissues than did $Sepp^{+/+}$ mice (37). This indicates that selenoprotein P is not necessary for cells to export selenium.

Selenium Supply to Cells

Cultured cells require selenium for growth (54). They can acquire it from serum or from forms such as selenite. Several reports have indicated that the serum component providing selenium to cultured cells is selenoprotein P. One group purified selenoprotein P from bovine serum using as a marker its activity as a survival-promoting factor for cultured rat central neurons (79). In their system, selenium in the form of their purified bovine selenoprotein P was six times more effective than was selenium as selenite. Moreover, boiling the purified protein did not abolish the protection, which suggests that the native structure of the selenoprotein was not required for the effect.

Takahashi's group addressed directly the question of selenium supply to cultured cells (66). Glutathione peroxidase activity was used as an index of the selenium status of Jurkat cells. Human selenoprotein P was approximately five times more effective in supplying selenium than was plasma glutathione peroxidase, selenocystine, and selenite. Selenomethionine was even less effective.

In a follow-up study, this group digested human selenoprotein P into *N*-terminal and *C*-terminal fragments (65). They showed that the *C*-terminal fragment, but not the *N*-terminal fragment, could supply selenium to cultured cells. However, the effectiveness of the *C*-terminal fragment was only about one-tenth that of the full-length protein. These findings suggest the selenium supplied by selenoprotein P is that in its *C* terminus, but the *N* terminus enhances uptake. This would speak for the binding properties of the *N*-terminal portion of the molecule (see "Heparin Binding" section above) playing a role in the selenium donation.

Defense Against Oxidative Injury

Several intracellular selenoproteins metabolize reactive oxygen intermediates and thereby defend the cell against oxidative injury. Selenoprotein P has been postulated to defend against oxidative injury in the extracellular space. Its phospholipid hydroperoxide thiol peroxidase activity and its ability to bind to cells are properties that might support such a function. In addition, in vitro incubation experiments showed that adding selenoprotein P delayed free radical–induced oxidative damage to low-density lipoproteins (75) and prevented nitrosylation by peroxynitrite (70).

In 1980, it was reported that selenium-deficient rats developed massive liver necrosis and lipid peroxidation following administration of small doses of the redox-cycling compound diquat (19). Injection of selenium ten hours before diquat injection, but not two hours before it, prevented the injury. It was postulated that synthesis of a selenoprotein was occurring that protected the liver against the reactive oxygen intermediates produced by diquat cycling. Further experiments, in which selenium doses were varied, associated selenoprotein P with that protection (13, 34).

Ultrastructural characterization of the diquat liver injury revealed that centrilobular sinusoidal endothelial cells were injured within minutes of diquat administration to selenium-deficient rats (4). The endothelial cells became detached within an hour, leaving the hepatocytes exposed to the blood. At two hours, the hepatocytes were necrotic. Based on these results and the report that selenoprotein P associates with endothelial cells, it was postulated that selenoprotein P protects the sinusoidal endothelial cells against oxidative molecules resulting from diquat cycling (4).

Similar studies were attempted in mice in anticipation of using *Sepp*$^{-/-}$ mice to test the hypothesis. However, because the severe and rapid liver necrosis observed in selenium-deficient rats given diquat did not occur in selenium-deficient mice (R.F. Burk, unpublished observations); mice cannot be used to evaluate this proposed function of selenoprotein P.

STUDIES IN HUMAN BEINGS

Human and rat selenoprotein P amino acid sequences are 72% identical and each contains ten selenocysteine residues (32). The first selenocysteine in each is residue 40 and it is paired with a cysteine at residue 43. However, the second selenocysteine, which delimits the selenium-rich *C*-terminal domain from the *N*-terminal domain, is residue 286 in the human sequence and residue 245 in the rat one. The *N*-terminal domain is thus longer in the human protein than in the rat protein and the selenium-rich *C*-terminal domain is only 22% of the human sequence compared with 33% of the rat sequence.

Human selenoprotein P has been purified by several groups, but only rudimentary characterization of it has been carried out. Two groups have found two protein bands on SDS-PAGE, which suggests the presence of isoforms (1, 55). Another group carried out purification in the presence of diisopropylfluorophosphate and found only one band (64). That group proposes that proteolysis generated the second band seen by the other groups and that isoforms are not present. Resolution of this point will require further work.

Early methods to quantitate selenoprotein P in plasma were cumbersome. One method relied on chromatographic separation of selenoprotein P, glutathione peroxidase, and albumin with subsequent determination of the selenium in each fraction (77). Although it provided some useful information, this method lacked specificity and was superseded by antibody-based assays. The first specific method employed was a radioimmunoassay that used a polyclonal antibody preparation (36). It relied on competition between the selenoprotein P in the plasma sample and ^{75}Se-labeled selenoprotein P. Production of the labeled protein required culturing human hepatoblastoma cells in the presence of ^{75}Se-labeled selenite. Because ^{75}Se has a relatively short half-life, this method could not be widely used.

ELISA assays that have the advantage of not requiring labeled selenoprotein P are now being used. Takahashi and colleagues have produced monoclonal antibodies suitable for accurate determination of human selenoprotein P (67). They reported a mean value $\pm$SD in the plasma of healthy Japanese subjects of

5.3 ± 1.1 mg per liter, $n = 73$. Using different monoclonal antibodies, our group has determined that our reference U.S. plasma contains 5.8 mg selenoprotein P per liter (78). Application of the ELISA should facilitate studies of selenoprotein P in human subjects.

Selenoprotein P in Populations

Åkesson's group has investigated selenoprotein P in Europe and Scandinavia (58b, 59). Both these regions have selenium intakes that are marginal with respect to maintenance of plasma glutathione peroxidase activity. Åkesson's studies showed that selenoprotein P concentration correlated with plasma glutathione peroxidase activity and selenium concentration (59).

A selenium supplementation trial was carried out in Finland before selenium was added to fertilizer there (49). Åkesson's group assayed stored plasma samples from that study for selenoprotein P (59). Pre-supplementation values were approximately 60% of the maximal values of selenoprotein P after supplementation (59). A study carried out in New Zealand, another low-selenium country, gave similar results (25). Thus, New Zealand and many countries in Scandinavia and Europe have plasma levels of selenoprotein P that are below the optimal value. This suggests that residents of those countries are mildly selenium deficient.

More severe selenium deficiency occurs in certain areas of China. A study in Sichuan Province revealed selenoprotein P levels in healthy men that were 13% of the U.S. standard (36). Plasma selenium concentration and glutathione peroxidase were similarly depressed. These determinations of selenoprotein P, and of other selenium biomarkers, demonstrate that large areas of the world have selenium intakes that are not adequate to optimize selenoproteins in the body. This implies that these subjects are selenium deficient.

Effect of Disease

Although other plasma biomarkers of selenium have been measured in a number of diseases, selenoprotein P has been assessed in detail only in cirrhosis (7). Selenoprotein P was depressed in cirrhotics in proportion to clinical severity of disease. Patients with severe disease had levels as low as 50% of the levels in healthy subjects. In the same study, plasma glutathione peroxidase activity was increased in proportion to clinical severity of disease. Thus, the two plasma selenoproteins responded to cirrhosis differently. Plasma selenoprotein P, much of which originates in the liver, was depressed, most likely because of impaired liver function. The rise in plasma glutathione peroxidase activity, however, may be a compensatory response to physiological factors in the kidney caused by the disease. In any case, it seems unlikely that patients with cirrhosis have nutritional selenium deficiency. It is likely, however, that cirrhosis alters selenium disposition in the body because of the central role of the liver in selenium homeostasis.

Depletion of selenoprotein P by apheresis treatment of hypercholesterolemia has been noted (60). Blood was passed through columns containing dextran sulfate cellulose and returned to the subjects. Selenoprotein P presumably bound to that substance because its plasma concentration was halved. Such treatment might affect biological functions dependent on selenoprotein P until normal levels are restored, but it is unlikely to deplete the body of selenium because only 1% of whole-body selenium was removed by a treatment (60).

Effect of Selenium Supplementation

In addition to the above-mentioned studies in Finland and New Zealand (25, 49), a recent trial in a low-selenium area of China assessed the response of selenoprotein P to 20 weeks of selenium supplementation (78). Plasma glutathione peroxidase activity increased to the level found in selenium-replete subjects with supplementation of 37 μg selenium daily, but selenoprotein P reached only 75% at the highest supplementation level, 61 μg (Figure 2). This indicates that optimization of selenium in all the tissues secreting selenoprotein P requires a greater selenium intake than does optimization of selenium in kidney, the organ that produces plasma glutathione peroxidase (5).

The major implication of this study is that selenoprotein P concentrations are a better biomarker than glutathione peroxidase for selenium in the whole body. Plasma glutathione peroxidase likely is a biomarker principally for selenium in the kidney. Thus, it can be recommended that selenoprotein P replace glutathione peroxidase as the indicator of selenium nutritional status in the healthy person.

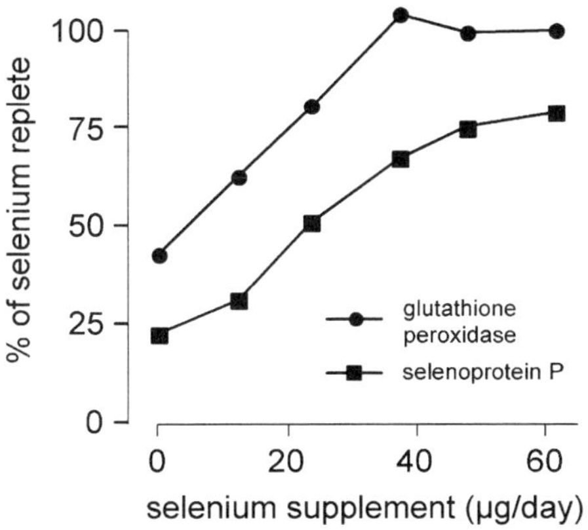

Figure 2 Response of plasma selenoproteins to selenium supplementation of selenium-deficient human subjects (78). Average dietary selenium intake was 10 μg per day. Each symbol represents the mean of ten subjects receiving selenium daily as selenomethionine for 16–20 weeks. Glutathione peroxidase reached its highest activity at a supplementation level of 37 μg. Selenoprotein P reached only 75% of the U.S. standard value at the highest supplementation level of 61 μg.

CONCLUSIONS

Selenoprotein P stands out, even among selenoproteins, for its unusual physical and metabolic characteristics. The *N*-terminal domain of its primary structure has a selenium-containing redox center, a pH-sensitive heparin-binding site, and two histidine-rich stretches. Thus, this part of the molecule has both enzymatic and binding capabilities as well as the capacity to localize the molecule to areas of low pH. The smaller *C*-terminal domain is selenium rich and contains some selenenylsulfide bonds. Thus, this part of the molecule provides selenium to cells and might be redox active.

Four isoforms that range from just the *N*-terminal domain to the full-length protein are present in rat plasma. Their presence implies that the *N*-terminal domain can function independently of the rest of the molecule but that the *C*-terminal domain needs the *N*-terminal domain for it to function.

The flux of selenium through selenoprotein P is very high. This indicates that the protein is turning over at a rapid rate. Reasons for this rapid turnover might be that the protein serves to transport selenium to all parts of the body and/or that it serves as an antioxidant molecule that cannot be reduced back to an active form. Mice with selenoprotein P deleted demonstrate that it is involved in the provision of selenium to the brain, testis, and fetus, but that it does not appear to be necessary for supply of selenium to most other tissues. The high turnover cannot be accounted for by supply of selenium to brain and testis. Thus, the purpose of this high turnover of selenium, and presumably of the entire protein, needs to be determined. It should provide important clues to selenoprotein P function.

Human selenoprotein P is an accessible index of selenium nutritional status that appears to be more useful than plasma glutathione peroxidase activity or selenium concentration. There are indications that selenium metabolism is altered in diseases such as cirrhosis, so study of selenoprotein P in these diseases can be expected to yield health benefits, as can studies of mutations affecting the protein. The investigation of selenoprotein P in humans is at an early stage, but work already done indicates that selenium and selenoprotein P are important to human health.

ACKNOWLEDGMENTS

The authors' research is supported by NIH grants ES02497 and DK58763.

The *Annual Review of Nutrition* is online at http://nutr.annualreviews.org

LITERATURE CITED

1. Åkesson B, Bellew T, Burk RF. 1994. Purification of selenoprotein P from human plasma. *Biochim. Biophys. Acta* 1204:243–49
2. Åkesson B, Martensson B. 1991. Chromatography of selenoproteins in human serum using matrix-bound heparin. *Int. J. Vitam. Nutr. Res.* 61:72–76
3. Arteel GE, Franken S, Kappler J, Sies H. 2000. Binding of selenoprotein P to

heparin: characterization with surface plasmon resonance. *Biol. Chem.* 381:265–68
4. Atkinson JB, Hill KE, Burk RF. 2001. Centrilobular endothelial cell injury by diquat in the selenium-deficient rat liver. *Lab. Invest.* 81:193–200
5. Avissar N, Ornt DB, Yagil Y, Horowitz S, Watkins RH, et al. 1994. Human kidney proximal tubules are the main source of plasma glutathione peroxidase. *Am. J. Physiol.* 266:C367–75
6. Böck A. 1994. Incorporation of selenium into bacterial selenoproteins. In *Selenium in Biology and Human Health*, ed. RF Burk, pp. 9–24. New York: Springer-Verlag
7. Burk RF, Early DS, Hill KE, Palmer IS, Boeglin ME. 1998. Plasma selenium in patients with cirrhosis. *Hepatology* 27:794–98
8. Burk RF, Foster KA, Greenfield PM, Kiker KW. 1974. Binding of simultaneously administered inorganic selenium and mercury to a rat plasma protein. *Proc. Soc. Exp. Biol. Med.* 145:782–85
9. Burk RF, Gregory PE. 1982. Some characteristics of ^{75}Se-P, a selenoprotein found in rat liver and plasma, and comparison of it with seleno-glutathione peroxidase. *Arch. Biochem. Biophys.* 213:73–80
10. Burk RF, Jordan HE, Kiker KW. 1977. Some effects of selenium status on inorganic mercury metabolism in the rat. *Toxicol. Appl. Pharmacol.* 40:71–82
11. Burk RF, Hill KE. 1994. Selenoprotein P. a selenium-rich extracellular glycoprotein. *J. Nutr.* 124:1891–97
12. Burk RF, Hill KE. 1999. Orphan selenoproteins. *BioEssays* 21:231–37
13. Burk RF, Hill KE, Awad JA, Morrow JD, Kato T, et al. 1995. Pathogenesis of diquat-induced liver necrosis in selenium-deficient rats. Assessment of the roles of lipid peroxidation by measurement of F_2 isoprostanes. *Hepatology* 21:561–69
14. Burk RF, Hill KE, Boeglin ME, Ebner FF, Chittum HS. 1997. Selenoprotein P associates with endothelial cells in rat tissues. *Histochem. Cell Biol.* 108:11–15
15. Burk RF, Hill KE, Motley AK. 2003. Selenoprotein metabolism and function: evidence for more than one function for selenoprotein P. *J. Nutr.* 133:1517–20S
16. Burk RF, Hill KE, Motley AK. 2003. Selenoprotein P and tissue distribution of selenium. In *BITREL 2002. Proceedings of International Symposium on Bio-Trace Elements 2002*, ed. S Enomoto, Y Seko, pp. 91–22. Wako, Japan: RIKEN
17. Burk RF, Hill KE, Motley AK, Hu M, Austin LM. 2004. Deletion of selenoprotein P disrupts selenium homeostasis in the mouse. *FASEB J.* 18:A849
18. Burk RF, Hill KE, Read R, Bellew T. 1991. Response of rat selenoprotein P to selenium administration and fate of its selenium. *Am. J. Physiol.* 261:E26–E30
19. Burk RF, Lawrence RA, Lane JM. 1980. Liver necrosis and lipid peroxidation in the rat due to paraquat and diquat administration. *J. Clin. Invest.* 65:1024–31
20. Carlson BA, Novoselov SV, Kumaraswamy E, Lee BJ, Anver MR, et al. 2004. Specific excision of the selenocysteine tRNA[Ser]Sec (Trsp) gene in mouse liver demonstrates an essential role of selenoproteins in liver function. *J. Biol. Chem.* 279:8011–17
21. Chittum HS, Himeno S, Hill KE, Burk RF. 1996. Multiple forms of selenoprotein P in rat plasma. *Arch. Biochem. Biophys.* 325:124–28
22. Conrad HE. 1998. *Heparin-Binding Proteins*. San Diego, CA: Academic
23. Dreher I, Jakobs TC, Köhrle J. 1997. Cloning and characterization of the human selenoprotein P promoter. *J. Biol. Chem.* 272:29364–71
24. Driscoll DM, Copeland PR. 2003. Mechanism and regulation of selenoprotein synthesis. *Annu. Rev. Nutr.* 23:17–40
25. Duffield AJ, Thomson CD, Hill KE, Williams S. 1999. An estimation of selenium requirements for New Zealanders. *Am. J. Clin. Nutr.* 70:896–903

26. Esaki N, Nakamura T, Tanaka H, Soda K. 1982. Selenocysteine lyase, a novel enzyme that specifically acts on selenocysteine. Mammalian distribution and purification and properties of pig liver enzyme. *J. Biol. Chem.* 257:4386–91
27. Feldhoff RC, Taylor JM, Jefferson LS. 1977. Synthesis and secretion of rat albumin in vivo, in perfused liver, and in isolated hepatocytes. Effects of hypophysectomy and growth hormone treatment. *J. Biol. Chem.* 252:3611–16
28. Flohé L, Gunzler WA, Schock HH. 1973. Glutathione peroxidase: a selenoenzyme. *FEBS Lett.* 32:132–34
29. Fomenko DE, Gladyshev VN. 2003. Identity and functions of CxxC-derived motifs. *Biochemistry* 42:11214–25
30. Gladyshev VN, Khangulov SV, Stadtman TC. 1994. Nicotinic acid hydroxylase from *Clostridium barkeri*: electron paramagnetic resonance studies show that selenium is coordinated with molybdenum in the catalytically active selenium-dependent enzyme. *Proc. Natl. Acad. Sci. USA* 91:232–36
31. Herrman JL. 1977. The properties of a rat serum protein labelled by the injection of sodium selenite. *Biochim. Biophys. Acta* 500:61–70
32. Hill KE, Lloyd RS, Burk RF. 1993. Conserved nucleotide sequences in the open reading frame and 3′-untranslated region of selenoprotein P. *Proc. Natl. Acad. Sci. USA* 90:537–41
33. Hill KE, Lloyd RS, Yang J-G, Read R, Burk RF. 1991. The cDNA for rat selenoprotein P contains ten TGA codons in the open reading frame. *J. Biol. Chem.* 266:10050–53
34. Hill KE, McCollum GW, Boeglin ME, Burk RF. 1997. Thioredoxin reductase activity is decreased by selenium deficiency. *Biochem. Biophys. Res. Commun.* 234:293–95
35. Hill KE, Motley AK, Hu M, Austin LM, Burk RF. 2004. Deletion of selenoprotein P in female mice results in poor selenium status of their fetuses and neonates. *FASEB J.* 18:A849
36. Hill KE, Xia Y, Åkesson B, Boeglin ME, Burk RF. 1996. Selenoprotein P concentration in plasma is an index of selenium status in selenium-deficient and selenium-supplemented Chinese subjects. *J. Nutr.* 126:138–45
37. Hill KE, Zhou J, McMahan WJ, Motley AK, Atkins JF, et al. 2003. Deletion of selenoprotein P alters distribution of selenium in the mouse. *J. Biol. Chem.* 278:13640–46
38. Hill KE, Zhou J, McMahan WJ, Motley AK, Burk RF. 2004. Neurological dysfunction occurs in mice with targeted deletion of selenoprotein P gene. *J. Nutr.* 134:157–61
39. Himeno S, Chittum HS, Burk RF. 1996. Isoforms of selenoprotein P in rat plasma. Evidence for a full-length form and another form that terminates at the second UGA in the open reading frame. *J. Biol. Chem.* 271:15769–75
40. Hoekstra WG. 1975. Biochemical function of selenium and its relation to vitamin E. *Fed. Proc.* 34:2083–89
41. Hondal RJ, Ma S, Caprioli RM, Hill KE, Burk RF. 2001. Heparin-binding histidine and lysine residues of rat selenoprotein P. *J. Biol. Chem.* 276:15823–31
42. Kato T, Read R, Rozga J, Burk RF. 1992. Evidence for intestinal release of absorbed selenium in a form with high hepatic extraction. *Am. J. Physiol.* 262:G854–58
43. Koeman JH, Peeters WH, Koudstaal-Hol CH, Tjioe PS, de Goeij JJ. 1973. Mercury-selenium correlations in marine mammals. *Nature* 245:385–86
44. Kryukov GV, Castellano S, Novoselov SV, Lobanov AV, Zehtab O, et al. 2003. Characterization of mammalian selenoproteomes. *Science* 300:1439–43
45. Kryukov GV, Gladyshev VN. 2000. Selenium metabolism in zebrafish: multiplicity of selenoprotein genes and expression of a protein containing seventeen selenocysteine residues. *Genes Cells* 5:1049–60

46. Kryukov GV, Kryukov VM, Gladyshev VN. 1999. New mammalian selenocysteine-containing proteins identified with an algorithm that searches for selenocysteine insertion sequence elements. *J. Biol. Chem.* 274:33888–97
47. Lescure A, Fagegaltier D, Carbon P, Krol A. 2002. Protein factors mediating selenoprotein synthesis. *Curr. Protein Pept. Sci.* 3:143–51
48. Lescure A, Gautheret D, Carbon P, Krol A. 1999. Novel selenoproteins identified in silico and in vivo by using a conserved RNA structural motif. *J. Biol. Chem.* 274: 38147–54
49. Levander OA, Alfthan G, Arvilommi H, Gref CG, Huttunen JK, et al. 1983. Bioavailability of selenium to Finnish men as assessed by platelet glutathione peroxidase activity and other blood parameters. *Am. J. Clin. Nutr.* 37:887–97
50. Low SC, Grundner-Culemann E, Harney JW, Berry MJ. 2000. SECIS-SBP2 interactions dictate selenocysteine incorporation efficiency and selenoprotein hierarchy. *EMBO J.* 19:6882–90
51. Ma SG, Caprioli RM, Hill KE, Burk RF. 2003. Loss of selenium from selenoproteins: conversion of selenocysteine to dehydroalanine in vitro. *J. Am. Soc. Mass Spectrom.* 14:593–600
52a. Ma SG, Hill KE, Burk RF, Caprioli RM. 2003. Mass spectrometric identification of N- and O-glycosylation sites of full-length rat selenoprotein P and determination of selenide-sulfide and disulfide linkages in the shortest isoform. *Biochemistry* 42:9703–11
52b. Ma SG, Hill KE, Burk RF, Caprioli RM. 2005. Determination of selenide-sulfide (selenenylsulfide) linkages in a selenopeptide from rat selenoprotein P. *J. Mass Spectrom.* e-print ahead of publication
53. Ma SG, Hill KE, Caprioli RM, Burk RF. 2002. Mass spectrometric characterization of full-length rat selenoprotein P and three isoforms shortened at the C terminus. Evidence that three UGA codons in the mRNA open reading frame have alternative functions of specifying selenocysteine insertion or translation termination. *J. Biol. Chem.* 277:12749–54
54. McKeehan WL, Hamilton WG, Ham RG. 1976. Selenium is an essential trace nutrient for growth of WI-38 diploid human fibroblasts. *Proc. Natl. Acad. Sci. USA* 73: 2023–27
55. Mostert V, Lombeck I, Abel J. 1998. A novel method for the purification of selenoprotein P from human plasma. *Arch. Biochem. Biophys.* 357:326–30
56. Mostert V, Wolff S, Dreher I, Köhrle J, Abel J. 2001. Identification of an element within the promoter of human selenoprotein P responsive to transforming growth factor-beta. *Eur. J. Biochem.* 268:6176–81
57. Motsenbocker MA, Tappel AL. 1982. A selenocysteine-containing selenium-transport protein in rat plasma. *Biochim. Biophys. Acta* 719:147–53
58a. Olson GE, Winfrey VP, NagDas SK, Hill KE, Burk RF. 2005. Selenoprotein P is required for mouse sperm development. *Biol. Reprod.* In press
58b. Persson-Moschos M. 2000. Selenoprotein P. *Cell. Mol. Life Sci.* 57:1836–45
59. Persson-Moschos M, Alfthan G, Åkesson B. 1998. Plasma selenoprotein P levels of healthy males in different selenium status after oral supplementation with different forms of selenium. *Eur. J. Clin. Nutr.* 52:363–67
60. Persson-Moschos M, Bonnefont-Rousselot D, Assogba U, Bruckert E, Jaudon MC, et al. 1995. Preferential depletion of selenoprotein P in hypercholesterolaemic patients treated by LDL-apheresis. *Clin. Chim. Acta* 240:209–12
61. Read R, Bellew T, Yang J-G, Hill KE, Palmer IS, Burk RF. 1990. Selenium and amino acid composition of selenoprotein P, the major selenoprotein in rat serum. *J. Biol. Chem.* 265:17899–905
62. Rotruck JT, Pope AL, Ganther HE,

Swanson AB, Hafeman D, Hoekstra WG. 1973. Selenium: biochemical role as a component of glutathione peroxidase. *Science* 179:588–90
63. Saijoh K, Saito N, Lee MJ, Fujii M, Kobayashi T, Sumino K. 1995. Molecular cloning of cDNA encoding a bovine selenoprotein P-like protein containing 12 selenocysteines and a (His-Pro) rich domain insertion, and its regional expression. *Mol. Brain Res.* 30:301–11
64. Saito Y, Hayashi T, Tanaka A, Watanabe Y, Suzuki M, et al. 1999. Selenoprotein P in human plasma as an extracellular phospholipid hydroperoxide glutathione peroxidase. *J. Biol. Chem.* 274:2866–71
65. Saito Y, Sato N, Hirashima M, Takebe G, Nagasawa S, Takahashi K. 2004. Domain structure of bi-functional selenoprotein P. *Biochem. J.* 381:841–46
66. Saito Y, Takahashi K. 2002. Characterization of selenoprotein P as a selenium supply protein. *Eur. J. Biochem.* 269:5746–51
67. Saito Y, Watanabe Y, Saito E, Honjoh T, Takahashi K. 2001. Production and application of monoclonal antibodies to human selenoprotein P. *J. Health Sci.* 47:346–52
68. Schomburg L, Schweizer U, Holtmann B, Flohé L, Sendtner M, Köhrle J. 2003. Gene disruption discloses role of selenoprotein P in selenium delivery to target tissues. *Biochem. J.* 370:397–402
69. Schweizer U, Michaelis M, Köhrle J, Schomburg L. 2004. Efficient selenium transfer from mother to offspring in selenoprotein-P-deficient mice enables dose-dependent rescue of phenotypes associated with selenium deficiency. *Biochem. J.* 378:21–26
70. Sies H, Arteel GE. 2000. Interaction of peroxynitrite with selenoproteins and glutathione peroxidase mimics. *Free Radic. Biol. Med.* 28:1451–55
71. Steinert P, Bächner D, Flohé L. 1998. Analysis of the mouse selenoprotein P gene. *Biol. Chem.* 379:683–91
72. Suzuki KT, Sasakura C, Yoneda S. 1998. Binding sites for the (Hg-Se) complex on selenoprotein P. *Biochim. Biophys. Acta* 1429:102–12
73. Takebe G, Yarimizu J, Saito Y, Hayashi T, Nakamura H, et al. 2002. A comparative study on the hydroperoxide and thiol specificity of the glutathione peroxidase family and selenoprotein P. *J. Biol. Chem.* 277:41254–58
74. Thisse C, Degrave A, Kryukov GV, Gladyshev VN, Obrecht-Pflumio S, et al. 2003. Spatial and temporal expression patterns of selenoprotein genes during embryogenesis in zebrafish. *Gene Expr. Patterns* 3:525–32
75. Traulsen H, Steinbrenner H, Buchczyk DP, Klotz LO, Sies H. 2004. Selenoprotein P protects low-density lipoprotein against oxidation. *Free Radic. Res.* 38:123–28
76. Tujebajeva RM, Harney JW, Berry MJ. 2000. Selenoprotein P expression, purification, and immunochemical characterization. *J. Biol. Chem.* 275:6288–94
77. Whanger PD, Xia Y, Thomson CD. 1994. Protein technics for selenium speciation in human body fluids. *J. Trace Elem. Electrolytes Health Dis.* 8:1–7
78. Xia Y, Hill KE, Byrne DW, Xu J, Burk RF. 2005. Effectiveness of selenium supplements in a low-selenium area of China. *Am. J. Clin. Nutr.* In press
79. Yan J, Barrett JN. 1998. Purification from bovine serum of a survival-promoting factor for cultured central neurons and its identification as selenoprotein P. *J. Neurosci.* 18:8682–91
80. Yang J-G, Hill KE, Burk RF. 1989. Dietary selenium intake controls rat plasma selenoprotein P concentration. *J. Nutr.* 119:1010–12
81. Yang J-G, Morrison-Plummer J, Burk RF. 1987. Purification and quantitation of a rat plasma selenoprotein distinct from glutathione peroxidase using monoclonal antibodies. *J. Biol. Chem.* 262:13372–75
82. Yasui Y, Hasada K, Yang J-G, Koiwai O. 1996. Structure and organization of

the gene encoding human selenoprotein P. *Gene* 175:260–70

83. Yoneda S, Suzuki KT. 1997. Detoxification of mercury by selenium by binding of equimolar Hg-Se complex to a specific plasma protein. *Toxicol. Appl. Pharmacol.* 143:274–80

84. Zhong L, Arner ES, Holmgren A. 2000. Structure and mechanism of mammalian thioredoxin reductase: The active site is a redox-active selenolthiol/selenenylsulfide formed from the conserved cysteine-selenocysteine sequence. *Proc. Natl. Acad. Sci. USA* 97:5854–59

Annu. Rev. Nutr. 2005. 25:237–60
doi: 10.1146/annurev.nutr.25.050304.092526

First published online as a Review in Advance on March 7, 2005

ENERGY INTAKE, MEAL FREQUENCY, AND HEALTH: A Neurobiological Perspective*

Mark P. Mattson
Laboratory of Neurosciences, National Institute on Aging Intramural Research Program, Baltimore, Maryland 21224, and Department of Neuroscience, Johns Hopkins University School of Medicine, Baltimore, Maryland 21205; email: mattsonm@grc.nia.nih.gov

Key Words BDNF, caloric restriction, insulin resistance, obesity, serotonin

■ **Abstract** The size and frequency of meals are fundamental aspects of nutrition that can have profound effects on the health and longevity of laboratory animals. In humans, excessive energy intake is associated with increased incidence of cardiovascular disease, diabetes, and certain cancers and is a major cause of disability and death in industrialized countries. On the other hand, the influence of meal frequency on human health and longevity is unclear. Both caloric (energy) restriction (CR) and reduced meal frequency/intermittent fasting can suppress the development of various diseases and can increase life span in rodents by mechanisms involving reduced oxidative damage and increased stress resistance. Many of the beneficial effects of CR and fasting appear to be mediated by the nervous system. For example, intermittent fasting results in increased production of brain-derived neurotrophic factor (BDNF), which increases the resistance of neurons in the brain to dysfunction and degeneration in animal models of neurodegenerative disorders; BDNF signaling may also mediate beneficial effects of intermittent fasting on glucose regulation and cardiovascular function. A better understanding of the neurobiological mechanisms by which meal size and frequency affect human health may lead to novel approaches for disease prevention and treatment.

CONTENTS

*The US Government has the right to retain a nonexclusive, royalty-free license in and to any copyright covering this paper.

FOOD INTAKE AND LIFE SPAN

More than 70 years ago, it was discovered that reducing energy intake during adult life can increase the life span of laboratory rodents (87). The ability of caloric restriction (CR) during adult life to lengthen life span has been observed consistently in many different species of mammals (134). In all such energy-restriction studies described in this chapter the control group was fed ad libitum and the CR diet group received amounts of micronutrients equivalent to those consumed by the control group. It should therefore be kept in mind that, with regard to food intake, ad libitum feeding in the laboratory is not the norm for rodents in the wild. Instead, the control animals are overfed and overweight. Both the amount of the energy restriction and the duration of restriction period influence the extent to which life span is increased (134). Reductions in energy intake of 30%–40% below the ad libitum level increase both the average and maximum life span of mice and rats by 30%–40%. Maximum extension of life span is achieved when CR is initiated in young adult animals, with diminishing extension as the time of onset of energy restriction is delayed. The amount by which CR extends life span in rodents also depends upon the baseline energy intake of the control group and the magnitude of CR; life span is progressively increased with progressive reductions in energy intake from the ad libitum amount up to approximately 50% reduction, beyond which further CR results in increased mortality. A study of the effects of CR (30% reduction in calories) on the life span of rhesus monkeys was initiated in 1987. The data obtained to date suggest that the health of the monkeys on CR is improved and their life span is increased compared with the monkeys on the control diet (82). In humans, overeating promotes diseases in multiple organ systems that usually shorten life. In the United States, overeating is now considered a leading cause of morbidity and mortality (13, 16). Particularly disturbing is the rapid increase in overweight children with insulin resistance who are at very high risk for diabetes and vascular diseases that shorten life (94).

By comparison with the intense interest in the quantity (and quality) of food intake on health and longevity, the influence of meal frequency has been under-studied. Intermittent fasting regimens, such as every-other-day fasting (EODF, the most commonly employed protocol in animal studies), can increase the life span of rats and mice (19, 45, 47). Both mean and maximum life spans are increased by EODF in different species and in most (but not all) strains of rodents (134). The relationship of the age of initiation of intermittent fasting and life span was studied in Wistar rats. Increases in life span were obtained by EODF during all or part of the life span, but there was not a strong correlation between the effects of EODF on growth and body composition and its effect on life span (10). Life span extension by EODF is associated with improved glucose metabolism and cardiovascular function, and increased function and resilience of the brain (4, 84, 130).

In contrast to animal studies, the results of human studies that have attempted to determine the effects of CR and meal frequency on health have been difficult to interpret because of their design. The studies of starvation by Ancel Keys were perhaps the first to suggest that severe long-term CR may actually have health benefits in humans (67). More recently, participants in the Biosphere study who were forced to eat a low-calorie diet over a period of approximately two years exhibited highly significant decreases in blood pressure and insulin and cholesterol levels (129). Health benefits of smaller, more frequent meals are suggested from survey-based evaluations of the association between meal frequency and obesity, hypercholesterolemia, and glucose intolerance (35), and from the assessment of the effects of short-term (days to weeks) high and low meal-frequency diets on glucose regulation (65, 66). It has been suggested that skipping breakfast is unhealthy (66), but other findings indicate that skipping breakfast can decrease risk factors for cardiovascular disease and diabetes (80). Data from an epidemiological study of 6928 adults revealed no association between breakfast skipping and mortality (138). Studies of different populations of humans that periodically fast as part of their religion suggest health benefits of such reduced meal-frequency diets (2). Unfortunately, most of the studies on meal frequency and human health that have been performed were conducted over short time periods (days to weeks) with low numbers of subjects and did not control for calorie intake, exercise, and other important variables. However, in a recent study of nonobese human subjects maintained for 22 days on an EODF regimen, it was shown that this intermittent-fasting diet results in a highly significant decrease in insulin levels (57).

In principle, there should be a window of energy intake that promotes optimum health, and this should also be true for meal frequency (Figure 1). However, the actual values for optimum calorie intake and meal frequency may vary considerably among individuals because of factors such as their activity level, age, and sex. For example, a physician or dietician can be confident in recommending that a 30-year-old overweight sedentary female who consumes 3000 calories per day reduce her intake to 2000 calories per day. However, it is unclear to what extent (if any) a 30-year-old normal-weight active, but hypercholesterolemic, male who consumes 2300 calories per day would benefit from reducing his intake to 2000 calories per day. In regard to meal frequency, there are insufficient data from human studies to justify any recommendations.

GROWTH AND REPRODUCTION

As might be expected, CR and intermittent fasting can reduce body weight in adults, an effect that is often desirable. CR reduces body weight and retards body weight gain in adults of all species of organisms (134). The growth-retarding effect

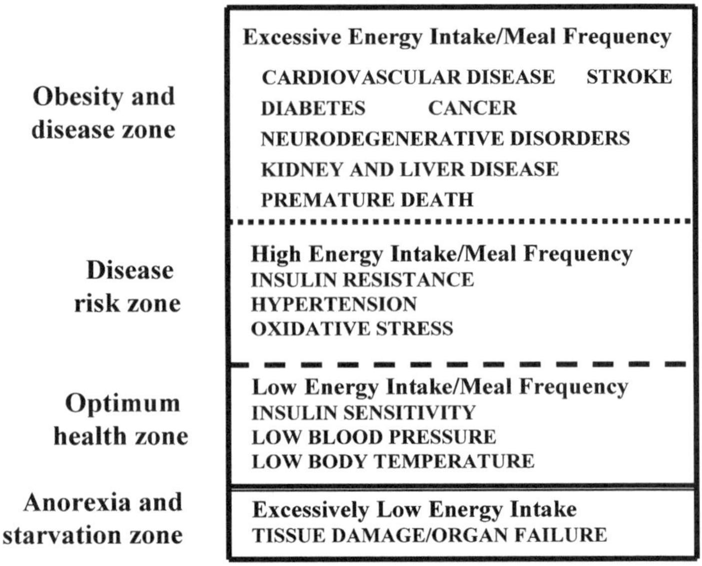

Figure 1 Influence of different levels of energy intake and meal frequency on health. Excessive energy intake results in obesity and a strong likelihood of morbidity and premature death. High levels of energy intake and meal frequency may increase the risk of diabetes, cardiovascular diseases, cancer, and neurodegenerative disorders. Moderate reductions in energy intake and meal frequency promote optimum health, whereas excessive dietary restriction, as in anorexia nervosa, can result in morbidity and mortality.

of CR was partially prevented by leptin administration in mice; this was associated with reduced insulin-like growth factor (IGF)-1 levels but increased levels of IGF-1 receptor (41). These findings suggest important roles for leptin and IGF-1 signaling mechanisms in the effects of CR on growth. Studies performed approximately 40 years ago demonstrated that intermittent fasting periods of days to weeks could be effective in the correction and control of obesity in humans (34, 121). In rodents, the effects of EODF on body weight differ among species and strains. For example, Wistar and Sprague-Dawley rats exhibit 20%–30% reductions in body weight (46, 130), whereas C57BL/6 and A/J mice show little reduction in body weight during periods of many months on EODF (4, 47). Interestingly, while the growth of young adult rats is retarded by EODF, regular exercise (treadmill running) enhanced the growth of the EODF rats (115). In a study of the eating patterns of children in the Bogalusa Heart Study, there was a marked increase in the percentage of children who skipped breakfast (from 8% to 30%) from 1973 to 1978, but there was no association between this change in meal pattern and overweight status (102).

The development of embryos, infants, and juveniles is very sensitive to energy intake. Accordingly, and in contrast to adults, it is critical that developing humans receive sufficient energy to permit normal growth and physical and cognitive development. Physiological adaptations can occur that modify the effects of CR on body weight and development. When pregnant Sprague-Dawley rats are maintained on CR (15%, 30%, or 50% restriction) during gestation, they continue to gain weight, in contrast to nonpregnant rats, which lose weight on the 30% and 50% CR diets (109). Moreover, the growth of the developing embryos was not reduced in the rats on the CR diets. These findings suggest that pregnant rats are able to modify their metabolism during pregnancy in ways that allow normal growth of their embryos. However, people who are undernourished during fetal and early postnatal development are at increased risk for developing type 2 diabetes as adults (51). An association between low birth weight and the risk of type 2 diabetes in adult life has been established in several different human studies. Maternal CR and maternal diabetes may alter the development of the endocrine pancreas in the developing fetus in ways that predispose the offspring to insulin resistance later in life (108). Male rats growth-retarded during fetal life and cross-fostered shortly after birth to normal lactating dams reach a normal weight by weaning but have a reduced longevity. Thus, energy restriction during embryonic and early postnatal life can promote disease in adult life and may reduce longevity. CR can have adverse effects on reproduction in women. For example, in one study of 47 women who were underweight because they practiced CR, 29 had unexplained infertility and 18 had menstrual dysfunction (8). When 36 of these women subsequently followed a dietary regimen to increase their weight, 19 of 26 infertile women conceived spontaneously, and 9 of 10 women with secondary amenorrhea resumed menstruation. Thus, the practice of CR in young women may be a cause of unexplained infertility and menstrual disorders. Studies of women with anorexia nervosa with or without amenorrhea, and similar in body mass index, showed that the eumenorrheic women had higher levels of body fat, leptin, and IGF-1 compared with the amenorrheic women (95). The latter findings suggest that interindividual differences in neuroendocrine responses to severe CR may determine whether women suffer reproductive abnormalities.

Animal studies have documented effects of CR on specific aspects of reproductive physiology in females and males. Rat pups whose mothers had been fed either ad libitum or 50% CR were maintained on ad libitum or CR diets. CR during embryonic development and during postnatal development significantly impaired reproduction and decreased milk yield (90). When young adult Kunmin mice were maintained on a 35% CR diet for three months, their maturation of reproductive function was delayed and their fertility was decreased (140). Sperm motility was reduced and numbers of abnormal sperm increased in mice on the CR diet. When young adult male Wistar rats were maintained on CR, there was a significant decrease in the size of their testis and epididymis, levels of circulating testosterone were reduced, and their copulatory efficiency was reduced (116). Although severe CR has adverse effects on fertility and reproduction, more moderate levels of CR can prolong the reproductive period in rodents (91). In a National Institute on Aging study of monkeys maintained on 30% CR for more than 15 years, the reproductive system of females did not appear to be adversely affected (82, 113). Collectively, the available data suggest that moderate levels of CR may not adversely affect growth and reproduction, whereas more severe energy restriction is detrimental. The effects of intermittent fasting on reproductive systems remain to be determined.

HEALTH INDICATORS

A large amount of information on the physiological effects of energy restriction and, to a lesser extent, reduced-meal-frequency diets has been collected from studies of rodents, monkeys, and humans (56, 82, 134). Examples of several reproducible changes documented in rodents and primates are presented in Table 1.

TABLE 1 Physiological changes associated with energy restriction and intermittent fasting in mammals

Variable	Energy restriction	Intermittent fasting
Blood	**(56*, 82*, 134*)[r,m,h]**	**(1, 3, 32, 37, 57, 83*)[r,h]**
Glucose	Decrease	Decrease
Insulin	Decrease	Decrease
IGF-1	Decrease	No change or increase
Triglycerides	Decrease	na
LDL cholesterol	Decrease or no change	Decrease or no change
HDL cholesterol	Increase	Increase or no change
Ketones	No change	Increase
Cardiovascular	**(39, 56*, 82*, 134*, 142)[r,m,h]**	**(112, 130)[r,h]**
Blood pressure	Decrease	Decrease
Heart rate	Decrease	Decrease
Atherosclerosis	Decrease	na
Muscle	**(56*, 133, 134*)[r,h]**	**(37)[r]**
Insulin sensitivity	Increase	Increase
Lipid accumulation	Decrease	Decrease
Brain	**(15, 27, 62, 81, 92)[r,m]**	**(71, 72, 75, 83*)[r]**
Cognition	Enhanced memory	Enhanced memory
Motor function	Improved	Improved
Neurogenesis	No change	Increase
Pain threshold	Increased	na
BDNF, GDNF	No change or increase	Increase

FOOTNOTES: r, rodents; m, monkeys; h, humans.

ABBREVIATIONS: BDNF, brain-derived neurotrophic factor; GDNF, glial cell line–derived neurotrophic factor; HDL, high-density lipoprotein; IGF, insulin-like growth factor; LDL, low-density lipoprotein; na, not assessed.

*References 56, 82, 83, and 134 are review articles that include references to the relevant primary studies.

A sustained reduction in body temperature occurs in mammals on CR diets, whereas in animals on EODF, body temperature is decreased during the fasting period and increases in the fed state (130). Rats and mice maintained on 40% CR or EODF exhibit reductions in circulating levels of insulin and glucose (4). Another highly reproducible effect of both CR and EODF is to decrease resting heart rate and blood pressure and to improve cardiovascular stress adaptation (39, 130, 142). Insulin resistance and hypertension are major risk factors for coronary and cerebrovascular artery disease, consistent with vasculoprotective effects of CR and intermittent fasting. Changes in blood lipids that occur in rodents, monkeys, and humans on CR [decreased low-density lipoprotein (LDL) cholesterol and triglycerides and increased levels of high-density lipoprotein (HDL) cholesterol] would also be expected to suppress atherosclerosis (39, 82). Consistent with a cardioprotective effect of regular fasting in humans, Moslems who fast during the month of Ramadan have reduced levels of LDL cholesterol and increased levels of HDL cholesterol (112).

CR and intermittent fasting have beneficial effects on immune function in adults. Data suggest that both reduced-energy and reduced-meal-frequency diets can reduce inflammatory responses, as indicated by reduced production of tumor necrosis factor by macrophages (127). T lymphocyte responses to concanavalin A and responses of B lymphocytes to pokeweed mitogen were reduced in obese subjects compared with normal weight controls, and these impairments in immune responsiveness were reversed by CR (123). On the other hand, the production of inflammatory cytokines and other mediators of inflammation are decreased in rodents on CR. In addition, allergic reactions to commonly encountered allergens, such as dust mite antigen, are decreased in rodents on CR (29). Overall, the effects of CR on the immune system appear to be beneficial, promoting the eradication of infectious agents while limiting tissue damage caused by inflammation. However, cell-mediated immune function is impaired in anorexia nervosa (79), which suggests that extreme CR has detrimental effects on the immune system. The effectiveness of the immune system in battling infection is also affected by meal frequency. When weanling mice were subjected to EODF, the responses of their leukocytes to immune challenge were reduced during the first month on the diet and recovered to normal levels by six months (78). In contrast, the immune responses of 17-month-old mice were improved by EODF. Collectively, the available data suggest that CR and intermittent fasting enhance immune function in adults but may compromise certain immune responses in infants and juveniles.

CR and intermittent fasting can influence indicators of health of the nervous system. CR (40%) in female mice during their adult life prevented age-related declines in learning and motor coordination (62). Analysis of the structure of dendrites in layer V pyramidal neurons in the parietal cortex of rats that had been maintained on either EODF or ad libitum diets revealed that EODF suppresses age-related loss of dendritic spines, a structural indicator of synapses (97). Such effects on the structure of neurons may underlie the beneficial effects of dietary restriction in preserving learning and memory and motor function in rodents.

Age-related alterations in neurotransmitter-synthesizing enzymes and neurotransmitter receptors in the brain were suppressed in rats that had been maintained on an EODF diet during their adult life compared with rats fed ad libitum (75). EODF was particularly effective in increasing cholinergic markers (choline acetyltransferase and muscarinic receptors). Another reported physiological effect of EODF on the nervous system is increased pain thresholds in mice (27); however, its implications for health are not clear. The influence of overeating on the health of the central and peripheral nervous systems are poorly understood, but it does appear to have numerous adverse effects that can lead to morbidity and mortality (84).

Energy restriction and reduced meal frequency can increase the resistance of organisms to various types of stress. For example, intermittent fasting increased the resistance of rats to cold stress and resulted in changes in collagen and bone consistent with an antiaging effect (60). Thermoregulation is compromised during aging in mice, resulting in reduced cold tolerance, and EODF ameliorates this age-related alteration (122). Mice subjected to 14 cycles of one day of fasting followed by two days of ad libitum feeding exhibited reduced energy expenditure in brown adipose tissue, an adaptation that may play a role in the conservation of energy during intermittent bouts of food deprivation (28). Adult male rats were maintained on an alternating schedule of three days fasting and three days refeeding for ten weeks, and several physiological responses to exercise were measured (37). In response to two hours of swimming, rats on the control diet exhibited hypoglycemia, whereas rats on the EODF diet were able to maintain blood glucose levels even though they had lower levels of liver glycogen and plasma free fatty acids. Thus, CR and intermittent fasting can enhance homeostatic mechanisms that counteract the potentially damaging effects of environmental stressors.

DISEASE

Overeating increases the risk of numerous diseases and shortens life span (13, 16). Accordingly, CR reduces disease risk in overweight individuals and may also have health benefits in those of normal weight (56). The influence of meal frequency on health and disease processes is not well known. However, studies of the physiological effects of long-term energy restriction and intermittent fasting in animals and humans are revealing possible mechanisms responsible for effects of meal size and frequency on health and disease processes.

Cancer

Studies of rodents have consistently shown that both CR and intermittent fasting can reduce the incidence of spontaneous tumors and can suppress the development and growth of induced cancers. When adult tumor-prone mice were maintained on either 40% energy restriction or a one-day-per-week fasting regimen, the onset of spontaneous tumors was significantly delayed (12). A "weight-cycling" regimen in which mice were fed a repeating cycle of three weeks at 50% of ad libitum intake followed by three weeks ad libitum during their adult life reduced both the incidence and latency of mammary tumors (20). When one-month-old Wistar rats were maintained on a schedule of 48 h of fasting per week for 48 weeks, they were more resistant to hepatocarcinogenesis induced by diethylnitrosamine compared with rats fed ad libitum (111). In another study, 40% energy restriction protected against carcinogen-induced tumor formation in mice, but an energy cycling diet (alternating two-day periods of 40% energy restriction and ad libitum feeding) was ineffective (55). CR also appears to decrease cancer incidence in monkeys (82). The mechanism by which energy restriction suppresses cancer formation may involve enhancement of apoptosis and inhibition of angiogenesis (98).

Type 2 Diabetes

The risk for type 2 diabetes is greatly increased by excessive weight gain attributable to long-term diets with energy intakes in excess of requirement (23), and CR is effective in improving glucose regulation in individuals with diabetes (135). Animal studies strongly support antidiabetic effects of CR and intermittent fasting diets. Both CR and EODF reduce blood glucose and insulin concentrations and improve glucose tolerance in rodents (4, 133, 136). The issue of whether it is healthier to eat small frequent meals or less-frequent larger meals is currently the subject of considerable debate (85). Although it has been reported that patients with diabetes are better able to "control" their blood glucose concentrations when they eat regular small meals, an intermittent very-low-calorie diet improved weight loss and glycemic control more effectively than did moderate CR in subjects with type 2 diabetes (135). Moreover, two different fasting regimens (EODF and fasting two days per week) reduced diabetes incidence in Brattleboro rats (106). Increased insulin sensitivity appears to be the major mechanism responsible for the antidiabetic effects of energy restriction and intermittent fasting (4, 48).

Cardiovascular Disease

Data from epidemiological studies have shown that low-energy diets reduce the risk of cardiovascular disease and stroke in humans (3). A recent study in humans provided strong evidence that long-term CR can reduce the risk of atherosclerosis (39). In addition to suppressing the process of atherosclerosis, energy restriction and regular fasting may more directly protect heart and brain cells against ischemic damage. Indeed, CR protected the heart against myocardial infarction in rats (24). When rats were maintained for three months on EODF, the extent of brain damage following a stroke was decreased and functional outcome improved (144). Thus, CR and intermittent fasting can counteract the processes that, over long periods, result in occlusion of blood vessels, and may also improve outcome in those who suffer a myocardial infarction or stroke.

Neurodegenerative and Psychiatric Disorders

By comparison with the large amount of data suggesting that reduced energy intake and meal frequency can protect against diabetes, cardiovascular disease, and cancers, relatively little is known of the influence of meal size and frequency on neurological disorders. Age-related deficits in motor function and cognition can be prevented or delayed in mice and rats maintained on 30%–40% CR or EODF (62, 92). Diabetic and prediabetic women have impaired cognitive performance and greater risk of developing cognitive impairment (141). When mice were maintained on EODF, the dopaminergic neurons in their brains were protected against dysfunction and degeneration induced by the toxin MPTP (1-methyl-4-phenyl-1,2,3,6-tetrahydropyridine), a model of Parkinson's disease (30). In a nonhuman primate model of Parkinson's disease, 30% CR was effective in reducing the severity of symptoms (81). EODF and CR can protect hippocampal neurons and basal forebrain cholinergic neurons against death induced by excitotoxins (18, 22). EODF in rats protected hippocampal neurons against degeneration induced by the amnestic excitotoxin kainic acid; memory impairment was preserved in the intermittent-fasted rats compared to the control rats fed ad libitum (18). EODF was also beneficial in a mouse model of Huntington's disease, delaying the neurodegenerative process and motor dysfunction and increasing survival (31). In contrast to the neuroprotective effects of EODF in the just-mentioned brain disorder models, EODF was not beneficial in a mouse model of amyotrophic lateral sclerosis, a motor neuron disorder (107). Thus, the influence of meal size and frequency on the development and progression of neurodegenerative disorders may depend upon the specific disorder.

Accumulating data suggest that meal size and frequency can affect mental health. There is an increased prevalence of insulin resistance in patients with schizophrenia and chronic depression compared with the general population (124). Overweight and insulin resistance have also been associated with bipolar disorder (88). The explanation(s) for these relationships might simply be that subjects with psychiatric disorders eat more and exercise less. However, it is also possible that overeating is a contributing factor to the development of psychiatric disorders. The latter possibility is supported by studies showing that CR improves mood in obese subjects (137). The mechanisms by which CR and intermittent fasting might affect the risk of psychiatric disorders are unknown but might involve changes in neurotransmitters and neurotrophic factors (see "Cellular and Molecular Mechanisms" and "The Brain Mediates Health Effects of Dietary Excesses and Frugality" sections below). Anorexia nervosa and binge eating are psychiatric conditions that fall within a broader spectrum of obsessive-compulsive disorders (54). These disorders are associated with considerable morbidity and mortality, and provide examples of the existence of a lower limit of energy intake and upper limits of meal size that, if exceeded, lead to disease (36).

Other Diseases

Meal size and frequency affect tissues throughout the body, and it is therefore not surprising that CR and fasting have been shown to influence disease processes in many different organ systems. Examples include the following. When mice and rats were maintained on CR during their adult life, the incidence of spontaneous cataracts was decreased (139). EODF improved renal function and reduced age-related glomerular lesions in rats (42). CR enhanced the regeneration of hepatocytes and prevented mortality in a rat model of liver injury (5). Patients with arthritis exhibited improved disease activity when they were maintained on CR (64). Considerable further work will be required to establish the full spectrum of diseases that may be subject to modification by energy intake and meal frequency.

CELLULAR AND MOLECULAR MECHANISMS

Studies of tissues from animals on CR and fasting diets have provided evidence for two major mechanisms by which meal size and frequency affect health and disease susceptibility. One mechanism involves the production and removal of free radicals, and the second involves stress resistance (84, 93, 134). Overeating increases oxidative stress in cells throughout the body as indicated by lipid peroxidation and the accumulation of oxidatively damaged proteins and DNA. Conversely, the amount of oxidative damage to cellular proteins, lipids, and nucleic acids is decreased in various tissues of rodents on CR (87). The vulnerability of cells to being damaged and killed by oxidative insults (radiation, mitochondrial toxins, ischemia, iron, etc.) is decreased in animals maintained on CR or EODF diets (18, 30, 40, 68). CR and EODF may suppress oxidative stress by reducing the amount of superoxide anion radical produced in the mitochondria and by stimulating the expression of genes that encode antioxidant enzymes and protein chaperones (49, 120).

When meal size and frequency are decreased in rats and mice, they become more resistant to being killed by severe stresses including exposure to toxins and high temperatures (5, 53, 119). Mice that had been maintained on EODF for one to six weeks exhibited increased resistance to death induced by gamma irradiation; the protective effect became maximal after two to three weeks of EODF (69). The stress resistance is manifest at the cellular level. For example, neurons in the brains of animals on CR and EODF diets exhibit increased resistance to being killed by neurotoxins (18, 22, 30), and heart and brain cells are more resistant to ischemic injury (1, 144).

Analyses of gene expression (and levels of the encoded proteins) reveal that CR and EODF increase the production of multiple cell survival–promoting proteins in tissues ranging from liver to brain. The stress proteins induced include protein chaperones such as heat-shock protein 70 and glucose-regulated protein 78 (30, 58, 144) and growth factors such as brain-derived neurotrophic factor (BDNF) and glial cell line–derived neurotrophic factor (GDNF) (31, 72, 81). The ability of cells

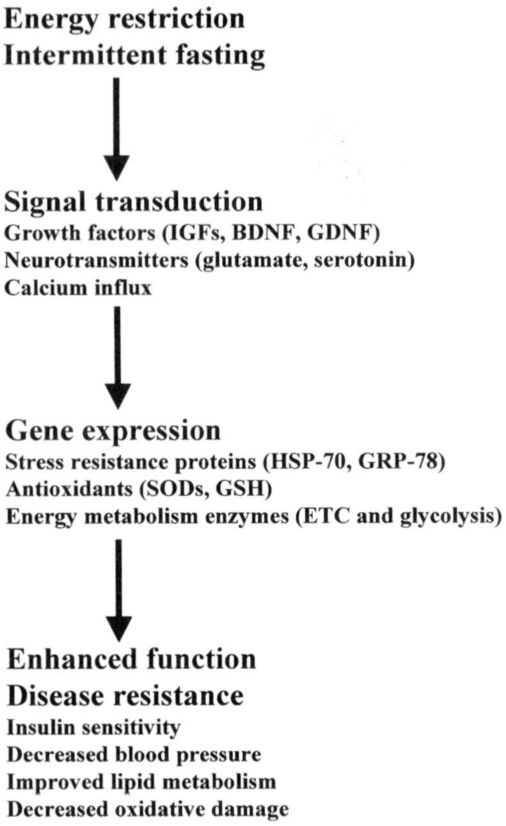

Figure 2 Mechanisms by which reduced energy intake and meal frequency may protect against disease. Dietary restriction results in the activation of signaling pathways that stimulate the expression of genes that encode proteins that help cells cope with stress and resist disease. BDNF, brain-derived neurotrophic factor; ETC, electron transport chain; GDNF, glial cell line–derived neurotrophic factor; GRP-78, glucose-regulated protein 78; GSH, glutathione; HSP-70, heat-shock protein 70; IGFs, insulin-like growth factors; SOD, superoxide dismutase.

to activate a stress response is enhanced in animals that have been maintained on CR (26, 58). Such enhanced stress resistance has been proposed as a major mechanism whereby energy restriction and intermittent fasting increase life span (Figure 2). On the other hand, overeating may foster disease by reducing the ability of cells to activate stress-resistance pathways. Recent studies of organisms from yeast to mammals have identified proteins called sirtuins (a type of histone deacetylase) that can increase cellular stress resistance and may be key mediators of the life span–extending effects of CR. For example, in rats, the sirtuin SIRT1 is induced by CR, and it increases the resistance of cells to stress-induced death (21).

THE BRAIN MEDIATES HEALTH EFFECTS OF DIETARY FRUGALITY AND EXCESSES

The brain evolved as the major regulator of food acquisition and energy metabolism (83). By direct innervation, and indirectly through the regulation of neuroendocrine systems, the brain controls the function and homeostasis of tissues and organs throughout the body. The brain is responsible for the behaviors involved in the identification and ingestion of food, and it regulates energy allocation and usage in various organs. The importance of the brain in energy regulation is underscored by its ability to perceive signals regarding energy intake and availability from peripheral organs and to modify behavior and cellular metabolism in adaptive ways. Nuclear magnetic resonance spectroscopy was used to measure adnosine triphosphate and phospocreatine levels in brain and liver of rats in the fasting and fed states and during intermittent feeding (14). The brain itself, in contrast to the liver, is able to maintain energy metabolism regardless of whether energy is supplied intermittently or continuously. The preservation of brain energy metabolism, at the expense of some peripheral tissues, is critical for the organism's ability to find food and replenish energy reserves.

The brain is also the master regulator of stress responses, which involve sensory inputs, and activation of neuroendocrine pathways involving the hypothalamus, which produces corticotrophin-releasing hormone, and the pituitary gland, which produces adrenocorticotrophin. Adrenocorticotrophin, in turn, stimulates production of glucocorticoids (cortisol in primates and corticosterone in rodents) in adrenocortical cells. Interestingly, basal levels of glucocorticoids are increased by CR and EODF, consistent with a mild stress response stimulated by such restricted diets (105, 130). It appears that the brain's perception of CR and intermittent fasting as stressors is central to activation of stress-resistance mechanisms that may protect against disease (11).

Lat & Holeckova (71) provided evidence that intermittent fasting results in increased excitability of the CNS. CR may reduce, and overeating increases, activity of the sympathetic nervous system, which likely contributes the opposite effects of CR and overeating on blood pressure (143). Levels of beta-adrenergic receptors increase in the liver during aging in rats fed ad libitum, but not in rats on EODF (25). The increased activity in nerve cell circuits in animals on energy restriction or intermittent fasting likely contributes to several beneficial effects of the reduced meal size and frequency within the brain. For example, CR and EODF enhance learning and memory ability in rodents (62). The production of new nerve cells in the brain is also influenced by meal size and frequency. The adult mammalian brain contains populations of self-renewing stem cells that are capable of forming new neurons and glial cells. EODF increases the survival of newly generated neurons in the dentate gyrus of the hippocampus in adult mice (72). On the other hand, CR did not increase hippocampal neurogenesis, but did enhance glial cell genesis by increasing the survival of newly generated glial cells (15).

BRAIN-DERIVED NEUROTROPHIC FACTOR

CR and intermittent fasting may affect health by activating signal transduction pathways in the brain that exert effects not only in the brain itself, but also in the periphery. Recent studies have shown that EODF can stimulate the production of BDNF in neurons in many different brain regions (31, 72). Other studies have shown that BDNF is a very important neurotrophic factor that plays roles in feeding, learning and memory, locomotion, stress responses, and affective behaviors (108). BDNF promotes neuronal differentiation and survival, synaptogenesis, and synaptic plasticity (43, 73, 114). BDNF may serve in adaptive responses of mammals to a variety of environmental stimuli because BDNF expression in the hippocampus increases in response to cognitive stimulation and EODF, but decreases under conditions of chronic uncontrollable stress (86, 89). Decreased BDNF levels occur in several neurodegenerative disorders including Alzheimer's, Parkinson's, and Huntington's diseases (38, 59, 61). BDNF suppresses feeding and improves glucose metabolism, as demonstrated in studies of BDNF+/− mice (32, 76). When BDNF+/− mice are maintained on an EODF diet, levels of BDNF increase in their brains and blood glucose levels and body weights are normalized (32).

The increased level of BDNF in the brain with regular exercise and intermittent fasting may be important in the improved glucose regulation because intracerebroventricular infusion of BDNF can increase peripheral insulin sensitivity in normal rodents (100) and ameliorates diabetes in mice (101). Moreover, mice in which BDNF was eliminated from the brain after birth were hypersensitive to stress, had elevated plasma glucose and insulin levels, and were obese (110). Thus, EODF and exercise enhance BDNF signaling, which, in turn, may stimulate signaling pathways that improve glucose metabolism and increase cellular stress resistance, thereby protecting against several different diseases.

Serotonin

Serotonin (5-hydroxytryptamine) is an evolutionarily conserved neurotransmitter that regulates the development and function of the mammalian brain and serves important roles in the regulation of energy metabolism in diverse organisms (7, 125). Serotonergic neurons in the raphe nucleus of the brain stem possess axons that form synapses in many different brain regions. Serotonin activates receptors coupled to GTP-binding proteins, most notably those that activate adenylate cyclase resulting in cyclic AMP production. Studies in which serotonin signaling was manipulated using pharmacological agents have provided evidence for important roles for this neurotransmitter in learning and memory, appetite regulation, neurogenesis, and affective behaviors (17). Reductions in serotonin signaling occur in several prominent psychiatric disorders, including depression and anxiety disorders (126), and in neurodegenerative disorders such as Alzheimer's disease (96).

Interestingly, serotonin may improve mood and protect neurons against degeneration by activating receptors coupled to cyclic AMP production and stimulation of BDNF production (114). BDNF, in turn, can enhance the survival and growth of serotonergic neurons (77).

Serotonin signaling can modify the risk of several major age-related disorders in both rodents and humans. Antidepressants that appear to act by increasing synaptic serotonin levels can improve risk factors for diabetes and cardiovascular disease. Patients with clinical depression have reduced insulin sensitivity compared with control subjects without depression, and the insulin sensitivity in the patients increases during treatment with serotonin-selective reuptake inhibitors (SSRIs) (103). Treatment with the SSRI paroxetine increased insulin sensitivity in depressed diabetic women (104), and when men with abdominal obesity were treated for six months with the SSRI citalopram, they showed improved glucose tolerance and their cardiovascular responses to stress were attenuated (74). Moreover, the disease process in the brain is suppressed and hyperglycemia is ameliorated by SSRI treatment in a murine model of Huntington's disease (33). The metabolic syndrome has been reported to be associated with suppressed neuroendocrine responses to serotonin (99), which suggests that a defect in serotonergic control of hypothalamic function may underlie the impaired ability of patients with insulin resistance to engage adaptive responses to stress.

Roles for serotonin in health effects of energy intake and meal frequency remain to be established. However, data are accumulating that suggest associations between food intake patterns, serotonin signaling, and disease risk. For example, using in vivo microdialysis methods, Gur et al. (50) provided evidence that serotonergic signaling is increased in the hypothalamus of female rats that had been maintained for four weeks on a food-restriction regimen. Serotonin turnover in the brain is affected by semi-starvation in rats, consistent with a role for this neurotransmitter in mediating responses to changes in meal frequency (118). Levels of serotonin are decreased in the brains of rats during aging, and treatment of the aged rats with the antioxidant alpha-lipoic acid increased serotonin levels, which suggests that serotonin depletion during aging may result, at least in part, from oxidative stress (6). These findings suggest that serotonin signaling in the brain can suppress a process, i.e., oxidative stress, which may be fundamental to the aging process. During normal aging in humans, levels of serotonin are relatively stable and levels of several serotonin receptors decrease; in contrast, patients with Alzheimer's disease exhibit degeneration of serotonergic neurons that, in combination with serotonin receptor loss, results in a severe functional serotonergic deficit (96). Positron emission tomography imaging of glucose metabolism in the brains of young and old control subjects and subjects treated with the SSRI citalopram suggests that age-related loss of serotonin innervation of the cerebral cortex can be compensated for in some brain regions (44). These kinds of data suggest a role for serotonin in aging and provide a rationale for direct tests of the effects of manipulations of serotonergic signaling on life span in rodents.

IMPLICATIONS FOR IMPROVING HEALTH

What are the implications of the findings described in this article for improving health? The data from the animal studies reviewed above suggest that reducing energy intake and intermittent fasting can have numerous health benefits, effectively reducing morbidity and mortality. Most adults and many children in industrialized countries could clearly benefit from reducing energy intake by decreasing meal size. The problem is how to accomplish this in an environment of an overabundance of continuously accessible high-energy foods and beverages and in the face of unavoidable advertisements from the food industry. To date, the majority of people who overeat have been unable to voluntarily limit their food intake, despite their knowledge of the health hazards of overeating. Primary care physicians are not trained in diet management and are not prepared to prescribe specific eating regimens on a case-by-case basis. This is unfortunate, as overeating is a major health problem and should be treated as such. Beyond simply reducing the amount of food consumed, CR can be accomplished by substituting foods with a low energy density (vegetables and fruits) for those with a high energy density (fried foods, fatty meats, etc.). The latter approach has the added benefit of including foods that contain higher amounts of vitamins and various other beneficial phytochemicals.

What strategies and interventions might be implemented to take advantage of the health benefits of CR and intermittent fasting? Physicians are trained to deal with extreme overeating and anorexia, disorders that can be considered psychiatric disorders that result from abnormalities in brain neurochemistry and can be treated with behavioral therapy and medications (128, 132). In contrast, most practicing physicians are not trained to make recommendations regarding the health benefits of dietary restriction in individuals who are not obese. Medical students and residents should be trained in the physiology of dietary restriction and its value in disease prevention for most individuals. Controlled human studies should be performed in order to establish the parameters of meal frequency and energy intake that are optimal for reducing the risk of major diseases. Patients would then be prescribed a dietary regimen that would be expected to result in health benefits. Because of the strong links between insulin sensitivity and blood pressure to diabetes and cardiovascular disease, these variables could be monitored in individual patients as surrogate measures of disease risk. The limited data available from human studies of meal frequency suggest that if the subjects can adhere to an intermittent fasting regimen for at least 10–14 days, it thereafter becomes relatively easy to continue on the diet (57; M.P. Mattson, unpublished data).

For those who are unable or unwilling to reduce their food intake to improve their health, emerging evidence suggests that it may be possible to develop dietary supplements and drugs that induce energy restriction by influencing hunger and appetite (9) or by mimicking the effects of CR (63). For example, drugs that increase serotonin and BDNF levels should be effective, in principle, in suppressing food intake. However, the use of serotonin reuptake inhibitors in obese patients has had mixed results. Drugs that target hypothalamic neuropeptide signaling pathways that control appetite hold considerable promise for the treatment of overeating as well as for anorexia, and the development of such drugs is under way (52).

Finally, it may be possible to activate the same cellular and molecular pathways that occur in various tissues in response to CR and intermittent fasting. For example, some of these pathways, which result in increased cellular stress resistance, can be activated by physical exercise and cognitive stimulation (84). Animal studies suggest that CR and intermittent-fasting pathways might also be activated with dietary supplements and drugs. For example, dietary supplementation with 2-deoxy-D-glucose has been shown to induce beneficial physiological effects similar to CR and intermittent fasting (63, 131). Another approach is to activate sirtuins. Recent studies have shown that resveratrol stimulates sirtuins and can exert antiaging effects at the cellular level; interestingly, resveratrol is thought to be a chemical responsible for the health benefits of consumption of red wine (70, 117). However, the long-term safety of such pharmacological approaches remains to be established. Nevertheless, future advances in understanding the mechanisms by which energy intake and meal frequency affect health and disease processes will lead to novel approaches for increasing both the quality and quantity of our lives.

The *Annual Review of Nutrition* is online at http://nutr.annualreviews.org

LITERATURE CITED

1. Abete P, Testa G, Ferrara N, De Santis D, Capaccio P. 2002. Cardioprotective effect of ischemic preconditioning is preserved in food-restricted senescent rats. *Am. J. Physiol. Heart Circ. Physiol.* 282:H1978–87
2. Adlouni A, Ghalim N, Benslimane A, Lecerf JM, Saile R. 1997. Fasting during Ramadan induces a marked increase in high-density lipoprotein cholesterol and decrease in low-density lipoprotein cholesterol. *Ann. Nutr. Metab.* 41:242–49
3. Altmann J, Kornhuber AW, Kornhuber HH. 1987. Stroke: cardiovascular risk factors and the quantitative effects of dietary treatment on them. *Eur. Neurol.* 26:90–99
4. Anson RM, Guo Z, de Cabo R, Iyun T, Rios M, et al. 2003. Intermittent fasting dissociates beneficial effects of dietary restriction on glucose metabolism and neuronal resistance to injury from calorie intake. *Proc. Natl. Acad. Sci. USA* 100:6216–20
5. Apte UM, Limaye PB, Desaiah D, Bucci TJ, Warbritton A, Mehendale HM. 2003. Mechanisms of increased liver tissue repair and survival in diet-restricted rats treated with equitoxic doses of thioacetamide. *Toxicol. Sci.* 72:272–82
6. Arivazhagan P, Panneerselvam C. 2002. Neurochemical changes related to ageing in the rat brain and the effect of DL-alpha-lipoic acid. *Exp. Gerontol.* 37:1489–94
7. Azmitia EC. 2001. Modern views on an ancient chemical: serotonin effects on cell proliferation, maturation, and apoptosis. *Brain Res. Bull.* 56:413–24
8. Bates GW, Bates SR, Whitworth NS. 1982. Reproductive failure in women who practice weight control. *Fertil. Steril.* 37:373–78
9. Bays H, Dujovne C. 2002. Pharmacotherapy of obesity: currently marketed and upcoming agents. *Am. J. Cardiovasc. Drugs* 2:245–53
10. Beauchene RE, Bales CW, Bragg CS, Hawkins ST, Mason RL. 1986. Effect of age of initiation of feed restriction on

growth, body composition, and longevity of rats. *J. Gerontol.* 41:13–19
11. Berner YN, Stern F. 2004. Energy restriction controls aging through neuroendocrine signal transduction. *Ageing Res. Rev.* 3:189–98
12. Berrigan D, Perkins SN, Haines DC, Hursting SD. 2002. Adult-onset calorie restriction and fasting delay spontaneous tumorigenesis in p53-deficient mice. *Carcinogenesis* 23:817–22
13. Bianchini F, Kaaks R, Vainio H. 2002. Overweight, obesity, and cancer risk. *Lancet Oncol.* 3:565–74
14. Bodoky G, Yang ZJ, Meguid MM, Laviano A, Szeverenyi N. 1995. Effects of fasting, intermittent feeding, or continuous parenteral nutrition on rat liver and brain energy metabolism as assessed by ^{31}P-NMR. *Physiol. Behav.* 58:521–27
15. Bondolfi L, Ermini F, Long JM, Ingram DK, Jucker M. 2004. Impact of age and caloric restriction on neurogenesis in the dentate gyrus of C57BL/6 mice. *Neurobiol. Aging* 25:333–40
16. Bray GA. 2004. Medical consequences of obesity. *J. Clin. Endocrinol. Metab.* 89:2583–89
17. Brezun JM, Daszuta A. 1999. Depletion in serotonin decreases neurogenesis in the dentate gyrus and the subventricular zone of adult rats. *Neuroscience* 89:999–1002
18. Bruce-Keller AJ, Umberger G, McFall R, Mattson MP. 1999. Food restriction reduces brain damage and improves behavioral outcome following excitotoxic and metabolic insults. *Ann. Neurol.* 45:8–15
19. Carlson AJ, Hoelzel F. 1946. Apparent prolongation of the life span of rats by intermittent fasting. *J. Nutr.* 31:363–77
20. Cleary MP, Jacobson MK, Phillips FC, Getzin SC, Grande JP, Maihle NJ. 2002. Weight-cycling decreases incidence and increases latency of mammary tumors to a greater extent than does chronic caloric restriction in mouse mammary tumor virus-transforming growth factor-alpha female mice. *Cancer Epidemiol. Biomarkers Prev.* 11:836–43
21. Cohen HY, Miller C, Bitterman KJ, Wall NR, Hekking B, et al. 2004. Calorie restriction promotes mammalian cell survival by inducing the SIRT1 deacetylase. *Science* 305:390–92
22. Contestabile A, Ciani E, Contestabile A. 2004. Dietary restriction differentially protects from neurodegeneration in animal models of excitotoxicity. *Brain Res.* 1002:162–66
23. Costacou T, Mayer-Davis EJ. 2003. Nutrition and prevention of type 2 diabetes. *Annu. Rev. Nutr.* 23:147–70
24. Crandall DL, Feirer RP, Griffith DR, Beitz DC. 1981. Relative role of caloric restriction and exercise training upon susceptibility to isoproterenol-induced myocardial infarction in male rats. *Am. J. Clin. Nutr.* 34:841–47
25. Dax EM, Ingram DK, Partilla JS, Gregerman RI. 1989. Food restriction prevents an age-associated increase in rat liver beta-adrenergic receptors. *J. Gerontol.* 44:B72–76
26. de Cabo R, Furer-Galban S, Anson RM, Gilman C, Gorospe M, Lane MA. 2003. An in vitro model of caloric restriction. *Exp. Gerontol.* 38:631–39
27. de los Santos-Arteaga M, Sierra-Dominguez SA, Fontanella GH, Delgado-Garcia JM, Carrion AM. 2003. Analgesia induced by dietary restriction is mediated by the kappa-opioid system. *J. Neurosci.* 23:11120–26
28. Desautels M, Dulos RA. 1988. Effects of repeated cycles of fasting-refeeding on brown adipose tissue composition in mice. *Am. J. Physiol.* 255:E120–28
29. Dong W, Kari FW, Selgrade MK, Gilmour MI. 2000. Attenuated allergic responses to house dust mite antigen in feed-restricted rats. *Environ. Health Perspect.* 108:1125–31
30. Duan W, Mattson MP. 1999. Dietary restriction and 2-deoxyglucose administration improve behavioral outcome and

reduce degeneration of dopaminergic neurons in models of Parkinson's disease. *J. Neurosci. Res.* 57:195–206
31. Duan W, Guo Z, Jiang H, Ware M, Li XJ, Mattson MP. 2003. Dietary restriction normalizes glucose metabolism and BDNF levels, slows disease progression, and increases survival in huntingtin mutant mice. *Proc. Natl. Acad. Sci. USA* 100:2911–16
32. Duan W, Guo Z, Jiang H, Ware M, Mattson MP. 2003. Reversal of behavioral and metabolic abnormalities, and insulin resistance syndrome, by dietary restriction in mice deficient in brain-derived neurotrophic factor. *Endocrinology* 144:2446–53
33. Duan W, Guo Z, Jiang H, Ladenheim B, Xu X, et al. 2004. Paroxetine retards disease onset and progression in huntingtin mutant mice. *Ann. Neurol.* 55:590–94
34. Duncan GG, Jenson WE, Fraser RI, Cristofori FC. 1962. Correction and control of intractable obesity. Practicable application of intermittent periods of total fasting. *JAMA* 181:309–12
35. Fabry P, Heil Z, Fodor J, Braun T, Zvolankova K. 1964. The frequency of meals and its relation to overweight, hypercholesterolemia and decreased glucose tolerance. *Lancet* 18:614–15
36. Fairburn CG, Harrison PJ. 2003. Eating disorders. *Lancet* 361:407–16
37. Favier RJ, Koubi HE. 1988. Metabolic and structural adaptations to exercise in chronic intermittent fasted rats. *Am. J. Physiol.* 254:R877–84
38. Ferrer I, Goutan E, Marin C, Rey MJ, Ribalta T. 2000. Brain-derived neurotrophic factor in Huntington disease. *Brain Res.* 866:257–61
39. Fontana L, Meyer TE, Klein S, Holloszy JO. 2004. Long-term calorie restriction is highly effective in reducing the risk for atherosclerosis in humans. *Proc. Natl. Acad. Sci. USA* 101:6659–63
40. Frame LT, Hart RW, Leakey JE. 1998. Caloric restriction as a mechanism mediating resistance to environmental disease. *Environ. Health Perspect.* 106:S313–24
41. Gat-Yablonski G, Ben-Ari T, Shtaif B, Potievsky O, Moran O, et al. 2004. Leptin reverses the inhibitory effect of caloric restriction on longitudinal growth. *Endocrinology* 145:343–50
42. Gehrig JJ Jr, Ross J, Jamison RL. 1988. Effect of long-term, alternate day feeding on renal function in aging conscious rats. *Kidney Int.* 34:620–30
43. Ghosh A. 1994. Requirement for BDNF in activity-dependent survival of cortical neurons. *Science* 263:1618–23
44. Goldberg S, Smith GS, Barnes A, Ma Y, Kramer E, et al. 2004. Serotonin modulation of cerebral glucose metabolism in normal aging. *Neurobiol. Aging* 25:167–74
45. Goodrick CL, Ingram DK, Reynolds MA, Freeman JR, Cider NL. 1982. Effects of intermittent feeding upon growth and life span in rats. *Gerontology* 28:233–41
46. Goodrick CL, Ingram DK, Reynolds MA, Freeman JR, Cider NL. 1983. Effects of intermittent feeding upon growth, activity, and lifespan in rats allowed voluntary exercise. *Exp. Aging Res.* 9:203–09
47. Goodrick CL, Ingram DK, Reynolds MA, Freeman JR, Cider NL. 1990. Effects of intermittent feeding upon body weight and lifespan in inbred mice: interaction of genotype and age. *Mech. Ageing Dev.* 55:69–87
48. Granberry MC, Fonseca VA. 1999. Insulin resistance syndrome: options for treatment. *South. Med. J.* 92:2–15
49. Guo Z, Ersoz A, Butterfield DA, Mattson MP. 2000. Beneficial effects of dietary restriction on cerebral cortical synaptic terminals: preservation of glucose and glutamate transport and mitochondrial function after exposure to amyloid beta-peptide, iron, and 3-nitropropionic acid. *J. Neurochem.* 75:314–20
50. Gur E, Newman ME, Avraham Y, Dremencov E, Berry EM. 2003. The differential effects of food restriction on

5-HT1A and 5-HT1B receptor mediated control of serotonergic transmission in the hippocampus and hypothalamus of rats. *Nutr. Neurosci.* 6:169–75

51. Hales CN, Ozanne SE. 2003. The dangerous road of catch-up growth. *J. Physiol.* 547:5–10
52. Halford JC, Cooper GD, Dovey TM. 2004. The pharmacology of human appetite expression. *Curr. Drug Targets* 5:221–40
53. Hall DM, Oberley TD, Moseley PM, Buettner GR, Oberley LW, et al. 2000. Caloric restriction improves thermotolerance and reduces hyperthermia-induced cellular damage in old rats. *FASEB J.* 14:78–86
54. Halmi KA, Sunday SR, Klump KL, Strober M, Leckman JF, et al. 2003. Obsessions and compulsions in anorexia nervosa subtypes. *Int. J. Eat. Disord.* 33:308–19
55. Harris SR, Brix AE, Broderson JR, Bunce OR. 1995. Chronic energy restriction versus energy cycling and mammary tumor promotion. *Proc. Soc. Exp. Biol. Med.* 209:231–36
56. Heilbronn LK, Ravussin E. 2003. Calorie restriction and aging: review of the literature and implications for studies in humans. *Am. J. Clin. Nutr.* 78:361–69
57. Heilbronn LK, Smith SR, Martin CK, Anton S, Ravussin E. 2005. Alternate-day fasting in nonobese subjects: effects on body weight, body composition, and energy metabolism. *Am. J. Clin. Nutr.* 81:69–73
58. Heydari AR, You S, Takahashi R, Gutsmann A, Sarge KD, Richardson A. 1996. Effect of caloric restriction on the expression of heat shock protein 70 and the activation of heat shock transcription factor 1. *Dev. Genet.* 18:114–24
59. Hock C, Heese K, Hulette C, Rosenberg C, Otten U. 2000. Region-specific neurotrophin imbalances in Alzheimer disease: decreased levels of brain-derived neurotrophic factor and increased levels of nerve growth factor in hippocampus and cortical areas. *Arch. Neurol.* 57:846–51
60. Holeckova E, Chvapil M. 1965. The effect of intermittent feeding and fasting and of domestication on biological age in the rat. *Gerontologia* 11:96–119
61. Howells DW, Porritt MJ, Wong JY, Batchelor PE, Kalnins R, et al. 2000. Reduced BDNF mRNA expression in Parkinson's disease substantia nigra. *Exp. Neurol.* 166:127–35
62. Ingram DK, Weindruch R, Spangler EL, Freeman JR, Walford RL. 1987. Dietary restriction benefits learning and motor performance of aged mice. *J. Gerontol.* 42:78–81
63. Ingram DK, Anson RM, de Cabo R, Mamczarz J, Zhu M, et al. 2004. Development of calorie restriction mimetics as a prolongevity strategy. *Ann. NY Acad. Sci.* 1019:412–23
64. Iwashige K, Kouda K, Kouda M, Horiuchi K, Takahashi M, et al. 2004. Calorie restricted diet and urinary pentosidine in patients with rheumatoid arthritis. *J. Physiol. Anthropol. Appl. Human Sci.* 23:19–24
65. Jenkins JD, Wolever TM, Vuksan V, Brighenti F, Cunnane SC, et al. 1989. Nibbling versus gorging: metabolic advantages of increased meal frequency. *N. Engl. J. Med.* 321:929–34
66. Keski-Rahkonen A, Kaprio J, Rissanen A, Virkkunen M, Rose RJ. 2003. Breakfast skipping and health-compromising behaviors in adolescents and adults. *Eur. J. Clin. Nutr.* 57:842–53
67. Keys A. 1994. 1944 symposium on convalescence and rehabilitation. *FASEB J.* 8:1201–2
68. Kim KY, Ju WK, Neufeld AH. 2004. Neuronal susceptibility to damage: comparison of the retinas of young, old and old/caloric restricted rats before and after transient ischemia. *Neurobiol. Aging* 25:491–500
69. Kozubik A, Pospisil M. 1982. Protective

effect of intermittent fasting on the mortality of gamma-irradiated mice. *Strahlentherapie* 158:734–38
70. Lamming DW, Wood JG, Sinclair DA. 2004. Small molecules that regulate lifespan: evidence for xenohormesis. *Mol. Microbiol.* 53:1003–9
71. Lat J, Holeckova E. 1971. The effect of intermittent feeding and fasting on the nonspecific excitability level of the central nervous system in the rat. *Physiol. Bohemoslov.* 20:441–45
72. Lee J, Duan W, Mattson MP. 2002. Evidence that brain-derived neurotrophic factor is required for basal neurogenesis and mediates, in part, the enhancement of neurogenesis by dietary restriction in the hippocampus of adult mice. *J. Neurochem.* 82:1367–75
73. Lindsay RM. 1994. Neurotrophins and receptors. *Prog. Brain Res.* 103:3–14
74. Ljung T, Ahlberg AC, Holm G, Friberg P, Andersson B, et al. 2001. Treatment of abdominally obese men with a serotonin reuptake inhibitor: a pilot study. *J. Intern. Med.* 250:219–24
75. London ED, Waller SB, Ellis AT, Ingram DK. 1985. Effects of intermittent feeding on neurochemical markers in aging rat brain. *Neurobiol. Aging* 6:199–204
76. Lyons WE, Mamounas LA, Ricaurte GA, Coppola V, Reid SW, et al. 1999. Brain-derived neurotrophic factor-deficient mice develop aggressiveness and hyperphagia in conjunction with brain serotonergic abnormalities. *Proc. Natl. Acad. Sci. USA* 96:15239–44
77. Mamounas LA, Blue ME, Siuciak JA, Altar CA. 1995. Brain-derived neurotrophic factor promotes the survival and sprouting of serotonergic axons in rat brain. *J. Neurosci.* 15:7929–39
78. Mann PL. 1978. The effect of various dietary restricted regimes on some immunological parameters of mice. *Growth* 42:87–103
79. Marcos A, Varela P, Santacruz I, Munoz-Velez A, Morande G. 1993. Nutritional status and immunocompetence in eating disorders. A comparative study. *Eur. J. Clin. Nutr.* 47:787–93
80. Martin A, Normand S, Sothier M, Peyrat J, Louche-Pelissier C, Laville M. 2000. Is advice for breakfast consumption justified? Results from a short-term dietary and metabolic experiment in young healthy men. *Br. J. Nutr.* 84:337–44
81. Maswood N, Young J, Tilmont E, Zhang Z, Gash DM, et al. 2004. Caloric restriction increases GDNF levels and attenuates neurochemical and behavioral deficits in a primate model of Parkinson's disease. *Proc. Natl. Acad. Sci. USA* 101:18171–76
82. Mattison JA, Lane MA, Roth GS, Ingram DK. 2003. Calorie restriction in rhesus monkeys. *Exp. Gerontol.* 38:35–46
83. Mattson MP. 2002. Brain evolution and lifespan regulation: conservation of signal transduction pathways that regulate energy metabolism. *Mech. Aging Dev.* 123:947–53
84. Mattson MP. 2003. Gene-diet interactions in brain aging and neurodegenerative disorders. *Ann. Intern. Med.* 139:441–44
85. Mattson MP. 2005. The need for controlled studies of the effects of meal frequency on health. *Lancet* 365:In press
86. Mattson MP, Chan SL, Duan W. 2002. Modification of brain aging and neurodegenerative disorders by genes, diet, and behavior. *Physiol. Rev.* 82:637–72
87. McCay CM, Crowell MF, Maynard LA. 1989. The effect of retarded growth upon the length of life span and upon the ultimate body size. *Nutrition* 5:155–71
88. McElroy SL, Kotwal R, Malhotra S, Nelson EB, Keck PE, Nemeroff CB. 2004. Are mood disorders and obesity related? A review for the mental health professional. *J. Clin. Psychiatry* 65:634–51
89. McEwen BS. 2002. Sex, stress and the hippocampus: allostasis, allostatic load and the aging process. *Neurobiol. Aging* 23:921–39
90. McGuire MK, Littleton AW, Schulze KJ,

Rasmussen KM. 1995. Pre- and post-weaning food restrictions interact to determine reproductive success and milk volume in rats. *J. Nutr.* 125:2400–6
91. McShane TM, Wise PM. 1996. Lifelong moderate caloric restriction prolongs reproductive life span in rats without interrupting estrous cyclicity: effects on the gonadotropin-releasing hormone/luteinizing hormone axis. *Biol. Reprod.* 54:70–75
92. Means LW, Higgins JL, Fernandez TJ. 1993. Mid-life onset of dietary restriction extends life and prolongs cognitive functioning. *Physiol. Behav.* 54:503–8
93. Merry BJ. 2004. Oxidative stress and mitochondrial function with aging—the effects of calorie restriction. *Aging Cell* 3:7–12
94. Miller J, Rosenbloom A, Silverstein J. 2004. Childhood obesity. *J. Clin. Endocrinol. Metab.* 89:4211–18
95. Miller KK, Grinspoon S, Gleysteen S, Grieco KA, Ciampa J, et al. 2004. Preservation of neuroendocrine control of reproductive function despite severe undernutrition. *J. Clin. Endocrinol. Metab.* 89:4434–38
96. Morgan DG, May PC, Finch CE. 1987. Dopamine and serotonin systems in human and rodent brain: effects of age and neurodegenerative disease. *J. Am. Geriatr. Soc.* 35:334–45
97. Moroi-Fetters SE, Mervis RF, London ED, Ingram DK. 1989. Dietary restriction suppresses age-related changes in dendritic spines. *Neurobiol. Aging* 10:317–22
98. Mukherjee P, Abate LE, Seyfried TN. 2004. Antiangiogenic and proapoptotic effects of dietary restriction on experimental mouse and human brain tumors. *Clin. Cancer Res.* 10:5622–29
99. Muldoon MF, Mackey RH, Williams KV, Korytkowski MT, Flory JD, Manuck SB. 2004. Low central nervous system serotonergic responsivity is associated with the metabolic syndrome and physical inactivity. *J. Clin. Endocrinol. Metab.* 89:266–71
100. Nakagawa T, Ono-Kishino M, Sugara E, Yamanaka M, Taiji M, Noguchi H. 2002. Brain-derived neurotrophic factor (BDNF) regulates glucose and energy metabolism in diabetic mice. *Diabetes Metab. Res. Rev.* 18:185–91
101. Nakagawa T, Tsuchida A, Itakura Y, Nonomura T, Ono M, et al. 2000. Brain-derived neurotrophic factor regulates glucose metabolism by modulating energy balance in diabetic mice. *Diabetes* 49:436–44
102. Nicklas TA, Morales M, Linares A, Yang SJ, Baranowski T, et al. 2004. Children's meal patterns have changed over a 21-year period: the Bogalusa Heart Study. *J. Am. Diet. Assoc.* 104:753–61
103. Okamura F, Tashiro A, Utumu A, Imai T, Suchi T, et al. 2000. Insulin resistance in patients with depression and its changes during the clinical course of depression: minimal model analysis. *Metabolism* 49:1255–60
104. Paile-Hyvarinen M, Wahlbeck K, Eriksson JG. 2003. Quality of life and metabolic status in mildly depressed women with type 2 diabetes treated with paroxetine: a single-blind randomised placebo controlled trial. *BMC Fam. Pract.* 4:7
105. Patel NV, Finch CE. 2002. The glucocorticoid paradox of restriction in slowing brain aging. *Neurobiol. Aging* 23:707–17
106. Pedersen CR, Hagemann I, Bock T, Buschard K. 1999. Intermittent feeding and fasting reduces diabetes incidence in BB rats. *Autoimmunity* 30:243–50
107. Pedersen WA, Mattson MP. 1999. No benefit of dietary restriction on disease onset or progression in ALS Cu/Zn-SOD mutant mice. *Brain Res.* 833:117–20
108. Reusens B, Remacle C. 2001. Intergenerational effect of an adverse intrauterine environment on perturbation of glucose metabolism. *Twin Res.* 4:406–11
109. Reynolds LK, Ho HP, Taper LJ. 1984.

Effect of caloric restriction during pregnancy on maternal and fetal body composition in the obese Sprague-Dawley rat. *J. Nutr.* 114:2247–55

110. Rios M, Fan G, Fekete C, Kelly J, Bates B, et al. 2001. Conditional deletion of brain-derived neurotrophic factor in the postnatal brain leads to obesity and hyperactivity. *Mol. Endocrinol.* 15:1748–57

111. Rocha NS, Barbisan LF, de Oliveira ML, de Camargo JL. 2002. Effects of fasting and intermittent fasting on rat hepatocarcinogenesis induced by diethylnitrosamine. *Teratog. Carcinog. Mutagen.* 22:129–38

112. Roky R, Houti I, Moussamih S, Qotbi S, Aadil N. 2004. Physiological and chronobiological changes during Ramadan intermittent fasting. *Ann. Nutr. Metab.* 48:296–303

113. Roth GS, Mattison JA, Ottinger MA, Chachich ME, Lane MA, Ingram DK. 2004. Aging in rhesus monkeys: relevance to human health interventions. *Science* 305:1423–26

114. Russo-Neustadt A. 2003. Brain-derived neurotrophic factor, behavior, and new directions for the treatment of mental disorders. *Semin. Clin. Neuropsychiatry* 8:109–18

115. Sakamoto K, Grunewald KK. 1987. Beneficial effects of exercise on growth of rats during intermittent fasting. *J. Nutr.* 117:390–95

116. Santos AM, Ferraz MR, Teixeira CV, Sampaio FJ, da Fonte Ramos C. 2004. Effects of undernutrition on serum and testicular testosterone levels and sexual function in adult rats. *Horm. Metab. Res.* 36:27–33

117. Sardi B. 2004. *The Anti-Aging Pill*. San Dimas, CA: Here & Now Books. 189 pp.

118. Schweiger U, Broocks A, Tuschl RJ, Pirke KM. 1989. Serotonin turnover in rat brain during semistarvation with high-protein and high-carbohydrate diets. *J. Neural Transm.* 77:131–39

119. Shaikh ZA, Jordan SA, Tang W. 1999. Protection against chronic cadmium toxicity by caloric restriction. *Toxicology* 133:93–103

120. Sreekumar R, Unnikrishnan J, Fu A, Nygren J, Short KR, et al. 2002. Effects of caloric restriction on mitochondrial function and gene transcripts in rat muscle. *Am. J. Physiol. Endocrinol. Metab.* 283:E38–43

121. Stewart WK, Fleming LW, Robertson PC. 1966. Massive obesity treated by intermittent fasting. A metabolic and clinical study. *Am. J. Med.* 40:967–86

122. Talan MI, Ingram DK. 1985. Effect of intermittent feeding on thermoregulatory abilities of young and aged C57BL/6J mice. *Arch. Gerontol. Geriatr.* 4:251–59

123. Tanaka S, Inoue S, Isoda F, Waseda M, Ishihara M, et al. 1993. Impaired immunity in obesity: suppressed but reversible lymphocyte responsiveness. *Int. J. Obes. Relat. Metab. Disord.* 17:631–36

124. Toalson P, Ahmed S, Hardy T, Kabinoff G. 2004. The metabolic syndrome in patients with severe mental illnesses. *Prim. Care Companion J. Clin. Psychiatry* 6:152–58

125. Van Kesteren RE, Spencer GE. 2003. The role of neurotransmitters in neurite outgrowth and synapse formation. *Rev. Neurosci.* 14:217–31

126. Vaswani M, Linda FK, Ramesh S. 2003. Role of selective serotonin reuptake inhibitors in psychiatric disorders: a comprehensive review. *Prog. Neuropsychopharmacol. Biol. Psychiatry* 27:85–102

127. Vega VL, De Cabo R, De Maio A. 2004. Age and caloric restriction diets are confounding factors that modify the response to lipopolysaccharide by peritoneal macrophages in C57BL/6 mice. *Shock* 22:248–53

128. Wadden TA, Butryn ML. 2003. Behavioral treatment of obesity. *Endocrinol. Metab. Clin. North Am.* 32:981–1003

129. Walford RL, Mock D, Verdery R, MacCallum T. 2002. Calorie restriction in

Biosphere 2: alterations in physiologic, hematologic, hormonal, and biochemical parameters in humans restricted for a 2-year period. *J. Gerontol. A Biol. Sci. Med. Sci.* 57:B211–24
130. Wan R, Camandola S, Mattson MP. 2003. Intermittent food deprivation improves cardiovascular and neuroendocrine responses to stress in rats. *J. Nutr.* 133: 1921–29
131. Wan R, Camandola S, Mattson MP. 2004. Dietary supplementation with 2-deoxy-D-glucose improves cardiovascular and neuroendocrine stress adaptation in rats. *Am. J. Physiol. Heart Circ. Physiol.* 287: H1186–93
132. Wang GJ, Volkow ND, Thanos PK, Fowler JS. 2004. Similarity between obesity and drug addiction as assessed by neurofunctional imaging: a concept review. *J. Addict. Dis.* 23:39–53
133. Wang ZO, Bell-Farrow AD, Sonntag W, Cefalu WT. 1997. Effect of age and caloric restriction on insulin receptor binding and glucose transporter levels in aging rats. *Exp. Gerontol.* 32:671–84
134. Weindruch R, Sohal RS. 1997. Seminars in medicine of the Beth Israel Deaconess Medical Center. Caloric intake and aging. *N. Engl. J. Med.* 337:986–94
135. Williams KV, Mullen ML, Kelley DE, Wing RR. 1998. The effect of short periods of caloric restriction on weight loss and glycemic control in type 2 diabetes. *Diabetes Care* 21:2–8
136. Wing RR, Blair EH, Bononi P, Marcus MD, Watanabe R, Bergman RN. 1994. Caloric restriction per se is a significant factor in improvements in glycemic control and insulin sensitivity during weight loss in obese NIDDM patients. *Diabetes Care* 17:30–36
137. Wing RR, Marcus MD, Blair EH, Burton LR. 1991. Psychological responses of obese type II diabetic subjects to very-low-calorie diet. *Diabetes Care* 14:596–99
138. Wingard DL, Berkman LF, Brand RJ. 1982. A multivariate analysis of health-related practices: a nine-year mortality follow-up of the Alameda County Study. *Am. J. Epidemiol.* 116:765–75
139. Wolf NS, Li Y, Pendergrass W, Schmeider C, Turturro A. 2000. Normal mouse and rat strains as models for age-related cataract and the effect of caloric restriction on its development. *Exp. Eye Res.* 70:683–92
140. Wu A, Wan F, Sun X, Liu Y. 2002. Effects of dietary restriction on growth, neurobehavior, and reproduction in developing Kunmin mice. *Toxicol Sci.* 70:238–44
141. Yaffe K, Blackwell T, Kanaya AM, Davidowitz N, Barrett-Connor E, Krueger K. 2004. Diabetes, impaired fasting glucose, and development of cognitive impairment in older women. *Neurology* 63:658–63
142. Young JB, Mullen D, Landsberg L. 1978. Caloric restriction lowers blood pressure in the spontaneously hypertensive rat. *Metabolism* 27:1711–14
143. Young JB, Landsberg L. 1982. Diet-induced changes in sympathetic nervous system activity: possible implications for obesity and hypertension. *J. Chronic Dis.* 35:879–86
144. Yu ZF, Mattson MP. 1999. Dietary restriction and 2-deoxyglucose administration reduce focal ischemic brain damage and improve behavioral outcome: evidence for a preconditioning mechanism. *J. Neurosci. Res.* 57:830–39

Annu. Rev. Nutr. 2005. 25:261–95
doi: 10.1146/annurev.nutr.25.050304.092633

First published online as a Review in Advance on April 15, 2005

REDOX REGULATION BY INTRINSIC SPECIES AND EXTRINSIC NUTRIENTS IN NORMAL AND CANCER CELLS

Archana Jaiswal McEligot,[1] Sun Yang,[2] and Frank L. Meyskens, Jr.[2,3]
Departments of Medicine ([1]Epidemiology and [2]Hematology/Oncology Divisions) and [3]Biological Chemistry, Chao Family Comprehensive Cancer Center, University of California, Irvine, Orange, California 92868; email: mceligot@uci.edu, syang2@uci.edu, flmeyske@uci.edu

Key Words antioxidant nutrients, TR/TRX, GSH/GSSG, transcription factors, apoptosis

■ **Abstract** Cells in multicellular organisms are exposed to both endogenous oxidative stresses generated metabolically and to oxidative stresses that originate from neighboring cells and from other tissues. To protect themselves from oxidative stress, cells are equipped with reducing buffer systems (glutathione/GSH and thioredoxin/thioredoxin reductase) and have developed several enzymatic mechanisms against oxidants that include catalase, superoxide dismutase, and glutathione peroxidase. Other major extrinsic defenses (from the diet) include ascorbic acid, β-carotene and other carotenoids, and selenium. Recent evidence indicates that in addition to their antioxidant function, several of these redox species and systems are involved in regulation of biological processes, including cellular signaling, transcription factor activity, and apoptosis in normal and cancer cells. The survival and overall well-being of the cell is dependent upon the balance between the activity and the intracellular levels of these antioxidants as well as their interaction with various regulatory factors, including Ref-1, nuclear factor-κB, and activating protein-1.

CONTENTS

INTRODUCTION

Reactive oxygen species (ROS), such as H_2O_2, superoxide anion ($O_2^{\bullet}$) and the hydroxyl radical ($^{\bullet}OH$), and anion (OH^-) are generated in cells by several pathways and have been implicated in a multitude of physiological processes including aging and immune function, and in disease initiation and progression, such as atherosclerosis and carcinogenesis. Earlier research on free radicals hypothesized that oxidative stress was the primary mechanism by which reactive oxygen species (ROS) influenced biological processes. An elevated oxidized state within a cell can be extremely harmful, resulting in radical generation that leads to lipid peroxidation, DNA cross-linking, and formation of disulfide bonds in proteins. Increased ROS production caused by exposure to carcinogens may result in human cancer and other degenerative diseases. In response to protection against elevated levels of oxidative stress and/or ROS, cells possess several intrinsic systems as well as extrinsic derived antioxidants/reductants, which maintain the intracellular environment in a highly reduced state (130). The major intrinsic systems emphasized in this review include glutathione/oxidized glutathione (GSH/GSSG) and thioredoxin reductase/thioredoxin (TR/TRX), while the extrinsic molecules (among many antioxidants) include vitamin C, carotenoids, and selenium. Other antioxidant enzyme species such as superoxide dismutase (SOD) and catalase also protect the cell against oxidative stress (111).

The study of redox-dependent regulation of molecular processes has gained attention recently (130). In addition to protecting against oxidative stress, research conducted primarily during the past decade has produced evidence of additional major biological functions of these intrinsic and extrinsic species, including regulation of transcription factors, complex cellular signaling pathways, and cell survival.

BIOCHEMISTRY OF REDOX METABOLISM

Redox Intrinsic Species/Systems

GSH/GSSG One of the major indicators of redox status in the cell is the GSH/GSSG system (159). GSH is a tripeptide of γ-glutamate, cysteine, and glycine and is the predominant low-molecular-weight intracellular thiol, maintained at high concentrations (1–10 mM) in the physiologic state. It is one of the major reductants found in eukaryotic cells. Because the normal cellular state exists primarily in favor of GSH, the intracellular environment is highly reducing, and under physiological conditions, ratios (GSH/GSSG) of 30:1 to 100:1 have been measured (77). The reduced status of the cell in this range protects the cell from oxidants produced during normal metabolism and makes possible reductive biosynthesis (159) (Figure 1).

Glutathione has several biological functions and forms (214). The various forms of the glutathione peroxidase enzymes, a selenium-dependent system, are involved in inactivating ROS, including H_2O_2 and other peroxides, via conversion of the GSH molecule to its oxidized form GSSG. Also, GSH in conjunction with glutathione-s-transferase interacts with various oxidized metabolites, including those produced by estrogen, melanin, prostaglandin, and leukotriene synthesis, as well as with xenobiotics in which GSH forms mercapturates.

TR/TRX The TR/TRX system is a ubiquitous redox couple endogenous within prokaryotic and eukaryotic cells (159). TR is an NADPH-dependent flavin adenine dinucleotide-containing flavoenzyme, and along with TRX plays a key role in maintaining a reduced intracellular environment (7). Interconversion between the oxidized and reduced form of TR requires transfer of electrons from NADPH. The flavin adenine dinucleotide prosthetic group of TR donates the electrons from NADPH to active-site cysteines, resulting in the catalytically active form of TR, which has the ability to reduce the active-site cystine bond of oxidized TRX (Figure 1). Gallegos and colleagues (55) have shown that selenium specifically increases the activity of TR, including stabilizing TRmRNA, which in turn leads to increased TR production and increased growth of normal and cancer cells.

OTHER INTRINSIC REDOX SPECIES Superoxide dismutase, a very important intrinsic enzyme, catalyzes the dismutation of the highly reactive superoxide anion to O_2 and to the less reactive species H_2O_2. Several forms of SOD are present in the human cell, including cytosolic Cu/Zn-SOD, mitochondrial SOD, and extracellular SOD (2) (Figure 1).

Hydrogen peroxide in animals is detoxified by catalase as well as by other intrinsic species (111). The enzymatic reaction involves the conversion of hydrogen

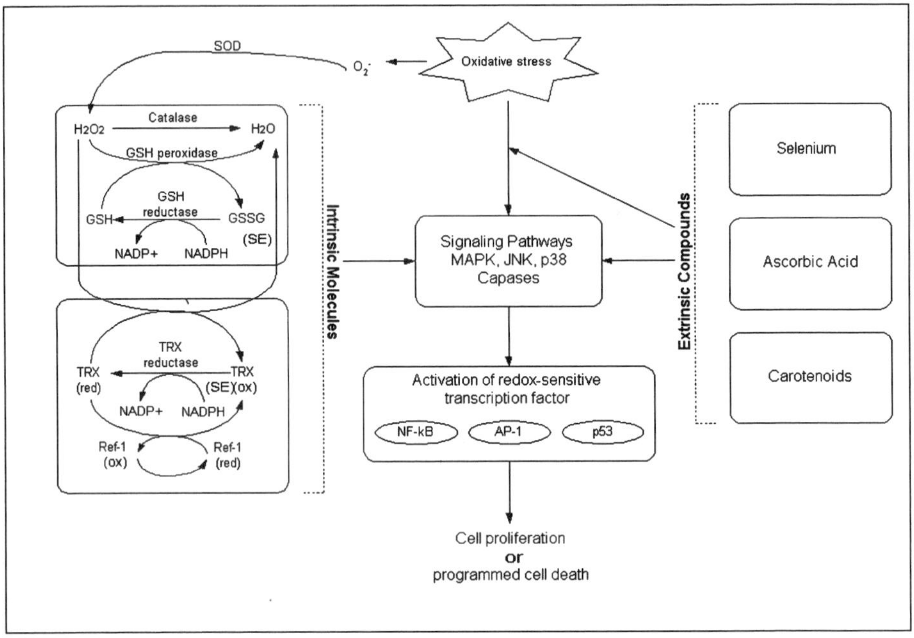

Figure 1 Redox regulation of cellular processes by intrinsic and extrinsic molecules. Various intrinsic redox systems, such as glutathione (GSH/GSSG) and thioredoxin and thioredoxin reductase (TRX/TR), regulate biological processes. Oxidative stress such as ultraviolet radiation results in formation of H_2O_2 and superoxides ($O_2^{\bullet}$). Superoxide dismutase (SOD) catalyzes the conversion of $O_2^{\bullet}$ to H_2O_2, which eventually is converted to water by GSH as well as by TRX. Both TRX and GSH reactions are selenium dependent. Extrinsic molecules, including selenium, ascorbic acid, and carotenoids, also affect cellular processes, including cell signaling, activation of transcription factors, and apoptosis. JNK, Jun N-terminal kinase; MAPK, mitogen-activated protein kinase; SE, selenium.

peroxide generated in normal cells to H_2O water by catalase. Even though catalase is not essential for some cell types under normal conditions, this enzyme plays a critical role in the acquisition of tolerance to oxidative stress.

Extrinsic Redox Species and Systems: Focus on Ascorbic Acid, Carotenoids, and Selenium

ASCORBIC ACID The antioxidant activity of vitamin C, primarily via its ability to donate electrons and therefore function as a reducing agent, has been studied extensively (80, 142). The primary dietary sources of vitamin C are fruits and vegetables (67). Specifically, dietary foods rich in vitamin C include grapefruit, honeydew, kiwi, mango, orange, papaya, strawberries, tangerine, and watermelon (67). The antioxidant mechanism of vitamin C occurs via the reduction of highly reactive radicals, such as hydroxyl, peroxyl, and superoxide radicals, as well as singlet oxygen and reactive peroxides, which can be internally generated via metabolic processes and externally derived from ultraviolet (UV) light and gamma-ray radiation (89). During this process, the relatively unreactive ascorbyl radical is formed (80). Many in vitro and in vivo studies have investigated the antioxidant function of ascorbic acid, which may reduce DNA damage (48, 142, 169, 181) and possibly reduce cancer risk.

CAROTENOIDS The antioxidant action of carotenoids, which protects the cell against oxidative stress (derived from everyday exposure to UV radiation and/or chemicals in the environment), occurs via several mechanisms. Dietary availability of carotenoids is from vegetables and fruits. Carrots are excellent sources of β- and α-carotene, tomatoes are rich in lycopene, dark green leafy vegetables are high in lutein, and orange fruits such as tangerines are rich in β-cryptoxanthin (33).

One of the main mechanisms of the antioxidant action of carotenoids is the ability to quench singlet oxygen ($^1O_2$) (50). Singlet oxygen, the electronically excited form of oxygen, is formed as a result of many reactions in the body, including reactions involving H_2O_2 and peroxide enzymes, but the primary source is exposure to UV light (89). Singlet oxygen is highly reactive and produces cellular damage by oxidizing amino acids found in proteins and nucleic acids, which may result in DNA strand breakage. Carotenoids (CAR, below) can quench these singlet oxygen species by reacting with them, and because of the long-chain hydrocarbon structure of carotenoids, these compounds can return to ground state by releasing a small amount of heat. Through this reaction, the highly reactive singlet oxygen species is also returned to ground state, becoming more stable.

$$^1O_2 + \text{CAR} \rightarrow {}^3O_2 + {}^3\text{CAR}$$

$$^3\text{CAR} \rightarrow \text{CAR} + \text{heat}$$

An additional antioxidant action of carotenoids is the ability to interact with free radicals, such as peroxyl or alkoxyl radicals. Carotenoids are capable of transferring electrons (acting as electron donors) and reducing free radicals to nonradical compounds, and in the process produce carotenoid radical cations (98). Thus, suboptimal intake of carotenoids may result in increased DNA damage and contribute to carcinogenesis via reduced action of these antioxidants on singlet oxygen quenching and free radicals.

SELENIUM Selenium has many biochemical roles, including antioxidant functions and regulation of thyroid metabolism, redox status, and immunity (95). Dairy, eggs, fish, meat, grains, and Brazil nuts are rich sources of selenium. Because selenium content and availability in food is highly dependent on the soil in the region, dietary selenium in food varies geographically (33).

Selenium, in the form of selenocysteine, is a major constituent of many antioxidant enzymes known as selenoproteins. Between 30 and 40 selenoproteins have been identified, and 21 have been further characterized by purification and cloning (114). Two of the selenoproteins identified, GPX and TR (described above), are intricately involved in intracellular redox regulation. The selenoproteins that have been characterized contain selenium at the active site, and therefore many redox reactions/functions are selenium dependent. In addition to regulation of biological processes via selenoproteins, selenium, as reviewed previously, also has direct effects on prevention of oxidative damage, gene expression, and apoptosis (95, 114).

REDOX REGULATION OF BIOLOGICAL PROCESSES IN NORMAL CELLS BY INTRINSIC SPECIES

Cellular Signaling

Cellular signaling involves many cytoplasmic protein kinase cascades (i.e., MAPKs, PI3K/AKT, PKCs) that form pathways connecting exogenous stimuli to the nucleus, resulting in transcription and synthesis of proteins. Cellular signaling activities and expression are very sensitive to both exogenous and intracellular redox status and respond to many exogenous pro-oxidative or oxidative stresses. Many studies demonstrate that multiple intracellular signaling pathways are activated by UV radiation (37, 58, 179, 180, 205), ionizing radiation (9), and heavy metals (105) with generation of ROS, or directly by H_2O_2 (93) and nitric oxide exposure (101), subsequently leading to the activation of nuclear transcription factors in normal cells.

GSH, TRX AND CELLULAR SIGNALING Cellular signaling is regulated by intracellular redox status maintained by reducing antioxidants and redox proteins. Intracellular GSH depletion by DL-buthionine-(S,R)-sulfoximine (BSO), a potent and specific inhibitor of gamma-glutamyl cysteine synthetase, leads to a decline in the levels of GSH. This is followed by an increase in ROS production in a dose- and time-dependent manner with the activation of extracellular signal–regulated kinases (ERK) 1/2 pathway (36). More specifically, protein kinase C (PKC), which has two pairs of zinc finger structures in its regulatory domain and several cysteines in its catalytic sites, has been shown to be sensitive to redox regulation (60). A study by Chu et al. (30) directly demonstrated that regulation of PKC is redox dependent. Purified, recombinant human PKC isoforms were differentially regulated by GSH or oxidized glutathione (GSSG), and cystine-induced inactivation of PKCγ and PKCϵ was rescued by exogenous dithiothreitol and thioredoxin. However, Ward et al. (206) observed an irreversible inactivation of PKC by GSH, suggesting that GSH depletion–mediated PKC activation might be due to the rescue of PKC from inhibition as well as through the induction of novel PKC isoforms and enhanced specific isoform activity (38, 39). Moreover, thioredoxin restored the catalytic activity of PKC-zeta in pulmonary artery endothelial cells in a thiol-reducing dependent mechanism (87). In addition, overexpression of manganese superoxide dismutase, an antioxidative enzyme, selectively inhibited PKC epsilon and prevented subsequent activation of c-Jun N-terminal kinase (JNK), thereby leading to delayed AP-1 transcriptional activation (222).

Cellular signaling such as PKC activation also influences intracellular redox status by affecting the expression or activity of certain redox-regulating proteins. The activity of TRX and TR in normal epidermis extracts was increased significantly with application of the PKC activator 12-O-tetradecanoylphorbol-13-acetate (TPA) (99), while Anema et al. (3) reported downregulation of TR expression via transiently exposing cells to TPA in cultured human umbilical-vein endothelial cells. In addition, TPA treatment increased PKC phosphorylation of the apurinic/apyrimidinic endonuclease 1 (APE/Ref-1) protein (75). APE/Ref-1 regulates the redox status of many transcription factors. Another study, conducted by Flaherty et al. (49), found that TPA in conjunction with granulocyte-macrophage colony-stimulating factor increased Ref-1 protein levels, but TPA alone produced no increase.

TRX, GSH, and Regulation of Transcription Factors

A growing body of literature suggests that regulation of gene expression by redox-sensitive transcription factors is dependent on the redox status of the cell (56). Two of the intrinsic redox elements discussed above (TRX and GSH), as well as extrinsic nutrients (vitamin C, carotenoids, and selenium), are involved in regulating the actions of various transcription factors, including nuclear factor-κB (NF-κB) and activator protein-1 (AP-1). The regulation of these transcription factors is complex. Studies have shown that under different conditions both antioxidants and oxidants activate AP-1 (121). In normal cells, both transcription factors induce gene regulation that influences inflammation, immune function, cell growth and survival, and stress responses (89).

TRX and GSH may have overlapping as well as compartmentalized functions in activation and regulation of transcription factors, including regulation of NF-κB and AP-1 in the cytoplasm and the nucleus (66, 71). Earlier studies showed that exogenous treatment or transient expression of TRX resulted in a dose-dependent downregulation/inhibition of NF-κB, while AP-1 activity was strongly upregulated and enhanced (121, 178). Galter and colleagues (56) showed that both NF-κB and AP-1 were activated upon treatment of cells with 1,3-bis-(2-chloroethyl)-1-nitrosourea, a compound that, among other functions, elevates intracellular levels of GSSG by inhibiting glutathione reductase. Gel shift assays and transfection studies with reporter constructs also showed that GSSG inhibited DNA-binding ability of NF-κB and AP-1. A more recent study provides evidence that TRX has a differential role in regulating NF-κB in the cytoplasm and nucleus (71). TRX inhibited NF-κB activity in the cytoplasm, while upregulating the ability of NF-κB to bind to DNA in the nucleus. Other studies have shown that TRX can also regulate several other transcriptional factors, including hypoxia-inducible factor-1 (HIF-1), Nrf-2, and cytochrome P450's (66, 76, 209). Hansen et al. (66) assessed the role of TRX and GSH in Nrf-2-dependent signaling. Nuclear translocation (which measures cytoplasmic activity) of Nrf-2 was regulated via GSH, whereas nuclear activity was primarily controlled by TRX.

Regulation of Apoptosis

ROS AND ANTIOXIDANTS IN APOPTOSIS Mitochondria are the specialized organelles that are involved in the control of apoptosis via production of ROS. Many studies have indicated a role for ROS in the regulation of apoptosis. This subject has been reviewed extensively (19, 64, 204). Generally, apoptosis can be induced by the addition of ROS such as H_2O_2 (63) or by depletion of cellular exogenous antioxidants such as GSH (6, 21, 31). In other instances, apoptosis is associated with stimulation and production of intracellular ROS (43, 224). It is reasonable to postulate that antioxidants might prevent apoptosis through a redox-based mechanism. Both intracellular and exogenous antioxidants such as GSH (188) and thioredoxin-1 (10) as well as N-acetylcysteine (176) protect cells from apoptosis or the activation of apoptosis-related signaling pathway. Furthermore, cells overexpressing the antioxidant enzyme SOD are relatively resistant to radiation-induced apoptosis (211). However, other studies have also revealed that the apoptosis response was conserved in mitochondrial DNA experimentally depleted cells, which were deficient in respiration; this finding suggests that mitochondrial oxidative phosphorylation is not essential or only attenuates related signals for apoptosis in certain cases (81, 85).

TRX AND REGULATION OF APOPTOSIS The role of the TRX/TR pathway in apoptosis has been investigated. Exogenous thioredoxin-1 prevented apoptosis of lymphoid cells induced by glutathione depletion (79) or of apoptosis in human neuroblastoma SH-SY5Y cells induced by a Parkinsonian-producing neurotoxin (2). Adding TRX to culture media significantly prolonged the survival of B-cell chronic lymphocytic leukemia cells, and release of an autocrine growth factor was observed, which suggests an increased cell survival (135). Overexpression of thioredoxin-1 protected cells not only from oxidative stress-induced apoptosis (137) but also from cytotoxic and DNA-damaging effects of many chemotherapeutic drugs such as cisplatin, mitomycin C, doxorubicin, etoposide, staurosporine, thapsigargin, and diepoxybutane (10, 174, 218). The mechanisms of action might be related to its regulation of NF-κB or AP-1 cell survival pathways (52, 112), as well as inhibition of tumor-suppressor protein PTEN (120) and proapoptotic proteins such as apoptosis signal-regulating kinase 1 (ASK1) (8, 175), which binds to thioredoxin directly in a redox-dependent manner and results in the loss of their kinase activities.

Mitochondria thioredoxin (thioredoxin-2, TRX-2) is a critical antioxidant in regulating mitochondrial ROS-induced cytotoxicity. TRX-2-deficient cells showed an accumulation of intracellular ROS and induced cytochrome c release into the cytosol, followed by mitochondria-dependent apoptosis (195). Similarly, Zhang

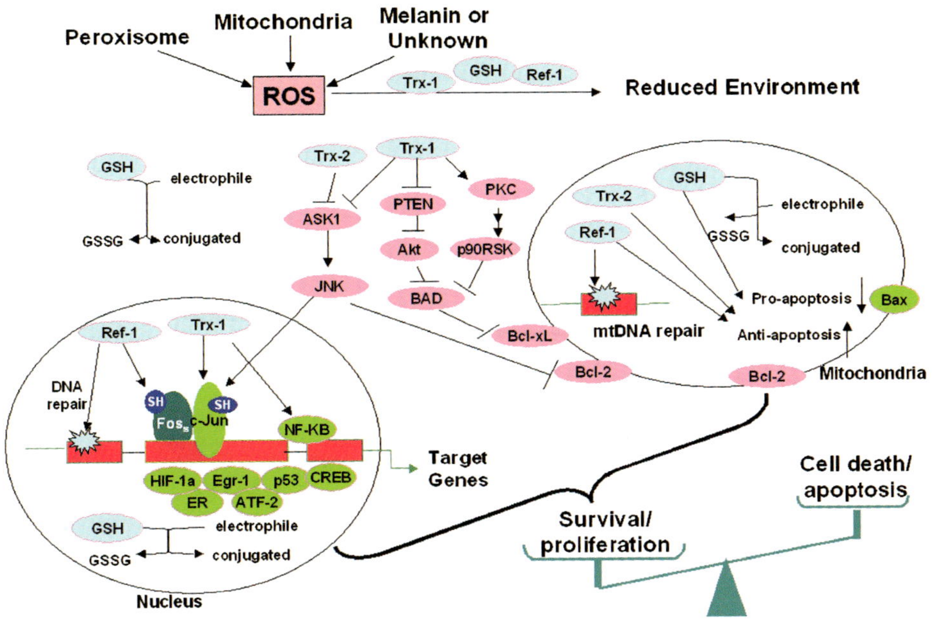

Figure 2 Abnormal redox-mediated signal regulation in cancer cells. The cumulative production of reactive oxygen species found in cancer cells is associated with altered redox regulation of signaling. In certain compartments, especially the nucleus and mitochondria, elevated levels of thioredoxin and apurinic/apyrimidinic endonuclease 1 as well as glutathione contributed to a reducing environment. This intracellular milieu not only facilitates escape from apoptosis but also produces an aggressive proliferation potential through activation of cell survival signals mediated by redox-sensitive nuclear transcription factors such as AP-1 and NF-κB, as well as by interfering with the cellular apoptosis pathway, both directly and indirectly. ASK1, apoptosis signal-regulating kinase 1; JNK, Jun N-terminal kinase; Akt, AKT8 virus oncogene cellular homolog; PTEN, phosphatase and tensin homologue deleted on chromosome 10; ER, estrogen receptor; HIF-1α, hypoxia inducible factor-1α; ATF-2, activating transcription factor-2; Egr-1, early growth response-1; CREB, cAMP response element-binding protein.

et al. (221) demonstrated that TRX-2 and TRX-1 cooperatively inhibited ASK1 activities. Overexpression of TRX-2 in endothelial cells blocked ASK1-induced apoptosis as well as oxidant-induced apoptosis in human osteosarcoma cells (27). However, Patenaude et al. (152) reported that the cellular responses to various pro-oxidant or nonoxidant apoptotic stimuli were quite similar between mitochondrial thioredoxin reductase-2 (TRX R2) or TRX-2 overexpressed cells and controls. The use of different cell lines in the respective studies may explain the divergence of these conclusions.

GSH AND REGULATION OF APOPTOSIS The protective role of GSH against apoptosis and cell death emanates from multifactorial mechanisms that involve detoxification and modulation of cellular redox state and the subsequent redox-sensitive cell-signaling pathways (115, 220), as well as the interaction with pro- and anti-apoptotic signals. Upon withdrawal of interleukin-3, cells overexpressing Bcl-xL (antiapoptosis member) failed to lose significant amounts of GSH and no apoptosis was evident, while GSH in Bax (proapoptosis member) overexpressing cells was significantly reduced and sensitive to apoptosis, indicating a possible role of GSH in Bcl-xL-mediated antiapoptosis mechanisms (15). Additionally, GSH depletion by BSO treatment significantly enhanced Bax-induced apoptosis in four non-small-cell lung cancer cell lines (74), suggesting that the redox status maintained by thiols may interfere with Bax-mediated apoptosis. Increased GSH levels were observed in melphalan-induced apoptosis in human melanoma cells by inhibition of Bax/cytochrome c redistribution (12). More importantly, increasing evidence has shown an intimate link between GSH and antiapoptotic Bcl-2 and Bcl-2-mediated apoptosis. The cells overexpressing Bcl-2 had significantly higher levels of GSH with translocation into the nucleus (200), but the increase in GSH content was not due to increased synthesis (119). Consistently, depletion of GSH within Bcl-2 high-expression cells resensitized them to apoptosis without alternating Bcl-2 protein levels (124, 213). GSH also prevented apoptosis through the inhibition of AP24, an apoptotic protease that transmits signals to induce DNA fragmentation (213). Therefore, GSH levels are an important factor in the efficacy of anticancer drug–induced apoptosis. It is well documented that depletion of GSH facilitates tumor treatment, with higher response to apoptosis induction.

REF-1 AND APOPTOSIS The human DNA repair enzyme APE/Ref-1 is a dual function protein that plays an important role in both DNA base excision repair and in transcriptional responses to oxidative stress (45, 53). Endogenous AP sites are produced through a variety of mechanisms, i.e., oxidative damage, resulting in mutations or genetic instability. APE/Ref-1 is one of the key enzymes involved in the repair process. Moreover, in addition to its DNA repair activity, APE/Ref-1 has also been found to facilitate the DNA-binding activity of several transcription factors, including AP-1, NF-κB, Myb, p53, and Pax, through both redox-dependent and redox-independent mechanisms.

The relationship of Ref-1 and apoptosis has been extensively studied. This protein has a dual function with overlapping endonuclease and redox properties. Many studies have revealed that upregulation of Ref-1 protects cells from various apoptosis stimuli, including oxidative stress, chemotherapeutic drugs, and radiation treatment, as well as tumor necrosis factor (TNF) superfamily receptor 6 (Fas)-mediated cell death signal (4, 61, 62, 170). In contrast, downregulation of Ref-1 expression is associated with apoptosis and sensitization of cells to induced apoptosis both in vitro (46, 171) and in vivo (91, 128). Most importantly, a cause-and-effect relationship between apoptosis and Ref-1 levels was first reported by Robertson et al. (171), who found that when apoptosis was blocked by Bcl-2 (anti-apoptosis member) overexpression, reduction of Ref-1 was no longer evident and cells underwent differentiation. Consistently, preventing the loss of Ref-1 by inhibiting protein synthesis rescued neurons from experimentally induced cell death (28). The possible mechanisms involved might be related to redox-activation by APE/Ref-1 of many cell survival signals, such as NF-κB and AP-1, and maintenance of genomic integrity through enhanced repair of cytotoxic DNA lesions (167), through serving as an adaptive response to apoptotic stimuli. However, Gaiddon et al. (54) reported that coexpression of Ref-1 potentiated p53-induced apoptosis in H1299 cells, and supported the conclusion drawn by Yao et al. (217) who showed a possible relationship between Ref-1 induction and the occurrence of hypoxia-induced apoptosis. The role of Ref-1 in contributing to apoptosis may depend on the different types of cell lines and the nature of the underlying stresses used for such studies.

MITOCHONDRIAL REDOX

Mitochondrial DNA (mtDNA) codes for 13 respiratory chain subunits and exhibits high susceptibility to mutation compared with nuclear genomic DNA (110). The presence of mtDNA mutations in many cancer cells has been demonstrated, including in solid tumors of breast, colon, stomach, liver, kidney, bladder, head/neck, and lung, as well as for hematologic diseases such as leukemia, myelodysplastic syndrome, and lymphoma [reviewed in depth by Copeland et al. (32) and Penta et al. (154)]. Wei & Lee (208) demonstrated that impairment in mitochondrial respiration and oxidative phosphorylation elicits an increase in oxidative stress that causes a host of mtDNA rearrangements and deletions. Vergani et al. (202) also found that mitochondrial DNA depletion resulted in an oxidized intracellular redox status. In addition, Carew et al. (23) reported that in human chronic lymphocytic leukemia, mtDNA mutations appeared to be associated with increased ROS generation. Patients who were refractory to conventional therapeutic agents tended to have higher mutation rates than did patients who responded to treatment. These observations suggest that normal mitochondrial function is not only essential for cellular biological activities but also is crucial for maintaining intracellular redox status.

Mitochondria are the most redox-active organelles. Maintaining mitochondrial redox status depends not only on total cellular redox environment but also on its own reduction capacities, including glutathione pools, antioxidant enzymes, and mitochondrial thioredoxins such as TRX-2 (177). Alterations in mitochondrial redox status significantly affected the apoptotic process. Experimentally induced GSH deficiency in newborn rats has been shown to result in striking enlargement and degeneration of mitochondria (82). Increasing evidence also has demonstrated that upregulation of mitochondrial antioxidant proteins such as TRX-2 and peroxiredoxin-3 (Prdx3) effectively protected cells from mitochondrial-mediated apoptosis (27, 136, 221). An antiapoptotic phenotype has been observed in drug-resistant cells with mitochondrial morphological alterations (42).

REDOX REGULATION OF BIOLOGICAL PROCESSES IN NORMAL CELLS BY EXTRINSIC NUTRIENT SPECIES

Vitamin C

VITAMIN C AND TRANSCRIPTION FACTORS The action of ascorbic acid (AA) on redox-dependent biological function is due to the direct redox role of AA and its metabolites as well as to generation of the ascorbate free radical. Recently, in vitro and in vivo studies have demonstrated the ability of AA to regulate factors that may influence gene expression, apoptosis, and other cellular functions (22, 24, 108, 125, 133, 160, 168). Carcamo and coworkers (22) loaded cells with AA and then induced oxidative stress, which generated dehydroascorbic acid. NF-κB binding was suppressed while IKB kinase beta was unaffected, which suggests that vitamin C plays a role to down-modulate cell signaling (Table 1).

Several studies investigated the mechanism by which ascorbic acid regulates the AP-1 complex, including the Fos (c-Fos, Fos B, and Fra-1) and Jun (c-Jun, Jun B, and Jun D) superfamilies (5, 25, 26) (Table 1). Catani and coworkers (26) examined the role of ascorbate in the regulation of several transcripts, including GST-pi, MLH1, and fra-1 (a member of the FOS family of transcription factors that regulate AP-1). After loading of vitamin C in normal human keratinocytes, fra-1 messenger RNA was induced within two hours. The same group showed that application of ascorbate inhibits expression of c-Jun and c-Fos, which are involved in AP-1 activity. Furthermore, after exposure to UV-B radiation, ascorbate-treated cells led to a 50% decrease in JNK phosphorylation (which activated AP-1), thus inhibiting the JNK/AP-1 signaling pathways.

Studies in healthy subjects have shown that supplementation with vitamin C can reduce oxidative protein damage and modulate expression of adhesion molecules, such as ICAM, which via various signaling pathways may be involved in carcinogenesis and atherosclerosis (24, 168, 212). One study supplemented 40 healthy subjects (half of the subjects had low plasma ascorbate levels) with 250 mg/day of ascorbate and measured modulation of ICAM-1 expression (168). Prior to

TABLE 1 Nutrients and their role in the regulation of biological processes*

Nutrient	Regulation of biological intermediates
Ascorbic acid	Regulation of transcription factors/transcripts NF-κB AP-1, fra-1 gene, Fos (c-Fos, Fos B, Fra-1) and Jun (c-Jun, Jun B and Jun D) superfamilies GST-pi MLH1 Regulation of apoptosis Fas induced Adhesion molecules, ICAM IL-1 downregulation
Carotenoids (β-carotene, α-carotene lutein, lycopene, β-cryptoxanthin)	Regulation of transcription factors Via RAR, RXR NF-κB Apoptosis Proinflammatory cytokines, IL-6, TNF-alpha BCL-2 Bax
Selenium	Regulation of transcription factors NF-kB AP-1 P53 Cell signaling intermediates MAPK, JNK, ERK p38 Regulation of apoptosis BCL-2 Bax

*Abbreviations: AP-1, activating protein-1; Bax, important proapoptosis mediator; BCL-2, an important antiapoptosis mediators; ERK, extracellular-signal-regulated kinase; Fas, TNF superfamily receptor 6; GST, glutathione-S-transferase; IL-1, interleukin-6; JNK, c-Jun amino-terminal kinase; MAPK, mitogen-activated protein kinase; NF-κB, nuclear factor-kappa-B; RAR, retinoic acid receptor; RXR, retinoid X receptor; TNF, tumor necrosis factor.

supplementation, subjects with low plasma ascorbate had higher levels of ICAM-1 mRNA, and after supplementation for six weeks, ICAM-1 mRNA was significantly reduced in those with low plasma levels. The results suggest that antioxidant supplementation can influence cellular response, including gene expression and cell signaling.

VITAMIN C AND APOPTOSIS In most studies, vitamin C, the major water-soluble antioxidant, inhibits cell death triggered by various stimuli, and much of this protection has been attributed to its antioxidant property (20, 98, 109, 155, 156, 193). Studies of the antiapoptotic activity of vitamin C in monocytes and thymocytes have provided evidence of a role of vitamin C in modulation of the immune system (109, 155). A recent study by Perez-Cruz et al. (155) investigated the role of vitamin C and FAS-induced apoptosis (155). Fresh human monocytes as well as U937 cells (of monocytic origin) were incubated with vitamin C. Accumulation of vitamin C inhibited FAS-mediated cell death, and apoptosis was associated with reduced levels of ROS; decrease in activity of capase 3, 8, and 10; and preservation of mitochondrial membrane integrity.

Studies using mouse models/cells as well as humans also have demonstrated the protective effect of ascorbate against UV damage or other stimuli promoting cell death (20, 156, 193, 198). Stewart and coworkers (193) showed that mouse keratinocytes preincubated with ascorbic acid exhibited a significant decrease in DNA adducts induced by UVB radiation. Another study tested whether mouse T-cells incubated with ascorbic acid reduced T-cell apoptosis (20). Both activated and resting T-cells responded to ascorbic acid, and T-cell apoptotic pathways induced by three different conditions were inhibited, including growth factor withdrawal and spontaneous and steroid-induced death, which suggests that vitamin C may protect the immune system from overproliferation via this mechanism. In human keratinocytes, cells incubated with ascorbate showed a substantial decrease in apoptosis induced by UV radiation; this protection by ascorbic acid was related to reduced lipid peroxidation as well as downregulation of proinflammatory cytokines, such as IL-1 (198). Therefore, in vitro and in vivo data suggest that vitamin C protects against cell death in cells exposed to UV-mediated cytotoxicity.

Carotenoids

CAROTENOIDS AND TRANSCRIPTION FACTORS Emerging evidence suggests that carotenoids or their derivatives, including retinoic acid (RA), interact and regulate transcription factors (134). It has been well established that retinoic acid, the parent compound of retinoids, produces multiple effects on cells, including inhibition of cell proliferation and enhanced cell differentiation. Via its interaction with two nuclear receptors—retinoic acid receptors and retinoid X receptors—RA regulates biological processes. The binding of the retinoic acid ligand to these receptors, located in the nucleus of the cell, mediates upregulation or inhibition of gene expression. Recently, studies have assessed whether lycopene may interact as a ligand with nuclear receptors and have found that the action of lycopene and other carotenoids either was similar to RA or substantially weaker (185).

CAROTENOIDS AND APOPTOSIS Studies assessing carotenoids and their effects on regulation of transcription factors and apoptosis have primarily investigated β-carotene. Tests conducted in acinar pancreatic cells from mice showed that cells under oxidative stress upregulated NF-κB and increased production of inflammatory cytokines (183). However, supplementation with β-carotene suppressed NF-κB activation and production of interleukin-6 (IL-6) and TNF-alpha inflammatory cytokines (184), which suggests that β-carotene has a protective effect. Additional in vivo studies reveal that normal cells supplemented with carotenoids are protected from programmed cell death (159, 161, 162). Prior to exposure to single-dose UVB radiation, Skh-1 mice were administered lutein plus zeaxanthin for two weeks (59). Supplementing with these carotenoids produced a significant decrease ($p < 0.05$) in proliferating cells and proliferating cell antigen. Also, signal transduction intermediates JNK and p-JNK were inhibited and antiapoptotic protein BCL-2 was upregulated by β-carotene supplementation, while the apoptotic BAX protein was downregulated after induction by external stimuli, which suggests that carotenoids appropriately attenuate apoptosis in normal cells (161, 162).

Selenium

SELENIUM AND TRANSCRIPTION FACTORS A majority of the action and regulation of transcription factors by selenium occurs via selenoproteins, including TR and GPX. Selenium as a constituent of TR can regulate DNA-binding ability of NF-κB and AP-1 as well as other transcription factors.

Selenite and selenodigulathione are effective oxidants of reduced thioredoxin and reduced TR, which diminishes the TR pool and may explain the inhibitory influence of selenium on cell growth and cancer progression (192). After incubation of lymphocytes with selenite and selenodigulathione, a 50% inhibition of AP-1 DNA binding was observed, which suggests a mechanism for the anticancer influence of selenium. Another study reported similar results, showing that selenite blocked AP-1 DNA binding by 50% and decreased expression of an AP-1-dependent gene (65). A more recent study in human leukocytes showed that selenomethionine and selenocysteine inhibited nuclear accumulation of AP-1 and NF-κB elicited by an exogenous oxidant (86).

Selenium has been shown to influence NF-κB activity (18, 97, 98, 109). The role of selenium in the regulation of NF-κB activity is supported by data showing that treatment of cell cultures with selenium alone and/or overexpression of seleno-dependent GPX reduce activation of NF-κB (18, 97, 98, 109). In human cells overexpressing GPX, exposure to H_2O_2 resulted in a reduction of intracellular ROS accumulation and decreased NF-κB activity (97).

Selenium and selenoproteins have also been shown to regulate p53 (131, 153, 189). It is well established that the tumor suppressor protein p53 has a multitude of cellular functions, from gene regulation to DNA repair. Several functions of p53 are redox regulated (150, 153). The ability of p53 to induce transcription was measured in yeast; p53 activity was suppressed in yeast deficient for the gene encoding TR (153). Furthermore, results showed that p53 functioned as a transcription factor only after reduction of disulfides, a finding that suggests activity of p53 is selenium dependent as well as redox related (153).

SELENIUM AND CELLULAR SIGNALING Selenium is involved in signal transduction via its activation of several intermediates, including mitogen-activated protein kinases (MAPKs) and transcription factors such as AP-1 and NF-κB (as discussed above), which influence gene expression and cell growth. Park and coworkers (149) assessed the molecular mechanism of selenium in cell signaling, and found that selenite inhibits both JNK and p38, which are subfamilies of the MAPK signaling pathway. In vitro studies showed that selenite directly regulated JNK, and upon addition of reductants, the inhibition of JNK by selenite was reversed, which suggests that a thiol redox mechanism was involved in the repression of JNK by selenite. Another report also found that ebselen, a seleno-organic compound, inhibited nitric oxide and NF-κB by suppressing phosphorylation of JNK; however, p38 was not modulated (186). These results suggest that selenium can regulate NF-κB and protooncogene expression via an effect on signal transduction intermediates. A more recent in vitro experiment demonstrated that selenium suppressed the p38 MAPK pathway and prevented lipopolysaccharide inflammatory response (94). Therefore, modulation of signaling cascades by selenium affects various cellular activities, including cell survival, apoptosis, and gene expression. In vivo studies are needed to confirm the importance of these observations.

SELENIUM AND APOPTOSIS A large body of evidence has shown that selenium is involved in the molecular processes leading to cell death. However, the role of selenium in apoptosis is complex because of its pro-oxidant as well as antioxidant functions (114). In normal cells, the activity of selenium as an antioxidant confers protection against cell death via regulation of cell-signaling molecules (166, 219). A study supplementing keratinocytes with 50 nM of selenomethionine conferred 95% protection against cell death induced by 960 J/m^2 UVB, while 100% of cells were rescued from apoptosis against 600 J/m^2 UVB (166). Recent studies from the same group further indicated that incubation of keratinocytes with selenomethionine and selenite protected cells against oxidative DNA damage, and supplementation of cells with selenocompounds reduced cellular apoptosis initiated by UV radiation by 71% (164, 165). Selenium also protected cells from UV radiation–induced apoptosis; however, selenium had minimal influence on p53 expression, which suggests that selenium protection against apoptosis is independent of the p53 pathway and may impact cellular survival via regulation of the Fas/Fas ligand or TNF-α pathways (164). In addition, it has been demonstrated (as shown above) that TRX and GPX—both selenoproteins—are involved in apoptosis; therefore, selenium as a component of these proteins indirectly affects apoptosis.

REDOX ABERRATIONS IN CANCER CELLS

General Aberrations

Much evidence has shown that redox balance is impaired in cancer cells compared with normal human cells (138, 194), which may be related to oncogenic stimulation (11) and/or mitochondrial malfunction. Altered levels of antioxidative enzymes (i.e., SOD, catalase, and glutathione peroxidase) and nonenzymic antioxidants (i.e., GSH; vitamins A, C, and E; thioredoxins; and Ref-1), as well as the related signal pathways, are evident in many human tumors and are fundamentally involved in carcinogenesis and tumor progression (Figure 2, see color insert).

Elevated levels of mRNA thioredoxin-1 have been reported and increased protein levels have been observed in many human primary tumors, including cervical cancer, non-small-cell lung cancer, pancreatic cancer, and hepatoma (extensively reviewed in 203). In addition, Lincoln et al. (104) found that in aggressive invasive mammary carcinomas and advanced malignant melanomas, TRX expression was substantially elevated compared with less aggressive tumors. TRX expression in neoplastic cells was also found in both the nucleus and cytoplasm of the neoplastic cells and was positively correlated with TR levels and localization. These observations suggested that increased TRX/TR regulates both nuclear and cytoplasmic redox status as well as activates nuclear transcription factors, facilitating a more aggressive potential for tumor cells. Elevated TRX-1 not only contributes to the development of tumor resistance (215, 218) but also is closely associated with patient outcome. A recent study of primary non-small-cell lung cancer found an association among TRX-1, regional lymph node involvement, and decreased patient survival (88). A study reported by Raffel et al. (163) also demonstrated a significant association between increased TRX-1 expression and colorectal cancer patient survival.

It is well documented that Ref-1 is involved in different stages of tumor development (initiation, promotion, and progression) through maintenance of intracellular redox status and activation of a cell survival signal, as well as through repair of damaged DNA lesions. Many tumors, including cervical, pediatric rhabdomyosarcomas, prostate, epithelial ovarian cancers, and germ cell, exhibit elevated Ref-1 expression in comparison with normal tissues (45). Recently, Orii et al. (141) also reported that a higher predominance of Ref-1 active-form expression was observed in almost all leiomyoma and leiomyosarcoma samples compared with that of normal myometrial cells; this might be related to the higher proliferative activity and could contribute to the selective growth advantage of these tumors. Additionally, as Ref-1 exhibits both cytoplasmic and nuclear enzymic activities, specific subcellular localization of Ref-1 has also been investigated in many human tumors. Epithelial ovarian cancers display both nuclear and cytoplasmic staining, with cytoplasmic localization predominating, whereas normal tissue exhibited strong nuclear staining without cytoplasmic staining (126). Tanner et al. (196) reported elevated nuclear APE/Ref-1 expression during the progression of ovarian carcinomas. Importantly, Ref-1 expression in tumor cells also was closely related to treatment resistance. Robertson et al. (170) demonstrated that higher levels of APE/Ref-1, observed in testicular cancer of various histologies, might be associated with their relative resistance to bleomycin and radiation. Hedley and collaborators (69) found highly significant increases in thioredoxin and Ref-1 expression within the hypoxic microenvironment of invasive cervical carcinomas. Herring et al. (70) also found that there was a correlation between intrinsic radiosensitivity and expression of Ref-1 in cervical carcinomas. Because cells exposed to hypoxia in tissue are resistant to radiation and are associated with poor prognosis (73), this observation leads to the conclusion that elevated thioredoxin and Ref-1 may act in a coordinated manner to promote cancer cell survival.

GSH, GSH-related Enzymes in Cancer Cells

Gamma-glutamyl cysteine synthetase (GCS), the rate-limiting enzyme in GSH biosynthesis, is highly expressed in most cases of malignant mesothelioma and inhibition of GCS by BSO potentiated cisplatin-induced cytotoxicity (83). In human colorectal carcinomas, strong cytoplasmic staining for GCS heavy subunit was detected with a higher frequency than in adenoma and was significantly correlated with multidrug-resistance protein 1 expression (197). Another GSH-related enzyme, glutathione-S-transferase (GST), was elevated in colonic neoplasia compared with adjacent normal mucosa (129), but only a marginal increase in breast cancer was noted compared with normal adjacent tissues (44). Nelson et al. (132) also observed that loss of GSTP1 expression in prostate cancer appeared to be characteristic for prostatic epithelial neoplasia lesions, and was most often associated with somatic "CpG island" DNA methylation changes. In human glioma cell lines, high levels of GST-pi protein expression correlated with enhanced sensitivity to vincristine-induced cell death (210).

Melanoma

The skin is chronically exposed to both endogenous and environmental pro-oxidant agents such as UV radiation, a well-known initiator and promoter of skin cancers (16). The imbalance between pro-oxidant and antioxidant activities in skin cells subsequently leads to ROS-mediated oxidative damage and might contribute to skin diseases (17). Our group (122) has intensively investigated the abnormal redox status in human melanoma compared with normal melanocytes. Melanin acts not only as an antioxidant to neutralize ROS (187) but also as a pro-oxidant (47, 191). We have proposed that continuously elevated intracellular ROS is caused, at least in part, by the presence of oxidized melanin functioning as a pro-oxidant that subsequently results in dysregulated nuclear transcription signals, including NF-κB (116, 117, 122) and AP-1 (216), leading to the transcription of genes related to melanoma tumorigenesis, promotion, and progression.

DIETARY NUTRIENTS AND INFLUENCE ON CANCER CELLS

Carotenoids

Several investigations have demonstrated the antiproliferative effect of carotenoids on various cancer cell lines (1, 14, 107, 151, 190). Inhibition of cell cycle progression by lycopene has been shown in breast, lung, and prostate cell lines (90, 107, 151). Human prostate cancer cell lines were incubated with either lycopene alone or with lycopene plus α-tocopherol (151). The combination of the two antioxidants strongly inhibited prostate cancer cell proliferation, whereas lycopene alone had very little effect. In contrast, lycopene alone was shown to regulate transcription factors (90). MCF7 mammary cancer cells supplemented with lycopene significantly reduced the insulin-like growth factor-I induction of cell signaling and inhibited AP-1 binding; these results suggest that lycopene has an inhibitory effect on mammary cancer cell growth.

Attenuation of apoptosis by carotenoids in cancer cells has been documented previously (144). Palozza and colleagues showed a proapoptotic effect of β-carotene in different cancer cell lines (including human colon and leukemic cancer cell lines), but the cell lines had varying degree of sensitivity to β-carotene (143, 145, 146). The same group investigated the role of β-carotene in attenuation of apoptosis via regulation of NF-κB in colon and leukemic cancer cell lines (148). The findings clearly showed that β-carotene, via a redox mechanism, increased ROS and GSSG/GSH ratio, and these results were associated with increased NF-κB binding ability, inhibition of cell growth, and enhanced proapoptotic activity in tumor cells (147). Cleavage products of β-carotene were also shown to regulate breast cancer cell proliferation, the effects of which may be mediated by regulation of AP-1 (199). Another study showed that carotenoids, by interacting with cell membrane molecules, activated the capase-8 cell-signaling pathway, which was pivotal for initiating apoptosis, in human colon, leukemic, and melanoma tumor cell lines (146). In congruence with these results, β-carotene has been shown to inhibit the expression of the antiapoptotic protein Bcl-2 in cancer cells, thereby reducing growth of cancer cells (144). These data suggest that carotenoids regulate proliferation and growth as well as apoptosis via attenuation of various transcription factors and signaling intermediates.

Selenium

From epidemiological to clinical to basic science data, selenium has been shown to have anticarcinogenic properties. Several studies have demonstrated the antigrowth effect of selenium in androgen-sensitive LnCAP cells as well as in androgen-resistant lines such as DU-145 and PC3 (118, 201, 207). Numerous mechanisms have been delineated for the anticarcinogenesis function of selenium, including antioxidant function, regulation of cell signaling, and proapoptotic influence in cancer cells (95).

Premalignant human breast cell lines were incubated with methylselenic acid, a form of selenium (40). Both cell lines exhibited growth inhibition and induction of apoptosis. Methylselenic acid altered the expression of 30 genes, which were categorized into cell-cycle regulators (include cyclin A and D1, p16, and p27) and apoptotic and signaling genes, such as MAPK and ERK (kinases) (40). Additional reports have suggested that the molecular basis for selenium in inducing apoptosis in cancer cells occurs via mediation of cell signaling targets, including caspase 8 and 9 pathways (41, 57, 78, 84).

The influence of selenium on molecular processes including cell signaling and apoptosis has been shown to occur (but not exclusively) via a redox-dependent mechanism (183, 223). Regulation of p53 by selenomethionine required redox-dependent Ref-1 (183). After sustained exposure to selenite, upregulation of redox-sensitive proteins, manganese superoxide dismutase and p21, was observed (223). These data suggest that selenium, in different forms, attenuates various targets and regulates apoptosis and cell signaling.

Other Dietary Compounds (Resveratrol, Epigallocatechin-3-Gallate, Isothiocynates)

Although the current review emphasizes carotenoids, selenium, and vitamin C, there is growing evidence that other dietary constituents, including resveratrol, epigallocatechin-3-gallate (EGCG), and isothiocynates function as chemopreventive agents and modulate cellular processes in cancer cells (13, 92, 100). Resveratrol is found in many plant species, including grapes, and therefore is a component of red wine (13). Resveratrol induces cell cycle arrest and apoptosis in many cancer cell lines. The proapoptotic action of resveratrol is associated with p53 and JNK activation. EGCG, a component of green and black tea, also exerts differential effects on cancer and normal cells, where cancer cells are more responsive to EGCG (202). Human colorectal cells treated with EGCG experienced cell death and exhibited nuclear condensation, DNA fragmentation, and caspase activation. Both resveratrol and EGCG also have been shown to affect NF-κB activation. Also, cruciferous vegetables, such as cabbage, broccoli, and cauliflower, are high in isothiocynates and demonstrate chemopreventive function (92). The anticarcinogenic function of isothiocynates can partially be explained via the upregulation of phase II detoxifying enzymes and inhibition of phase I carcinogen-activating enzymes by isothiocynates. Isothiocynates also induce cell cycle arrest and modulate NF-κB and AP-1, which elicit an apoptotic response in cancer cells.

POTENTIAL FOR INTERVENTION IN REDOX SYSTEMS AND SPECIES

Molecular Manipulation

Normally, topical application or oral administration of antioxidants to scavenge ROS or depletion of antioxidants to potentiate ROS damage are methods used to enhance, respectively, the preventive or chemotherapeutic effect (17, 115). Recently, extensive studies on the role of TRX, GSH, and Ref-1 in promotion, progression, and drug resistance have confirmed their potential as attractive targets for the development of new cancer-preventive and therapeutic strategies (45, 115, 158).

DRUGS THAT INTERACT WITH GSH IMPAIR INTRACELLULAR REDOX BUFFERING SYSTEM It is well established that elevated GSH renders cancer cells resistant against chemotherapy and radiation treatment; therefore, this compound might be a good candidate target for further manipulation. Many compounds that interfere with the GSH pathway through different mechanisms have exhibited promising antitumor activities, either by inducing apoptosis or by reversing drug resistance to chemotherapeutic agents in tumor cells.

BSO, which induces GSH depletion through inhibiting the synthesis of γ-glutamylcysteine, sensitizes HL-60 human leukemia cells as well as arsenic-resistant acute promyelocytic leukemia-derived cell lines to arsenic trioxide treatment (34, 35), and also restores the senescence of resistant tumor cells to melphalan both in vitro and in vivo (140, 182, 200). Cepsilon, isolated from the stem bark of *Magnolia sieboldii*, induces apoptosis in human promonocytic leukemia U937 cells by rapidly depleting the intracellular GSH and protein thiols (29). The growth-inhibitory effect of allicin, the major ingredient of crushed garlic, was also correlated with GSH levels (72). TER199, an analog of glutathione designed to be a specific inhibitor of GST P1-1, has also significantly reversed the multidrug-resistance protein 1-mediated drug resistance for vincristine, doxorubicin, etoposide, and mitoxantrone (139). TER286, a novel nitrogen mustard alkylating prodrug activated by GST, has selectively exhibited more toxicity to tumors expressing higher GST P1-1 levels (173).

DRUGS THAT INHIBIT TRX Elevated levels of TRX or TR have been found in many aggressive human tumors that exhibit a lower apoptosis rate, a higher growth potential, and an elevated invasion capacity, implicating the involvement of TRX/TR in different stages of tumor development (104). Based on the observations that the lower TRX content in SH-SY5Y neuroblastoma cells causes higher susceptibility to serum deprivation–induced apoptosis (2) and that TRX antisense effectively reduced the anchorage-independent potential of Smad7-overexpressing cells (8), it has been suggested that specific TRX inhibitors might exhibit inhibitory effects on cancer cell growth. 1-Methyl-propyl-2-imidazolozyl disulfide (PX-12), a TRX-1 inhibitor binding to the Cys73 residue, not only significantly potentiated the inhibitory effect of cisplatin on pancreatic cancer (8) but also exhibited promising antitumor activities among a variety of tumor cell lines both in vitro and in vivo (158).

DRUGS THAT INHIBIT REF-1 Ref-1 seems to be a central protein that regulates the action of many transcription factors and provides a unique link with oxidative stress, redox-activated transcription factors, and DNA base excision repair (45). The elevated Ref-1 in many cancers is always associated with aggressive proliferation, increased resistance to therapeutic agents and poor prognosis (as stated in the "Redox Aberrations in Cancer Cells" section above). Decreasing Ref-1 inhibited platelet-derived growth factor–induced proliferation as well as cell cycle progression from G0/G1 to S phase (68). In addition, Lau et al. (103) found that APE/Ref-1 antisense significantly potentiated the cytotoxity of gemcitabine in Panc-1 cells. These observations have supported further investigation of novel strategies for cancer treatments that target Ref-1, either by enhancing the sensitivity of tumor cells to chemotherapy or by inhibiting proliferation. By using sophisticated computer programs to model the three-dimensional structure of Ref-1/APE protein and virtual screening software to dock molecules from virtual drug libraries to the protein, our group has found several compounds that inhibit the endonuclease activity of Ref-1 in vitro (unpublished data). Preliminary data also showed that some of these compounds exhibit active antimelanoma activities and sensitize melanoma cells to dacarbazine treatment.

DIETARY INTERVENTION TRIALS AND FUTURE DIRECTION

Observational epidemiology studies have suggested that the consumption of fruits and vegetables and/or micronutrients, including carotenoids, vitamin E, selenium, folate, and polyphenols, is related to a reduction in cancer risk (51, 113). Nonetheless, case-control and cohort studies are subject to confounding and other biases; therefore, several randomized controlled trials have been conducted to test the effects of dietary supplementation with micronutrients on cancer risk (51). The Alpha-Tocopherol, Beta-Carotene (ATBC) Cancer Prevention Trial assessed the influence of supplementation with β-carotene and α-tocopherol on lung cancer risk in Finnish male smokers. The results of the ATBC trial showed that supplementation with β-carotene and α-tocopherol slightly increased the incidence of lung cancer in smokers. A subanalysis revealed that this increased risk was strongly associated with heavy smoking and drinking. Additional research conducted by the Beta-Carotene and Retinol Efficacy Trial, which tested a combination of β-carotene and retinol, showed a 28% increased risk in lung cancer in the group supplemented with β-carotene and retinol (51). Possibly the doses used in these studies were too high. Recent studies have also shown the pro-oxidant influence of high amounts of β-carotene in the presence of cigarette smoke in a ferret model (103, 106). Also, it may well be that β-carotene is not the only constituent in vegetables and fruits that confers anticarcinogenic effects.

Randomized clinical trials also have been conducted to assess the influence of fat, fiber, vegetable, and fruit intake on cancer risk (51). Several trials, including the Polyp Prevention Trial, investigated the effects of consuming a high-fiber, low-fat, high-vegetable and -fruit diet on adenomatous polyp recurrence. The trials followed participants for one to four years. Little to no significant reduction in polyp recurrence was observed. Possible contributors to the null results include a small sample size, insufficient follow-up time, and wrong endpoints, as well as the failure to assess other protective dietary sources and micronutrients in the trial. Currently, an intervention trial enrolling 3000 women is examining the influence of an overall dietary pattern of high fruit and vegetable intakes on breast cancer recurrence (157, 172).

The question of whether diet or dietary nutrients can reduce incidence of cancer and/or function in a chemopreventive manner has been the subject of much discussion. The limitations of randomized dietary clinical trials in which interventions were conducted with only a single nutrient are considerable. Supplementation with a single nutrient in prevention trials overlooks the pivotal impact that other micronutrients collectively assert. Many nutritional compounds and redox systems influence regulation of biological processes governing cellular signaling, transcription factor activity, and apoptosis, which are all intricately involved in determining whether a cell progresses from a normal cell to a cancer cell. However, because a number of extrinsic and intrinsic redox species regulate different and/or the same molecular targets, designing intervention studies that can effectively incorporate these numerous variables is complex. Nonetheless, randomized clinical trials are still the gold standard in investigating further the results derived from observational and laboratory studies on the association between nutrition and cancer prevention and control. Also, chemoprevention strategies and randomized clinical trials may require modulation/interventions of overall dietary patterns, such as increasing vegetable, fruit, and fiber intake and/or a "cocktail" of micronutrients working together in concert to introduce a sustained protection against cancer risk outcomes (123).

In addition, identifying appropriate molecular markers and targets is critical in the discovery of new therapies to reduce cancer risks. It is well established that TRX, Ref-1, and GSH do not act in isolation, but form an intricate network in the cell; therefore, blockade of one target alone might not be sufficient to achieve a clinical benefit. Thus, multitargeted compounds or targeted compounds used in combination likely are of more powerful and promising potential for cancer prevention and treatment, both with respect to efficacy and for prevention of resistance. Also, screening natural compounds or dietary components targeting these signals would shed new light on cancer chemoprevention, with high efficacy and low toxicity.

Redox regulation involves intrinsic components, including TRX, GSH, and extrinsic micronutrients, including selenium, vitamin C and carotenoids, which function in distinct, yet additive, synergistic and/or antagonist roles to control cellular processes. Because a multitude of molecules govern the same and/or different pathways, to move the field of redox regulation forward, expertise in various fields is required. Therefore, future clinical trials will need to include a multidisciplinary approach and include molecular biologists, nutritionists, biochemists, epidemiologists and clinicians to translate redox regulation of biological processes at the cellular level to humans in efforts to achieve the greatest public health benefit.

ACKNOWLEDGMENTS

Supported in part by CA62203 from the National Institutes of Health and a Sun Fellowship to S. Yang. We thank Sandy Schroeder for excellent administrative assistance.

The *Annual Review of Nutrition* is online at http://nutr.annualreviews.org

LITERATURE CITED

1. Amir H, Karas M, Giat J, Danilenko M, Levy R, et al. 1999. Lycopene and 1,25-dihydroxyvitamin D3 cooperate in the inhibition of cell cycle progression and induction of differentiation in HL-60 leukemic cells. *Nutr. Cancer* 33(1):105–12
2. Andoh T, Chock PB, Chiueh CC. 2002. The roles of thioredoxin in protection against oxidative stress-induced apoptosis in SH-SY5Y cells. *J. Biol. Chem.* 277: 9655–60
3. Anema SM, Walker SW, Howie AF, Arthur JR, Nicol F, Beckett GJ. 1999. Thioredoxin reductase is the major selenoprotein expressed in human umbilical-vein endothelial cells and is regulated by protein kinase C. *Biochem. J.* 342: 111–17
4. Angkeow P, Deshpande SS, Qi B, Liu YX YC, Park, et al. 2002. Redox factor-1: an extra-nuclear role in the regulation of endothelial oxidative stress and apoptosis. *Cell Death Differ.* 9:717–25
5. Deleted in proof
6. Armstrong JS, Steinauer KK, Hornung B, Irish JM, Lecane P, et al. 2002. Role of glutathione depletion and reactive oxygen species generation in apoptotic signaling in a human B lymphoma cell line. *Cell Death Differ.* 9:252–63
7. Arner ES, Holmgren A. 2000. Physiological functions of thioredoxin and thioredoxin reductase. *Eur. J. Biochem.* 267: 6102–9
8. Arnold NB, Ketterer K, Kleeff J, Friess H, Buchler MW, Korc M. 2004. Thioredoxin is downstream of Smad7 in a pathway that promotes growth and suppresses cisplatin-induced apoptosis in pancreatic cancer. *Cancer Res.* 64:3599–606
9. Azzam EI, De Toledo SM, Spitz DR, Little JB. 2002. Oxidative metabolism modulates signal transduction and micronucleus formation in bystander cells from alpha-particle-irradiated normal human fibroblast cultures. *Cancer Res.* 62:5436–42
10. Baker A, Payne CM, Briehl MM, Powis G. 1997. Thioredoxin, a gene found over-expressed in human cancer, inhibits apoptosis in vitro and in vivo. *Cancer Res.* 57: 5162–67
11. Benhar M, Dalyot I, Engelberg D, Levitzki A. 2001. Enhanced ROS production in oncogenically transformed cells potentiates c-Jun N-terminal kinase and p38 mitogen-activated protein kinase activation and sensitization to genotoxic stress. *Mol. Cell Biol.* 21:6913–26
12. Biroccio A, Benassi B, Fiorentino F, Zupi G. 2004. Glutathione depletion induced by c-Myc downregulation triggers apoptosis on treatment with alkylating agents. *Neoplasia* 6:195–206
13. Bode AM, Dong Z. 2004. Targeting signal transduction pathways by chemopreventive agents. *Mutat. Res.* 555:33–51
14. Boileau TW, Liao Z, Kim S, Lemeshow S, Erdman JW Jr, Clinton SK. 2003. Prostate carcinogenesis in N-methyl-N-nitrosourea (NMU)-testosterone-treated rats fed tomato powder, lycopene, or energy-restricted diets. *J. Natl. Cancer Inst.* 95:1578–86
15. Bojes HK, Datta K, Xu J, Chin A, Simonian P, et al. 1997. Bcl-xL overexpression attenuates glutathione depletion in FL5.12 cells following interleukin-3 withdrawal. *Biochem. J.* 325:315–19
16. Bowden GT. 2004. Prevention of non-melanoma skin cancer by targeting ultraviolet-B-light signalling. *Nat. Rev. Cancer* 4:23–35
17. Briganti S, Picardo M. 2003. Antioxidant activity, lipid peroxidation and skin diseases. What's new. *J. Eur. Acad. Dermatol. Venereol.* 17:663–69

18. Brigelius-Flohe R, Friedrichs B, Maurer S, Schultz M, Streicher R. 1997. Interleukin-1-induced nuclear factor kappa B activation is inhibited by overexpression of phospholipid hydroperoxide glutathione peroxidase in a human endothelial cell line. *Biochem. J.* 328(Pt. 1): 199–203
19. Cai J, Jones DP. 1999. Mitochondrial redox signaling during apoptosis. *J. Bioenerg. Biomembr.* 31:327–34
20. Campbell JD, Cole M, Bunditrutavorn B, Vella AT. 1999. Ascorbic acid is a potent inhibitor of various forms of T cell apoptosis. *Cell Immunol.* 194:1–5
21. Canals S, Casarejos MJ, de Bernardo S, Rodriguez-Martin E, Mena MA. 2001. Glutathione depletion switches nitric oxide neurotrophic effects to cell death in midbrain cultures: implications for Parkinson's disease. *J. Neurochem.* 79: 1183–95
22. Carcamo JM, Pedraza A, Borquez-Ojeda O, Zhang B, Sanchez R, Golde DW. 2004. Vitamin C is a kinase inhibitor: Dehydroascorbic acid inhibits IκBα kinase β. *Mol. Cell Biol.* 24:6645–52
23. Carew JS, Zhou Y, Albitar M, Carew JD, Keating MJ, Huang P. 2003. Mitochondrial DNA mutations in primary leukemia cells after chemotherapy: clinical significance and therapeutic implications. *Leukemia* 17:1437–47
24. Carty JL, Bevan R, Waller H, Mistry N, Cooke M, et al. 2000. The effects of vitamin C supplementation on protein oxidation in healthy volunteers. *Biochem. Biophys. Res. Commun.* 273:729–35
25. Catani MV, Costanzo A, Savini I, Levrero M, de Laurenzi V, et al. 2002. Ascorbate up-regulates MLH1 (Mut L homologue-1) and p73: implications for the cellular response to DNA damage. *Biochem. J.* 364:441–47
26. Catani MV, Rossi A, Costanzo A, Sabatini S, Levrero M, et al. 2001. Induction of gene expression via activator protein-1 in the ascorbate protection against UV-induced damage. *Biochem. J.* 356:77–85
27. Chen Y, Cai J, Murphy TJ, Jones DP. 2002. Overexpressed human mitochondrial thioredoxin confers resistance to oxidant-induced apoptosis in human osteosarcoma cells. *J. Biol. Chem.* 277:33242–48
28. Chiarini LB, Freitas FG, Petrs-Silva H, Linden R. 2000. Evidence that the bifunctional redox factor/AP endonuclease Ref-1 is an anti-apoptotic protein associated with differentiation in the developing retina. *Cell Death Differ.* 7:272–81
29. Choi JH, Ha J, Park JH, Lee JY, Lee YS, et al. 2002. Costunolide triggers apoptosis in human leukemia U937 cells by depleting intracellular thiols. *Jpn. J. Cancer Res.* 93:1327–33
30. Chu F, Ward NE, O'Brian CA. 2003. PKC isozyme S-cysteinylation by cystine stimulates the pro-apoptotic isozyme PKC delta and inactivates the oncogenic isozyme PKC epsilon. *Carcinogenesis* 24: 317–25
31. Chuang JI, Chang TY, Liu HS. 2003. Glutathione depletion-induced apoptosis of Ha-ras-transformed NIH3T3 cells can be prevented by melatonin. *Oncogene* 22: 1349–57
32. Copeland WC, Wachsman JT, Johnson FM, Penta JS. 2002. Mitochondrial DNA alterations in cancer. *Cancer Invest.* 20: 557–69
33. Cotton PA, Subar AF, Friday JE, Cook A. 2004. Dietary sources of nutrients among U.S. adults, 1994 to 1996. *J. Am. Diet. Assoc.* 104:921–30
34. Dai J, Weinberg RS, Waxman S, Jing Y. 1999. Malignant cells can be sensitized to undergo growth inhibition and apoptosis by arsenic trioxide through modulation of the glutathione redox system. *Blood* 93:268–77
35. Davison K, Mann KK, Waxman S, Miller WH Jr. 2004. JNK activation is a mediator of arsenic trioxide-induced apoptosis

in acute promyelocytic leukemia cells. *Blood* 103:3496–502
36. de Bernardo S, Canals S, Casarejos MJ, Solano RM, Menendez J, Mena MA. 2004. Role of extracellular signal-regulated protein kinase in neuronal cell death induced by glutathione depletion in neuron/glia mesencephalic cultures. *J. Neurochem.* 91:667–82
37. Devary Y, Gottlieb RA, Smeal T, Karin M. 1992. The mammalian ultraviolet response is triggered by activation of Src tyrosine kinases. *Cell* 71:1081–91
38. Domenicotti C, Marengo B, Verzola D, Garibotto G, Traverso N, et al. 2003. Role of PKC-delta activity in glutathione-depleted neuroblastoma cells. *Free Radic. Biol. Med.* 35:504–16
39. Domenicotti C, Paola D, Vitali A, Nitti M, d'Abramo C, et al. 2000. Glutathione depletion induces apoptosis of rat hepatocytes through activation of protein kinase C novel isoforms and dependent increase in AP-1 nuclear binding. *Free Radic. Biol. Med.* 29:1280–90
40. Dong Y, Ip C, Ganther H. 2002. Evidence of a field effect associated with mammary cancer chemoprevention by methylseleninic acid. *Anticancer Res.* 22:27–32
41. Dong Y, Zhang H, Hawthorn L, Ganther HE, Ip C. 2003. Delineation of the molecular basis for selenium-induced growth arrest in human prostate cancer cells by oligonucleotide array. *Cancer Res.* 63:52–59
42. Dvorakova K, Payne CM, Tome ME, Briehl MM, Vasquez MA, et al. 2002. Molecular and cellular characterization of imexon-resistant RPMI8226/I myeloma cells. *Mol. Cancer Ther.* 1:185–95
43. Eisler H, Frohlich KU, Heidenreich E. 2004. Starvation for an essential amino acid induces apoptosis and oxidative stress in yeast. *Exp. Cell. Res.* 300:345–53
44. El-Rayes BF, Ali S, Heilbrun LK, Lababidi S, Bouwman D, et al. 2003. Cytochrome p450 and glutathione transferase expression in human breast cancer. *Clin. Cancer Res.* 9:1705–9
45. Evans AR, Limp-Foster M, Kelley MR. 2000. Going APE over ref-1. *Mutat. Res.* 461:83–108
46. Fan Z, Beresford PJ, Zhang D, Xu Z, Novina CD, et al. 2003. Cleaving the oxidative repair protein Apel enhances cell death mediated by granzyme A. *Nat. Immunol.* 4:145–53
47. Farmer PJ, Gidanian S, Shahandeh B, Di Bilio AJ, Tohidian N, Meyskens FL Jr. 2003. Melanin as a target for melanoma chemotherapy: pro-oxidant effect of oxygen and metals on melanoma viability. *Pigment Cell Res.* 16:273–79
48. Fenech M. 2001. Recommended dietary allowances (RDAs) for genomic stability. *Mutat. Res.* 480–481:51–54
49. Flaherty DM, Monick MM, Carter AB, Peterson MW, Hunninghake GW. 2001. GM-CSF increases AP-1 DNA binding and Ref-1 amounts in human alveolar macrophages. *Am. J. Respir. Cell Mol. Biol.* 25:254–59
50. Foote CS. 1968. Mechanisms of photosensitized oxidation. There are several different types of photosensitized oxidation which may be important in biological systems. *Science* 162:963–70
51. Forman MR, Hursting SD, Umar A, Barrett JC. 2004. Nutrition and cancer prevention: a multi-disciplinary perspective on human trials. *Annu. Rev. Nutr.* 24:223–54
52. Freemerman AJ, Gallegos A, Powis G. 1999. Nuclear factor κB transactivation is increased but is not involved in the proliferative effects of thioredoxin overexpression in MCF-7 breast cancer cells. *Cancer Res.* 59:4090–94
53. Fritz G. 2000. Human APE/Ref-1 protein. *Int. J. Biochem. Cell Biol.* 32:925–29
54. Gaiddon C, Moorthy NC, Prives C. 1999. Ref-1 regulates the transactivation and pro-apoptotic functions of p53 in vivo. *EMBO J.* 18:5609–21
55. Gallegos A, Berggren M, Gasdaska JR,

Powis G. 1997. Mechanisms of the regulation of thioredoxin reductase activity in cancer cells by the chemopreventive agent selenium. *Cancer Res.* 57:4965–70

56. Galter D, Mihm S, Droge W. 1994. Distinct effects of glutathione disulphide on the nuclear transcription factor κB and the activator protein-1. *Eur. J. Biochem.* 221:639–48
57. Ghosh J. 2004. Rapid induction of apoptosis in prostate cancer cells by selenium: reversal by metabolites of arachidonate 5-lipoxygenase. *Biochem. Biophys. Res. Commun.* 315:624–35
58. Gonzales M, Bowden GT. 2002. The role of PI 3-kinase in the UVB-induced expression of c-fos. *Oncogene* 21:2721–28
59. Gonzalez S, Astner S, An W, Goukassian D, Pathak MA. 2003. Dietary lutein/zeaxanthin decreases ultraviolet B-induced epidermal hyperproliferation and acute inflammation in hairless mice. *J. Invest. Dermatol.* 121:399–405
60. Gopalakrishna R, Jaken S. 2000. Protein kinase C signaling and oxidative stress. *Free Radic. Biol. Med.* 28:1349–61
61. Haga S, Terui K, Zhang HQ, Enosawa S, Ogawa W, et al. 2003. Stat3 protects against Fas-induced liver injury by redox-dependent and -independent mechanisms. *J. Clin. Invest.* 112:989–98
62. Hall JL, Wang X, Van Adamson, Zhao Y, Gibbons GH. 2001. Overexpression of Ref-1 inhibits hypoxia and tumor necrosis factor-induced endothelial cell apoptosis through nuclear factor-κB-independent and -dependent pathways. *Circ. Res.* 88: 1247–53
63. Hampton MB, Orrenius S. 1997. Dual regulation of caspase activity by hydrogen peroxide: implications for apoptosis. *FEBS Lett.* 414:552–56
64. Hampton MB, Orrenius S. 1998. Redox regulation of apoptotic cell death. *Biofactors* 8:1–5
65. Handel ML, Watts CK, deFazio A, Day RO, Sutherland RL. 1995. Inhibition of AP-1 binding and transcription by gold and selenium involving conserved cysteine residues in Jun and Fos. *Proc. Natl. Acad. Sci. USA* 92:4497–501
66. Hansen JM, Watson WH, Jones DP. 2004. Compartmentation of nrf-2 redox control: regulation of cytoplasmic activation by glutathione and DNA binding by thioredoxin-1. *Toxicol. Sci.* 82:308–17
67. Haytowitz DB. 1995. Information from USDA's Nutrient Data Bank. *J. Nutr.* 125(7):1952–55
68. He T, Weintraub NL, Goswami PC, Chatterjee P, Flaherty DM, et al. 2003. Redox factor-1 contributes to the regulation of progression from G0/G1 to S by PDGF in vascular smooth muscle cells. *Am. J. Physiol. Heart Circ. Physiol.* 285:H804–12
69. Hedley D, Pintilie M, Woo J, Nicklee T, Morrison A, et al. 2004. Upregulation of the redox mediators thioredoxin and apurinic/apyrimidinic excision (APE)/Ref-1 in hypoxic microregions of invasive cervical carcinomas, mapped using multispectral, wide-field fluorescence image analysis. *Am. J. Pathol.* 164:557–65
70. Herring CJ, West CM, Wilks DP, Davidson SE, Hunter RD, et al. 1998. Levels of the DNA repair enzyme human apurinic/apyrimidinic endonuclease (APE1, APEX, Ref-1) are associated with the intrinsic radiosensitivity of cervical cancers. *Br. J. Cancer* 78:1128–33
71. Hirota K, Murata M, Sachi Y, Nakamura H, Takeuchi J, et al. 1999. Distinct roles of thioredoxin in the cytoplasm and in the nucleus. A two-step mechanism of redox regulation of transcription factor NF-κB. *J. Biol. Chem.* 274:27891–97
72. Hirsch K, Danilenko M, Giat J, Miron T, Rabinkov A, et al. 2000. Effect of purified allicin, the major ingredient of freshly crushed garlic, on cancer cell proliferation. *Nutr. Cancer* 38:245–54
73. Hockel M, Schlenger K, Mitze M, Schaffer U, Vaupel P. 1996. Hypoxia and

radiation response in human tumors. *Semin. Radiat. Oncol.* 6:3–9
74. Honda T, Coppola S, Ghibelli L, Cho SH, Kagawa S, et al. 2004. GSH depletion enhances adenoviral Bax-induced apoptosis in lung cancer cells. *Cancer Gene Ther.* 11:249–55
75. Hsieh MM, Hegde V, Kelley MR, Deutsch WA. 2001. Activation of APE/Ref-1 redox activity is mediated by reactive oxygen species and PKC phosphorylation. *Nucleic Acids Res.* 29:3116–22
76. Husbeck B, Powis G. 2002. The redox protein thioredoxin-1 regulates the constitutive and inducible expression of the estrogen metabolizing cytochromes P450 1B1 and 1A1 in MCF-7 human breast cancer cells. *Carcinogenesis* 23:1625–30
77. Hwang C, Sinskey AJ, Lodish HF. 1992. Oxidized redox state of glutathione in the endoplasmic reticulum. *Science* 257:1496–502
78. Ip C, Thompson HJ, Zhu Z, Ganther HE. 2000. In vitro and in vivo studies of methylseleninic acid: evidence that a monomethylated selenium metabolite is critical for cancer chemoprevention. *Cancer Res.* 60:2882–86
79. Iwata S, Hori T, Sato N, Hirota K, Sasada T, et al. 1997. Adult T cell leukemia (ATL)-derived factor/human thioredoxin prevents apoptosis of lymphoid cells induced by L-cystine and glutathione depletion: possible involvement of thiol-mediated redox regulation in apoptosis caused by pro-oxidant state. *J. Immunol.* 158:3108–17
80. Jacob RA. 1999. Vitamin C. In *Modern Nutrition in Health and Disease*, ed. ME Shils, JA Olson, M Shike, pp. 467–83. Philadelphia, PA: Lea & Febiger. 9th ed.
81. Jacobson MD, Burne JF, King MP, Miyashita T, Reed JC, Raff MC. 1993. Bcl-2 blocks apoptosis in cells lacking mitochondrial DNA. *Nature* 361:365–69
82. Jain A, Martensson J, Stole E, Auld PA, Meister A. 1991. Glutathione deficiency leads to mitochondrial damage in brain. *Proc. Natl. Acad. Sci. USA* 88:1913–17
83. Jarvinen K, Soini Y, Kahlos K, Kinnula VL. 2002. Overexpression of gamma-glutamylcysteine synthetase in human malignant mesothelioma. *Hum. Pathol.* 33:748–55
84. Jiang C, Hu H, Malewicz B, Wang Z, Lu J. 2004. Selenite-induced p53 Ser-15 phosphorylation and caspase-mediated apoptosis in LNCaP human prostate cancer cells. *Mol. Cancer Ther.* 3:877–84
85. Jiang S, Cai J, Wallace DC, Jones DP. 1999. Cytochrome c-mediated apoptosis in cells lacking mitochondrial DNA. Signaling pathway involving release and caspase 3 activation is conserved. *J. Biol. Chem.* 274:29905–11
86. Jozsef L, Filep JG. 2003. Selenium-containing compounds attenuate peroxynitrite-mediated NF-κB and AP-1 activation and interleukin-8 gene and protein expression in human leukocytes. *Free Radic. Biol. Med.* 35:1018–27
87. Kahlos K, Zhang J, Block ER, Patel JM. 2003. Thioredoxin restores nitric oxide-induced inhibition of protein kinase C activity in lung endothelial cells. *Mol. Cell. Biochem.* 254:47–54
88. Kakolyris S, Giatromanolaki A, Koukourakis M, Powis G, Souglakos J, et al. 2001. Thioredoxin expression is associated with lymph node status and prognosis in early operable non-small cell lung cancer. *Clin. Cancer Res.* 7:3087–91
89. Kamata H, Hirata H. 1999. Redox regulation of cellular signalling. *Cell. Signal.* 11:1–14
90. Karas M, Amir H, Fishman D, Danilenko M, Segal S, et al. 2000. Lycopene interferes with cell cycle progression and insulin-like growth factor I signaling in mammary cancer cells. *Nutr. Cancer* 36: 101–11
91. Kawase M, Fujimura M, Morita-Fujimura Y, Chan PH. 1999. Reduction of apurinic/apyrimidinic endonuclease expression after transient global cerebral

ischemia in rats: implication of the failure of DNA repair in neuronal apoptosis. *Stroke* 30:441–48

92. Keum YS, Jeong WS, Kong AN. 2004. Chemoprevention by isothiocyanates and their underlying molecular signaling mechanisms. *Mutat. Res.* 555:191–202
93. Kim BY, Han MJ, Chung AS. 2001. Effects of reactive oxygen species on proliferation of Chinese hamster lung fibroblast (V79) cells. *Free Radic. Biol. Med.* 30: 686–98
94. Kim SH, Johnson VJ, Shin TY, Sharma RP. 2004. Selenium attenuates lipopolysaccharide-induced oxidative stress responses through modulation of p38 MAPK and NF-κB signaling pathways. *Exp. Biol. Med. (Maywood)* 229:203–13
95. Klein EA. 2004. Selenium: epidemiology and basic science. *J. Urol.* 171:S50–53
96. Kretz-Remy C, Arrigo AP. 2001. Selenium: a key element that controls NF-κB activation and IκBα half life. *Biofactors* 14(1–4):117–25
97. Kretz-Remy C, Mehlen P, Mirault ME, Arrigo AP. 1996. Inhibition of I κB-α phosphorylation and degradation and subsequent NF-κB activation by glutathione peroxidase overexpression. *J. Cell Biol.* 133:1083–93
98. Krinsky NI. 1994. The biological properties of carotenoids. *Pure Appl. Chem.* 66:1003–10
99. Kumar S, Holmgren A. 1999. Induction of thioredoxin, thioredoxin reductase and glutaredoxin activity in mouse skin by TPA, a calcium ionophore and other tumor promoters. *Carcinogenesis* 20:1761–67
100. Kwak MK, Wakabayashi N, Kensler TW. 2004. Chemoprevention through the Keap1-Nrf2 signaling pathway by phase 2 enzyme inducers. *Mutat. Res.* 555:133–48
101. Lander HM, Sehajpal PK, Novogrodsky A. 1993. Nitric oxide signaling: a possible role for G proteins. *J. Immunol.* 151: 7182–87
102. Deleted in proof
103. Lau JP, Weatherdon KL, Skalski V, Hedley DW. 2004. Effects of gemcitabine on APE/ref-1 endonuclease activity in pancreatic cancer cells, and the therapeutic potential of antisense oligonucleotides. *Br. J. Cancer* 91:1166–73
104. Lincoln DT, Ali Emadi EM, Tonissen KF, Clarke FM. 2003. The thioredoxin-thioredoxin reductase system: over-expression in human cancer. *Anticancer Res.* 23:2425–33
105. Liu C, Russell RM, Wang XD. 2004. Low dose beta-carotene supplementation of ferrets attenuates smoke-induced lung phosphorylation of JNK, p38 MAPK, and p53 proteins. *J. Nutr.* 134(10):2705–10
106. Liu C, Wang XD, Bronson RT, Smith DE, Krinsky NI, Russell RM. 2000. Effects of physiological versus pharmacological beta-carotene supplementation on cell proliferation and histopathological changes in the lungs of cigarette smoke-exposed ferrets. *Carcinogenesis* 21:2245–53
107. Liu Y, Chang RL, Cui XX, Newmark HL, Conney AH. 1997. Synergistic effects of curcumin on all-trans retinoic acid- and 1 alpha,25-dihydroxyvitamin D3-induced differentiation in human promyelocytic leukemia HL-60 cells. *Oncol. Res.* 9(1):19–29; erratum 9(2):99
108. Deleted in proof
109. Makropoulas V, Bruning T, Schulze-Osthoff K. 1996. Selenium-mediated inhibition of transcription factor NF-κB and HIV LTR promoter activity. *Arch. Toxicol.* 70(5):277–83
110. Mandavilli BS, Santos JH, Van Houten B. 2002. Mitochondrial DNA repair and aging. *Mutat. Res.* 509:127–51
111. Mates JM, Perez-Gomez C, Nunez de Castro I. 1999. Antioxidant enzymes and human diseases. *Clin. Biochem.* 32:595–603
112. Matthews JR, Wakasugi N, Virelizier JL, Yodoi J, Hay RT. 1992. Thioredoxin

regulates the DNA binding activity of NF-κB by reduction of a disulphide bond involving cysteine 62. *Nucleic Acids Res.* 20:3821–30

113. McCullough ML, Giovannucci EL. 2004. Diet and cancer prevention. *Oncogene* 23:6349–64
114. McKenzie RC, Arthur JR, Beckett GJ. 2002. Selenium and the regulation of cell signaling, growth, and survival: molecular and mechanistic aspects. *Antioxid. Redox Signal.* 4:339–51
115. McLellan LI, Wolf CR. 1999. Glutathione and glutathione-dependent enzymes in cancer drug resistance. *Drug Resist. Updat.* 2:153–64
116. McNulty SE, del Rosario R, Cen D, Meyskens FL Jr., Yang S. 2004. Comparative expression of NFκB proteins in melanocytes of normal skin vs. benign intradermal naevus and human metastatic melanoma biopsies. *Pigment Cell Res.* 17: 173–80
117. McNulty SE, Tohidian NB, Meyskens FL Jr. 2001. RelA, p50 and inhibitor of κBα are elevated in human metastatic melanoma cells and respond aberrantly to ultraviolet light B. *Pigment Cell Res.* 14:456–65
118. Menter DG, Sabichi AL, Lippman SM. 2000. Selenium effects on prostate cell growth. *Cancer Epidemiol. Biomarkers Prev.* 9:1171–82
119. Meredith MJ, Cusick CL, Soltaninassab S, Sekhar KS, Lu S, Freeman ML. 1998. Expression of Bcl-2 increases intracellular glutathione by inhibiting methionine-dependent GSH efflux. *Biochem. Biophys. Res. Commun.* 248:458–63
120. Meuillet EJ, Mahadevan D, Berggren M, Coon A, Powis G. 2004. Thioredoxin-1 binds to the C2 domain of PTEN inhibiting PTEN's lipid phosphatase activity and membrane binding: a mechanism for the functional loss of PTEN's tumor suppressor activity. *Arch. Biochem. Biophys.* 429:123–33
121. Meyer M, Schreck R, Baeuerle PA. 1993. H_2O_2 and antioxidants have opposite effects on activation of NF-κB and AP-1 in intact cells: AP-1 as secondary antioxidant-responsive factor. *EMBO J.* 12:2005–15
122. Meyskens FL Jr, Farmer P, Fruehauf JP. 2001. Redox regulation in human melanocytes and melanoma. *Pigment Cell Res.* 14:148–54
123. Meyskens FL Jr, Szabo E. 2004. How should we move the field of chemopreventive agent development forward in a productive manner? *Recent Results Cancer Res.* 166:113–24
124. Mirkovic N, Voehringer DW, Story MD, McConkey DJ, McDonnell TJ, Meyn RE. 1997. Resistance to radiation-induced apoptosis in Bcl-2-expressing cells is reversed by depleting cellular thiols. *Oncogene* 15:1461–70
125. Mistry P, Herbert KE. 2003. Modulation of hOGG1 DNA repair enzyme in human cultured cells in response to pro-oxidant and antioxidant challenge. *Free Radic. Biol. Med.* 35:397–405
126. Moore DH, Michael H, Tritt R, Parsons SH, Kelley MR. 2000. Alterations in the expression of the DNA repair/redox enzyme APE/ref-1 in epithelial ovarian cancers. *Clin. Cancer Res.* 6:602–9
127. Deleted in proof
128. Nagano I, Murakami T, Manabe Y, Abe K. 2002. Early decrease of survival factors and DNA repair enzyme in spinal motor neurons of presymptomatic transgenic mice that express a mutant SOD1 gene. *Life Sci.* 72(4–5):541–48
129. Naidu KA, Nasir A, Pinkas H, Kaiser HE, Brady P, Coppola D. 2003. Glutathione-S-transferase pi expression and activity is increased in colonic neoplasia. *In Vivo* 17:479–82
130. Nakamura H, Nakamura K, Yodoi J. 1997. Redox regulation of cellular activation. *Annu. Rev. Immunol.* 15:351–69
131. Nelson KK, Bacon B, Christensen MJ. 1996. Selenite supplementation decreases expression of MAZ in HT29 human

colon adenocarcinoma cells. *Nutr. Cancer* 26(1):73–81

132. Nelson WG, De Marzo AM, Deweese TL, Lin X, Brooks JD, et al. 2001. Preneoplastic prostate lesions: an opportunity for prostate cancer prevention. *Ann. NY Acad. Sci.* 952:135–44
133. Nespereira B, Perez-Ilzarbe M, Fernandez P, Fuentes AM, Paramo JA, Rodriguez JA. 2003. Vitamins C and E downregulate vascular VEGF and VEGFR-2 expression in apolipoprotein-E-deficient mice. *Atherosclerosis* 171:67–73
134. Niles RM. 2004. Signaling pathways in retinoid chemoprevention and treatment of cancer. *Mutat. Res.* 555:81–96
135. Nilsson J, Soderberg O, Nilsson K, Rosen A. 2000. Thioredoxin prolongs survival of B-type chronic lymphocytic leukemia cells. *Blood* 95:1420–26
136. Nonn L, Berggren M, Powis G. 2003. Increased expression of mitochondrial peroxiredoxin-3 (thioredoxin peroxidase-2) protects cancer cells against hypoxia and drug-induced hydrogen peroxide-dependent apoptosis. *Mol. Cancer Res.* 1: 682–89
137. Nordberg J, Arner ES. 2001. Reactive oxygen species, antioxidants, and the mammalian thioredoxin system. *Free Radic. Biol. Med.* 31:1287–312
138. Oberley TD, Oberley LW. 1997. Antioxidant enzyme levels in cancer. *Histol. Histopathol.* 12:525–35
139. O'Brien ML, Vulevic B, Freer S, Boyd J, Shen H, Tew KD. 1999. Glutathione peptidomimetic drug modulator of multidrug resistance-associated protein. *J. Pharmacol. Exp. Ther.* 291:1348–55
140. O'Dwyer PJ, Hamilton TC, LaCreta FP, Gallo JM, Kilpatrick D, et al. 1996. Phase I trial of buthionine sulfoximine in combination with melphalan in patients with cancer. *J. Clin. Oncol.* 14:249–56
141. Orii A, Masutani H, Nikaido T, Zhai YL, Kato K, et al. 2002. Altered post-translational modification of redox factor 1 protein in human uterine smooth muscle tumors. *J. Clin. Endocrinol. Metab.* 87:3754–59
142. Padayatty SJ, Katz A, Wang Y, Eck P, Kwon O, et al. 2003. Vitamin C as an antioxidant: evaluation of its role in disease prevention. *J. Am. Coll. Nutr.* 22:18–35
143. Palozza P, Calviello G, Serini S, Maggiano N, Lanza P. 2001. β-Carotene at high concentrations induces apoptosis by enhancing oxy-radical production in human adenocarcinoma cells. *Free Radic. Biol. Med.* 30:1000–7
144. Palozza P, Serini S, Di Nicuolo F, Calviello G. 2004. Modulation of apoptotic signalling by carotenoids in cancer cells. *Arch. Biochem. Biophys.* 430:104–9
145. Palozza P, Serini S, Maggiano N, Angelini M, Boninsegna A, et al. 2002a. Induction of cell cycle arrest and apoptosis in human colon adenocarcinoma cell lines by beta-carotene through down-regulation of cyclin A and Bcl-2 family proteins. *Carcinogenesis* 23:11–18
146. Palozza P, Serini S, Torsello A, Boninsegna A, Covacci V, et al. 2002b. Regulation of cell cycle progression and apoptosis by beta-carotene in undifferentiated and differentiated HL-60 leukemia cells: possible involvement of a redox mechanism. *Int. J. Cancer* 97:593–600
147. Palozza P, Serini S, Torsello A, Di Nicuolo F, Maggiano N, et al. 2003b. Mechanism of activation of caspase cascade during beta-carotene-induced apoptosis in human tumor cells. *Nutr. Cancer* 47:76–87
148. Palozza P, Serini S, Torsello A, Di Nicuolo F, Piccioni E, et al. 2003a. Beta-carotene regulates NF-κB DNA-binding activity by a redox mechanism in human leukemia and colon adenocarcinoma cells. *J. Nutr.* 133:381–88
149. Park HS, Park E, Kim MS, Ahn K, Kim IY, Choi EJ. 2000. Selenite inhibits the c-Jun N-terminal kinase/stress-activated protein kinase (JNK/SAPK) through a

thiol redox mechanism. *J. Biol. Chem.* 275:2527–31

150. Parks D, Bolinger R, Mann K. 1997. Redox state regulates binding of p53 to sequence-specific DNA, but not to non-specific or mismatched DNA. *Nucleic Acids Res.* 25:1289–95
151. Pastori M, Pfander H, Boscoboinik D, Azzi A. 1998. Lycopene in association with alpha-tocopherol inhibits at physiological concentrations proliferation of prostate carcinoma cells. *Biochem. Biophys. Res. Commun.* 250:582–85
152. Patenaude A, Ven Murthy MR, Mirault ME. 2004. Mitochondrial thioredoxin system: effects of TRX R2 overexpression on redox balance, cell growth, and apoptosis. *J. Biol. Chem.* 279:27302–14
153. Pearson GD, Merrill GF. 1998. Deletion of the *Saccharomyces cerevisiae* TRR1 gene encoding thioredoxin reductase inhibits p53-dependent reporter gene expression. *J. Biol. Chem.* 273:5431–34
154. Penta JS, Johnson FM, Wachsman JT, Copeland WC. 2001. Mitochondrial DNA in human malignancy. *Mutat. Res.* 488:119–33
155. Perez-Cruz I, Carcamo JM, Golde DW. 2003. Vitamin C inhibits FAS-induced apoptosis in monocytes and U937 cells. *Blood* 102:336–43
156. Pfeffer F, Casanueva E, Kamar J, Guerra A, Perichart O, Vadillo-Ortega F. 1998. Modulation of 72-kilodalton type IV collagenase (matrix metalloproteinase-2) by ascorbic acid in cultured human amnion-derived cells. *Biol. Reprod.* 59:326–29
157. Pierce JP, Faerber S, Wright FA, Newman V, Flatt SW, et al. 1997. Feasibility of a randomized trial of a high-vegetable diet to prevent breast cancer recurrence. *Nutr. Cancer* 28:282–88
158. Powis G, Montfort WR. 2001. Properties and biological activities of thioredoxins. *Annu. Rev. Pharmacol. Toxicol.* 41:261–95
159. Powis G, Briehl M, Oblong J. 1995. Redox signalling and the control of cell growth and death. *Pharmacol. Ther.* 68(1):149–73
160. Puskas F, Gergely P, Niland B, Banki K, Perl A. 2002. Differential regulation of hydrogen peroxide and Fas-dependent apoptosis pathways by dehydroascorbate, the oxidized form of vitamin C. *Antioxid. Redox Signal.* 4:357–69
161. Qin F, Rounds NK, Mao W, Kawai K, Liang CS. 2001. Antioxidant vitamins prevent cardiomyocyte apoptosis produced by norepinephrine infusion in ferrets. *Cardiovasc. Res.* 51:736–48
162. Qin F, Shite J, Liang CS. 2003. Antioxidants attenuate myocyte apoptosis and improve cardiac function in CHF: association with changes in MAPK pathways. *Am. J. Physiol. Heart Circ. Physiol.* 285(2):H822–32
163. Raffel J, Bhattacharyya AK, Gallegos A, Cui H, Einspahr JG, et al. 2003. Increased expression of thioredoxin-1 in human colorectal cancer is associated with decreased patient survival. *J. Lab. Clin. Med.* 142:46–51
164. Rafferty TS, Beckett GJ, Walker C, Bisset YC, McKenzie RC. 2003b. Selenium protects primary human keratinocytes from apoptosis induced by exposure to ultraviolet radiation. *Clin. Exp. Dermatol.* 28: 294–300
165. Rafferty TS, Green MH, Lowe JE, Arlett C, Hunter JA, et al. 2003a. Effects of selenium compounds on induction of DNA damage by broadband ultraviolet radiation in human keratinocytes. *Br. J. Dermatol.* 148:1001–9
166. Rafferty TS, McKenzie RC, Hunter JA, Howie AF, Arthur JR, et al. 1998. Differential expression of selenoproteins by human skin cells and protection by selenium from UVB-radiation-induced cell death. *Biochem. J.* 332:231–36
167. Ramana CV, Boldogh I, Izumi T, Mitra S. 1998. Activation of apurinic/apyrimidinic endonuclease in human cells by reactive oxygen species and its correlation with their adaptive response to genotoxicity of

free radicals. *Proc. Natl. Acad. Sci. USA* 95:5061–66

168. Rayment SJ, Shaw J, Woollard KJ, Lunec J, Griffiths HR. 2003. Vitamin C supplementation in normal subjects reduces constitutive ICAM-1 expression. *Biochem. Biophys. Res. Commun.* 308:339–45
169. Rehman A, Collis CS, Yang M, Kelly M, Diplock AT, et al. 1998. The effects of iron and vitamin C co-supplementation on oxidative damage to DNA in healthy volunteers. *Biochem. Biophys. Res. Commun.* 246:293–98
170. Robertson KA, Bullock HA, Xu Y, Tritt R, Zimmerman E, et al. 2001. Altered expression of Ape1/ref-1 in germ cell tumors and overexpression in NT2 cells confers resistance to bleomycin and radiation. *Cancer Res.* 61:2220–25
171. Robertson KA, Hill DP, Xu Y, Liu L, Van Epps S, et al. 1997. Down-regulation of apurinic/apyrimidinic endonuclease expression is associated with the induction of apoptosis in differentiating myeloid leukemia cells. *Cell Growth Differ.* 8:443–49
172. Rock CL, Flatt SW, Wright FA, Faerber S, Newman V, et al. 1997. Responsiveness of carotenoids to a high vegetable diet intervention designed to prevent breast cancer recurrence. *Cancer Epidemiol. Biomarkers Prev.* 6:617–23
173. Rosario LA, O'Brien ML, Henderson CJ, Wolf CR, Tew KD. 2000. Cellular response to a glutathione S-transferase P1-1 activated prodrug. *Mol. Pharmacol.* 58: 167–74
174. Ruppitsch W, Meisslitzer C, Hirsch-Kauffmann M, Schweiger M. 1998. Overexpression of thioredoxin in Fanconi anemia fibroblasts prevents the cytotoxic and DNA damaging effect of mitomycin C and diepoxybutane. *FEBS Lett.* 422:99–102
175. Saitoh M, Nishitoh H, Fujii M, Takeda K, Tobiume K, et al. 1998. Mammalian thioredoxin is a direct inhibitor of apoptosis signal-regulating kinase (ASK) 1. *EMBO J.* 17:2596–606
176. Samuni AM, Degraff W, Cook JA, Krishna MC, Russo A, Mitchell JB. 2004. The effects of antioxidants on radiation-induced apoptosis pathways in TK6 cells. *Free Radic. Biol. Med.* 37:1648–55
177. Schafer FQ, Buettner GR. 2001. Redox environment of the cell as viewed through the redox state of the glutathione disulfide/glutathione couple. *Free Radic. Biol. Med.* 30:1191–212
178. Schenk H, Klein M, Erdbrugger W, Droge W, Schulze-Osthoff K. 1994. Distinct effects of thioredoxin and antioxidants on the activation of transcription factors NF-κB and AP-1. *Proc. Natl. Acad. Sci. USA* 91:1672–76
179. Schieven GL, Kirihara JM, Myers DE, Ledbetter JA, Uckun FM. 1993. Reactive oxygen intermediates activate NF-κB in a tyrosine kinase-dependent mechanism and in combination with vanadate activate the p56lck and p59fyn tyrosine kinases in human lymphocytes. *Blood* 82:1212–20
180. Schieven GL, Mittler RS, Nadler SG, Kirihara JM, Bolen JB, et al. 1994. ZAP-70 tyrosine kinase, CD45, and T cell receptor involvement in UV- and H2O2-induced T cell signal transduction. *J. Biol. Chem.* 269:20718–26
181. Schneider M, Diemer K, Engelhart K, Zankl H, Trommer WE, Biesalski HK. 2001. Protective effects of vitamins C and E on the number of micronuclei in lymphocytes in smokers and their role in ascorbate free radical formation in plasma. *Free Radic. Res.* 34:209–19
182. Schnelldorfer T, Gansauge S, Gansauge F, Schlosser S, Beger HG, Nussler AK. 2000. Glutathione depletion causes cell growth inhibition and enhanced apoptosis in pancreatic cancer cells. *Cancer* 89:1440–47
183. Seo JY, Kim H, Seo JT, Kim KH. 2002. Oxidative stress induced cytokine production in isolated rat pancreatic acinar cells: effects of small-molecule antioxidants. *Pharmacology* 64:63–70

184. Seo YR, Kelley MR, Smith ML. 2002. Selenomethionine regulation of p53 by a ref1-dependent redox mechanism. *Proc. Natl. Acad. Sci. USA* 99:14548–53
185. Sharoni Y, Danilenko M, Dubi N, Ben-Dor A, Levy J. 2004. Carotenoids and transcription. *Arch. Biochem. Biophys.* 430:89–96
186. Shimohashi N, Nakamuta M, Uchimura K, Sugimoto R, Iwamoto H, et al. 2000. Selenoorganic compound, ebselen, inhibits nitric oxide and tumor necrosis factor-alpha production by the modulation of jun-N-terminal kinase and the NF-κB signaling pathway in rat Kupffer cells. *J. Cell Biochem.* 78:595–606
187. Sichel G, Corsaro C, Scalia M, Sciuto S, Geremia E. 1987. Relationship between melanin content and superoxide dismutase (SOD) activity in the liver of various species of animals. *Cell Biochem. Funct.* 5:123–28
188. Slater AF, Stefan C, Nobel I, van den Dobbelsteen DJ, Orrenius S. 1995. Signalling mechanisms and oxidative stress in apoptosis. *Toxicol. Lett.* 82–83:149–53
189. Smith ML, Lancia JK, Mercer TI, Ip C. 2004. Selenium compounds regulate p53 by common and distinctive mechanisms. *Anticancer Res.* 24:1401–8
190. Sokoloski JA, Hodnick WF, Mayne ST, Cinquina C, Kim CS, Sartorelli AC. 1997. Induction of the differentiation of HL-60 promyelocytic leukemia cells by vitamin E and other antioxidants in combination with low levels of vitamin D3: possible relationship to NF-κB. *Leukemia* 11:1546–53
191. Sotomatsu A, Tanaka M, Hirai S. 1994. Synthetic melanin and ferric ions promote superoxide anion-mediated lipid peroxidation. *FEBS Lett.* 342:105–8
192. Spyrou G, Bjornstedt M, Kumar S, Holmgren A. 1995. AP-1 DNA-binding activity is inhibited by selenite and selenodiglutathione. *FEBS Lett.* 368:59–63
193. Stewart MS, Cameron GS, Pence BC. 1996. Antioxidant nutrients protect against UVB-induced oxidative damage to DNA of mouse keratinocytes in culture. *J. Invest. Dermatol.* 106:1086–89
194. Szatrowski TP, Nathan CF. 1991. Production of large amounts of hydrogen peroxide by human tumor cells. *Cancer Res.* 51:794–98
195. Tanaka T, Hosoi F, Yamaguchi-Iwai Y, Nakamura H, Masutani H, et al. 2002. Thioredoxin-2 (TRX-2) is an essential gene regulating mitochondria-dependent apoptosis. *EMBO J.* 21:1695–703
196. Tanner B, Grimme S, Schiffer I, Heimerdinger C, Schmidt M, et al. 2004. Nuclear expression of apurinic/apyrimidinic endonuclease increases with progression of ovarian carcinomas. *Gynecol. Oncol.* 92:568–77
197. Tatebe S, Unate H, Sinicrope FA, Sakatani T, Sugamura K, et al. 2002. Expression of heavy subunit of γ-glutamylcysteine synthetase (γ-GCSh) in human colorectal carcinoma. *Int. J. Cancer* 97:21–27
198. Tebbe B, Wu S, Geilen CC, Eberle J, Kodelja V, Orfanos CE. 1997. L-ascorbic acid inhibits UVA-induced lipid peroxidation and secretion of IL-1α and IL-6 in cultured human keratinocytes in vitro. *J. Invest. Dermatol.* 108:302–6
199. Tibaduiza EC, Fleet JC, Russell RM, Krinsky NI. 2002. Excentric cleavage products of β-carotene inhibit estrogen receptor positive and negative breast tumor cell growth in vitro and inhibit activator protein-1-mediated transcriptional activation. *J. Nutr.* 132:1368–75
200. Vahrmeijer AL, van Dierendonck JH, Schutrups J, van de Velde CJ, Mulder GJ. 1999. Effect of glutathione depletion on inhibition of cell cycle progression and induction of apoptosis by melphalan (L-phenylalanine mustard) in human colorectal cancer cells. *Biochem. Pharmacol.* 58:655–64
201. Venkateswaran V, Klotz LH, Fleshner

NE. 2002. Selenium modulation of cell proliferation and cell cycle biomarkers in human prostate carcinoma cell lines. *Cancer Res.* 62(9):2540–45

202. Vergani L, Floreani M, Russell A, Ceccon M, Napoli E, et al. 2004. Antioxidant defences and homeostasis of reactive oxygen species in different human mitochondrial DNA-depleted cell lines. *Eur. J. Biochem.* 271:3646–56
203. Voehringer DW, McConkey DJ, McDonnell TJ, Brisbay S, Meyn RE. 1998. Bcl-2 expression causes redistribution of glutathione to the nucleus. *Proc. Natl. Acad. Sci. USA* 95:2956–60
204. Voehringer DW, Meyn RE. 2000. Redox aspects of Bcl-2 function. *Antioxid. Redox Signal.* 2:537–50
205. Wan YS, Wang ZQ, Shao Y, Voorhees JJ, Fisher GJ. 2001. Ultraviolet irradiation activates PI 3-kinase/AKT survival pathway via EGF receptors in human skin in vivo. *Int. J. Oncol.* 18:461–66
206. Ward NE, Pierce DS, Chung SE, Gravitt KR, O'Brian CA. 1998. Irreversible inactivation of protein kinase C by glutathione. *J. Biol. Chem.* 273:12558–66
207. Webber MM, Perez-Ripoll EA, James GT. 1985. Inhibitory effects of selenium on the growth of DU-145 human prostate carcinoma cells in vitro. *Biochem. Biophys. Res. Commun.* 130:603–9
208. Wei YH, Lee HC. 2002. Oxidative stress, mitochondrial DNA mutation, and impairment of antioxidant enzymes in aging. *Exp. Biol. Med.* (*Maywood*) 227:671–82
209. Welsh SJ, Bellamy WT, Briehl MM, Powis G. 2002. The redox protein thioredoxin-1 (TRX-1) increases hypoxia-inducible factor 1α protein expression: TRX-1 overexpression results in increased vascular endothelial growth factor production and enhanced tumor angiogenesis. *Cancer Res.* 62:5089–95
210. Winter S, Strik H, Rieger J, Beck J, Meyermann R, Weller M. 2000. Glutathione S-transferase and drug sensitivity in malignant glioma. *J. Neurol. Sci.* 179:115–21
211. Wong GH. 1995. Protective roles of cytokines against radiation: induction of mitochondrial MnSOD. *Biochim. Biophys. Acta* 1271:205–9
212. Woollard KJ, Loryman CJ, Meredith E, Bevan R, Shaw JA, et al. 2002. Effects of oral vitamin C on monocyte: endothelial cell adhesion in healthy subjects. *Biochem. Biophys. Res. Commun.* 294: 1161–68
213. Wright SC, Wang H, Wei QS, Kinder DH, Larrick JW. 1998. Bcl-2-mediated resistance to apoptosis is associated with glutathione-induced inhibition of AP24 activation of nuclear DNA fragmentation. *Cancer Res.* 58:5570–76
214. Wu G, Fang YZ, Yang S, Lupton JR, Turner ND. 2004. Glutathione metabolism and its implications for health. *J. Nutr.* 134:489–92
215. Yamada M, Tomida A, Yoshikawa H, Taketani Y, Tsuruo T. 1996. Increased expression of thioredoxin/adult T-cell leukemia-derived factor in cisplatin-resistant human cancer cell lines. *Clin. Cancer Res.* 2:427–32
216. Yang S, McNulty S, Meyskens FL Jr. 2004. During human melanoma progression AP-1 binding pairs are altered with loss of c-Jun in vitro. *Pigment Cell Res.* 17:74–83
217. Yao KS, Clayton M, O'Dwyer PJ. 1995. Apoptosis in human adenocarcinoma HT29 cells induced by exposure to hypoxia. *J. Natl. Cancer Inst.* 87:117–22
218. Yokomizo A, Ono M, Nanri H, Makino Y, Ohga T, et al. 1995. Cellular levels of thioredoxin associated with drug sensitivity to cisplatin, mitomycin C, doxorubicin, and etoposide. *Cancer Res.* 55: 4293–96
219. Yoon SO, Kim MM, Chung AS. 2001. Inhibitory effect of selenite on invasion of HT1080 tumor cells. *J. Biol. Chem.* 276:20085–92

220. Zhang K, Mack P, Wong KP. 1998. Glutathione-related mechanisms in cellular resistance to anticancer drugs. *Int. J. Oncol.* 12:871–82
221. Zhang R, Al-Lamki R, Bai L, Streb JW, Miano JM, et al. 2004. Thioredoxin-2 inhibits mitochondria-located ASK1-mediated apoptosis in a JNK-independent manner. *Circ. Res.* 94:1483–91
222. Zhao Y, Kiningham KK, Lin SM, St Clair DK. 2001. Overexpression of MnSOD protects murine fibrosarcoma cells (FSa-II) from apoptosis and promotes a differentiation program upon treatment with 5-azacytidine: involvement of MAPK and NFκB pathways. *Antioxid. Redox Signal.* 3:375–86
223. Zhong W, Oberley TD. 2001. Redox-mediated effects of selenium on apoptosis and cell cycle in the LNCaP human prostate cancer cell line. *Cancer Res.* 61:7071–78
224. Zhou Y, Hileman EO, Plunkett W, Keating MJ, Huang P. 2003. Free radical stress in chronic lymphocytic leukemia cells and its role in cellular sensitivity to ROS-generating anticancer agents. *Blood* 101:4098–104

Annu. Rev. Nutr. 2005. 25:297–315
doi: 10.1146/annurev.nutr.25.050304.092639

First published online as a Review in Advance on April 1, 2005

REGULATION OF GENE TRANSCRIPTION BY BOTANICALS: Novel Regulatory Mechanisms

Neil F. Shay
Department of Biological Sciences, University of Notre Dame, Notre Dame, Indiana 46556; email: nshay1@nd.edu

William J. Banz
Department of Animal Science, Food & Nutrition, Southern Illinois University, Carbondale, Illinois 62901; email: banz@siu.edu

Key Words transcription, hyperforin, isoflavones, resveratrol, epigallocatechin gallate, sirtuins

■ **Abstract** Early investigations of gene regulation revealed that nutrients could modulate gene expression, an example being the discovery of metal-regulated gene transcription (11, 19, 44). Only more recently have we focused on the ability of non-nutritional botanicals or functional food components to affect gene expression at the transcriptional level. Significant findings include the discovery that hyperforin is an active ingredient of the herbal remedy St. John's wort, and activates gene transcription of cytochrome p450-3A4, causing significant botanical-drug interactions. Recently, the lipid-regulating peroxisome proliferator-activated receptors have been studied as receptors activated by soy isoflavones, perhaps explaining the lipid-lowering effect of soy intake. Epigallocatechin gallate has been shown to be an inhibitor of the protealytic activity of the proteasome; this inhibition has a significant implication for cell proliferation and the stability of transcription factors in the nucleus. Very recently, the effects of botanicals have been studied as activators of sirtuins, important deacetylation enzymes that have been shown to enhance lifespan in a variety of organisms. Sirtuins have been implicated in the lifespan-enhancing effect of caloric restriction. Originally presumed to act mainly on compaction or accessibility of DNA, recent evidence shows important activity of sirtuins as controllers of transcriptional coactivator availability. This review focuses on novel mechanisms by which botanical products regulate cell function via gene transcription. Investigating these newly appreciated mechanisms will assist with the characterization and clarification of specific effects of botanicals on gene expression.

CONTENTS

INTRODUCTION

The ability to control the expression of gene products is essential for single-celled and multicellular organisms dealing with a changing environment. Multicellular organisms must also be able to regulate gene expression to successfully complete the complex process of development. When considering mammalian physiology, homeostasis must be maintained despite constantly changing conditions related to diurnal, dietary, and other environmental challenges. At the level of the individual cell, maintenance of homeostasis is due in part to the ability of gene expression to be regulated. Simply put, at various times, proteins may need to be present or absent, their relative level increased or decreased, or receptor or enzyme activity altered by covalent modification such as phosphorylation or by the binding of regulatory proteins that may have positive or negative activity on target of interest. Genes may be regulated at many different levels, including transcription, mRNA processing, export from the nucleus, rate of translation, and half-life of both mRNA and polypeptide products (27, 57). Despite the wide array of regulatory mechanisms that control gene expression, it is gene transcription that is most often regarded as the most important aspect of genetic regulation. This role is due to at least two different factors. First, transcription is an initial event and therefore should be properly considered an initiating or committing step in the multistep process that is gene expression. Second, basal levels of gene transcription are often quite low in comparison with the elevated levels produced by the interaction of gene-specific activators and gene-specific DNA elements within the promoter regions of genes. This difference in magnitude between basal and elevated levels of transcription is often the most dramatic mechanism involved in the regulation of most genes. Although other factors such as mRNA turnover or translational efficiency also contribute to regulation, we most often see these mechanisms play a lesser role in regulation. Notable exceptions in nutrient regulation of gene expression do exist, e.g., the translational and post-translational control of transferrin and transferrin receptor by cellular iron concentrations is a hallmark example of post-transcriptional regulation (10, 60).

The activators of gene expression may serve to either inhibit or stimulate transcription by RNA polymerase II. Typically, activators have common structural features that contain activities such as DNA binding, transcription activation, and dimerization domains that may allow activators to bind as either homo- or heterodimers. The DNA-binding domains of transcriptional activators may fall into one of at least three different categories, including zinc-containing domains, homeodomains, and leucine zippers (bZIP) or helix-loop-helix (bHLH) motifs. The transcriptional activating portions of activators are most often described as acidic, glutamine-rich, or proline-rich domains. Binding of activators to their regulatory sequences in DNA may be affected by availability of the activators themselves (i.e., levels of the activator are changed via either enhanced synthesis, increased import into the nucleus, or by dissociation from inhibitory factors that serve to sequester an activator). The activator may also be covalently modified, gaining enhanced activity as an activator (i.e., via cell signaling processes that may ultimately result in phosphorylation or ubiquitination of the activator). Ligand activation has the ability to modify dramatically the capability of activators to stimulate gene transcription; a notable example is the thyroid hormone receptor. Thyroid hormone (TH) has the ability to bind to regulatory sequences within the promoter of TH-regulated genes. The receptor may bind with its heterodimer partner, the retinoic acid X receptor (RXR) at regulatory sequences, serving as a repressor of transcription until the TH-receptor is activated by binding of TH to the receptor. This ligand-binding event may induce changes in other proteins surrounding the TH-receptor/RXR dimer that subsequently enhances RNA polymerase II binding and transcription (24).

The nuclear receptors are a family of zinc-containing proteins that interact with steroids, hydrophobic hormone molecules, or xenobiotics. The ability of nuclear receptors to bind to these ligands suggests that these proteins have an additional domain—a hormone-binding or ligand-binding domain. The structure of nuclear receptors includes an amino-terminus ligand-independent activation function; a DNA-binding domain containing two highly conserved zinc finger motifs that target the receptor to specific hormone response elements, and a large carboxy terminus region that includes a ligand-binding domain and ligand-dependent activation function (35). The steroid receptors were the first nuclear receptors to be cloned. Since then, a set of 48 related human genes have been identified, which is thought to represent the set of human nuclear receptors (46). The nuclear receptor family includes one set of receptors for which there is a high-affinity ligand-receptor interaction; examples include the estrogen, androgen, and vitamin D receptors. Another set of receptors within the nuclear receptor family include receptors that have a lower affinity for ligand. This class includes receptors that bind dietary or intracellular lipids, such as the liver X receptors (LXRs), the farnesoid X receptor (FXR), and the peroxisome proliferator-activated receptors (PPARs). Importantly, this set of nuclear receptors also includes the pregnane X receptor (PXR), sometimes also called the steroid xenobiotic receptor (SXR). The PXR receptor is among the more "promiscuous" nuclear receptors, allowing it to bind to steroids, toxic bile acids, environmental contaminants, and prescription drugs. Among the set of PXR ligands are many relatively hydrophobic botanical compounds. A third set of nuclear receptors are called the "orphan receptors." Orphan receptors by definition are the group of nuclear receptors for which a specific receptor ligand has not yet been identified. Some orphan receptors may in fact not have a ligand that will activate them.

Although the nuclear receptors offer an immediate model for how botanical products may interact with transcription machinery to affect gene expression, certainly several other mechanisms do exist that would permit botanical compounds to affect gene regulation. In addition to ligand activation, other processes have been implicated in the regulation of transcription factors: phosphorylation state, ubiquitin-dependent changes in protein half-life, and "SUMOlation" (small ubiquitin-related modifiers) of transcription factors (28). For example, SUMOlation may target transcription factors to inactive regions of the nucleus called "PML bodies," so named after localization of the promyelocytic leukemia protein to these poorly understood nuclear structures. The PML bodies have been proposed to serve a role as the storage site or reserve for transcription factors (52). Other covalent modifications of transcriptional machinery include methylation and acetylation. Some of these examples may have been caused by the activation of specific signal transduction pathways. Thus, there are many levels at which botanical compounds may be interacting with the process of transcription. The focus of this review is to provide a small set of examples of how botanical compounds may affect biological function by affecting the process of gene regulation. Our attempt here is to provide readers with a limited set of examples, and to focus on newer, less-reviewed topics rather than on more-documented or frequently summarized research areas.

BOTANICALS AND NUCLEAR RECEPTOR REGULATION

At present, the most information available regarding the specific regulation of gene transcription by botanical compounds may be as ligands or regulators of nuclear receptors. Among the best described examples are those of PXR activation by hyperforin, an active ingredient of the herbal St. John's wort (SJW), and the regulation of cholesterol and bile acid metabolism by the Ayurvedic medication, guggulsterone. As the latter was the exclusive focus of two recent reviews (53, 54), including one in this journal, we follow below with a discussion of hyperforin as a botanical product with activity as a nuclear receptor ligand.

The Pregnane X Receptor and Hyperforin

The herbal remedy SJW has long been touted as a natural antidepressant. As an herbal product, the extensive clinical testing associated with the drug development process was not required. Recently, clinical reports suggested that use of SJW was accelerating the metabolism of prescription drugs used concomitantly, such as the antiviral protease inhibitor indinavir (41), used in the treatment of AIDS; the immunosuppressant cyclosporine, administered to organ transplant recipients (48); and oral contraceptives (2). Because these drugs are metabolized by hepatic cytochrome P450-3A4 (CYP3A4), Kliewer and colleagues (22, 32) set out to determine if hyperforin, the active ingredient in SJW suggested to have the antidepressant activity, could in fact be an activator of CYP3A4, a monooxygenase that hydroxylates many xenobiotics, a committing step in the oxidation and elimination of hydrophobic compounds. Estimates suggest that 60% or more of prescription drugs are metabolized and excreted by a CYP3A4-dependent pathway. A chloramphenicol reporter-based assay was performed in CV-1 cells to compare the ability of three different commercial SJW products with purified hyperforin and other compounds isolated from SJW. Testing also included the specific pregnane X receptor (PXR) ligand, SR12813, and a hallmark inducer of CYP3A4, the antibiotic rifampicin. The cell-based reporter assay demonstrated that extracts prepared from SJW products, SR12813, rifampicin, and hyperforin isolated from SJW were all potent inducers of the PXR-regulated murine CYP3A1-tk-CAT reporter. When used to compare activation of the 3A1 promoter in a dose-response study, hyperforin was found to be ~100-fold more potent than rifampicin. Rifampicin has been a well-studied inducer of CYP3A4 because of interactions known to be associated with antibiotic and other drug therapies. Kliewer and colleagues (22, 32) then demonstrated that hyperforin and SR12813 were nearly identical in their ability to act as a specific ligand for the PXR ligand-binding domain, as verified in a competition binding assay. A K_i for hyperforin was measured at 27 nM. Further proof was provided by demonstrating increased levels of the CYP3A4 mRNA in human hepatocytes treated with extracts from commercially available SJW products along with both rifampicin and hyperforin. These data demonstrate the caution that must be exercised when using nonprescription botanical products. The combination of reporter-based assays, a direct assay of receptor binding, and the subsequent analysis of gene expression in human cells provided a clear picture of PXR activation along with a model for assessment of other botanicals suspected of PXR activation. Following these studies from Moore et al. (32), Watkins et al. (55) demonstrated that hyperforin could indeed bind to the ligand-binding domain of human PXR and was able to crystallize a PXR-hyperforin complex, the structure of which was determined at 2.1 Å resolution. Other groups (59) have confirmed results shown by Moore et al. (32) and Watkins et al. (55).

Peroxisome Proliferator-Activated Receptors, Soy Isoflavones, and Resveratrol

Soy intake has long been recognized to favorably affect circulating cholesterol levels, especially in hypercholesterolemic individuals (1). Various components of soy have been investigated in an attempt to determine if one or more components might be hypocholesterolemic, including soy protein, soy lipids, the presence of bioactive peptides (or their production during the digestive process), and phytochemicals that include soy sterols, saponins, and isoflavones. Among the community of nutrition researchers, the mechanism responsible for improvements in lipid profiles due to soy intake is still debated. Our own working hypothesis is that there is likely more than one bioactive component in soy, and that the soy isoflavones have a bioactivity that affects lipid metabolism. A recent meta-analysis points to isoflavone intake as a factor related to improvements in blood lipids (62), although other analyses have not confirmed this relationship (58). Isoflavones are particularly abundant in soy and in clover. In soy, the predominant isoflavones are genistein, daidzein, and glycitein. Metabolic conversion of daidzein into another isoflavone, equol, may be of particular importance because equol may have an unusually high bioactivity (50). The isoflavones were one of the first confirmed examples of an ingredient in a food source being an endocrine disruptor. Early studies identifying isoflavones as bioactive agents determined that clover isoflavones were agonists of estrogenic activity, interrupting the estrus cycle of sheep feeding exclusively on isoflavone-containing red clover (37). Starting with these early findings, a significant amount of research has been directed toward understanding soy isoflavones as phytoestrogens, especially in the context of bone metabolism, cancer, and reproductive function. Because there is a large body of research investigating the estrogenic action of isoflavones, we chose not to discuss them here, but we refer the reader to several reviews that provide a starting point for information on the important topic of isoflavones as phytoestrogens (3, 7, 49).

Although the evidence had become clear that soy isoflavones acted as phytoestrogens, the prospect of isoflavones acting as ligands or activators of other nuclear receptors had not been investigated until recently. Potential candidates would include receptors involved in lipid metabolism that display promiscuous ligand-binding capability. Such candidates would be the PPARs, the LXR, and the FXR. Mangelsdorf and colleagues (43) demonstrated how receptor ligands for the PPARs (fibrates or glitazones), LXR (oxysterols), or FXR (bile acids) could activate gene transcription and alter liver lipid levels, bile acid synthesis, net cholesterol absorption, and lipoprotein metabolism. Known effects of soy intake on blood lipids and lipid metabolism resembled some of the actions caused by activation of these lipid-regulating nuclear receptors. At a qualitative level, it appears that the space-filling chemical structure of isoflavones is similar to that of the fibrates, agonists of PPARα used to treat hyperlipidemia and type 2 diabetes (8). Thus, in our own laboratories, we formulated the hypothesis that one effect of soy intake on lipid metabolism may be due to isoflavones acting as activators of PPARs. We began a variety of studies utilizing PPARα and PPARγ expression vectors in a murine macrophage model and completed metabolic studies in the obese Zucker rat (29). Further, we used a panel of chimeric nuclear receptors in HepG2 cells to screen isoflavones and other soy components to determine which compounds might indeed be serving as ligands of nuclear receptors (45).

Two studies published in 2003 indicated that isoflavones are activating PPAR-directed gene transcription. Focusing on effects related to osteogenesis and the effects of the soy isoflavone genistein as an activator of the estrogen receptor and PPARs, Dang et al. (6) studied the effects of genistein on osteogenesis in KS483 and mouse bone marrow cells. Genistein was found to have a biphasic activity on markers of osteogenesis, peaking at a concentration of $\sim$1 μM in a cell culture trial. However, when following markers for adipogenesis, the dose-dependent effects of genistein were quite different, as the $\sim$1 μM concentration of genistein that produced a maximal effect on osteogenic parameters was found to produce a negligible stimulation of adipogenesis. At higher concentrations of genistein, adipogenesis was promoted. When tested in combination with antiestrogen ICI 164,382, the osteogenic activity of genistein at ~1 μM was reduced, whereas the adipogenic activity of genistein at the higher dose was not blocked by the antiestrogen. Dang and colleagues (6) hypothesized that the adipogenic activity of genistein was caused by activation of PPARγ in the adipocyte. They subsequently performed a PPAR-directed luciferase test and a direct-competition binding assay using genistein as a competitor of radiolabeled rosiglitazone. Genistein dose-dependently stimulated PPAR-directed gene expression in the micromolar range, and binding tests indicated that genistein bound to the PPARγ receptor and measured a K_i for genistein of 5.7 μM. This important study was to our knowledge the first demonstration of genistein as a ligand for a PPAR receptor. Furthermore, the data from this report indicate that the bioactivity of genistein is likely mediated at least in part by activation of more than one nuclear receptor. At a given circulating concentration of genistein, the effect may be different from tissue to tissue depending on the relative expression of nuclear receptors within each tissue. The in vitro results of Dang et al. (6) predict an osteogenic effect of genistein at low concentrations resembling the effects of estrogen; while higher concentrations of genistein may more resemble the action of the antidiabetic medications, the glitazones. Glitazones are ligands for PPARγ and improve insulin sensitivity; however, they also stimulate adipogenesis (26).

Another study combining in vivo and in vitro trials demonstrated effects of an isoflavone-containing soy extract and the individual soy isoflavones genistein and daidzein as activators of both PPARα and PPARγ (29). Male and female obese Zucker rats (OZRs) were fed diets with either casein or soy as the source of protein. Two different soy diets were used, with low or high content of isoflavones. Both male and female OZRs treated with high-isoflavone soy protein had reduced liver weight compared with the other diet groups. This reduced liver weight may have been due to reduced hepatic cholesterol and triglyceride content. Compared with casein-fed OZRs, male and female rats fed high-isoflavone soy had reduced levels of plasma cholesterol. Plasma triglycerides were not affected by diet treatment except for an unexplained rise in plasma triglyceride levels in female rats fed the high-isoflavone soy diet. The reduction in hepatic weight and lipid content is consistent with the effect of fibrates, agonists of the PPARα receptor (25). In vivo studies also determined that the consumption of only the high-isoflavone diet improved glucose tolerance in female OZRs. In contrast to lipid weight and blood lipid changes resembling the action of PPARα, the latter findings are consistent with the effect of glitazones on PPARγ. In vitro studies utilizing RAW264.7 cells determined that treatment with a mixture of unconjugated soy isoflavones (isoflavones without any covalently attached carbohydrate) and the isoflavones genistein and daidzein positively influenced both PPARα- and PPARγ-directed gene expression. A third soy isoflavone, glycitein, did not share the same potent effect exhibited by the other two isoflavones. Taken together, the work of Dang et al. (6) and Mezei et al. (29) provide strong evidence that soy isoflavones have action as PPAR activators.

Other studies provide supporting evidence for a relationship between isoflavones and PPARs. Iqbal et al. (17) performed a genetic screen examining gene expression patterns in the liver of female OZRs that were provided diets that contained casein, low-isoflavone soy, or high-isoflavone soy as the source of protein. Interestingly, one of the hepatic mRNAs confirmed to be induced in rats fed a soy-containing diet was carnitine palmitoyl transferase-I (CPT-I). CPT-I is a hepatic gene involved in the transfer of fatty acids into the mitochondria, promoting β-oxidation, and is known to be strongly induced by PPARα (16). Another genetic screen identified a set of hepatic mRNAs regulated by the presence of high levels of dietary isoflavones provided to gerbils (30). Two mRNAs, encoding transferrin and phosphoenolpyruvate carboxykinase, were found in this screen to be down-regulated after consumption of high-isoflavone-containing soy. These two genes have been shown previously to be down-regulated by PPAR agonists (13, 56).

More recent confirmatory results were published by Kim et al. (21). A set of PPAR-regulated genes involved in the β-oxidation pathway were studied by real-time PCR after exposing HepG2 cells to 10 μM genistein for up to 48 hours. For the first 24 hours of treatment, relative mRNA levels for acyl CoA synthase, CPT-I, medium-chain acyl-CoA dehydrogenase, hydroxymethylglutaryl-CoA synthase, acyl CoA oxidase (isoforms 1 and 2), and enoyl-CoA hydratase were all found to be induced in HepG2 cells exposed to 10 μM genistein using a real-time PCR method. Protein levels for CPT-I were also measured by immunoblotting and found to be similarly elevated by the genistein treatment. Kim and colleagues then treated HepG2 cells simultaneously with genistein and the estrogen receptor inhibitor ICI182780. The concurrent treatment of HepG2 cells with genistein and antiestrogen on CPT-I induction resembled the effect of genistein alone, and they concluded that induction of CPT-I is mediated by PPARs and is independent of estrogen action. PPARα receptor levels were also induced during exposure to genistein. It is not clear at present whether increases in PPAR-directed gene expression are occurring mainly due to genistein serving as a PPAR agonist or by enhancing PPAR responsiveness due to increased receptor number. In HepG2- and CV-1-based transfection assays, genistein was able to induce PPARα-directed luciferase expression when cells were exposed to concentrations of genistein as low as 0.1 μM.

Additional support indicating actions of isoflavones on PPARs comes from a very recent report (45) utilizing chimeric transcription factors containing nuclear receptor ligand-binding domains and Gal4 DNA-binding domains. These chimeras were transfected into HepG2 cells along with a Gal4-directed luciferase reporter. After exposure of HepG2 cells to various treatments for 24 hours, cell lysates were collected and luciferase expression measured as an indicator of transactivation. These studies confirmed many previous reports demonstrating activity of isoflavones as activators of estrogen receptors (ERs). A mixture of unconjugated isoflavones, genistein alone, and daidzein alone were all able to induce estrogen receptor-dependent gene expression. However, when tested simultaneously in the presence of 1 μM estradiol, the presence of isoflavones did not stimulate estrogen-dependent gene expression to any greater degree. This was thought to be a result of the much higher affinity of estradiol for its receptor compared with the ability of isoflavones to bind to ERs. Aside from studies using the ERα-Gal4 chimeric receptor, a panel of nine other chimeric receptors was tested to determine which receptors might be activated by isoflavones. Exposure to isoflavones produced significant induction when chimeras based on the PPARα, PPARγ, PXR, and TRβ were used in conjunction with a Gal4-luciferase reporter. The individual isoflavones genistein and daidzein appeared to significantly induce these receptors as did a mixture of unconjugated isoflavones. A mixture of conjugated isoflavones was generally a less potent inducer, especially for PPARγ. Other receptors that were unresponsive to isoflavones or marginally responsive were vitamin D, glucocorticoid, liver X, and farnesoid X. Soy saponin, a nonisoflavone soy compound, was generally not able to transactivate any nuclear receptor-Gal4 chimera. Paralleling the first study from Ricketts et al. (45), further tests were conducted to evaluate the ability of isoflavones to transactivate chimeric receptors in the presence of known agonists for each receptor. For the case of ERα mentioned above, no synergy of action was noted when cells were concurrently exposed to estradiol and an isoflavone. However, when cells transfected with PPARα-, PPARγ-, or TRβ-Gal4 chimeras were concurrently exposed to an isoflavone and the specific receptor agonist, there appeared to be enhanced luciferase expression compared with that observed in cells treated with agonist or isoflavone alone. This synergy was hypothesized to be caused by one of at least two different mechanisms. First, it may be that the specific receptor agonist and isoflavone form a duplex of sorts in the ligand-binding domain of the receptor. It has been determined previously that for at least one PPARγ ligand, two agonist molecules bind simultaneously in the ligand-binding pocket (47). An alternative to this explanation would be that isoflavones are acting through a second, nonligand-dependent mechanism, e.g., by altering the phosphorylation state of coactivators or corepressors, or by enhancing the effective half-life of nuclear receptors in the nucleus caused by a reduction in proteasome activity. Other evidence has demonstrated that the presence of isoflavones with clofibrate have a synergistic effect on PPARα-directed luciferase expression (31). Taken together, the data from several different research groups appear to point to an in vitro activity of isoflavones on PPAR-directed gene expression. Some of the trials demonstrating positive effects on PPAR-directed gene expression in cell culture systems used concentrations of isoflavones entirely consistent with blood levels reported in clinical studies. In vivo results described above demonstrate changes in lipid metabolism and glucose tolerance resembling the effects of fibrate and/or glitazone therapy. Taken together, it appears that soy isoflavones do have an in vivo activity on PPAR receptors.

A recent study completed to evaluate the effect of resveratrol as a PPAR activator suggests a rethinking of the bioactive role assigned to resveratrol. Resveratrol, the polyphenol abundant in grape skins and consumed in grape juice and wine, among other products, has been thought to be a bioactive compound largely by virtue of its antioxidant and anti-inflammatory activities. Resveratrol has protective effects on the cardiovascular system including inhibition of platelet aggregation, it promotes vasodilation, and it reduces atherosclerosis. Many consider resveratrol the active ingredient associated with the cardioprotective effect of red wine consumption (9, 38). Although a wide-ranging number of studies of resveratrol have characterized the effects of this compound on cell proliferation, protection against oxidative damage, and several different cell signaling pathways, to our knowledge, the work of Inoue et al. (18) was the first to examine the potential of resveratrol to act as a PPAR agonist. Using a chimeric reporter system similar to that used by Ricketts et al. (45), resveratrol was found to selectively transactivate PPARα- and PPARγ-Gal4 chimeras by 15- to 30-fold above control levels compared with 15 other nuclear receptor chimeras in which no appreciable degree of transactivation was noted. This increase was evaluated at 10, 50, and 100 μM and found to be dose-dependent at those concentrations. These effects were observed in the CV-1 cell line and in a number of blood vessel endothelial cells. In testing in vivo, treatment with resveratrol and PPARα agonists reduced brain infarct volume in a mouse model for stroke. This attenuation was not observed when the same treatments were given to PPARα-knockout mice, which suggests that the protective effect of resveratrol may specifically involve PPARα. As we gain a greater appreciation of the interaction between cellular regulatory mechanisms and botanical compounds or food ingredients, a few principles are becoming clear. First, as with resveratrol, it is possible that one ingested dietary compound may interact with a number of systems such as PPAR regulation, antioxidative protection, and effects on cell signaling processes. Second, the promiscuous nature of nuclear receptors allows for the interaction of many different ingested compounds with the detoxification and lipid-regulating systems of the body. A diet high in phytochemical content may be providing a total input to a variety of promiscuous nuclear receptors that cannot be estimated by following only one food or botanical.

UBIQUITINATION, THE PROTEASOME, AND EPIGALLOCATECHIN GALLATE

A somewhat recent interest in the study of gene regulation is the interaction of the proteolytic activity of proteasomes with the process of transcription. Proteasomal action may modify the half-life and environment of transcription factors and coactivators. Proteasomes are described as "chambered proteases" that consist of an array of polypeptide subunits with a variety of enzymatic activities arranged in a barrel-shaped or cylindrical configuration. A capped or gated pore allows access to the interior of the proteasome, in which proteolysis occurs. The eukaryotic 26S proteasome is among the best characterized. Within the interior of the proteasome, substrate degradation occurs in a processive manner and substrate unfolding must occur prior to proteolysis. Associated with proteasomes are chaperone complexes that regulate access to the proteasome after an appropriate substrate (e.g., an unfolded protein) is recognized. Recognition and proteolysis are two separate events at the proteosome. The 26S proteasome typically recognizes substrates that have been tagged with a polymer assembled from ubiquitin subunits. It is recognized that there is a wide variety of enzymes that regulate the process of polyubiquitin tagging. Some of the events involved in ATP-requiring proteosome-mediated proteolysis include recognition of polypeptide substrates, unfolding of the polypeptide, and control of polypeptide entry into the protease-containing chamber. Another regulatory activity of the proteasome is removal of polypeptide-bound polyubiquitin chains. After deubiquitination, ubiquitin is released intact and may participate in further cycles of ubiquitination and targeting of polypeptides to proteasomes. Polyubiquitin removal has been shown to be tightly linked to subsequent events at the proteasome to ensure that proteolysis of the tagged substrates will occur. A recent review of the proteasome and its regulation provides additional detail (40).

What roles then does the proteasome serve in cells and how might proteasome activity be regulated by dietary components to affect gene expression? Proteasomal activity contributes to the amino acid pool to allow normal protein synthesis rates. Enzyme activity may be regulated by degradation. Importantly, proteasomal activity may be a most important mechanism for the removal of transcription factors that are no longer needed. Proteasomes are involved in the degradation of cyclins, and thus are critically involved in cell cycle regulation. The proteasome is a site for turnover of foreign proteins encoded by viruses or other invasive pathogens and is also the site of turnover of proteins that are folded incorrectly because of translation errors or mutations. A notable example of a direct disease link to proteasomal activity is in cystic fibrosis. Many cases of cystic fibrosis are thought to be caused by the accelerated degradation of a mutant version of the cystic fibrosis transmembrane conductance regulator chloride transporter. An example of proteasomal regulation of transcription factors has been studied for PPARγ (12). In 3T3-F442A cells, PPARγ levels were shown to be dependent on the specific PPAR ligand and also the concentration of the ligand. Unexpectedly, along with greater transcriptional activation by PPARγ at higher agonist concentrations, it was determined that the overall amount of the receptor was decreased. This reduction in the level of the receptor was determined to be post-translational in nature and mediated by the AF-2 region of PPARγ. Inhibitors of proteasome activity blocked the ligand-dependent decrease in receptor levels. Finally, it was determined that ubiquitination of PPARγ was enhanced by the presence of ligand.

Several studies have begun to associate a biological activity of the polyphenols present in green tea, such as epigallocatechin-3-gallate (EGCG) to inhibition of proteasome activity. Nam et al. (36) found that EGCG, at concentrations typically observed in the serum of green tea drinkers, inhibited proteasome activity and caused growth arrest in the G1 phase of cell cycle in several tumor cell and transformed cell lines. In vitro analyses of proteolytic activity of the purified 20S portion of the proteasome were measured at various concentrations of EGCG and other similar compounds. EGCG was found to inhibit the chymotrypsin-like activity of the 20S subunit at a concentration of ~100 nM. Other in vitro assays confirmed this inhibitory effect of EGCG on proteolytic action. Proteasomal activity was also reduced by EGCG in intact Jurkat cells. During treatment with EGCG, the accumulation of proteasomal target proteins p27, IκB-α, and other ubiquitinated proteins was observed. These decreases in proteasomal activity and increases in substrate were found to be independent of protein synthesis. Further, EGCG treatment caused Jurkat T and LNCaP cancer cells to enter growth arrest while in the G1 phase of the cell cycle. SV-40-transformed fibroblasts were more susceptible to EGCG compared with normal fibroblasts, as determined by relative entry into growth arrest during treatment. Subsequently, this same research group evaluated chemical modifications of ECGC and determined that enantiomeric analogs of EGCG were potent proteasome inhibitors, whereas modification of the hydroxyl groups of EGCG obliterated proteasomal inhibition (51). Most recently, it was found that EGCG acts to facilitate covalent modification of an amino-terminal threonine on the chymotrypsin-like β5 subunit of the proteasome.

In addition to playing a role in cell cycle regulation that may reduce the risk of certain cancers, consumption of EGCG-containing teas has also been shown to lessen the risk of atherosclerosis and to improve blood lipid levels (33). It may turn out that these clinically observed improvements are due to an effect of EGCG on the proteasome. However, rather than modifying targets of the cell cycle, in this case the target of proteasomal regulation may be sterol regulatory element–binding proteins (SREBPs) (14, 42). The SREBPs were discovered to be the pivotal regulatory proteins that allow cells to regulate intracellular cholesterol concentrations. Although not members of the nuclear receptor family, SREBPs are membrane-bound and normally localized to the endoplasmic reticulum. However, during times of low intracellular cholesterol concentrations, SREBPs are escorted to the golgi and are subsequently cleaved by a two-step process involving two separate golgi-specific proteases. These proteolytic events release a ~68 kDa N-terminal portion of the protein from the golgi. This processed protein has the bHLH structure characteristic of many transcription factors, and after cleavage, these "mature" SREBPs migrate to the nucleus, where they regulate a set of 30 or more genes involved in lipid and carbohydrate metabolism. Two SREBP genes encode three different isoforms; the isoform most directly related to cholesterol regulation is SREBP-2. Genes regulated by SREBP-2 include the LDL receptor and genes encoding enzymes of the cholesterol biosynthetic pathway, such as HMG-CoA reductase. Thus, activation or maturation of SREBP-2 leads to enhanced transcription and synthesis of receptors that will enhance uptake of cholesterol-containing lipoproteins; concurrently, intracellular cholesterol synthesis will be enhanced by increased levels of the biosynthetic enzymes.

Recently, Dou and colleagues (23) tested the hypothesis that EGCG affects lipid metabolism by controlling SREBP-regulated gene expression through inhibition of the proteasome. HepG2 cells were treated with 30 μM ECGC for 24 hours and cell protein was isolated at intervals during the treatment. Immunoblotting demonstrated that ubiquitination of protein was transient, with a maximal amount of ubiquitination observed 2 hours after first exposure to EGCG. Levels of the known target proteins of the proteasome, p27 and IκB-α, were elevated after 2 hours of exposure to EGCG and stayed at these elevated levels for the remainder of the 24-hour treatment period. The levels of 68 kDa mature SREBP-2 (mSREBP-2) increased up to sevenfold 8 hours after the onset of exposure to EGCG and remained at this elevated level of expression throughout the rest of the 24-hour treatment period. Along with other proteasomal markers proteins, SREBP-2 levels were increased dose-dependently after 10 hours of exposure to 0, 1, and 10 μM EGCG. A target of mSREBP-2 regulation, the LDL receptor, was similarly up-regulated by EGCG. As described above, the ester bond in EGCG and related compounds was shown to be a requisite for ubiquitination and accumulation of proteasomal target proteins. Expression of mSREBP-2 and the LDL-receptor followed this pattern exactly. Regulation of proteasomal activity and protein levels were then evaluated in HeLa cells, and expression patterns paralleled those observed in HepG2 cells. In HeLa cells, the inhibitory effect of EGCG was determined to be on the chymotrypsin-like rather than trypsin-like activity of the proteasome. Immunostaining of both HepG2 and HeLa cells provided visual confirmation of immunoblotting experiments: LDL-receptor levels are increased in cells treated with EGCG or inhibitors of the proteasome such as LLnL.

Interestingly, Dou and colleagues have asked if the reported antiproliferative effects of isoflavones may be mediated through proteasomal inhibition (20). Computational modeling of the 20S proteasome predicts that genistein could bind to the chymotrypsin-like site of the 20S proteasome. Unlike prior studies indicating a possible covalent modification of the proteasome by EGCG (describe above), modeling of genistein to the proteasome predicts a steric block of Thr1. Energy calculations indicating a less stable genistein-proteasome interaction compared with EGCG-proteasome binding led to the prediction of weaker proteasome inhibition by genistein compared with EGCG. In vitro testing determined that genistein could inhibit activity of the 20S proteasome with an IC_{50} of 26 μM. Inhibition of proteasomal chymotrypsin-like activity was also observed in cell extracts derived from LNCaP and MCF-7 solid tumor cells, with genistein being a more potent inhibitor than daidzein. Genistein was able to induce levels of ubiquitinated proteins and levels of proteasome target proteins at concentrations of genistein ranging from 50 to 200 μM. Protein markers of apoptosis and flow cytometry studies indicated induction of apoptosis by genistein at 50 to 100 μM. Following the previously discussed study (23), one might ask whether lipid-regulating proteins such as SREBP-2 would be affected if genistein was indeed inhibiting the activity of the proteasome. Recently, SREBP-2 levels were evaluated in HepG2 cells (34), and genistein treatment was observed to up-regulate mSREBP-2 and HMG-CoA reductase levels, although at lower doses than those tested by Kazi et al. (20). It remains to be seen if isoflavone up-regulation of mSREBP-2 levels is occurring via proteasomal inhibition, a second mechanism, or some combination of multiple mechanisms.

SIRTUINS: DEACETYLASES AND CONTROLLERS OF TRANSCRIPTION COFACTORS

A short set of reports from just the past few years illustrates another pathway by which dietary compounds may interact with the process of gene transcription. As an introduction to this topic, we describe some of the findings of Sinclair and colleagues (5, 15), who investigated the connection between caloric restriction and increases in longevity. In vivo studies have shown that caloric restriction is the only dietary treatment that has produced the most consistently even lifespan-increasing results across species. Studies have documented the increase in lifespan due to caloric restriction in both yeast and *Caenorhabditis elegans*, mediated by extra copies of genes of specific deacetylases called sirtuins or by small-molecule agonists of the sirtuins. A set of plant polyphenols were identified that had a significant stimulatory effect on SIRT1 catalytic rate, mediated by increases in K_m rather than V_{max} for the enzyme. The sirtuin-activating compounds (STACs) resveratrol, butein, piceatannol, quercetin, and others were shown to have a stimulatory effect on SIRT1 ranging from ~5- to ~13-fold. When tested using *Saccharomyces cerevisiae*, resveratrol at 2–5 μM activated the yeast sirtuin Sir2 by approximately twofold, and butein, fisetin, and resveratrol increased lifespan by 31%, 55%, and 70%, respectively. The ability of Sir2 to extend lifespan in yeast is thought to be due to a role in the stabilization of repetitive DNA sequences. Assays quantifying extrachromosomal DNA indicated resveratrol was able to reduce levels of these potentially toxic molecules. A further assay evaluated the effect of STACs on human sirtuin SIRT1. The molecules tested included those from the stilbene, chalcone, flavone, isoflavone, flavanone, and anthocyanidin families. Among all compounds, the stilbenes resveratrol, butein, and piceatannol, and the flavones fisetin, luteolin, and quercetin were among the best activators of human SIRT1 when tested at 100 μM. In parallel with this in vitro testing was an in vivo test evaluating cell survival in response to ionizing radiation. Even in doses as low as 250–500 nM, the presence of resveratrol was found to be protective and dependent on active SIRT1. A subsequent study confirmed the effect of STACs in *C. elegans* and *Drosophila melanogaster* (61).

The ability of resveratrol to interact with sirtuins was followed up with a second report (15). Cohen et al. (5) demonstrated the increase in sirtuin SIRT1 levels in tissues from calorically restricted rats. When FaO cells were treated with serum obtained from ad libitum–fed or food-restricted rats, SIRT1 levels were increased in the cells exposed to serum derived from the food-restricted rats. This serum also was observed to decrease apoptosis in 293T cells. Addition of insulin and/or IGF-1 to the serum obtained from calorically restricted rats eliminated the ability of the serum to decrease apoptosis. These 293T cells, when treated with resveratrol or transfected with a SIRT1 expression vector, demonstrated suppression of Bax-mediated apoptosis within 24 hours; this decrease in apoptosis corresponds to a presumably longer lifespan for cells. Transfection of a dominant-negative form of SIRT1 increased susceptibility of cells to apoptosis. Speculation regarding common responses in plant and animal stress situations include the suggestion that molecules indicating stress conditions within the plant may be utilized by fungal or animal cells as a signal of deteriorating environment and/or food supply. Further study of STACs, which are perhaps serving to enhance deacetylation of nuclear proteins and in turn help compact or condense regions of chromosomes, should prove to be a fascinating course of study and provide additional information on the ability of plant compounds to regulate mammalian processes. Other recent data provides support for a role for mammalian Sirt1 protein in helping mediate a response to caloric restriction in adipocytes by binding to PPARγ cofactors NCoR and SMRT. This association between Sirt1 and these cofactors serves to repress PPARγ activity. This response is attenuated in Sirt1 knockout mice (39). This

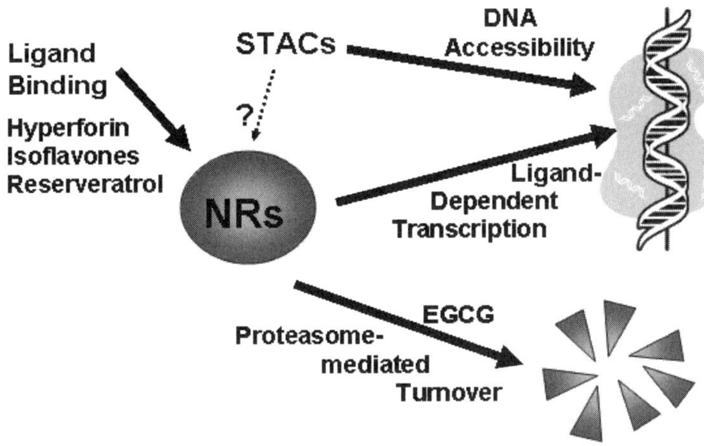

Figure 1 Selected actions of botanical compounds on gene transcription. Botanical compounds may affect gene expression by more than one mechanism. In the case of hyperforin and probably other compounds, including isoflavones and resveratrol, these molecules are likely acting directly on nuclear receptors as ligands, thus promoting transcription of genes with specific promoter elements. In the case of hyperforin, activated pregnane X receptor/retinoic acid X receptor heterodimers bound to such target sequences enhance transcription rates. A second mechanism may be via the inhibition of proteasome-mediated turnover of nuclear receptors (NRs) or other transcription factors. In the presence of a hypothesized inhibitor such as epigallocatechin-3-gallate (EGCG), turnover of regulatory proteins may be reduced. This in turn will produce a greater effect on transcription by the given factors "spared" from the proteasome. Finally, sirtuin-activating compounds (STACs) may be regulated by plant polyphenols, including resveratrol. Regulation of sirtuins or other related enzymes may limit accessibility of transcriptional machinery to DNA. Some limited evidence suggests STACs may also be regulating cofactor interactions with nuclear receptors, indicated here as a question mark.

finding may help explain the recent discovery that longevity in mice is controlled within adipose tissue (4).

SUMMARY

In this review, we have outlined three general mechanisms by which botanical products have been shown to regulate cell function by altering gene expression. These include activation of nuclear receptors, inhibition of the proteasome, and activation of sirtuins. These processes act directly on the process of gene transcription by controlling or influencing the processes of nuclear receptor activation, by controlling the half-life of transcription factors, and by regulating accessibility of condensed DNA or stabilization of coactivators. An overview of these mechanisms is presented in Figure 1. Just five to ten years ago, the prospect of recognizing the influence of botanicals on these processes would have been difficult to imagine. Although it is unclear if the immediate future will provide us with additional new mechanisms of control determined to be affected by botanicals, it is certain that these newly appreciated mechanisms will be investigated further to clarify the specific effects of botanicals on gene expression.

The *Annual Review of Nutrition* is online at http://nutr.annualreviews.org

LITERATURE CITED

1. Anderson JW, Johnstone BM, Cook-Newell ME. 1995. Meta-analysis of the effects of soy protein intake on serum lipids. *N. Engl. J. Med.* 333(5):276–82
2. Barnes J, Anderson LA, Phillipson JD. 2001. St John's wort (*Hypericum perforatum* L.): a review of its chemistry, pharmacology and clinical properties. *J. Pharm. Pharmacol.* 53(5):583–600
3. Barnes S. 2004. Soy isoflavones—phytoestrogens and what else? *J. Nutr.* 134(5):1225–28S
4. Bluher M, Kahn BB, Kahn CR. 2003. Extended longevity in mice lacking the insulin receptor in adipose tissue. *Science* 299(5606):572–74
5. Cohen HY, Miller C, Bitterman KJ, Wall NR, Hekking B, et al. 2004. Calorie restriction promotes mammalian cell survival by inducing the SIRT1 deacetylase. *Science* 305(5682):390–92
6. Dang ZC, Audinot V, Papapoulos SE, Boutin JA, Lowik CW. 2003. Peroxisome proliferator-activated receptor gamma (PPARgamma) as a molecular target for the soy phytoestrogen genistein. *J. Biol. Chem.* 278(2):962–67
7. Duncan AM, Phipps WR, Kurzer MS. 2003. Phyto-oestrogens. *Best Pract. Res. Clin. Endocrinol. Metab.* 17(2):253–71
8. Elisaf M. 2002. Effects of fibrates on serum metabolic parameters. *Curr. Med. Res. Opin.* 18(5):269–76
9. Fremont L. 2000. Biological effects of resveratrol. *Life Sci.* 66(8):663–73
10. Gebauer F, Hentze MW. 2004. Molecular mechanisms of translational control. *Nat. Rev. Mol. Cell Biol.* 5(10):827–35
11. Hamer DH, Walling M. 1982. Regulation in vivo of a cloned mammalian gene: Cadmium induces the transcription of a mouse metallothionein gene in SV40 vectors. *J. Mol. Appl. Genet.* 1(4):273–88

12. Hauser S, Adelmant G, Sarraf P, Wright HM, Mueller E, Spiegelman BM. 2000. Degradation of the peroxisome proliferator-activated receptor gamma is linked to ligand-dependent activation. *J. Biol. Chem.* 275:18527–33
13. Hertz R, Seckbach M, Zakin MM, Bar-Tana J. 1996. Transcriptional suppression of the transferrin gene by hypolipidemic peroxisome proliferators. *J. Biol. Chem.* 271(1):218–24
14. Horton JD. 2002. Sterol regulatory element-binding proteins: transcriptional activators of lipid synthesis. *Biochem. Soc. Trans.* 30(Pt. 6):1091–95
15. Howitz KT, Bitterman KJ, Cohen HY, Lamming DW, Lavu S, et al. 2003. Small molecule activators of sirtuins extend *Saccharomyces cerevisiae* lifespan. *Nature* 425(6954):191–96
16. Hsu MH, Savas U, Griffin KJ, Johnson EF. 2001. Identification of peroxisome proliferator-responsive human genes by elevated expression of the peroxisome proliferator-activated receptor alpha in HepG2 cells. *J. Biol. Chem.* 276(30): 27950–58
17. Iqbal MJ, Yaegashi S, Ahsan R, Lightfoot DA, Banz WJ. 2002. Differentially abundant mRNAs in rat liver in response to diets containing soy protein isolate. *Physiol. Genomics* 11(3):219–26
18. Inoue H, Jiang XF, Katayama T, Osada S, Umesono K, Namura S. 2003. Brain protection by resveratrol and fenofibrate against stroke requires peroxisome proliferator-activated receptor alpha in mice. *Neurosci. Lett.* 352:203–6
19. Karin M, Andersen RD, Slater E, Smith K, Herschman HR. 1980. Metallothionein mRNA induction in HeLa cells in response to zinc or dexamethasone is a primary induction response. *Nature* 286(5770):295–97
20. Kazi A, Daniel KG, Smith DM, Kumar NB, Dou QP. 2003. Inhibition of the proteasome activity, a novel mechanism associated with the tumor cell apoptosis-inducing ability of genistein. *Biochem. Pharmacol.* 66(6):965–76
21. Kim S, Shin HJ, Kim SY, Kim JH, Lee YS, et al. 2004. Genistein enhances expression of genes involved in fatty acid catabolism through activation of PPAR-alpha. *Mol. Cell. Endocrinol.* 220(1–2):51–58
22. Kliewer SA. 2003. The nuclear pregnane X receptor regulates xenobiotic detoxification. *J. Nutr.* 133(7 Suppl.):2444–47S
23. Kuhn DJ, Burns AC, Kazi A, Dou QP. 2004. Direct inhibition of the ubiquitin-proteasome pathway by ester bond-containing green tea polyphenols is associated with increased expression of sterol regulatory element-binding protein 2 and LDL receptor. *Biochim. Biophys. Acta* 1682(1–3):1–10
24. Lazar MA. 2003. Thyroid hormone action: a binding contract. *J. Clin. Invest.* 112(4):497–99
25. Lee SS, Pineau T, Drago J, Lee EJ, Owens JW, et al. 1995. Targeted disruption of the alpha isoform of the peroxisome proliferator-activated receptor gene in mice results in abolishment of the pleiotropic effects of peroxisome proliferators. *Mol. Cell. Biol.* 15(6):3012–22
26. Lehmann JM, Moore LB, Smith-Oliver TA, Wilkison WO, Willson TM, et al. 1995. An antidiabetic thiazolidinedione is a high affinity ligand for peroxisome proliferator-activated receptor gamma (PPAR gamma). *J. Biol. Chem.* 270(22):12953–56
27. Lodish H, Berk A, Matsudaira P, Kaiser CA, Scott MP, et al. 2003. *Molecular Cell Biology*. New York: Freeman. 5th ed.
28. Melchior F. 2000. SUMO—nonclassical ubiquitin. *Annu. Rev. Cell Dev. Biol.* 16: 591–626
29. Mezei O, Banz WJ, Steger RW, Peluso MR, Winters TA, et al. 2003. Soy isoflavones exert antidiabetic and hypolipidemic effects through the PPAR pathways in obese Zucker rats and murine RAW 264.7 cells. *J. Nutr.* 133(5):1238–43
30. Mezei O, Chou CN, Kennedy KJ,

Tovar-Palacio C, Shay NF. 2002. Hepatic cytochrome p450-2A and phosphoribosylpyrophosphate synthetase-associated protein mRNA are induced in gerbils after consumption of isoflavone-containing protein. *J. Nutr.* 132(9):2538–44
31. Mezei O, Shay NF. 2004. Soy isoflavones potentiate the effect of clofibrate and pioglitazone on PPAR-mediated activity in RAW264.7 cells. 2004 Experimental Biology Meeting abstracts. *FASEB* 19, Abstr. 361.7. http://select.biosis.org/faseb
32. Moore LB, Goodwin B, Jones SA, Wisely GB, Serabjit-Singh CJ, et al. 2000. St. John's wort induces hepatic drug metabolism through activation of the pregnane X receptor. *Proc. Natl. Acad. Sci. USA* 97(13):7500–2
33. Mukhtar H, Ahmad N. 2000. Tea polyphenols: prevention of cancer and optimizing health. *Am. J. Clin. Nutr.* 71:1698–702S; discussion 1703–4S
34. Mullen E, Brown RM, Osborne TF, Shay NF. 2004. Soy isoflavones affect sterol regulatory element binding proteins (SREBPs) and SREBP-regulated genes in HepG2 cells. *J. Nutr.* 134:2942–47
35. Nagy L, Schwabe JW. 2004. Mechanism of the nuclear receptor molecular switch. *Trends Biochem. Sci.* 29(6):317–24
36. Nam S, Smith DM, Dou QP. 2001. Ester bond-containing tea polyphenols potently inhibit proteasome activity in vitro and in vivo. *J. Biol. Chem.* 276(16):13322–30
37. Obst JM, Seamark RF. 1975. Hormone studies on ewes grazing an oestrogenic (Yarloop clover) pasture during the reproductive cycle. *Aust. J. Biol. Sci.* 28(3):279–90
38. Pervaiz S. 2003. Resveratrol: from grapevines to mammalian biology. *FASEB J.* 17(14):1975–85
39. Picard F, Kurtev M, Chung N, Topark-Ngarm A, Senawong T, et al. 2004. Sirt1 promotes fat mobilization in white adipocytes by repressing PPAR-gamma. *Nature* 429(6993):771–76
40. Pickart CM, Cohen RE. 2004. Proteasomes and their kin: proteases in the machine age. *Nat. Rev. Mol. Cell Biol.* 5:177–87
41. Piscitelli SC, Burstein AH, Chaitt D, Alfaro RM, Falloon J. 2000. Indinavir concentrations and St John's wort. *Lancet* 355(9203):547–48
42. Rawson RB. 2003. The SREBP pathway—insights from Insigs and insects. *Nat. Rev. Mol. Cell Biol.* 4(8):631–40
43. Repa JJ, Turley SD, Lobaccaro JA, Medina J, Li L, et al. 2000. Regulation of absorption and ABC1-mediated efflux of cholesterol by RXR heterodimers. *Science* 289(5484):1524–29
44. Richards MP, Cousins RJ. 1977. Isolation of an intestinal metallothionein induced by parenteral zinc. *Biochem. Biophys. Res. Commun.* 75(2):286–94
45. Ricketts ML, Moore DD, Banz WJ, Mezei O, Shay NF. 2005. Molecular mechanisms of action of the soy isoflavones includes activation of promiscuous nuclear receptors. *J. Nutr. Biochem.* In press
46. Robinson-Rechavi M, Escriva Garcia H, Laudet V. 2003. The nuclear receptor superfamily. *J. Cell Sci.* 116(Pt. 4):585–86
47. Rocchi S, Picard F, Vamecq J, Gelman L, Potier N, et al. 2001. A unique PPARgamma ligand with potent insulin-sensitizing yet weak adipogenic activity. *Mol. Cell* 8(4):737–47
48. Ruschitzka F, Meier PJ, Turina M, Luscher TF, Noll G. 2000. Acute heart transplant rejection due to Saint John's wort. *Lancet* 355(9203):548–49
49. Setchell KD, Lydeking-Olsen E. 2003. Dietary phytoestrogens and their effect on bone: evidence from in vitro and in vivo, human observational, and dietary intervention studies. *Am. J. Clin. Nutr.* 78:593–609S
50. Setchell KD, Brown NM, Lydeking-Olsen E. 2002. The clinical importance of the metabolite equol—a clue to the effectiveness of soy and its isoflavones. *J. Nutr.* 132(12):3577–84
51. Smith DM, Wang Z, Kazi A, Li LH, Chan

TH, et al. 2002. Synthetic analogs of green tea polyphenols as proteasome inhibitors. *Mol. Med.* 8(7):382–92
52. Takahashi Y, Lallemand-Breitenbach V, Zhu J, de The H. 2004. PML nuclear bodies and apoptosis. *Oncogene* 23(16):2819–24
53. Urizar NL, Liverman AB, Dodds DT, Silva FV, Ordentlich P, et al. 2002. A natural product that lowers cholesterol as an antagonist ligand for FXR. *Science* 296(5573):1703–6
54. Urizar NL, Moore DD. 2003. Gugulipid: a natural cholesterol-lowering agent. *Annu. Rev. Nutr.* 23:303–13
55. Watkins RE, Maglich JM, Moore LB, Wisely GB, Noble SM, et al. 2003. 2.1 Å crystal structure of human PXR in complex with the St. John's wort compound hyperforin. *Biochemistry* 42(6):1430–38
56. Way JM, Harrington WW, Brown KK, Gottschalk WK, Sundseth SS, et al. 2001. Comprehensive messenger ribonucleic acid profiling reveals that peroxisome proliferator-activated receptor gamma activation has coordinate effects on gene expression in multiple insulin-sensitive tissues. *Endocrinology* 142(3):1269–77
57. Weaver RF. 2003. *Molecular Biology*. New York: McGraw-Hill. 3rd ed.
58. Weggemans RM, Trautwein EA. 2003. Relation between soy-associated isoflavones and LDL and HDL cholesterol concentrations in humans: a meta-analysis. *Eur. J. Clin. Nutr.* 57(8):940–46
59. Wentworth JM, Agostini M, Love J, Schwabe JW, Chatterjee VK. 2000. St John's wort, a herbal antidepressant, activates the steroid X receptor. *J. Endocrinol.* 166(3):R11–16
60. Wilkie GS, Dickson KS, Gray NK. 2003. Regulation of mRNA translation by 5'- and 3'-UTR-binding factors. *Trends Biochem. Sci.* 28(4):182–88
61. Wood JG, Rogina B, Lavu S, Howitz K, Helfand SL, et al. 2004. Sirtuin activators mimic caloric restriction and delay ageing in metazoans. *Nature* 430(7000):686–89
62. Zhuo XG, Melby MK, Watanabe S. 2004. Soy isoflavone intake lowers serum LDL cholesterol: a meta-analysis of 8 randomized controlled trials in humans. *J. Nutr.* 134(9):2395–400

Annu. Rev. Nutr. 2005. 25:317–40
doi: 10.1146/annurev.nutr.25.051804.101917

First published online as a Review in Advance on April 4, 2005

POLYUNSATURATED FATTY ACID REGULATION OF GENES OF LIPID METABOLISM

Harini Sampath
Department of Nutritional Sciences, University of Wisconsin-Madison, Madison, Wisconsin 53706; email: Sampath@nutrisci.wisc.edu

James M. Ntambi
Departments of Biochemistry and Nutritional Sciences, University of Wisconsin-Madison, Madison, Wisconsin 53706; email: ntambi@biochem.wisc.edu

Key Words LXR, SREBP, PPAR, HNF-4α, NF-κB

■ **Abstract** Apart from being an important macronutrient, dietary fat has recently gained much prominence for its role in regulating gene expression. Polyunsaturated fatty acids (PUFAs) affect gene expression through various mechanisms including, but not limited to, changes in membrane composition, intracellular calcium levels, and eicosanoid production. Furthermore, PUFAs and their various metabolites can act at the level of the nucleus, in conjunction with nuclear receptors and transcription factors, to affect the transcription of a variety of genes. Several of these transcription mediators have been identified and include the nuclear receptors peroxisome proliferator-activated receptor (PPAR), hepatocyte nuclear factor (HNF)-4α, and liver X receptor (LXR) and the transcription factors sterol-regulatory element binding protein (SREBP) and nuclear factor-κB (NFκB). Their interaction with PUFAs has been shown to be critical to the regulation of several key genes of lipid metabolism. Working out the mechanisms by which these interactions and consequent effects occur is proving to be complicated but is invaluable to our understanding of the role that dietary fat can play in disease management and prevention.

CONTENTS

INTRODUCTION

Due to the recent spike in lipid-related disorders such as obesity and diabetes, dietary fat has been relegated to the darkest depths of our collective fears. Despite this, as our understanding of molecular mechanisms and biochemical pathways increases, we find that fatty acids are no longer just sources of energy, but also fine modulators of cellular signaling and metabolism.

The first and most obvious role of fat is as an essential nutrient; the well-characterized effects of essential fatty acid deficiency include flaky skin, diarrhea, and ultimately, death. Also, due to its energy density, it is the ideal storage form of excess energy. At the cellular level, fatty acids form an essential part of the phospholipid bilayer of membranes and serve as the precursors to signaling molecules such as steroids and prostaglandins. Apart from these established roles for fatty acids, it has now become increasingly clear that polyunsaturated fatty acids can specifically and rapidly effect changes in cellular metabolism, differentiation, and growth through alterations in gene expression patterns (96). This review sorts through some of the recent evidence implicating a role for polyunsaturated fatty acids (PUFAs) in affecting gene expression, with a special focus on genes of lipid metabolism.

Linoleic (n-6) and linolenic (n-3) acids cannot be synthesized de novo by mammals and are hence essential in the diet. The n-3 fatty acids, especially eicosapentanoic acid (20:5) and docosahexanoic acid (22:6) can be obtained from high-fat fish and marine mammals, while the n-6 fatty acids are concentrated in organ meats and vegetable oils. n-3 and n-6 PUFAs have been known to confer various health benefits, including increased insulin signaling (110), enhanced immune response (48, 80), decreased plasma lipid levels (40, 88), and decreased incidence of lung disease (100) and coronary heart disease (106, 107, 117). In addition, consumption of PUFAs is beneficial in certain cancers, including breast, prostate, and colorectal (24, 93). PUFAs have also been shown to be essential to the developing brain (1). At the same time, there is some concern over the consumption of n-6 fatty acids because of their known proinflammatory and proaggregatory effects. Thus, further understanding of the cellular processes affected by these fatty acids will be invaluable in increasing our present nutrition knowledge (96).

CELLULAR FATTY ACID METABOLISM

The fatty acid composition of a meal directly parallels the plasma fatty acid composition in the postabsorptive state. Following a meal, more than 95% of dietary fat (85%–90% in infants) is absorbed through the small intestine and channeled through the portal (fatty acids with less than 10 carbons) or lymphatic systems to form chylomicrons (CMs), the largest of the circulating lipoprotein classes. Along with chylomicrons, very-low-density lipoproteins (VLDLs) packaged in the liver also contribute to the plasma fatty acid profile. Apolipoproteins on the surface of CMs and VLDLs allow for their recognition by two different lipases (hepatic and lipoprotein) so that complex lipids carried in the lipoprotein can be hydrolyzed to free fatty acids (FFAs). Although there is still some discussion about whether subsequent cellular uptake of FFA occurs solely through diffusion or via transporter-mediated uptake, considerable evidence exists for a saturable transporter for long-chain fatty acids (LCFAs) in several tissues, such as intestine, heart, adipose, and liver (45a, 59). Several proteins have been identified as candidates for mediating fatty acid uptake in these tissues, including CD36 fatty acid transporter, caveolin, and fatty acid transport proteins (59).

Once within the cell, LCFAs are rapidly converted to fatty acyl-CoA thioesters by acyl-CoA synthetases (ACSs), six of which have been characterized (21). Fatty acyl-CoAs can then be sequestered through binding to acyl-CoA binding proteins (35). Alternately, fatty acyl-CoAs are channeled to various fates (Figure 1, see color insert); they can be incorporated into complex lipids such as triglycerides (TGs) and phospholipids (PLs) or further oxidized into metabolites such as epoxy- and hydroxy-fatty acids. These metabolites, in turn, have profound effects on gene regulation and cell-signaling pathways (Figure 1). For example, phosphatidylinositols, a class of phospholipids, serve as substrates for phospholipase-C (PLC) and are cleaved to inositol-triphosphate (IP_3) and diacylglycerol (DAG) in response to hormones such as vasopressin. The water-soluble IP_3 then translocates to the endoplasmic reticulum (ER) membrane where it promotes Ca^{2+} release from the ER, thereby activating various signaling pathways (Figure 1). Sphingolipids such as sphingomyelin and ceramide are yet other examples of complex lipids that can serve as cellular signaling molecules (76).

Another pathway for fatty acid metabolism is through their oxidation via the cyclooxygenase (COX) or lipooxygenase (LOX) pathways (76). Arachidonic acid is metabolized through these pathways to give rise to prostaglandins and thromboxanes (COX pathway) or to leukotrienes (LOX pathway) that can then act locally through G-protein mechanisms to increase cellular Ca^{2+} and cAMP levels (Figure 1). Changes in concentrations of these intracellular second messengers have been linked to changes in gene expression patterns (23, 34).

FATTY ACID REGULATION OF GENE EXPRESSION: BACTERIA AND YEAST

Regulation of genes of lipid metabolism by fatty acids has been documented in unicellular as well as more complex organisms. In *Escherichia coli*, the bacterial enzyme FadD, which is analogous to mammalian ACS, catalyzes the conversion of free fatty acids to fatty acyl-CoAs (8). Once activated, these CoAs have been shown to bind to the transcription factor FaDR and sequester it from its response element on various genes including fabA, fadL, fadD, fadE, fabB, and fadH. This results in downregulation of fatty acid synthesis via fabA and upregulation of fatty acid transport and metabolism (8).

Yeasts are capable of thriving entirely on LCFAs as their sole carbon source. When grown on LCFAs, there is an increase in peroxisomal proliferation, which indicates that fatty acids are capable of altering structural components in yeast (8). Faa1p and Faa4p, the yeast acyl-CoA synthetases, are responsible for the activation of LCFAs to acyl-CoAs. These acyl-CoAs can then be used for energy or stored as complex lipids. Furthermore, they can affect the transcription of various genes apart from those involved in peroxisome proliferation. Regulation of genes in the yeast seems to occur through the specific transcription factors Oaf1p/Pip1p and Oaf2p/Pip2p (8). Oaf1p and Oaf2p have been shown to form a heterodimer in response to exogenous fatty acids and bind to a cis element in the DNA promoter, termed the oleate responsive element (ORE), with the sequence CGGNNNTNA(N9–12)CCG. More than 40 yeast genes have been shown to contain this ORE in their promoter regions and are therefore good candidates for Oaf1p/Oaf2p-mediated regulation by fatty acids.

One key gene involved in lipid metabolism in the yeast is the OLE1 yeast Δ-9 desaturase, analogous to the mammalian stearoyl CoA desaturase (SCD) gene (8). The OLE1 gene has been shown to be repressed by both mono- and polyunsaturated fatty acids; however, this repression seems to be independent of Oaf1p/Oaf2p. Recently, an ER membrane protein, Mga2p, has been identified as a key player in the transcriptional and post-transcriptional mechanisms regulating the destabilization of OLE1 mRNA upon exposure to unsaturated fatty acids (16).

FATTY ACID REGULATION OF MAMMALIAN GENE EXPRESSION

The role of polyunsaturated fatty acids in the regulation of mammalian gene expression has been well characterized and is the focus of the remainder of this review. Some of the first reports of direct regulation of lipogenesis by fatty acids came from Allman & Gibson (2), who described the upregulation of fatty acid–synthesizing enzymes in the liver and epididymal fat pads of mice on high-carbohydrate diets. The authors showed that supplementation of a fat-free diet with either saturated fatty acids or cholesterol had no effect, but supplementation with linoleic acid greatly reduced ^{14}C-acetate incorporation into LCFAs within four days of feeding (2). Enzyme activities of fatty acid synthase (FAS), malic enzyme, and glucose-6-phosphate dehydrogenase (G6PD) were decreased, demonstrating rapid, direct, and specific regulation of enzymes of lipid metabolism by a particular fatty acid (2). These results were independently confirmed by various groups that showed decreases in hepatic lipogenic capacity upon linoleic acid feeding in wild-type (52) as well as genetically obese fa/fa rats (118). However, it was not until 1982 that a specific mechanism of action for this effect was suggested. Schwartz & Abraham (101a) used a specific antibody assay to show that corn oil supplementation of a high-carboyhydrate diet reduced the rate of synthesis of FAS protein in mouse liver. The question of whether the changes observed were effected directly by the fatty acid or by one of its metabolites was settled by the demonstration that columbinic acid, a PUFA that is not further metabolized to a prostaglandin, was equally capable of reducing FAS protein synthesis as linoleic acid (101a). However, while these authors suggested that the effect of linoleic acid on FAS protein synthesis was due to its desaturated nature, it has since been shown that several fatty acids as well as their various metabolites are capable of specifically effecting changes in gene expression patterns in liver, adipose, and other tissues.

While dietary fat could certainly affect cell signaling and gene expression by affecting membrane phospholipid content or through production of eicosanoids (Figure 1), it was the discovery of nuclear receptors capable of binding fatty acids that established a direct role for fatty acids in gene regulation (36). Within hours of feeding animals diets rich in PUFAs, there is a rapid and sustained activation of genes of lipid oxidation and a decrease in genes encoding enzymes of lipid synthesis (20, 55, 56, 62, 122). The result of this twofold action of PUFAs is a negative fat balance, thereby making PUFAs a good candidate for the dietary management of hyperlipidemia. Although the nuclear actions of PUFAs were first studied in hepatic cells, their actions have since been confirmed in 3T3-L1 cultured adipocytes (68, 103, 112) as well as in various tissues, including small intestine (77), pancreas (12), the immune system (111), and neonatal mouse brain (26).

Repression of Gene Expression by PUFAs

The inhibition of lipogenic genes in the liver by PUFAs is a very strong signal that overrides even the prolipogenic capacity of insulin and carbohydrates, which also tend to be highest postprandially. PUFA-rich diets in rodents have been shown to repress a variety of genes, including stearoyl CoA desaturase 1(SCD1), acetyl CoA carboxylase (ACC), FAS, L-type pyruvate kinase (L-PK), Δ-5 and Δ-6 desaturases, G6PD, and insulin-sensitive glucose transporter (GLUT)-4 in the liver (17–19, 54, 78, 95, 103, 112, 119). SCD1, L-PK, ACC, and FAS repression by PUFAs occurs at the level of transcription, whereas G6PD is controlled via post-transcriptional mechanisms (54, 95). Many of these genes are repressed by both n-3 and n-6 PUFAs. This seems to be a direct effect of the fatty acids themselves since addition of prostaglandin (PG) inhibitors does not abolish the effects of PUFAs on these genes (28, 119).

The findings in liver are quite different from what has been seen in adipose tissue (119). The suppression of genes such as FAS in adipose tissue of rat seems to be site-specific. PUFA-rich diets elicit this response in retroperitoneal but not in subcutaneous fat depots (86), perhaps due to known differences in site-specific metabolism of fatty acids (102). Also, unlike in liver, many adipose tissue genes seem to respond specifically to n-3 PUFAs (86). An exception to this generality is the regulation of SCD1 in adipose tissue by n-6 PUFAs (102). Obese animals show dramatically higher levels of SCD1 in both liver and adipose tissue. However, feeding both genetically obese (fa/fa) and lean Zucker rats a high n-6 fatty acid diet results in suppression of lipid synthesis (53, 118). This is consistent with the findings of Sessler & Ntambi (102) that addition of arachidonic acid, linoleic acid (n-6), and eicosapentanoic acid (n-3) to 3T3-L1 adipocytes all result in repression of SCD1 mRNA in a dose-dependent manner through alterations in mRNA stability.

Also unlike in liver, PUFA-mediated repression of lipogenic genes in adipose tissue involves eicosanoid production (54). As described above, eicosanoids are oxidative derivatives of PUFAs released from the phospholipids of plasma membranes that are capable of eliciting both acute changes in proteins as well as long-term changes in mRNA abundance (54). It has been shown, for example, that arachidonate suppresses FAS and S14 mRNA in 3T3-adipocytes. Inhibition of the COX pathway in these cells abolished the effect of arachidonate (68). In this study, the prostaglandins PGE2 and PGF2α were shown to function via a pertussis-sensitive G-protein coupled receptor (68), but G-protein-independent mechanisms for prostanoid inhibition of gene expression have also been described (54).

More recently, one of the key examples of PUFA regulation of lipogenesis comes from its effects on leptin, an adipose-derived hormone. Leptin has gained much attention due to its role in the prevention of obesity; high plasma leptin levels are closely associated with increased adiposity and obesity, and weight loss results in attenuation of these high plasma leptin levels (32). Although a high-fat diet in humans has been associated with high plasma leptin levels, substitution of PUFAs for saturated fat in the diet results in decreased leptin levels independent from changes in body mass (91). Raclot et al. (86) showed that n-3 PUFA [especially docosahexanoic acid (DHA)] feeding in rats resulted in decreased leptin mRNA in retroperitoneal fat, but not in subcutaneous fat, independent of plasma insulin levels. Reseland et al. (92) showed that addition of eicosapentanoic acid (EPA) and DHA but not saturated or monounsaturated fatty acids to human trophoblasts (BeWo) in culture resulted in decreased transcription of a transfected human leptin promoter. This was accompanied by decreased levels of peroxisome-proliferator receptor (PPAR)-γ and sterol-regulatory element-binding protein (SREBP)-1 mRNA levels, providing insight into the mechanisms by which n-3 PUFAs exert their effects on leptin (92). However, given the role of leptin in appetite suppression and repression of lipogenic genes such as SCD1, the physiological significance of PUFA-mediated repression of leptin remains to be determined.

Another adipose-derived hormone, resistin, has recently been reported to be inhibited by PUFAs. Resistin belongs to the resistin-like molecules (RELM) gene family. In the mouse, resistin is mainly expressed in adipose tissue, whereas RELMα, β, and γ are expressed in adipose tissue and lung, intestine, and hematopoietic tissues, respectively. The human homologs of resistin and RELMβ are expressed in macrophages and small intestine, respectively. There is evidence that resistin functions to inhibit glucose uptake in 3T3-L1 adipocytes (108) as well as L6 rat skeletal muscle cells (74). Thiazolidinediones, ligands for the nuclear receptor PPARγ discussed below, have previously been shown to repress resistin mRNA levels, at least in 3T3-L1 cells (108). Haugen et al. (41) have recently shown that the same effect is seen when 3T3-L1 cells are treated with EPA or arachidonic acid. At 60–250 uM quantities, arachidonic acid was especially effective in reducing resistin mRNA levels by about 80%. Inhibition of the COX-1 and mitogen-activated protein kinase pathways as well as actinomycin D and cycloheximide treatments resulted in attenuation of the PUFA response, which suggests that transcriptional and translational regulation of resistin by PUFAs occurs through a metabolite of arachidonic acid. The authors suggest that this regulation is not mediated by SREBP, but through a decrease in resistin mRNA stability (41).

Upregulation of Gene Expression by Fatty Acids

Fatty acids are key regulators of adipocyte differentiation; thus, they are potent activators of genes and proteins involved in adipogenesis. However, in contrast to their role in gene repression, saturated as well as unsaturated LCFAs seem to be equally effective in upregulating genes involved in adipogenesis (28). Mechanistically, nonmetabolizable fatty acids such as α-bromopalmitate are also capable of effecting changes (37), a finding that indicates a direct role for fatty acids in upregulation of these genes. It is possible that fatty acids directly upregulate gene expression, but in the case of certain genes such as ap2, this is unlikely since upregulation in response to fatty acids is not rapid and is inhibited by cycloheximide, an inhibitor of protein synthesis (3, 4). It is therefore more likely that fatty acids function by affecting the abundance of a transcription factor that mediates the regulation of these genes (28); further studies are required to understand the mechanism by which such regulation occurs.

In adipose tissue, phosphoenolpyruvate carboxykinase (PEPCK) is responsible for supplying glycerophosphate for triglyceride synthesis (Table 1) and is upregulated in response to PUFAs. While glucose inhibits PEPCK in adipose and liver, PUFAs induce PEPCK mRNA in 3T3 adipocytes (31). It seems clear that the induction of PEPCK by fatty acids in adipose tissue does not require protein synthesis or fatty acid metabolism to eicosanoids. This inhibition is specific to adipose tissue; the same response is not seen in the liver, where PEPCK serves in a gluconeogenic capacity (31).

In the liver, several genes have been demonstrated to be upregulated by fatty acids (Table 1); these include apolipoproteins AI and AII (6), acyl-CoA synthetase (28), acyl-CoA oxidase (6), liver fatty acid–binding protein (L-FABP) (71), carnitine palmitoyl transferase (CPT-1) (15), and cytochrome P450 A1 (28). CPT-1 and L-FABP are also upregulated in response to fatty acids in other tissues and

TABLE 1 Effects of polyunsaturated fatty acids on expression of genes involved in lipid metabolism*

Pathway gene	Transcription factor	Effect of PUFAs	References
Lipogenesis			
Stearoyl CoA desaturase 1	SREBP-1c, LXRα	↓	81
Sterol-regulatory element binding protein-1c	LXRα, PPARα	↓	85, 122, 125, 126
Fatty acid synthase	SREBP-1c, LXRα	↓	19, 122
Acetyl CoA carboxylase	SREBP-1c, LXRα	↓	95
Phosphoenol pyruvate carboxykinase (adipose)	PPARα	↓	114, 115
S14	SREBP-1c	↓	19
Fatty acid transport/metabolism			
Acyl CoA synthetase	PPARα	↑	99
Fatty acid transport protein	PPARα	↑	33
Energy utilization/fatty acid oxidation			
Carnitine palmitoyl transferase-1	PPARα	↑	9
Uncoupling protein-1	PPARα	↑	101b
Acyl CoA oxidase	PPARα	↑	6
Cholesterol metabolism			
Cyp7α hydroxylase	HNF-4α, LXR	↓	66
HMG CoA synthase	SREBP	↑	121
ApoCIII	HNF-4α	↓	42
TNFα	NF-κB	↓	128

*Abbreviations: Apo, apolipoprotein; Cyp, cytochrome P; HMG, hydroxymethylglutaryl; HNF-4α, hepatocyte nuclear factor-4 alpha; LXRα, liver X receptor alpha; NF-κB, nuclear factor-kappa B; PPARα, peroxisome proliferator receptor alpha; PUFA, polyunsaturated fatty acid; SREBP-1c, sterol-regulatory element binding protein-1c; TNFα, tumor necrosis factor alpha.

cell culture models, such as the small intestine (FABP) (77) and INS-1 pancreatic β-cell line (CPT-1) (5a).

MECHANISMS FOR PUFA-MEDIATED CHANGES IN GENE EXPRESSION

PUFAs have been shown to affect gene expression through at least three different nuclear receptors, PPAR, liver X receptor (LXR), and hepatocyte nuclear factor-4 alpha (HNF-4α), and through the transcription factors, SREBP, and nuclear factor-κB (NF-κB) (57). Along with various ancillary proteins and partners, several isoforms of each of these mediators interact with PUFAs and with each other to weave a complex pattern of regulation by fatty acids (Figure 2, see color insert).

Peroxisome Proliferator-Activated Receptors

STRUCTURE AND FUNCTION PPARs belong to the steroid hormone nuclear receptor superfamily of ligand-activated transcription factors that also includes the retinoic acid receptor (RAR), LXR, and the ubiquitous retinoid X receptor (RXR). Three different isoforms of PPAR, PPARα, PPARβ/δ, and PPARγ, have been identified and are encoded by three different genes; they all function by dimerizing with RXR and binding to a prescribed DNA sequence, termed the PPAR response element (PPRE) (Figure 2) (25). The PPRE comprises direct repeat sequences separated by a single nucleotide spacer (AGGNCA_AGGTCA), and the binding of the PPAR/RXR heterodimer to the PPRE affects transcription of the target gene (50).

PPARα is the major PPAR subtype found in hepatocytes and is involved in regulation of genes of lipid and carbohydrate metabolism. It is required for the clofibrate induction of peroxisomal and microsomal enzymes such as acyl-CoA oxidase (AOX) and CYP4A in the liver (64), CPT-1, the rate-limiting enzyme for β-oxidation of fatty acids (9, 38), as well as fatty acid translocases and transport proteins (75).

PPAR LIGANDS A wide range of structurally diverse natural and synthetic compounds have been shown to bind the various isoforms of PPAR, and because of their role in insulin sensitivity and lipid metabolism, much effort has been directed towards the identification and development of novel PPAR ligands. In general, all the n-3 and n-6 fatty acids activate the three PPAR isoforms. However, their affinities for the receptor vary, which suggests a role for site-specific availability and metabolism of particular fatty acids and differences in their affinity for specific PPAR subtypes. For example, EPA is a much more potent activator of PPARα in primary hepatocytes as compared with arachidonic acid (89). Kliewer et al. (65) showed through transactivation assays that polyunsaturated fatty acids such as linoleic, linolenic, and arachidonic acids were able to activate PPARα at a concentration of 100 uM. Since the concentration of these free fatty acids in human adult serum can be over 1 mM, it was concluded that these fatty acids are potent endogenous ligands of PPARα. Furthermore, these PUFAs were also found to activate PPARγ potently. The authors also demonstrated through transactivation and competitive binding assays that metabolites of PUFAs, such as the naturally occurring eicosanoids 8-HETE and 15 D-J2, were also able to activate PPARα and PPARγ. In fact, these eicosanoids showed more specificity and subtype selectivity than their fatty acid precursors in activating either PPARα or PPARγ more potently (65).

More recently, it has been shown that conjugated linoleic acids (CLA) are also capable of activating PPARγ. Feeding pigs CLA before perturbation of their gastrointestinal system with enteric bacteria markedly upregulated PPARγ and resulted in decreased mucosal inflammation (45b). These results have been confirmed in the RAW264.7 mouse macrophage cell line, where CLA supplementation results in decreased interferon-γ expression, mediated by upregulation of PPARγ.

Despite this abundance of endogenous ligands for PPARs, of greater therapeutic and commercial value in recent years has been the development of synthetic ligands for the different PPAR isoforms (51). Fibrates, a class of lipid-lowering drugs, are being used to manage high plasma cholesterol levels. Fibrates such as clofibrate and WY 14643 are potent activators of PPARα. Additionally, the insulin-sensitizing thiazolidinedione (TZD) class of drugs is used clinically to manage type II diabetes mellitus; these TZDs, which include the compound troglitazone, preferentially bind to and activate PPARγ. In addition to these ligands, PPARs, like some other nuclear receptors, can also be activated via phosphorylation, for example as induced by insulin through the mitogen-activated protein kinase pathway (25).

REGULATION OF GENES BY PPAR The effect of long-chain PUFAs on expression of a number of genes has been shown to be mediated through PPARs. These include, but are not limited to, acyl-CoA synthase (99), FATP (33), CPT1 (9), PEPCK (114, 115), UCP1 (101b), and SCD1 (73). PPARα is also required for the fish oil–mediated induction of AOX mRNA as well as CYP4A2 mRNA (6). However, the development of the PPARα-null mouse has shown that not all regulation of genes by PUFAs is mediated by PPARα. Bing et al. (7) showed that fish oil, a rich source of n-3 PUFAs, upregulated genes of β-oxidation in wild-type but not in PPARα-null mice. Although this was expected, the authors also observed that fish oil suppressed lipogenic genes such as S14 and FAS (7) in both wild-type and mutant mice, which suggests that the effects of PUFA on lipid oxidation and synthesis were not likely to be mediated by a common transcription factor, i.e., PPARα. The resultant search for a novel transcription factor regulated by PUFAs led to the identification of the SREBPs, discussed below, as key candidates.

In humans, the precise role of PPARα in liver is less clear; it is only weakly expressed and several splice variants of the isoform have been characterized (54, 84a). While the fibrate class of drugs is commonly used clinically as a lipid-lowering agent, there is not much evidence of upregulation of peroxisomal proliferation in human liver. It therefore has been suggested that the actions of fibrates in humans could be mediated through the actions of PPARα in nonhepatic tissues (54).

There is some evidence for PPAR mediated repression of genes through mechanisms involving competition, with the thyroid receptor (TR), for the RXR partner or competitive binding to response elements of other transcription factors such as HNF-4α, discussed further below (43). There is clear evidence, for example, that in the absence of excess RXR, the actions of the thyroid receptor (TR) are mitigated by PPARs. However, a lot of the suppression of lipogenic genes by fatty acids seems to be mediated via the actions of a different transcription factor, SREBP.

Sterol-Regulatory Element Binding Protein

STRUCTURE, FUNCTION AND ISOFORMS SREBPs belong to the helix-loop-helix family of transcription factors and were first identified through their ability to bind to a sterol response element found on genes involved in cholesterolgenesis (82). Three isoforms of SREBP have thus far been identified; SREBP-1a and SREBP-1c are important to regulation of genes of lipid synthesis, while SREBP-2 has been shown to control genes important to cholesterol homeostasis. SREBP-1a and SREBP-1c are transcribed from the same gene locus and differ only at their N-termini; SREBP-2 is encoded by a separate gene. While SREBP-1a is the predominant isoform in sterol-depleted cell lines, SREBP-1c is the major isoform in rodent and human liver and is now recognized as a key regulator of fatty acid and triglyceride synthesis (82).

SREBPs are synthesized as large proteins (125 kDa) and inserted into the ER membrane with two membrane-spanning domains and with their C-terminal end bound to the SREBP cleavage-activating protein (SCAP). When cellular sterol levels drop, the SREBP-SCAP complex moves to the Golgi apparatus, where it undergoes two proteolytic events, giving rise to the smaller (65 kDa), mature form of the protein. The mature protein then transits to the nucleus, where it binds to *cis* elements, termed sterol regulatory elements (SREs), in the promoters of target genes and induces transcription of a variety of genes involved in cholesterol, triglyceride, and fatty acid synthesis (11).

SREBPs themselves are not very potent activators of transcription and require the actions of ancillary proteins to affect transcription of target genes (67). Several such proteins have been identified, including the Sp1 transcription factor in the LDL promoter (97) and the CCAAT-binding factor/nuclear factor-Y (CBF/NF-Y) in the promoters of HMGCoA synthase (27) and farnesyl diphosphate synthase in cholesterol metabolism (29). Teran-Garcia and coworkers (113) have recently shown that mutation of the SREBP1 site in the promoter of the FAS gene results in only a 25% loss of PUFA repression of FAS. Conversely, mutation of the NF-Y site in the FAS promoter decreases PUFA repression of FAS by almost 50%.

EFFECTS OF POLYUNSATURATED FATTY ACIDS There is convincing in vitro (121) as well as in vivo (62, 122) evidence implicating a role for PUFAs in inhibiting maturation of SREBP in a post-translational manner, thereby repressing lipogenic gene expression. Incubation of CHO, HepG2, and CV-1 cells with micromolar quantities of PUFAs resulted in a decrease in transcription of SRE-containing genes in a dose-dependent manner. This regulation by PUFAs was absent in a defective CHO cell line that exhibited loss of SREBP regulation by sterols or in cells transfected with promoters containing mutant SREs. This suggests that PUFAs do not function at the level of SREBP binding to the SRE but rather through modulating intracellular regulatory sterol levels (121). Fasting-refeeding experiments in rodents have established that caloric intake is directly parallel to SREBP nuclear content (46); this trend is consistent with observations that lipogenic gene expression is greatly reduced during fasting and increased upon refeeding. These findings led to the hypothesis that the inhibitory effect of PUFAs on lipogenic gene expression could occur via repression of SREBP mRNA or inhibition of SREBP maturation. Rats fed fat-free diets supplemented with n-3 or n-6 PUFAs greatly reduce nuclear content of SREBP protein as well as expression of SREBP target genes (62, 122). Also, SREBP overexpression in transgenic mice leads to decreased sensitivity to PUFA-mediated repression of target genes (123). We have shown that while cholesterol feeding does not alter SREBP mRNA levels, it causes an increase in nuclear levels of SREBP protein. Supplementation of the diet with PUFA decreases the nuclear content of SREBP without affecting mRNA levels (61). These findings suggest that PUFAs function by inhibiting maturation of the precursor form of the SREBP protein (Figure 2).

Several mechanisms have been suggested whereby PUFAs can alter the maturation of SREBPs. Since increased intracellular sterol levels seem to result in a decline in SREBP maturation/transit, PUFAs could function by raising cellular cholesterol levels. Indeed, unsaturated fatty acids have been shown to increase sphingomyelinase activity, resulting in increased hydrolysis of sphingomyelin contained in the plasma membrane and increased cholesterol levels in the ER. This results in decreased maturation of SREBP-1 and SREBP-2 but does not affect SREBP mRNA levels (120).

Unsaturated fatty acids have also been shown to affect the hepatic abundance of SREBP-1a and SREBP-1c mRNA, but not that of SREBP-2, which is mainly regulated by sterols (57, 62, 69, 122, 123). This inhibition is dependent on chain length and degree of desaturation, with eicosapentanoate and arachidonate being more potent inhibitors than linoleic or oleic acids. Both reductions in SREBP-1 mRNA stability and decreased transcription of the SREBP-1 gene (Figure 2) have been suggested as possible mechanisms for this inhibition (57).

In HepG2 cells, arachidonic, linoleic, and eicosapentanoic acids all repress transcription of the SCD1 gene, which is known to have an SRE in its promoter region. However, overexpression of a mature SREBP in these cells does not prevent this repression by PUFAs, which suggests an SREBP-independent mechanism in the regulation of SCD1 gene expression (79); one possible candidate mediating this effect is another member of the nuclear receptor superfamily, LXR.

Liver X Receptors

STRUCTURE AND FUNCTION As mentioned above, LXRs are a set of nuclear receptors that have been recently identified as candidates for mediating gene regulation by fatty acids (39, 83). LXRs α and β have been well characterized for their ability to bind oxysterols such as 24, 25-epoxycholesterol as endogenous ligands. They have been shown to regulate diverse processes such as bile acid synthesis and lipogenesis (66, 90). LXRα is expressed mainly in liver, kidneys, intestine, adipose, and adrenal glands, while LXRβ is more ubiquitously expressed (66). LXRs function by heterodimerizing with RXRα and binding to direct repeats with four nucleotide spacers (DR4 elements), termed LXR response elements (LXREs), in the promoter regions of target genes (Figure 2).

REGULATION BY POLYUNSATURATED FATTY ACIDS Oxysterols are the natural endogenous ligands of LXRs α and β. Binding of oxysterols to LXRs has been shown to affect transcription of a variety of genes involved in cholesterol, lipid, and bile acid metabolism (Table 1). These include 7α-hydroxylase (Cyp7α), the rate-limiting enzyme in bile acid synthesis (66), lipoprotein lipase, FAS, ACC, SCD1, and the lipogenic transcription factor, SREBP1c (66, 90).

It has been shown that PUFAs inhibit the prolipogenic actions of LXRs through various mechanisms. One possibility is that competitive binding of PUFAs to LXRs prevents oxysterol binding, thereby antagonizing induction of target genes, notably SREBP1c, and consequently genes containing either LXREs or SREs in their promoter elements (39, 126). Yoshikawa et al. (127) showed that in HEK293 cells, unsaturated fatty acids resulted in decreased SREBP-1c promoter activity, with the order of potency being arachidonic acid > EPA > DHA > linoleic acid. Deletion of the two LXREs in the SREBP-1c promoter abolished the effects of PUFAs on SREBP-1c (127), suggesting an interaction between LXR and SREBP-1c. However, in direct contrast to this study, there is now evidence that repression of SREBP-1c mRNA levels by PUFAs is independent of LXRs. Pawar et al. (85) have shown that treatment of HEK293 cells with EPA results in inhibition of SREBP-1c mRNA in the presence and absence of an LXR agonist. Also, while fish oil enrichment of the diet resulted in repression of SRE-containing genes and induction of PPRE-containing genes in rats, neither EPA (in HEK293 cells) nor fish oil (in the diet) had any effect on classical LXR target genes such as CYP7A1 and ABCG5. The authors suggest that although PUFAs do in fact regulate SREBP-1c levels and consequently SRE-containing genes, this regulation does not extend to LXRE-containing genes and is therefore unlikely to involve an interaction between LXR and SREBP-1c.

Another mechanism that has recently been suggested is the inhibition of LXRs by PUFAs through activation of PPARα and PPARγ. PUFAs, as discussed above, are potent activators of PPARα and PPARγ. It was recently shown that overexpression of PPARα and PPARγ in HEK-293 cells inhibits SREBP-1c promoter activity in a dose-dependent manner (125). Mutation of the two LXREs in the SREBP-1c promoter abolished this effect of PPARs, and gel mobility shift assays showed that the activation of PPARs in fact reduced the binding of the LXR/RXR heterodimer to the LXRE (Figure 2). Supplementation with RXR decreased the repression observed, which suggests that competition between PPAR and LXR for the RXR partner could play a role in the inhibitory effects (125).

Hepatocyte Nuclear Factor-4α

HNF-4α is a member of the hepatocyte nuclear factor family that includes six different isoforms (42). HNF-4α is a highly conserved nuclear receptor that binds to DR1 elements as a homodimer and seems to be indispensable to hepatocyte differentiation and hepatic functions such as cholesterol and lipoprotein secretion. It is expressed mainly in liver, kidney, intestine, and pancreas and is capable of activating target genes even in the absence of ligand. It has been shown that PUFAs, in their CoA form, can affect HNF-4α activity; fatty acids can also affect HNF-4α activity via PKA-mediated phosphorylation (42). The importance of HNF-4α to glucose and lipid metabolism is underscored by the observation that mutations in the promoter of the HNF-4α gene lead to a form of maturity onset diabetes of the young (MODY1) (124). The development of a liver-specific HNF-4α knockout mouse has provided much insight into the role that this nuclear receptor plays in fatty acid mediated–regulation of hepatic genes (57).

Using mainly cell culture models, it has been demonstrated that HNF-4α is important to the activation of various genes involved in lipid and cholesterol metabolism, including ApoA-I, ApoA-II, ApoB, ApoC-II, ApoE, and ApoC-III (discussed below), as well as CYP7A1 (Table 1). HNF-4α has also been implicated in the regulation of iron metabolism by transferrin, carbohydrate metabolism through PEPCK and L-PK, as well as the cytochrome P450 system (42).

It has been reported that fatty acyl-CoAs are able to bind HNF-4α directly at physiological concentrations; binding of saturated fatty acids like palmitoyl CoA (16:0) and myristoyl-CoA (14:0) results in activation of HNF-4α while the binding of unsaturated fatty acids like α-linolenic acid (18:3n3), EPA (20:5n-3) and docosahexanoic acid (22:6n6) results in repression of HNF-4α (43). Furthermore, Hertz, Bar-Tana, and colleagues (44) have recently shown that the fibrate class of drugs are converted to fatty acyl-CoA thioesters within cells and are then able to repress the HNF-4α nuclear receptor and target genes such as Cyp7A1. In the case of the ApoCIII gene, fibrates also function by activating PPARα, which then competes with HNF-4α for binding to the promoter (44). Ongoing research will no doubt further strengthen the role of HNF-4α in mediating some of the hypolipidemic effects of the increasingly popular fibrate compounds.

Inhibitor-κB/Nuclear Factor-κB

Many other mechanisms of PUFA-mediated gene regulation have also been suggested; one of them includes the regulation of the transcription factor nuclear factor-κB (NF-κB). Inhibitor κB (I-κB) and NF-κB are present in the cytoplasm of cells, in their inactive form, as a heterodimer. Phosphorylation of I-κB degrades it, thereby allowing NF-κB to separate from I-κB, translocate to the nucleus, and affect the transcription of a variety of genes, including Cox2 and interleukin-6 (13, 60). The translocation of NF-κB has been shown to be regulated both positively and negatively by various PUFAs. While arachidonate stimulates NF-κB translocation and thus has a positive effect on the transcription of its target genes, EPA inhibits NF-κB translocation, resulting in lower transcription of NF-κB target genes (14, 128). Fish oil supplementation in humans has been shown to decrease levels of NF-κB target genes such as TNFα (128) by decreasing I-κB phosphorylation and consequent NF-κB translocation. The mechanisms by which EPA inhibits NF-κB translocation are as yet unclear. It has been suggested that because EPA is not readily metabolized through the COX pathway (63), it could function by inhibiting arachidonic acid metabolism rather than by forming eicosanoid mediators of its own (54). In fact, the addition of an arachidonate metabolism inhibitor, ETYA, to cells mimicked the effects of EPA (109). However, because both EPA and ETYA are also capable of inducing PPARα (65), it has been suggested that the effects observed with fish oil or ETYA treatment could be mediated by PPARα activation (54).

IMPLICATIONS TO HUMAN HEALTH

In the period between 1999 and 2000, an estimated 31% of the U.S. population was classified as obese, as defined by a body mass index of 30 or above. The monetary costs of this epidemic translated to 9.1% of total healthcare spending, a staggering sum of $92.6 billion (30). The effects of this rapidly rising epidemic stem not only from obesity itself, but also from related complications such as diabetes, hyperlipidemia, cardiovascular disease, and stroke. An indication of this is the fact that between the years 1999 and 2000, drugs targeting cardiovascular disease topped the list of pharmaceutical sales, at an estimated $43 billion.

Dietary PUFAs have long been shown to be effective in managing lipid levels and are consequently of benefit in preventing and treating lipid-related disorders. n-3 PUFA feeding has been clearly linked to decreased plasma triglyceride levels as well as decreased VLDL secretion (40, 54, 88). This seems to be controlled at the level of the ApoB and ApoCIII lipoproteins. ApoCIII synthesis has been shown to be modulated by HNF-4α activation; this could occur either through stimulation or inhibition of HNF-4α by saturated or unsaturated fatty acids, respectively, or through competition between PPARα and HNF-4α for binding to the ApoCIII promoter (43). Another mechanism proposed is the modulation of LDL receptor activity by fatty acids (94, 116), which results in decreased levels of ApoB; however, the generation of the LDL-receptor knockout mouse has created some controversy around this hypothesis (72). A recent study (84b) has shown that ApoB degradation is affected not only by n-3 PUFAs, as previously suggested, but also by n-6 PUFAs, and lipid peroxidation of these fatty acids is required for the effect. This study provides new insight into the role that dietary PUFAs could play in regulating ApoB secretion and preventing hyperlipidemia.

The identification and characterization of transcription factors such as SREBP-1c provide further insight into the role that dietary fat may play in the development of obesity and other lipid-related complications. As discussed above, SREBP-1c, which is downregulated in response to PUFAs, binds to response elements in the promoter regions of key lipogenic genes, including FAS, ACC, and SCD-1. Overexpression of SREBP-1a, -1c, -2, or SCAP results in increased lipid synthesis as well as increased liver and plasma lipid levels. Conversely, liver-specific knockouts of SCAP show decreased lipid synthesis and content and decreased expression of SREBP target genes (47). The implication of changes in SREBP target genes is strengthened further by the observation that global deletion of the SCD1 gene in mice results in the generation of lean mice (81). These mice show increased insulin sensitivity and decreased plasma and liver lipids (87). Furthermore, the SCD1 knockout mice also have increased rates of fatty acid oxidation, decreased fat pad weight, and are protected from diet-induced obesity (81). There are already some initial clues as to the translatability of this evidence from mice to human subjects. It has been shown, for example, that in human subjects with triglycerides ranging from 0.3 to 20 mM, SCD activity in liver, as measured by the plasma desaturation ratio, accounts for one-third of the variance in plasma triglyceride levels (5b).

Also of great importance to human health is the role that PUFAs play in the activation of the PPARs and the consequent increases in lipid clearance and oxidation. In addition to using fibrates and TZDs to clinically lower lipid levels and increase insulin sensitivity, PUFAs could represent a plausible dietary approach to the prevention of lipid-induced chronic disease.

CONCLUSIONS

In recent years, the understanding that fat is more than just a static store of energy has led to the discovery of various pathways whereby fatty acids affect gene expression. This review, although certainly not conclusive, has attempted to sort through the effects that various dietary fats have on some of these genes, especially those involved in lipid metabolism. As discussed, the effects that fatty acids exert differ based on their chain length, degree of desaturation, and extent of cellular metabolism. They can affect gene expression at the nuclear level either directly or through one of their metabolites, or they can alter various signaling cascades within the cell, thereby raising second messenger concentrations and thus affecting gene expression. Some of the well-characterized mediators of fatty acid–induced changes in gene expression include the nuclear receptors PPAR, HNF-4α, and LXR, as well as the transcription factors SREBP and NF-κB. Not only do these factors mediate the effects of fatty acids, there are also examples of crosstalk between them, making fatty acid regulation of gene expression a much more complicated story. The field is not without discrepancies, and it is probable that novel transcription factors and signaling mechanisms will be identified as our understanding of the topic grows.

The research on nuclear effects of fatty acids has certainly progressed well beyond its infancy. However, the increasing prevalence of obesity and lipid-related disorders such as diabetes and cardiovascular disease has no doubt intensified the search for new compounds, both pharmacological and nutritional, to manage these conditions. Now more than ever, there is a need to understand the changes that contribute to the development of metabolic disease. The coming years should bring a greater understanding of the mechanisms and pathways involved in the development of such diseases and an unraveling of the roles of various dietary fats in promoting or abating diet-induced disease.

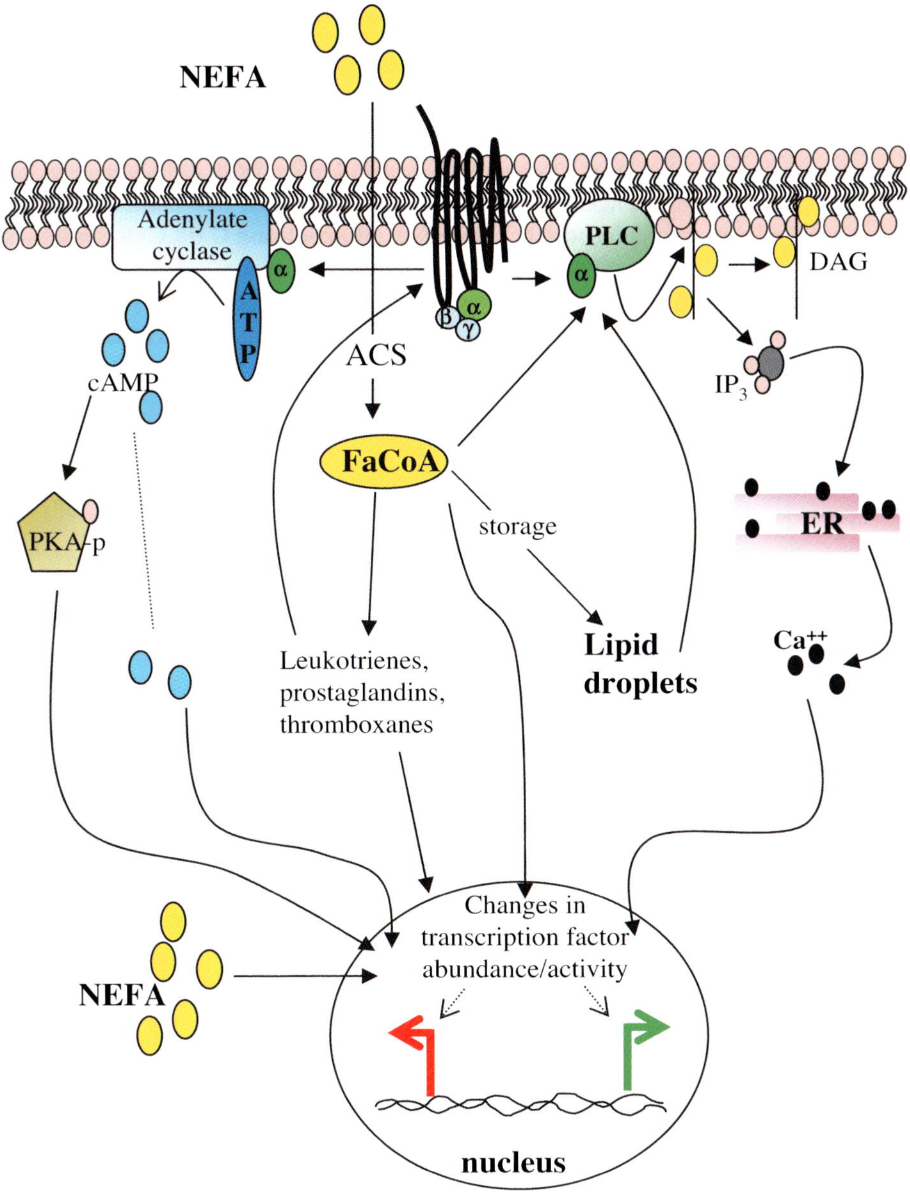

See legend on next page

Figure 2 Nuclear effects of fatty acids. Nonesterified fatty acids (NEFAs) interact with various transcription mediators through several mechanisms to change gene expression patterns. Fatty acids inhibit proteolytic maturation of SREBP-1 from the ER/Golgi (*a*) and subsequent binding of SREBP and coactivators such as NF-Y to SREs (*b*), thereby decreasing transcription of SRE-containing genes (*c*). Fatty acids also compete with oxysterols for binding to LXRα (*d*), thus decreasing transcription of LXR target genes (*e*), including SREBP-1 (*f*). Fatty acids also bind to and activate PPARα (*g*), thereby inducing transcription of PPRE-containing genes (*h*). PPARα activation has also been shown to inhibit LXR binding to the LXRE (*i*), which represents another level of regulation in the transcription of SREBP-1 and LXR target genes. Fatty acids have been shown to inhibit I-κB degradation (*j*), thereby preventing NF-κB translocation to the nucleus (*k*) and subsequent transactivation of NF-κB target genes (*l*). Abbreviations: ER, endoplasmic reticulum; I-κB, inhibitor κB; LXRα, liver X receptor α; LXRE, LXR response element; NF-κB, nuclear factor-κB; NF-Y, nuclear factor-Y; PPARα, peroxisome proliferator-activated receptor-α; PPRE, PPAR response element; RXRα, retinoid X receptor α; SRE, sterol response element; SREBP-1, sterol regulatory element-binding protein-1c.

ACKNOWLEDGMENTS

We thank Drs. Agnieszka Dobrzyn and Makoto Miyazaki for critical review of the manuscript. This work was supported by NIH grant NIDDK-R0162388 (J.M.N.) and American Heart Association Predoctoral fellowship 0415001Z (H.S.).

The *Annual Review of Nutrition* is online at http://nutr.annualreviews.org

LITERATURE CITED

1. Agostoni C, Trojan S, Bellu R, Riva E, Giovannini M. 1995. Neurodevelopment quotient of healthy long term infants at 4 months and feeding practice: the role of long-chain polyunsaturated fatty acids. *Pediatr. Res.* 38:262–66
2. Allman DW, Gibson DM. 1965. Fatty acid synthesis during early linoleic acid deficiency in the mouse. *J. Lipid Res.* 79:51–62
3. Amri EZ, Ailhaud G, Grimaldi P. 1991. Regulation of adipose cell differentiation. II. Kinetics of induction of the aP2 gene by fatty acids and modulation by dexamethasone. *J. Lipid Res.* 32:1457–63
4. Amri EZ, Bertrand B, Ailhaud G, Grimaldi P. 1991. Regulation of adipose cell differentiation. I. Fatty acids are inducers of the aP2 gene expression. *J. Lipid Res.* 32:1449–56

5a. Assimacopoulos-Jeannet F, Thumelin S, Roche E, Esser V, McGarry JD, Prentki M. 1997. Fatty acids rapidly induce the carnitine palmitoyltransferase I gene in the pancreatic beta-cell line INS-1. *J. Biol. Chem.* 272:1659–64

5b. Attie AD, Krauss RM, Gray-Keller MP, Brownlie A, Miyazaki M, et al. 2002. Relationship between stearoyl-CoA desaturase activity and plasma triglycerides in human and mouse hypertriglyceridemia. *J. Lipid Res.* 43:1899–907

6. Berthou L, Saladin R, Yaqoob P, Branellec D, Calder P, et al. 1995. Relation of rat liver apolipoprotein A-I, apolipoprotein A-II and acyl-coenzyme A oxidase gene expression by fibrates and dietary fatty acids. *Eur. J. Biochem.* 232:179–87
7. Bing R, Thelen A, Peters JM, Gonzalez FJ, Jump DB. 1997. Polyunsaturated fatty acid suppression of hepatic fatty acid synthase and S14 gene expression does not required peroxisome proliferator activated receptor α. *J. Biol. Chem.* 272:26827–32
8. Black PN, Faergeman NJ, DiRusso CC. 2000. Long-chain acyl-CoA-dependent regulation of gene expression in bacteria, yeast and mammals. *J. Nutr.* 130:305–9S
9. Brandt JM, Djouadi F, Kelly DP. 1998. Fatty acids activate transcription of the muscle carnitine palmitoyltransferase I gene in cardiac myocytes via the peroxisome proliferator-activated receptor-α. *J. Biol. Chem.* 273:23786–92
10. Deleted in proof
11. Brown MS, Goldstein JL. 1997. The SREBP pathway: regulation of cholesterol metabolism by proteolysis of a membrane-bound transcription factor. *Cell* 89:331–40
12. Brun T, Assimacopoulos-Jeannet F, Crokey BE, Prentki M. 1997. Long-chain fatty acids inhibit acetyl CoA carboxylase gene expression in pancreatic beta-cell line INS-1. *Diabetes* 46:393–400
13. Calder PC. 1997. n-3 Polyunsaturated fatty acids and cytokine production in health and disease. *Ann. Nutr. Metab.* 41:203–34
14. Camandola S, Leonarduzzi G, Musso T, Varesio L, Carini R, et al. 1996. Nuclear

factor κB is activated by arachidonic acid but not by eicosapentanoic acid. *Biochem. Biophys. Res. Commun.* 229: 643–47
15. Chatelain F, Kohl C, Esser V, McGarry JD, Girard J, Pegorier JP. 1996. Cyclic AMP and fatty acids increase carnitine palmitoyltransferase I gene transcription in cultured fetal rat hepatocytes. *Eur. J. Biochem.* 235:789–98
16. Chellappa R, Kandasamy P, Oh CS, Jiang Y, Vemula M, Martin CE. 2001. The membrane proteins, Spt23p and Mga2p, play distinct roles in the activation of *Saccharomyces cerevisiae* OLE1 gene expression. Fatty acid-mediated regulation of Mga2p activity is independent of its proteolytic processing into a soluble transcription activator. *J. Biol. Chem.* 276:43548–56
17. Cho HP, Nakamura MT, Clarke SD. 1999. Cloning, expression and fatty acid regulation of the human delta-5-desaturase. *J. Biol. Chem.* 274:37335–39
18. Cho HP, Nakamura MT, Clarke SD. 1999. Cloning, expression and nutritional regulation of the mammalian delta-6-desaturase. *J. Biol. Chem.* 274: 471–77
19. Clarke SD, Armstrong MK, Jump DB. 1990. Dietary PUFA uniquely suppress rat liver FAS and S14 mRNA content. *J. Nutr.* 120:225–31
20. Clarke SD, Turini M, Jump DB. 1997. Polyunsaturated fatty acids regulate lipogenic and peroxisomal gene expression by independent mechanisms. *Prostaglandins Leukot. Essent. Fatty Acids* 57:65–69
21. Coleman RA, Lwein TM, Muoio DM. 2000. Physiological and nutritional regulation of enzymes of triacylglycerol synthesis. *Annu. Rev. Nutr.* 20:77–103
22. Deleted in proof
23. Daniel PB, Walker WH, Habener JF. 1998. Cyclic AMP signaling and gene regulation. *Annu. Rev. Nutr.* 18:353–83
24. de Deckere EA. 1999. Possible beneficial effect of fish and fish n-3 polyunsaturated fatty acids in breast and colorectal cancer. *Eur. J. Cancer Prev.* 8:213–21
25. Desvergne B, Wahli W. 1999. Peroxisome proliferator-activated receptors: nuclear control of metabolism. *Endocr. Rev.* 20:649–88
26. DeWille JW, Farmer SJ. 1993. Linoleic acid controls neonatal tissue-specific stearoyl CoA desaturase mRNA levels. *Biochim. Biophys. Acta* 1170:291–95
27. Dooley KA, Millinder S, Osborne TF. 1998. Sterol regulation of 3-hydroxy-3-methylglutaryl-coenzyme A synthase gene through a direct interaction between sterol regulatory element binding protein and the trimeric CCAAT-binding factor/nuclear factor Y. *J. Biol. Chem.* 273:1349–56
28. Duplus E, Glorian M, Forest C. 2000. Fatty acid regulation of gene transcription. *J. Biol. Chem.* 275:30749–52
29. Ericsson J, Jackson SM, Edwards PA. 1996. Synergistic binding of sterol regulatory element-binding protein and NF-Y to the farnesyl diphosphate synthase promoter is critical for sterol-regulated expression of the gene. *J. Biol. Chem.* 271:24359–64
30. Finkelstein EA, Fiebelkorn IC, Wang G. 2003. National medical spending attributable to overweight and obesity: How much, and who's paying? *Health Aff.* W3:219–26
31. Forest C, Franckhauser S, Glorian M, Antras-Ferry J, Robin D, Robin P. 1997. Regulation of gene transcription by fatty acids, fibrates and prostaglandins: the phosphoenolpyruvate carboxykinase gene as a model. *Prostaglandins Leukot. Essent. Fatty Acids* 57:47–56
32. Friedman JM. 2002. The function of leptin in nutrition, weight, and physiology. *Nutr. Rev.* 60:S1–14
33. Frohnert BI, Hui TY, Bernlohr DA. 1999. Identification of a functional peroxisome proliferator-responsive element

in the murine fatty acid transport protein gene. *J. Biol. Chem.* 27:3970–77
34. Gabellini N. 2004. Transcriptional regulation by cAMP and Ca^{2+} links the Na^{+}/Ca^{2+} exchanger 3 to memory and sensory pathways. *Mol. Neurobiol.* 30:91–116
35. Gossett RE, Frolov AA, Roths JB, Behnke WD, Kier AB, Schroeder F. 1996. Acyl-CoA binding proteins: multiplicity and function. *Lipids* 31:895–918
36. Gottlicher M, Widmark E, Li Q, Gustafson JA. 1992. Fatty acids activate a chimera of the clofibric acid-activated receptor and the glucocorticoid receptor. *Proc. Natl. Acad. Sci. USA* 89:4653–57
37. Grimaldi PA, Knobel SM, Whitesell RR, Abumrad NA. 1992. Induction of aP2 gene expression by nonmetabolized long-chain fatty acids. *Proc. Natl. Acad. Sci. USA* 89:10930–34
38. Gulick T, Cresci S, Caira T, Moore DD, Kelly DP. 1994. The peroxisome proliferator-activated receptor regulates mitochondrial fatty acid oxidative enzyme gene expression. *Proc. Natl. Acad. Sci. USA* 91:11012–16
39. Hannah VC, Ou J, Luong A, Goldstein JL, Brown MS. 2001. Unsaturated fatty acids downregulate SREBP isoforms 1a and 1c by two mechanisms in HEK293 cells. *J. Biol. Chem.* 276:4365–72
40. Harris WS. 1997. Influence of n-3 fatty acid supplementation on the endogenous activities of plasma lipases. *Am. J. Clin. Nutr.* 65:1645–54S
41. Haugen F, Zahid N, Dalen KT, Hollung K, Nebb HI, Drevon CA. 2005. Resistin expression in 3T3-L1 adipocytes is reduced by arachidonic acid. *J. Lip. Res.* 46:143–53
42. Hayhurst GP, Lee YH, Lamber G, Ward JM, Gonzalez FJ. 2001. Hepatocyte nuclear factor 4α is essential for maintenance of hepatic gene expression and lipid homeostasis. *Mol. Cell. Biol.* 21:1393–403
43. Hertz R, Magenheim J, Berman I, Bar-Tana J. 1998. Fatty acyl-CoA thioesters are ligands of hepatic nuclear receptor 4-alpha. *Nature* 392:512–16
44. Hertz R, Sheena V, Kalderon B, Berman I, Bar-Tana J. 2001. Suppression of hepatic nuclear factor 4-alpha by acyl-CoA thioesters of hypolipidemic peroxisome proliferators. *Biochem. Pharmacol.* 61:1057–62
45a. Hirsch D, Stahl A, Lodish HF. 1998. A family of fatty acid transporters conserved from mycobacterium to man. *Proc. Natl. Acad. Sci. USA* 95:8625–29
45b. Hontecillas R, Wannemeulher MJ, Zimmerman DR, Hutto DL, Wilson JH. 2002. Nutritional regulation of porcine bacterial-induced colitis by conjugated linoleic acid. *J. Nutr.* 132:2019–27
46. Horton JD, Bashmakov Y, Shimomura I, Shimano H. 1998. Regulation of sterol regulatory element binding proteins in livers of fasted and refed mice. *Proc. Nat. Acad. Sci. USA* 95:5987–92
47. Horton JD, Goldstein JL, Brown MS. 2002. SREBPs: activators of the complete program of cholesterol and fatty acid synthesis in the liver. *J. Clin. Invest.* 109:1125–31
48. Hwang D. 2000. Fatty acids and immune responses—a new perspective in searching for clues to mechanism. *Annu. Rev. Nutr.* 20:431–56
49. Deleted in proof
50. Ijpenberg A, Jeannin E, Wahli W, Desvergne B. 1997. Polarity and specific sequence requirements of peroxisome proliferator-activated receptor (PPAR)/retinoid X, receptor heterodimer binding to DNA. A functional analysis of the malic enzyme gene PPAR response element. *J. Biol. Chem.* 272:20108–17
51. Issemann I, Green S. 1990. Activation of a member of the steroid hormone receptor superfamily by peroxisome proliferators. *Nature* 347:645–50
52. Jeffcoat R, James AT. 1978. The control of stearoyl-CoA desaturase by dietary linoleic acid. *FEBS Lett.* 85:114–18

53. Jones B, Maher MA, Banz WJ, Zemel MB, Whelan J, et al. 1996. Adipose tissue stearoyl CoA desaturase mRNA is increased by obesity and decreased by polyunsaturated fatty acids. *Am. J. Physiol.* 34:E44–49
54. Jump DB, Clarke SD. 1999. Regulation of gene expression by dietary fat. *Annu. Rev. Nutr.* 19:63–90
55. Jump DB, Clarke SD, MacDougald OA, Thelen AT. 1993. Polyunsaturated fatty acids inhibit S14 gene transcription in rat liver and cultured hepatocytes. *Proc. Natl. Acad. Sci. USA* 90:8454–58
56. Jump DB, Clarke SD, Thelen AT, Liimata M. 1994. Coordinate regulation of glycolytic and lipogenic gene expression by polyunsaturated fatty acids. *J. Lipid Res.* 35:1076–84
57. Jump DB. 2002. Dietary polyunsaturated fatty acids and regulation of gene transcription. *Curr. Opin. Lipidol.* 13:155–64
58. Deleted in proof
59. Kalant D, Cianflone K. 2004. Regulation of fatty acid transport. *Curr. Opin. Lipidol.* 15:309–14
60. Khalfoun B, Thibault F, Waitier H, Bardos P, Lebranchu Y. 1997. Docosahexanoic acid and eicosapentanoic acids inhibit in vitro human endothelial cell production of interleukin-6. *Adv. Exp. Med. Biol.* 400B:589–97
61. Kim HJ, Miyazaki M, Man WC, Ntambi JM. 2002. Sterol regulatory element-binding proteins (SREBPs) as regulators of lipid metabolism: Polyunsaturated fatty acids oppose cholesterol-mediated induction of SREBP-1 maturation. *Ann. NY Acad. Sci.* 967:34–42
62. Kim JH, Takahashi M, Ezaki O. 1999. Fish oil feeding decreases mature sterol regulatory element-binding protein 1 (SREBP-1) by down-regulation of SREBP1c mRNA in mouse liver. *J. Biol. Chem.* 274:25892–98
63. Kinsella JE, Broughton KS, Whelan JW. 1990. Dietary unsaturated fatty acids: interactions and possible needs in relation to eicosanoids synthesis. *J. Nutr. Biochem.* 1:123–41
64. Lee SS, Pineau T, Drago J, Lee EJ, Owens JW, et al. 1995. Targeted disruption of the α isoform of the peroxisome proliferator-activated receptor gene in mice results in abolishment of the pleiotropic effects of peroxisome proliferators. *Mol. Cell. Biol.* 15:3012–22
65. Lehmann JM, Lenhard JM, Oliver BB, Ringold GM, Kliewer SA. 1997. Peroxisome proliferator-activated receptors α and γ are activated by indomethacin and other non-steroidal anti-inflammatory drugs. *J. Biol. Chem.* 272:3406–10
66. Lu TT, Repa JJ, Mangelsdorf DJ. 2001. Orphan nuclear receptors as eLiXiRs and FiXeRs of sterol metabolism. *J. Biol. Chem.* 276:37735–38
67. Magaña MM, Koo SH, Towle HC, Osborne TF. 2000. Different sterol regulatory element-binding protein-1 isoforms utilize distinct co-regulatory factors to activate the promoter for fatty acid synthase. *J. Biol. Chem.* 275:4726–33
68. Mater MK, Pan D, Bergen WG, Jump DB. 1998. Arachidonic acid inhibits lipogenic gene expression in 3T3-L1 adipocytes through a prostanoid pathway. *J. Lipid Res.* 39:1327–34
69. Mater MK, Thelen A, Pan D, Jump DB. 1999. Sterol response element-binding protein 1c (SREBP1c) is involved in polyunsaturated fatty acid suppression of hepatic S14 gene transcription. *J. Biol. Chem.* 274:32725–32
70. Deleted in proof
71. Meunier-Durmort C, Poirier H, Niot I, Forest C, Besnard P. 1996. Up-regulation of the expression of the gene for liver fatty acid-binding protein by long-chain fatty acids. *Biochem. J.* 319:483–87
72. Millar JS, Maugeais C, Fuki IV, Rader DJ. 2002. Normal production rate of

apolipoprotein B in LDL receptor-deficient mice. *Arterioscler. Thromb. Vasc. Biol.* 22:989–94

73. Miller CW, Ntambi JM. 1996. Peroxisome proliferators induce mouse liver stearoyl-CoA desaturase 1 gene expression. *Proc. Natl. Acad. Sci. USA* 93:9443–48
74. Moon B, Kwan JJ, Sweeney DG, Begum N. 2003. Resistin inhibits glucose uptake in L6 cells independently of changes in insulin signaling and GLUT4 translocation. *Am. J. Physiol. Endocrinol. Metab.* 285:E106–15
75. Motojima K, Passilly P, Peters JM, Gonzalez FJ, Latruffe N. 1998. Expression of putative fatty acid transporter genes are regulated by peroxisome proliferators activated receptor alpha and gamma activators in a tissue- and inducer-specific manner. *J. Biol. Chem.* 273:16710–14
76. Nelson DL, Cox MM. 2005. *Lehninger Principles of Biochemistry*. New York: Freeman. 4th ed.
77. Niot I, Poirier H, Besnard P. 1997. Regulation of gene expression by fatty acids: special reference to fatty acid-binding protein (FABP). *Biochimie* 79:129–33
78. Ntambi JM. 1992. Dietary regulation of stearoyl-CoA desaturase-1 gene expression in mouse liver. *J. Biol. Chem.* 267:10925–30
79. Ntambi JM, Bene H. 2001. Polyunsaturated fatty acid regulation of gene expression. *J. Mol. Neurosci.* 16:273–78
80. Ntambi JM, Choi Y, Park Y, Peters JM, Pariza MW. 2002. Effects of conjugated linoleic acid (CLA) on immune responses, body composition and stearoyl-CoA desaturase. *Can. J. Appl. Physiol.* 27:617–28
81. Ntambi JM, Miyazaki M, Stoehr JP, Lan H, Kendziorski CM, et al. 2002. Loss of stearoyl-CoA desaturase-1 function protects mice against adiposity. *Proc. Natl. Acad. Sci. USA* 99:11482–86
82. Osborne TF. 2000. Sterol regulatory element-binding proteins (SREBPs): key regulators of nutritional homeostasis and insulin action. *J. Biol. Chem.* 275: 32379–82
83. Ou J, Tu H, Shan B, Luk A, DeBose-Boyd RA, et al. 2001. Unsaturated fatty acids inhibit transcription of sterol regulatory element-binding protein 1c (SREBP1c) gene by antagonizing ligand-dependent activation of LXR. *Proc. Natl. Acad. Sci. USA* 98:6027–32

84a. Palmer CN, Hsu MH, Griffin KJ, Rauchy JL, Johnson EF. 1998. Peroxisome proliferators activated receptor-alpha expression in human liver. *Mol. Pharmacol.* 53:14–22

84b. Pan M, Cederbaum AI, Zhang YL, Ginsberg HN, Williams KJ, Fisher EA. 2004. Lipid peroxidation and oxidant stress regulate hepatic apolipoprotein B degradation and VLDL production. *J. Clin. Invest.* 113:1277–87

85. Pawar A, Botolin D, Mangelsdorf DJ, Jump DB. 2003. The role of liver X receptor-α in the fatty acid regulation of hepatic gene expression. *J. Biol. Chem.* 278:40736–43
86. Raclot T, Groscolas R, Langin D, Ferre P. 1997. Site-specific regulation of gene expression by n-3 polyunsaturated fatty acids in rat white adipose tissues. *J. Lipid Res.* 38:1963–72
87. Rahman SM, Dobrzyn A, Dobrzyn P, Lee SH, Miyazaki M, et al. 2003. Stearoyl-CoA desaturase 1 deficiency elevates insulin-signaling components and down-regulates protein-tyrosine phosphatase 1B in muscle. *Proc. Natl. Acad. Sci. USA* 100:11110–15
88. Rambjor GS, Walen AI, Windson SL, Harris WS. 1996. Eicosapentaenoic acid is primarily responsible for hypotriglyceridemic effect of fish oil in humans. *Lipids* 31:S45–49
89. Ren B, Thelen AP, Peters JM, Gonzalez FJ, Jump DB. 1997. Polyunsaturated fatty acid suppression of hepatic fatty acid synthase and S14 gene expression does not require peroxisome

proliferator-activated receptor α. *J. Biol. Chem.* 272:26827–32

90. Repa JJ, Liang G, Ou J, Bashmakov Y, Lobaccaro JM, et al. 2000. Regulation of mouse sterol regulatory element binding protein-1c gene (SREBP-1c) by oxysterol receptors, LXRα and LXRβ. *Genes Dev.* 14:2819–30
91. Reseland JE, Anderssen SA, Solvoll K, Hjerman I, Urdal P, et al. 2001. Effect of long-term changes in diet and exercise on plasma leptin concentrations. *Am. J. Clin. Nutr.* 73:240–45
92. Reseland JE, Haugen F, Hollung K, Solvoll K, Halvorsen B, et al. 2001. Reduction of leptin gene expression by dietary polyunsaturated fatty acids. *J. Lipid Res.* 42:743–50
93. Rose DP. 1997. Effects of dietary fatty acids on breast and prostate cancers: evidence from in vitro experiments and animal studies. *Am. J. Clin. Nutr.* 66S: 1513–22S
94. Rumsey SC, Galeano NF, Lipschitz B, Deckelbaum RJ. 1995. Oleate and other long chain fatty acids stimulate low density lipoprotein receptor activity by enhancing acyl coenzyme A: cholesterol acyltransferase activity and altering intracellular regulatory cholesterol pools in cultured cells. *J. Biol. Chem.* 270:10008–16
95. Salati LM, Clarke SD. 1986. Fatty acid inhibition of hormonal induction of acetyl-Co enzyme A carboxylase in hepatocyte monolayers. *Arch. Biochem. Biophys.* 246:82–90
96. Sampath H, Ntambi JM. 2004. Polyunsaturated fatty acid regulation of gene expression. *Nutr. Rev.* 62:333–39
97. Sanchez HB, Yieh L, Osborne TF. 1995. Cooperation by sterol regulatory element-binding protein and sp1 in sterol regulation of low density lipoprotein receptor gene. *J. Biol. Chem.* 270:1161–69
98. Deleted in proof
99. Schoonjans K, Watanabe M, Suzuki H, Mahfoudi A, Krey G, Wahli W, et al. 1995. Induction of the acyl-coenzyme A synthetase gene by fibrates and fatty acids is mediated by a peroxisome proliferator response element in the C promoter. *J. Biol. Chem.* 270:19269–76
100. Schwartz J. 2000. Role of polyunsaturated fatty acids in lung disease. *Am. J. Clin. Nutr.* 71:393–96

101a. Schwartz RS, Abraham S. 1982. Effect of dietary polyunsaturated fatty acids on the activity and content of fatty acid synthetase in mouse liver. *Biochim. Biophys. Acta* 711:316–26

101b. Sears IB, MacGinnitie MA, Kovacs LG, Graves RA. 1996. Differentiation-dependent expression of the brown adipocyte uncoupling protein gene: regulation by peroxisome proliferator-activated receptor gamma. *Mol. Cell. Biol.* 16:3410–19

102. Sessler AM, Kaur N, Palta JP, Ntambi JM. 1996. Regulation of stearoyl CoA desaturase 1 mRNA stability by polyunsaturated fatty acids in 3T3-L1 adipocytes. *J. Biol. Chem.* 271:29854–58
103. Sessler AM, Ntambi JM. 1998. Polyunsaturated fatty acid regulation of gene expression. *J. Nutr.* 128:923–26
104. Deleted in proof
105. Deleted in proof
106. Siscovick DS, Raghunathan TE, King I, Weinmann S, Bovbjerg VE, et al. 2000. Dietary intake of long-chain polyunsaturated fatty acids and the risk of primary cardiac arrest. *Am. J. Clin. Nutr.* 71:208–12
107. Skerrett PJ, Hennekens CH. 2003. Consumption of fish and fish oils and decreased risk of stroke. *Prev. Cardiol.* 6:38–41
108. Steppan CM, Bailey ST, Bhat S, Brown EJ, Banerjee RR, et al. 2001. The hormone resistin links obesity to diabetes. *Nature* 409:307–12
109. Stuhlmeier KM, Kao JJ, Bach FH. 1997. Arachidonic acid influences proinflammatory gene induction by stabilizing the

inhibitor-κBα/nuclear factor-κB (NF-κB) complex by suppression of the nuclear translocation of NF-κB. *J. Biol. Chem.* 272:24679–83
110. Suresh Y, Das UN. 2003. Long-chain polyunsaturated fatty acids and chemically induced diabetes mellitus. Effect of omega-3 fatty acids. *Nutrition* 19:213–28
111. Tebbey PW, Buttke TM. 1993. Independent arachidonic acid-mediated gene regulatory pathways in lymphocytes. *Biochem. Biophys. Res. Commun.* 194:862–86
112. Tebbey PW, McGowan KM, Stephens JM, Buttke TM, Pekala PH. 1994. Arachidonic acid downregulates the insulin-dependent glucose transporter (GLUT-4) gene in 3T3-L1 adipocytes by inhibiting transcription and enhancing mRNA turnover. *J. Biol. Chem.* 269:639–44
113. Teran-Garcia M, Rufo C, Nakamura MT, Osborne TF, Clarke SD. 2002. NF-Y involvement in the polyunsaturated fat inhibition of fatty acid synthase gene transcription. *Biochem. Biophys. Res. Commun.* 290:1295–99
114. Tontonoz P, Hu E, Devine J, Beale EG, Spiegelman BM. 1995. PPAR gamma 2 regulates adipose expression of the phosphoenolpyruvate carboxykinase gene. *Mol. Cell Biol.* 15:351–57
115. Tontonoz P, Hu E, Graves RA, Budavari AI, Spiegelman BM. 1994. mPPAR 2: tissue-specific regulator of an adipocyte enhancer. *Genes Dev.* 8:1224–34
116. Ventura MA, Woollett LA, Spady DK. 1989. Dietary fish oil stimulates hepatic low density lipoprotein transport in the rat. *J. Clin. Invest.* 84:528–37
117. von Schacky C. 2000. n-3 Fatty acids and the prevention of coronary atherosclerosis. *Am. J. Clin. Nutr.* 71:224–27
118. Wahle KW, Radcliffe JD. 1977. Effect of a diet rich in sunflower oil on aspects of lipid metabolism in the genetically obese rat. *Lipids* 12:135–39
119. Wahle KW, Rotondo D, Heys SD. PUFA and gene expression in mammalian systems. *Proc. Nutr. Soc.* 62:349–60
120. Worgall TS, Johnson RA, Seo T, Gierens H, Deckelbaum RJ. 2002. Unsaturated fatty acid-mediated decreases in sterol regulatory element-mediated gene transcription are linked to cellular sphingolipid metabolism. *J. Biol. Chem.* 277:3878–85
121. Worgall TS, Sturley SL, Soe T, Osborne TF, Deckelbaum RJ. 1998. Polyunsaturated fatty acids decrease expression of promoters with sterol regulatory elements by decreasing levels of sterol regulatory element-binding protein. *J. Biol. Chem.* 273:23537–40
122. Xu J, Nakamura MN, Cho HP, Clarke S. 1999. Sterol regulatory element binding protein-1 expression is suppressed by dietary polyunsaturated fatty acids. *J. Biol. Chem.* 274:23577–83
123. Yahagi N, Shimano H, Hasty AH, Amemiya-Kudo M, Okazaki H, et al. 1999. A crucial role of sterol regulatory element-binding protein-1 in the regulation of lipogenic gene expression by polyunsaturated fatty acids. *J. Biol. Chem.* 274:35840–44
124. Yamagata K, Furuta H, Oda N, Kaisaki PJ, Menzel S, et al. 1996. Mutations in the hepatocyte nuclear factor-4α gene in maturity-onset diabetes of the young (MODY1). *Nature* 384:458–60
125. Yoshikawa T, Ide T, Shimano H, Yahagi N, Amemiya-Kudo M, et al. 2003. Cross-talk between peroxisome proliferator-activated receptor (PPAR) alpha and liver X receptor (LXR) in nutritional regulation of fatty acid metabolism. I. PPARs suppress sterol regulatory element binding protein-1c promoter through inhibition of LXR signaling. *Mol. Endocrinol.* 17:1240–54
126. Yoshikawa T, Shimano H, Amemiya-Kudo M, Yahagi N, Hasty AH, et al. 2001. Identification of liver X receptor-retinoid X receptor as an activator of the

sterol regulatory element binding protein 1c gene promoter. *Mol. Cell. Biol.* 21:2991–3000

127. Yoshikawa T, Shimano H, Yahagi N, Ide T, Amemiya-Kudo M, et al. 2002. Polyunsaturated fatty acids suppress sterol regulatory element binding protein 1c promoter activity by inhibition of liver X receptor (LXR) binding to LXR response elements. *J. Biol. Chem.* 277:1705–11

128. Zhao Y, Joshi-Barve S, Barve S, Chen LH. 2004. Eicosapentaenoic acid prevents LPS-induced TNF-alpha expression by preventing NF-κB activation. *J. Am. Coll. Nutr.* 23:71–78

Annu. Rev. Nutr. 2005. 25:341–90
doi: 10.1146/annurev.nutr.25.050304.092656

SINGLE NUCLEOTIDE POLYMORPHISMS THAT INFLUENCE LIPID METABOLISM: Interaction with Dietary Factors

Dolores Corella[1,2] and Jose M. Ordovas[1]
[1]Nutrition and Genomics Laboratory, Jean Mayer–U.S. Department of Agriculture Human Nutrition Research Center on Aging at Tufts University, Boston, Massachusetts 02111, and the [2]Genetic and Molecular Epidemiology Unit, School of Medicine, University of Valencia, Valencia 46010 Spain; email: dolores.corella@uv.es, jose.ordovas@tufts.edu

Key Words cholesterol, genes, nutrition, prevention, cardiovascular

■ **Abstract** Cardiovascular disease (CVD) risk is the result of complex interactions between genetic and environmental factors. During the past few decades, much attention has focused on plasma lipoproteins as CVD risk factors. The current evidence supports the concept that gene-environment interactions modulate plasma lipid concentrations and potentially CVD risk. The findings from studies examining gene-diet interactions and lipid metabolism have been highly promising. Several loci (i.e., APOA1, APOA4, APOE, and LIPC) are providing proof-of-concept for the potential application of genetics in the context of personalized nutritional recommendations for CVD prevention. However, the incorporation of these findings to the clinical environment is not ready for prime time. There is a compelling need for replication using a higher level of scientific evidence. Moreover, we need to evolve from the simple scenarios examined nowadays (i.e., one single dietary component, single nucleotide polymorphism, and risk factor) to more realistic situations involving interactions between multiple genes, dietary components, and risk factors. In summary, there is need for both large population studies and well-standardized intervention studies.

CONTENTS

0199-9885/05/0714-0341$20.00

INTRODUCTION

Lipoprotein metabolism comprises complex biological pathways. Their homeostasis is achieved by the coordinated action of a large number of nuclear factors, binding proteins, apolipoproteins, enzymes, and receptors (Figure 1). These pathways are also intertwined with energy metabolism and are subjected to hormonal controls that are essential for adjustment to environmental and internal conditions. Lipoprotein metabolism is commonly subdivided into three components: the exogenous pathway, the endogenous pathway, and the reverse cholesterol transport.

Figure 1 Human lipoprotein metabolism. Abbreviations: AI, apolipoprotein A-I; AII, apolipoprotein A-II; AIV, apolipoprotein A-IV; AV, apolipoprotein A-V; ABCA1, ATP-binding cassette, subfamily A, member 1; ABCG5, ATP-binding cassette, subfamily G, member 5; ABCG8, ATP-binding cassette, subfamily G, member 8; ACAT2, cytosolic acetoacetyl-CoA thiolase; apo, apolipoprotein; APOBEC1, apolipoprotein B mRNA editing enzyme; B48, apolipoprotein B-48; B100, apolipoprotein B-100; CII, apolipoprotein C-II; CIII, apolipoprotein C-III; CD36, CD36 antigen; CE, cholesteryl esters; CETP, cholesteryl ester transfer protein; chylos, chylomicron; chylo-R, chylomicron remnants; CYP7A1, cholesterol-7-alpha-hydroxylase; E, apolipoprotein E; FA, fatty acid; FABP2, intestinal fatty acid–binding protein; FFA, free fatty acid; HDL, high-density lipoprotein; HMGCR, 3-hydroxy-3-methylglutaryl-CoA reductase; HTGL, hepatic triglyceride lipase; IDL, intermediate density lipoproteins; LDL, low-density lipoprotein; LDLR, LDL receptor; Lp(a), lipoprotein a; LPL, lipoprotein lipase; mmLDL, minimally modified LDL; MTP, microsomal triglyceride transfer protein; NPC1L1, Niemann-Pick C1-like 1; oxLDL, oxidized LDL; PLTP, phospholipid transfer protein; SCARB1, scavenger receptor type I B; Sit, sitosterol; TG, triglycerides; UC, unesterified cholesterol; VLDL, very-low-density lipoprotein.

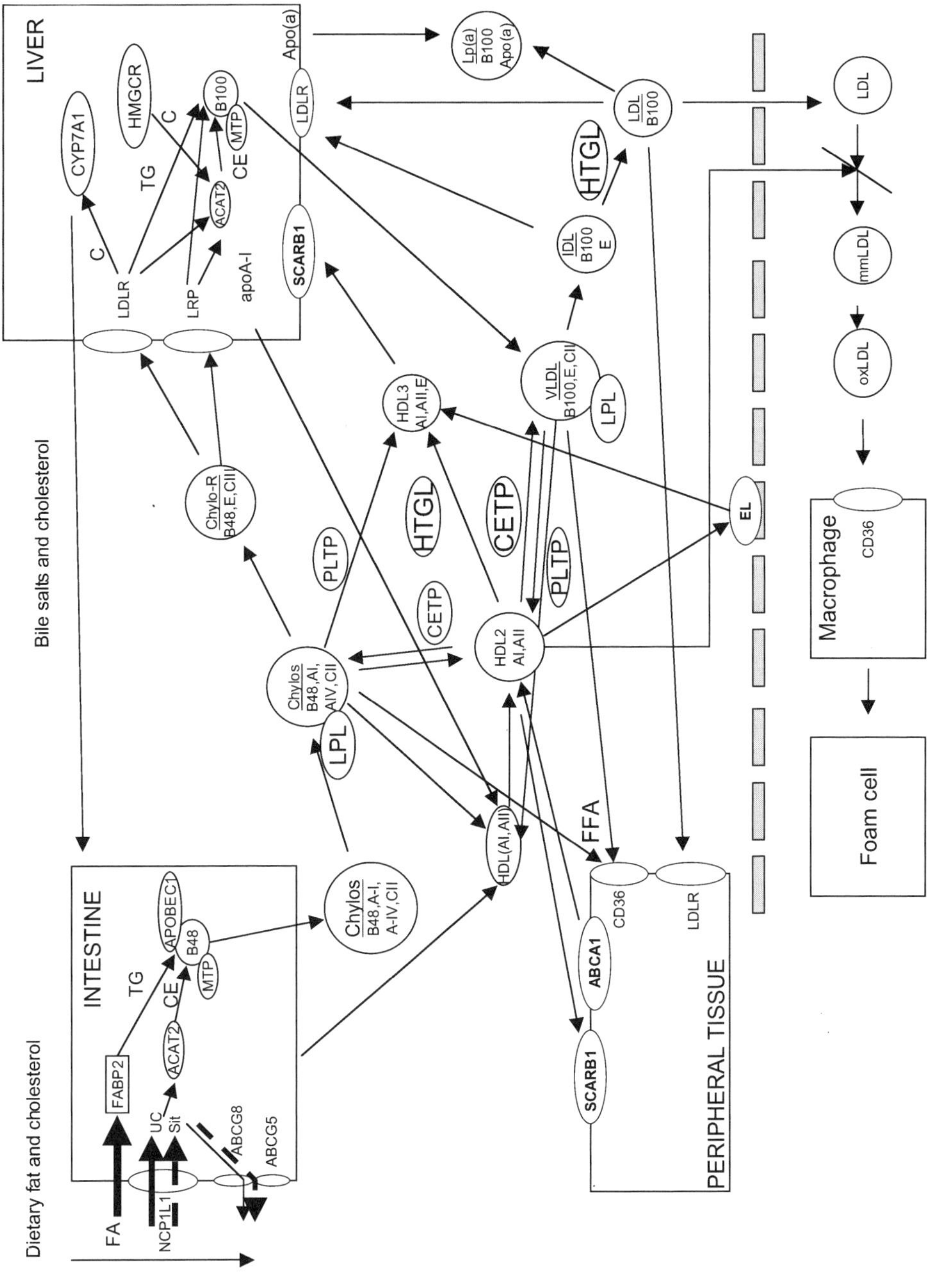
Dietary fat and cholesterol
Bile salts and cholesterol
LIVER
CYP7A1
HMGCR
C
TG
C
ACAT2
CE
MTP
B100
LDLR
LRP
apoA-I
SCARB1
LDLR
Apo(a)
Lp(a) B100 Apo(a)
LDL B100
HTGL
IDL B100 E
VLDL B100,E,CII
LPL
HDL3 AI,AII,E
HTGL
CETP
PLTP
CETP
PLTP
HDL2 AI,AII
Chylo-R B48,E,CII
Chylos B48,AI, AIV,CII
LPL
HDL(AI,AII)
EL
FFA
LDL
mmLDL
oxLDL
Macrophage
CD36
Foam cell
INTESTINE
TG
CE
APOBEC1
B48
MTP
ACAT2
FABP2
UC
Sit
ABCG8
ABCG5
FA
NCP1L1
Chylos B48,A-I, A-IV,CII
CD36
LDLR
ABCA1
SCARB1
PERIPHERAL TISSUE

Metabolism of Lipoproteins Carrying Exogenous Lipids

Most of our knowledge about the relation between plasma lipid concentrations and cardiovascular disease (CVD) risk comes from studies in the fasting state. However, humans are almost continuously in the postprandial state. The increased awareness of the atherogenic properties of postprandial triglyceride-rich lipoproteins (TRLs) and the dramatic interindividual variability in the postprandial lipoprotein response have stimulated research to gain more in-depth knowledge about the genetic and nongenetic factors modulating absorption, transport, and catabolism of dietary lipids (46, 50, 81). Dietary fats represent 30%–40% of the energy intake in the Western world, mostly in the form of triacylglycerols (TAGs) (~100 g per day). Under normal circumstances, the digestive system is very efficient in both digesting and absorbing the TAGs. Several enzymes contribute to the degradation, with most of the activity being driven by pancreatic lipase in the duodenum. Following its absorption into the enterocyte, fatty acids are transported intracellularly by the intestinal fatty acid–binding protein (IFBP). Then the resynthesis of TAGs for assembly of chylomicrons (CMs) occurs predominantly in the *sn*2-monoacylglycerol pathway and (in a lesser amount) in the glycerol-3-phosphate pathway. TAG synthesis occurs primarily in the smooth endoplasmic reticulum (SER) (76).

Cholesterol is another major dietary lipid absorbed in the enterocyte. Its homeostasis is maintained by a delicate equilibrium between dietary cholesterol absorption, de novo synthesis, and fecal excretion (46). The process of intestinal cholesterol absorption from foods has been difficult to understand, and only very recently, specific sterol carriers have been identified and characterized, such as the Niemann-Pick C1-like 1 (NPC1L1) (1, 29). In addition, other proteins, such as the scavenger receptor type I B (SCARB1) (61) and the ABC transporters (ABCG5 and ABCG8) (87), have been implicated in cholesterol absorption.

Both dietary TAG and cholesterol are secreted into the bloodstream as part of CM particles (101). The apolipoproteins associated with nascent CMs are apoB48, apoA-I, apoA-IV, apoC-II, and apoC-III. CM synthesis requires apoB48, which is translated from an apoB100 mRNA that is post-transcriptionally edited to end protein synthesis at codon 2153. This involves enzymatic deamination through the action of apoB mRNA editing enzyme (APOBEC1) (33). Microsomal triglyceride transfer protein (MTP) plays an important role in this process by binding to apoB and determining the complete synthesis and lipidation of nascent apoB when enough lipids are available (49). CMs are secreted into lymph vessels and then enter the blood circulation. Once the intestinal lipoproteins are in contact with other plasma lipoproteins [i.e., high-density lipoproteins (HDLs)], there is rapid transfer of proteins and lipid subfractions in order to facilitate their metabolic fate, which occurs in two main steps. First, the TAGs of CMs are hydrolyzed by lipoprotein lipase (LPL) in extrahepatic tissues to form CM remnants. CM remnants are removed from the plasma by hepatic receptors that bind to the apoE present in the particle (101).

Endogenous Lipoprotein Metabolism

The liver is the central organ for endogenous lipoprotein metabolism, beginning with the synthesis of very-low-density lipoproteins (VLDLs). As early as 1976, Havel & Kane (40) provided the basis for our understanding of VLDL assembly and secretion by proposing a mechanism involving the fusion of newly synthesized apoB with a droplet of TAG produced in the SER compartment. Most of the TAG utilized for the assembly of VLDL in the secretory apparatus of the hepatocyte is mobilized by lipolysis of the cytosolic TAG pool, followed by re-esterification. The lipases involved include arylacetamide deacetylase and/or TAG hydrolase. Some of the re-esterified products of lipolysis gain access to an apoB-rich VLDL precursor to form mature VLDL. Some, however, are returned to the cytosolic pool in a process that is stimulated by insulin and inhibited by MTP. Phospholipids also contribute to VLDL TAG in a process that involves ADP-ribosylation factor-1 (ARF-1)-mediated activation of phospholipase D. Phospholipases may prime membrane transport steps required for second-step fusion and/or channel phospholipids into a pathway for VLDL triglyceride production. VLDL production is controlled primarily at the level of presecretory degradation. Recently, it was discovered that the LDL receptor modulates VLDL production through its interactions with nascent VLDL in the secretory pathway (36). VLDL particles are precursors of intermediate-density lipoproteins and finally of LDL particles. LDL is known to be heterogeneous, comprising a number of distinct subpopulations defined on the basis of a number of characteristics, including particle density, size, charge, and chemical composition (60).

Reverse Cholesterol Transport

The classical HDL-dependent protective mechanism involves promoting efflux of excess cholesterol from cells in the arterial wall and returning it to the liver for excretion into the bile, a process known as reverse cholesterol transport. HDL is synthesized by both the liver and the intestine. Its precursor form is discoidal in shape and matures in circulation as it picks up unesterified cholesterol, and probably phospholipids, from cell membranes by a mechanism mediated by the ATP-binding cassette, subfamily A, member 1 (ABCA1) transporter. Unesterified cholesterol is esterified to cholesteryl ester within the HDL particle by the enzyme lecithin-cholesterol acyltransferase (LCAT) and the small HDL3 particle becomes a larger HDL2 particle. HDL cholesteryl ester can be taken up selectively by the liver or by organs synthesizing steroid hormones, such as the adrenals, through the action of the scavenger receptor class B type I (SCARB1). Cholesteryl ester can also be selectively transferred to apoB-containing lipoproteins in exchange for TAG through the action of cholesteryl ester transfer protein (CETP). Conversely, phospholipid transfer protein (PLTP) mediates transfer of phospholipids from apoB-containing lipoproteins to HDL. The TAG received by HDL2 is hydrolyzed by hepatic lipase and the particle is converted back to HDL3, completing the HDL cycle in plasma. Other members of the family of triglyceride lipase genes also influence the metabolism of HDL (3, 4, 22).

CANDIDATE GENES FOR LIPID METABOLISM

Genetic variability has been identified in humans for all the known lipid-related genes, and some of those variants have been studied for the past two decades, resulting in a plethora of reports and associations with abnormal lipid metabolism and plasma lipoprotein profiles. A detailed description of the biological role of each of the products from those candidate genes is beyond the scope of this review; they have been the focus of other publications (13, 69, 82). Some of the most important known genes involved in lipoprotein metabolism are ABCA1; ATP-binding cassette, subfamily G, member 5 (ABCG5); ATP-binding cassette, subfamily G, member 8 (ABCG8); acetylcholesterol acyltransferase 1 (ACAT1); cytosolic acetoacetyl-CoA thiolase (ACAT2); APOA1; APOA2; APOA4; APOA5; APOB; APOBEC1; APOCI; APOC2; APOC3; APOC4; APOE; APOH; APOJ; APOL1–APOL6; putative low-density lipoprotein (LDL) receptor adaptor protein (ARH); CD36 antigen (CD36); CCAAT/enhancer-binding protein-alpha (CEBPA); CETP; cubilin (CUBN); cholesterol-7-alpha-hydroxylase (CYP7A1); estrogen receptor 1 (ERS1); intestinal fatty acid binding protein (FABP2); 3-hydroxy-3-methylglutaryl-CoA reductase (HMGCR); LCAT; hepatic lipase (LIPC); hormone-sensitive lipase (LIPE); endothelial lipase (LIPG); lipoprotein a (LPA); LDL receptor (LDLR); lipoprotein lipase (LPL); low-density lipoprotein receptor-related protein 1 (LRP1); LRP2; LRP5; liver X receptor-alpha (LXRA); MTP; NPC1L1; low-density lipoprotein, oxidized, receptor 1 (OLR1); perilipin (PLIN); phospholipid transfer protein (PLTP); paroxonase 1 and 2 (PON1 and PON2); peroxisome-proliferator activator receptor-alpha (PPARA); PPAR-delta (PPARD); PPAR-gamma (PPARG); SCARB1; retinoid X receptor-alpha (RXRA); SREBP cleavage-activating protein (SCAP); sterol regulatory element–binding protein 1 (SREBP1); upstream stimulatory factor protein 1 (USF1), and VLDL receptor (VLDLR). This list is not, by any means, closed. In fact, its ranks are being continuously populated with new candidate genes emerging from the active research ongoing in this area. When it comes to the associations of genetic variants at these loci with plasma lipid levels in the general population, the genes with findings that are more consistent are the APOE in terms of associations with total cholesterol and LDL-C concentrations (38, 86), CETP with HDL-C levels (80), and the LPL and APOA5 loci with TAG levels (47, 91, 118). Most other loci have shown significant associations with different plasma lipids; however, for many of them there is lack of replication, producing doubts about their significance as global genetic markers. Moreover, most of them have to be tested in the context of gene-environment interactions.

There is still some confusion concerning the nomenclature of the identified gene variants (mutations or polymorphisms). To prevent this confusion some authors

(2) recommend using the terms "sequence variant" or "allelic variant" for any genomic change regardless of their frequency of phenotypic effects. However, in large epidemiological studies, the term "polymorphism" is still used as it was originally defined (a locus in which the least common allele occurs with a frequency of at least 1%). Thus, polymorphisms can be caused by mutations ranging from a single nucleotide base change to variations in several hundred bases, such as large deletions and/or insertions. The simpler and most common type of polymorphism, known as single nucleotide polymorphism (SNP), results from a single base mutation replacing one base for another. SNPs are estimated to represent about 90% of all human DNA polymorphisms. SNPs occur with a very high frequency, with estimates ranging from about 1 in 1000 bases to 1 in 100–300. Overall, it has been estimated that the human genome contains about ten million SNPs (18). Not long ago, the number of identified polymorphisms in candidate genes for lipid metabolism was small and there were dozens of studies focusing on a very limited number of specific genetic variants in different populations. This provided the opportunity to check the replication of the observed associations and potentially to increase the level of evidence, as in the case of the association between the *APOE* polymorphism and plasma LDL-C (86).

Currently, the vast number of SNPs available for candidate genes adds a level of complexity to the data interpretation as more investigators may focus their association studies on different SNP sets even for a single locus. In this regard, Humphries et al. (48) have strongly recommended making a distinction between functional SNPs (i.e., those altering an amino sequence or a transcription factor-binding element) and nonfunctional SNPs to avoid the use of nonfunctional genetic variants in association studies. They suggested that before SNPs are included in an epidemiological study, their functionality should be supported by good in vitro data. However, as these in vitro data may be difficult to obtain, some researchers have proposed the use of bioinformatic tools to infer functionality (100). One of the problems with the results obtained from association studies using apparently nonfunctional SNPs (that in some cases act as markers of the unknown functional variant) is their different degree of linkage disequilibrium with the true functional SNP among different populations (78). Thus, a nonfunctional variant may have a different impact in association studies depending on the linkage disequilibrium with the functional polymorphism and thus would contribute to the lack of replication of these studies in different populations. Lack of replication is the most excruciating problem in the hundreds of published reports of gene-lipid associations involving lipid metabolism (51). However, an important cause of variability is the potential influence of environmental factors. Moreover, taking into account the classical definition of phenotype (observable physical or biochemical characteristics of an organism, determined by both genetic makeup and environmental influences), an important reason to explain the controversial findings from studies involving genotype-phenotype association is that the majority of initial studies analyzing the association between SPNs and lipid traits did not consider the potential gene-environment interactions.

REGULATION OF LIPID METABOLISM: GENES VERSUS ENVIRONMENT

The homeostasis of lipid metabolism is the result of interactions between multiple genes and environmental (nongenetic) factors. Although currently there are no precise estimates about the specific contribution of genetic and environmental factors (tobacco smoking, alcohol consumption, dietary intake, physical activity, etc.) to dyslipidemia, it is thought that there are very few cases in which alterations of lipid metabolism are induced by genetic variation that will develop regardless of environmental factors. Even in those cases, environmental factors may affect the age of onset and severity of the disease (8). Overall, gene-environment interaction refers to the differential phenotypic effects of different environments on individuals with the same genotype or to the differential effects of the same environment on individuals with different genotypes (88). Genetic variation and the different individuals' responses to environmental factors present an opportunity and a challenge to cardiovascular prevention. On the other hand, some researchers prefer to use the concept of "context-dependent" genetic effect that involves gene-gene interactions (epistasis) as well as gene-environment interactions (56). Whether as a specific term, or integrated in the context-dependent concept, the study of gene-environment interactions will largely contribute to deciphering the underlying mechanisms for lipid-related disorders and to facilitating cardiovascular disease prevention. Along these lines, from a public health perspective, nutrition is the most important environmental factor interacting with our genes to increase or decrease the likelihood of developing lipid disorders.

The interactions involving dietary factors are called gene-diet interactions. Although the presence of a genetic component determining the differences in interindividual dietary response to specific nutritional recommendations and dietary interventions has been proposed for several decades (44), it has not been until recent years that researchers began to explore its molecular basis. In the next sections, a detailed description of the fundamentals and the main recent examples of gene-diet interactions involving lipid metabolism is provided.

GENE-DIET INTERACTIONS

Interindividual Variability

It is well known that the effect of dietary changes on plasma lipid concentrations differs significantly between individuals (53, 58). Some individuals (hyporesponders) appear to be relatively insensitive to dietary intervention, whereas others (hyperresponders) have enhanced sensitivity (57). In assessing the impact of these different interindividual responses to the same diet, Schaefer et al. (106) reported the effects of National Cholesterol Education Program (NCEP) Step 2 diets on plasma lipoprotein profiles in 72 men and 48 women. Compared with the baseline diet (an average American diet), consumption of an NCEP Step 2 diet was associated with significant decreases in LDL-C and HDL-C in both men and women. However, a large variability in lipid response to the diet was observed, with changes in LDL cholesterol ranging from +3% to −55% in men and from +13% to −39% in women. On average, such diets do achieve significant reductions of LDL-C concentrations; however, the magnitude of change varies substantially among individuals, with many showing either little change or even increases in LDL-C. From these data, it is clear that what is good at the population level is not necessarily good at the individual level. Moreover, low-fat diets can also result in reduced plasma HDL and/or increased TAG concentrations (58) that may be particularly harmful for some subjects. For example, it has been shown that individuals with a predominance of small, dense LDL particles (subclass pattern B), a phenotype that is associated with an increased risk of coronary heart disease, benefit more from a low-fat diet (59, 60) than do those with the subclass pattern A (larger LDL). Indeed, the latter group exhibited a more atherogenic pattern B subclass after consuming a low-fat diet. Currently there is still substantial controversy about what is the best diet to prevent heart diseases: the traditionally recommended low-fat diet, the Mediterranean diet based on a relatively high contribution of monounsaturated fatty acids (MUFAs), or even the emerging low-carbohydrate diet (20). However, although the general dietary recommendations have partially addressed the problem of special populations (i.e., children, pregnant women, elderly subjects), a key factor that has not been taken into account is the individual variation concerning such general recommendations. In this regard, increasing numbers of intervention studies are focusing on the interindividual differences in response to diet rather than showing the mean effect. The results of these studies show repeatedly the aforementioned dramatic variability in responses to diets designed to change plasma lipid profile. Moreover, increasing evidence supports that this variability in response is an intrinsic characteristic of the individual rather than the result of different dietary compliance with the experimental protocols. One of these studies, recently published by Jacobs et al. (52), demonstrates that individual TAG responses to a high-fat or to a low-fat diet are vastly different. Whereas some subjects have distinctly lower plasma TAG concentrations after consuming a high-fat diet, others had clearly lower TAG concentrations after consuming a low-fat diet. The authors suggest that many patients with hypertriglyceridemia are not treated optimally if general advice for either a low-fat or a high-fat diet is given; they conclude that the most beneficial alternative is to fit a dietary recommendation to each patient individually based on the patient's response to a low-fat or a high-fat diet (52). Therefore, studying the reasons for this variation in response to diet will allow us to better identify individuals who can benefit from a particular dietary intervention. Obviously, this is not an easy task. Parks et al. (90) proposed the use of an algorithm (discriminant function analysis) to predict which patients would experience significant elevations in plasma TAG after consuming a very low-fat, high-carbohydrate diet. Although three variables (baseline body mass index, fasting TAG, and insulin concentrations) accurately classified 90% of those who would experience an elevation in TAG $\geq$ 10% ($P < 0.05$) and 67% of those who experienced no change in the Parks et al. study (90), the predictive algorithm was not useful in subsequent studies (52).

Currently, considerable support exists for the notion that the interindividual variability in response to dietary modification is determined by genetic factors, especially for lipid and lipoprotein phenotypes (65). Indirect evidence supporting this hypothesis comes from the general observation that the phenotypic response to diet is determined partly by the baseline value of the phenotype that is itself affected by genetic factors (5, 58). However, taking into account the complexity of lipid metabolism, the main problem is how to uncover and elucidate the many potential gene-diet interactions.

Measurement of Gene-Diet Interaction

The nature versus nurture controversy in lipid metabolism is being replaced by systematic evaluation of nature-nurture interaction. Methods used in genetics and epidemiology to study gene-environment interaction continue to evolve, and both unmeasured genotype approach (genetic epidemiology) and measured genotype approach (molecular epidemiology) have been used to detect gene-environment interactions in humans. The unmeasured genotype approach is based on statistical analysis of the distribution of phenotypes in individuals and families and does not rely on any direct measure of DNA variation (30). The purpose of such studies is to provide clues to the importance of genetic factors embodied in the concept of heritability and measured by analysis of variance or correlation. No specific genes are measured at this stage. Heritability is defined as the proportion of phenotypic variance attributable to genetic variance. A value of 1.0 indicates that all of the population variation is attributable to genetic variation. A value of 0.0 indicates that genes do not contribute at all to phenotypic individual differences. The quantity (1.0 minus heritability) gives the environmental contribution to the trait, and it is the proportion of phenotypic variance attributable to environmental variance or the extent to which individual differences in the environment contribute to individual differences in behavior. Several twin and family studies have analyzed the genetic and environmental influence on lipid traits (42).

With advances in molecular genetics, the study of gene-environment interactions is now performed at the gene level. With this approach, genetic variation in one or in various candidate genes is investigated to discern the role of these candidate genes in determining gene-diet interactions. Direct measurement of DNA variants (i.e., SNPs) is needed to give precision and meaning to the genetic effects in gene-diet interactions. The concept of gene-diet interactions can be used in several different ways (37, 105). For example, statistical interaction exists if the degree or direction of the effect of one dietary factor (e.g., dietary fat) differs according to values of a second factor (gene variants). In recent years, an epidemiologic framework for evaluating gene-diet interaction has been proposed (9). In a simple gene-diet interaction model, in which both the susceptibility genotype at a single locus and the dietary exposure are considered dichotomous, one can construct an extended 2-by-2 table incorporating genetic and environment factors in studying disease etiology (e.g., hypercholesterolemia). The interaction of these two factors can be measured as a departure from a multiplicative model of disease risk (12, 105). Using such an approach, it is relatively easy to find parsimonious models by keeping statistical interactions to a minimum. However, in the study of lipid metabolism, rather than dichotomous traits, it is common to predict continuous variables such as plasma cholesterol concentrations as well as to analyze continuous variables to measure dietary intake. Then, in addition to a logistic regression model, covariance regression models with interaction terms are needed (12). Hierarchical multilevel interaction models then can be fitted, and the presence of a gene-diet interaction is identified by the detection of a statistically significant interaction term between the dietary exposure and the corresponding genetic variable. However, from a strict point of view it is not clear what ultimately constitutes interaction or synergy on the biological level; any statistical approach is inherently arbitrary and model-dependent (37).

Methodological Issues in Assessing Gene-Diet Interaction

Gene-diet interactions in epidemiological studies are currently detected based on the statistical significance of the interaction terms. Taking into account that a statistically significant association does not imply causality, special attention to bias is required. This issue is crucial and determines the study design as well as adequate control of misspecification. In terms of study design, intervention studies—mainly randomized controlled trials—offer the highest level of evidence (62). In intervention studies, as opposed to observational studies, the study conditions are controlled directly by the investigators, including the amount of food or nutrient administered as well as the time period. This control minimizes the possibility of bias and increases the level of causality. However, in observational studies (i.e., cohort, case-control, cross-sectional), the researcher does not provide food to study participants and obtains information about the type and amount of food consumed by dietary questionnaires, a method that increases the likelihood of confounding and decreases the level of evidence provided. However, some authors have pointed out the importance of Mendelian randomization (the random assortment of genes from parents to offspring that occurs during gamete formation and conception) in increasing the level of evidence provided by observational studies in which genetic polymorphisms are determined and dietary intake is estimated (28). Mendelian randomization can increase the level of evidence of observational studies because it results in population distributions of genetic variants that are generally independent of environmental factors that typically confound epidemiological associations between putative risk factors and disease. In some circumstances, this can provide a study design akin to randomized comparisons. In fact, Tobin et al. (114) have suggested that the approach should be termed "Mendelian deconfounding."

Misclassification of Dietary Exposures

Precise measurement of an individual's exposure to dietary factors is often difficult because of the individual's poor recall or ignorance of previous exposures, the complex pattern of nutrient intake, and the lack of good biological indicators of exposure levels for many nutrients. Therefore, in the study of gene-diet interaction, the consequences of a dietary mismeasurement can lead to bias in the estimation associated with interaction effects and possible loss of precision and power in the estimation of interactions. Nondifferential misclassification usually leads to biases of interaction toward the null value, and differential misclassification may produce biased interactions in either direction (increasing or decreasing risk). Therefore, high-quality dietary information in epidemiological studies is a key factor for establishing causality. More information about validity of the specific dietary instruments (i.e., diet records, 24-hour recalls, food-frequency questionnaires) can be found in Reference (83). In addition, another important question to be raised relates to which type of dietary information is more relevant in gene-diet interaction studies. Should we be using nutrients, foods, or dietary patterns? There is not a unique response, and it depends on the aims of the study and on the specific hypothesis that is under investigation. Each one of these approaches has advantages and methodological limitations (83).

Misclassification of Genetic Data

When measuring individuals' genotypes at the DNA level, misclassification can occur as the result of several factors. One of them is error in the laboratory determination. With the application of high-throughput methods, a number of which are under development, quality control procedures in the laboratory are particularly important. A misclassification of the genotype (i.e., a data set containing less than 95% reproducibility) can bias the measure of the association and largely affect gene-nutrient interactions. Quality control measures include internal validation, blinding, duplicates, test failure rate, inspection of whether genotype frequencies conform to Hardy-Weinberg equilibrium, and blinding of data entry (64). Another factor that may contribute to misclassification of genetic data is linkage disequilibrium. In addition to these factors, in the last few years it has been proposed that individual SNPs are not the best approach to measure the individual's genotype; the simultaneous analysis of different genetic variants (haplotypic approach) has been suggested as more appropriate (102). Moreover, Neale et al. (78) propose a shift toward a gene-based approach in which all genetic variants in the intragenic and regulatory regions of a candidate gene are considered jointly.

Sample Size Considerations

One of the most frequent errors in epidemiological studies aimed at investigating gene-diet interactions in lipid metabolism is the lack of statistical power (Type II error). In an epidemiological study of a given sample size, the power to detect statistical interactions is less than the power to detect main effects, and the variance of the interaction estimate also will be greater than the variance of the main effects estimate under a no-interaction model. More information about sample size and power calculation needed to detect gene-environment interaction for categorical and continuous variables can be found in Reference (35).

Nutrigenetics and Nutrigenomics

In the field of gene-diet interactions, two different concepts have emerged: nutrigenetics and nutrigenomics. Nutrigenetics examines the effect of genetic variation (mainly SNPs) on the interaction between diet and specific phenotypes. This includes the identification of gene variants associated with differential responses to nutrients. The goal of nutrigenetics is to generate recommendations regarding the risks and benefits to the individual of specific dietary components. It has been also termed "personalized nutrition." Nutrigenomics focuses on the effect of nutrients on the genome, proteome, and metabolome. Nutrigenomics involves the characterization of gene products and the physiological function and interactions of these products, promoting an increased understanding of how nutrition influences metabolic pathways and homeostatic control (77, 119). Several approaches are available for analyzing the effects of dietary factors, including differential gene expression, as well as proteomic methods to determine changes in protein levels and protein modifications (116). The role of genes implicated in lipid metabolism may be further studied by developing transgenic and gene-targeted animals treated with different diets, as well as by using other gene expression strategies. The combination of these technologies will contribute to the study of the function and nutritional regulation of different lipid metabolism–related genes as well as to the identification of new targets for therapeutic approaches (77).

LESSONS FROM MONOGENIC DISORDERS

Monogenic disorders are highly penetrant; however, even for these diseases there is evidence of dietary modulation having significant effects over the expression of the mutation and the disease risk associated with the genetic defect. The classical example involves familial hypercholesterolemia (FH). FH is a codominant inherited disorder of lipid metabolism characterized by very high concentrations of LDL-C, tendon xanthomas, *arcus lipoides corneae*, and increased risk of premature coronary heart disease (7). The clinical phenotype is more severe for homozygotes than for heterozygotes. Fortunately, homozygotes are rare (~1 per million) and the term FH is usually applied to the more common heterozygous condition (1 per 500 individuals in most countries). It has been known since the 1970s that the FH phenotype results from mutations in the LDLR gene, resulting in defective uptake of plasma LDL and dramatic elevation in plasma LDL-C levels (14). To date, more than 800 mutations have been reported to cause FH (http://www.ucl.ac.uk/fh; http://www.umd.necker.fr). Despite its mostly monogenic basis, the phenotypic expression in FH subjects varies dramatically (117). One obvious explanation is that this variability may be due to the severity of the specific mutation within the LDLR gene. Mutations have been categorized into five different classes. The so-called null-alleles result in failure to produce any protein, whereas other mutations lead to impairments in binding capacity, in post-translational processing, or in recycling (31).

The effects of mutation type on lipoprotein levels and on the risk for CVD have been studied extensively, with controversial results (10). However, the clinical presentation differs substantially even among individuals who share an identical LDLR mutation (120). Therefore, additional factors are presumed to influence the course of FH and lead to the dramatic variation in clinical manifestations. In a recent work, Bertolini et al. (11) investigated the presence of modifying genes affecting lipoprotein metabolism as a possible explanation of these differences. They found a significant modulation of common polymorphisms on clinical phenotypes of FH such as (*a*) plasma LDL-C (APOE, MTP, and APOB); (*b*) plasma HDL-C (LIPC, FABP-2, and LPL); (*c*) plasma TAG (APOE and APOA4), and (*d*) coronary artery disease (CAD) (FABP-2). In addition, Bertolini et al. (11) also suggested an important contribution of dietary factors to the variability in the FH phenotypes. There is indirect and direct evidence that diet modifies the effect of the genetic variation on FH phenotypes. This evidence comes from observational studies in the United States (123), Europe (108), and Asia (96, 109). In the United States, Williams et al. (123) screened 1134 individuals from 18 pedigrees in large families from Utah. In four pedigrees with FH, male heterozygotes had a mean serum cholesterol level of 352 mg/dL, myocardial infarction at an average age of 42 years, and coronary death at an average age of 45 years. However, the four ancestral males born before 1880 who were the known founders of the LDLR mutations for each of the pedigrees survived to ages 62, 68, 72, and 81 years. This suggests that some healthy lifestyle factors protected these men against the expression of a mutation that has led to coronary disease by age 45 years in all of their heterozygous great-grandsons. Specifically, the previous generations of these families consumed diets that were lower in total fat—particularly saturated fat—than the diets of their contemporary descendants. These findings were corroborated in the Netherlands (108) in a large Dutch pedigree. Similar observations, using a different approach, were made in Asian populations (95, 109).

Direct evidence that diet modulates the effect of LDLR mutations in FH patients came from experimental studies involving dietary modifications. However, in a systematic review that included published and unpublished randomized controlled trials from 1978 to 2000 in which a cholesterol-lowering diet in children and adults with FH was compared to other forms of dietary treatment or to no dietary intervention, Poustie et al. (98) concluded that there is a lack of adequate data to demonstrate that dietary intervention modulates clinical phenotypes. Nevertheless, scores of individual studies show significant differences (41). One of the main limitations of the systematic review by Poustie et al. (98) is the limited number of included studies owing to the strict inclusion criteria. Although pharmacological treatment with statins is currently the most potent intervention to reduce LDL-C concentrations in FH patients (21, 122), consensus panels from several Western countries recommend a healthy diet to decrease LDL-C concentrations and reduce CAD risk in these patients. In addition, it has been reported that a healthy diet can increase the LDL-C-lowering efficacy of hypocholesterolemic drugs (21). Moreover, it has been recommended that prevention of CAD in FH patients should be initiated in childhood. However, because treatment with statins has several limitations in patients younger than age 18 in most countries, a dietary approach is most important in the treatment of children with FH. An NCEP-ATPIII diet, supplemented with plant stanols/sterols (121), has a very appropriate nutrient composition, and according the current dietary guidelines can be recommended for all FH subjects, including children over age 2 (21). This dietary intervention to lower LDL-C concentrations is a good example of how diet can help to modify a genetically determined trait and it provides a strong basis to propose that other gene-dietary interactions can be detected in subjects whose genetic disease predisposition is due to common genetic SNPs in genes related to lipid metabolism.

COMMON GENETIC VARIANTS AND THEIR INTERACTION WITH DIETARY FACTORS

The evidence for gene-diet interactions between common SNPs at candidate genes and dietary factors in the field of lipid metabolism is continuously increasing. This evidence is presented below, following a discussion about the significance of statistical interactions and biological interactions.

Biological Interactions Versus Statistical Interactions

As pointed out for monogenic diseases, diet can play a pivotal role in the expression of the final phenotype. Understanding these simpler monogenic-nutrient interactions should help us to gain further insight into the more complex interactions for common genetic variants involved on the phenotypic expression of common lipid disorders. However, it should be noted that the term "gene-diet interactions" could be used in different ways (105): as biological interaction and as statistical interaction. The term "biological interaction" is commonly applied in monogenic diseases and is currently used in some dietary interventions in clinical practice to prevent the disease. For example, in subjects with mutations in the phenylketonuria gene, dietary restriction of the harmful nutrient (phenylalanine) has been successfully implemented in clinical practice for many years (19). Therefore, biological interaction exists when two or more factors influence a phenotype at the same time, and it does not necessarily entail statistical interaction (113). Apart from biological interactions, the primary interest of researchers nowadays has focused on statistical interactions. A statistical interaction exists if the degree or direction of the effect of one factor (e.g., an SNP) differs according to values of a second factor (e.g., a nutrient). Accordingly, the vast majority of reports examining gene-diet interactions involving common genetic variants and plasma lipid variables focus on statistically significant interactions (10, 12). However, biological interaction needs to be taken into consideration when designing preventive and therapeutic dietary interventions to modify specific phenotypes in genetically susceptible individuals. To illustrate the differences between statistical and biological interactions, two examples in the framework of the Framingham Study are presented. A classical example of gene-diet statistical interaction is the one found between the –75G/A polymorphism of the APOA1 gene and polyunsaturated fatty acid (PUFA) intake in the Framingham Study (85). In women, a statistically significant gene-diet interaction ($P < 0.05$) was found between PUFA intake (<4% of energy from fat, 4%–8%, and >8%) and the APOA1 SNP in determining plasma HDL-C concentrations (Figure 2). This interaction shows that PUFA intake modulates the effect of the –75A/G SNP on HDL-C concentrations. Thus, in carriers of the A allele, higher PUFA intakes were associated with higher HDL-C, whereas the opposite effect was observed in G/G homozygotes.

On the other hand, an example of a biologically significant but statistically insignificant interaction was found between the CETP TaqIB polymorphism and

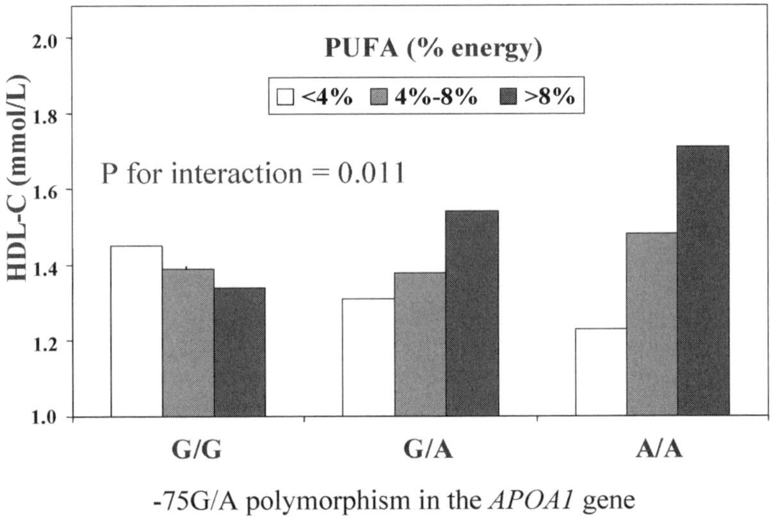

Figure 2 Statistical interaction between the –75G/A polymorphism in the APOA1 gene promoter and polyunsaturated fatty acid (PUFA) intake (<4%, 4%–8% and >8% of energy) in determining plasma HDL-C concentrations in women participating in the Framingham Study. Means of HDL-C were adjusted by age, body mass index, alcohol consumption, tobacco smoking, energy, and saturated fat and monounsaturated fat consumption. The reported P value was obtained for the interaction term between APOA1 genotype and PUFA in the multivariate lineal regression model including the covariates.

alcohol consumption in determining plasma HDL-C concentrations (D. Corella & J.M. Ordovas, unpublished data). We genotyped a population-based sample of 1411 men and 1505 women from the Framingham Study. B1B1 individuals had lower HDL-C concentrations compared with B1B2 and B2B2 individuals ($P < 0.001$) (82). Three categories of alcohol intake were considered according to reported daily intake: no alcohol intake, moderate intake, and high intake. No statistically significant interaction between the CETP-TaqIB genotype and alcohol intake was found. However, as observed in Figure 3, a biologically significant gene-diet interaction was observed. Thus, B1B1 subjects could have higher HDL-C concentrations when consuming alcohol than B2 carriers who do not consume alcohol. Taking into account that low HDL-C concentrations are considered a

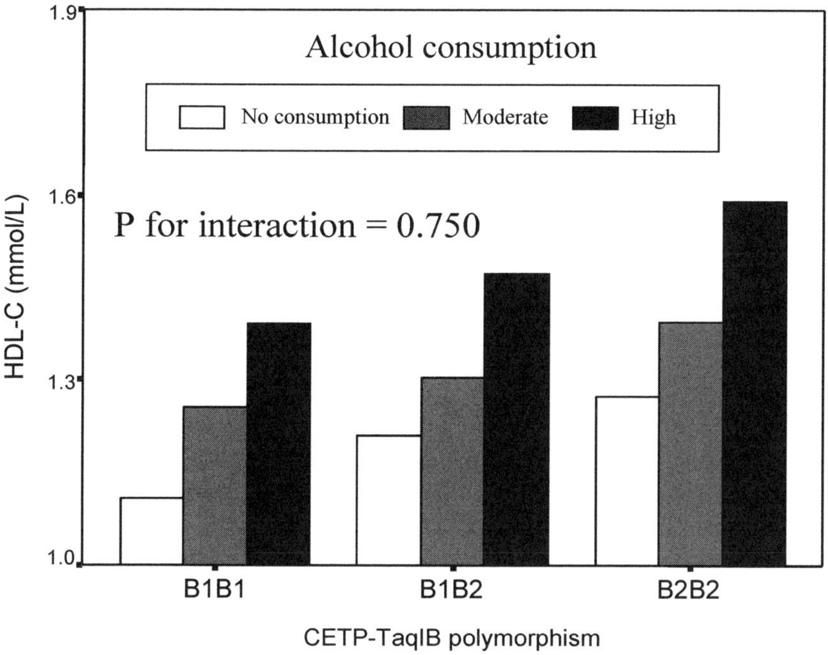

Figure 3 Biological interaction between the TaqIB polymorphism in the cholesteryl ester transfer protein (CETP) gene and alcohol intake in determining plasma high-density lipoprotein cholesterol (HDL-C) concentrations the Framingham Study. Three groups of alcohol intake were defined according to the reported amount of alcohol consumed per day: no consumption (alcohol consumption = 0 g/day), moderate (<26.4 g alcohol/day for men, <13.2 g/day for women), and high consumption (>26.4 g alcohol/day for men, >13.2 g alcohol/day for women). Means of HDL-C were adjusted by gender age, body mass index, tobacco smoking, and energy intake. The reported P value was obtained for the interaction term between the CETP genotype and alcohol intake in the multivariate lineal regression model including the covariates.

cardiovascular risk factor, dietary interventions aimed at increasing HDL-C in genetically susceptible B1B1 individuals could be a preventive measure. Our results clearly show that alcohol consumption can increase HDL-C concentrations in B1B1 individuals in a dose-dependent manner.

Gene-Diet Interactions Modulating Plasma Lipoprotein Concentrations

We summarize below the current evidence for gene-diet interactions in the field of lipid metabolism using as outcomes plasma lipid concentrations but also disease phenotypes such as obesity, cardiovascular diseases, and diabetes. Among dietary factors, total fat, specific fatty acids, carbohydrates, total energy intake, and alcohol intake are discussed. The evidence from observational as well as intervention studies is presented. Moreover, differences between studies in the fasting state as well as in the postprandial state are considered.

RESULTS FROM INTERVENTION STUDIES Intervention studies in which subjects receive a controlled dietary intake provide the best approach to ascertain true dietary intake under highly controlled conditions. However, these well-controlled feeding studies have several important logistic limitations, including the small number of participants and the brief duration of the interventions. Hundreds of intervention studies have examined gene-diet interactions on different parameters of lipid metabolism. However, the level of replication among studies that analyze the same genetic variation tends to be low. Potential reasons for the lack of replication are the different characteristics of study subjects, length of intervention, sample size limitation, and heterogeneity in the design. In a systematic review of literature published from 1966 to 2002, Masson et al. (72) identified 17 reviews on gene-diet interactions and 74 relevant articles that included dietary intervention studies in which measurements were taken of the lipid and lipoprotein response to diet in different genotype groups. They analyzed the published articles according to seven groups of genetic loci: APOA1, APOC3, and APOA4 cluster; APOB; APOE; enzymes (LPL, LIPC, and CYPA7); LDLR; other genes, including CETP, FABP; and neuropeptide Y. At each locus, one or more polymorphisms were included and the mainly short-term response to a defined dietary intervention [i.e., high-fat diet versus a low-fat diet, high saturated fatty acid (SFA) versus high PUFA, high MUFA versus low MUFA, etc.] was examined. After a comparative analysis of the individual findings, Masson et al. (72) concluded that there is evidence to suggest that variations in *APOA1*, *APOA4*, *APOB*, and *APOE* contribute to the heterogeneity in the lipid response to dietary intervention. However, the effects of the reported gene-diet interactions are not consistently seen and are sometimes conflicting. For example, for the *APOE* locus, 46 studies were analyzed. Of those, significantly different LDL-C responses to changes in the fat content of the diet by *APOE* genotype were reported in 11 studies. Table 1 includes a summary of this

TABLE 1 Summary of studies examining gene-diet interactions modulating fasting plasma lipid responses in intervention trials*

Gene/polymorphism	Population	Dietary factors examined	Conclusions	Reference
Apolipoprotein A-I (APOA1)				
APOA1 (−75G/A)	Systematic review	Various interventions	Thirteen reports have been published. Five found that the presence of the A allele was associated with greater LDL-C responses to changes in dietary fat.	(72)
Apolipoprotein A-IV (APOA4)				
APOA4 Gln360His	Systematic review	Various interventions	In general, *Gln/Gln* subjects show significantly greater total and LDL-C responses and *Gln/His* subjects show greater HDL-cholesterol responses to changes in dietary fat, cholesterol, or both. One study found no significant differences in LDL-C responses between genotypes. However, dense LDL decreased more in subjects carrying the *His* allele when PUFAs replaced SFAs in the diet. In the same study, there was a significant difference in HDL-C responses between genotype groups such that concentrations decreased in *Gln/Gln* subjects and increased in *Gln/His* subjects.	(72)
APOA4 Thr347Ser	Systematic review	Various interventions	The Ser allele was associated with increased total and LDL-cholesterol responsiveness when subjects switched from a high-SFA diet to the NCEP Step I diet. When the same subjects	(72)

(Continued)

TABLE 1 (*Continued*)

Gene/polymorphism	Population	Dietary factors examined	Conclusions	Reference
			changed from the NCEP Step I diet to a high-MUFA diet, subjects with the *Thr/Thr* genotype had a 1% decrease in total cholesterol concentrations, whereas subjects with the *Ser* allele had a 5% increase in total cholesterol concentrations. When the Thr347Ser and the apoA-I–75 (*G/A*) genotypes were combined, carriers of the *A* and *Ser* alleles showed greater LDL-C responses to changes in dietary fat. However, a study in FH subjects investigating both the Gln360His and Thr347Ser polymorphisms found no gene-diet or haplotype-diet interactions.	
APOA4 (Gln360His, Thr347Ser), CETP (TaqIB), SCARB1 (Exon 8), 3-hydroxy-3-methylglutaryl-coenzyme A reductase (HMGCR, VNTR) and APOE (E2/E3/E4)	41 males and 71 females (mean BMI 23, mean age 33 years)	Plant stanol ester consumption	No significant differences between the polymorphisms and dietary responsiveness to plant stanol ester consumption could be found, which indicates that it is unlikely that one of the single polymorphisms analyzed in this study is a major factor in explaining the variation in serum LDL cholesterol responses.	(97)

APOA4 (Thr347Ser), APOB (−516C > T), APOC3 (3175C > G), APOE (E2/E3/E4), CETP (TaqIB), FABP (Ala54Thr), LIPC (−480C > T), LPL (Asn291Ser)	The intervention study (RIVAGE) in Marseille. 300 patients randomized into two groups over periods of 3 and 12 months. Data obtained in about 100 patients after three months of dietary change.	Mediterranean or low-fat types versus standard Western type	The preliminary findings show interactions for APOE and LDL-cholesterol and TAG, APOA4 and LDL-C, MTP and LDL-C, and FABP2 and TAG.	(120)
Apolipoprotein B (APOB)				
APOB (XbaI)	Systematic review	Various interventions	Based on meta-analyses (see Reference 98a), X−X+ subjects had greater LDL-C responses that did X+X+ subjects.	(72)
APOB (EcoRI)	Systematic review	Various interventions	Based on meta-analyses (see Reference 98a), R−R− subjects had greater LDL-C and total cholesterol responses that did R+R+ subjects.	(72)
APOB (MspI)	Systematic review	Various interventions	Based on meta-analyses (see Reference 98a), M+M+ subjects had greater LDL-C and triglyceride responses that did M+M− subjects.	(72)
APOB (Ins/Del signal peptide)	Systematic review	Various interventions	Ten intervention studies found no significant effects of this polymorphism on dietary responsiveness, whereas two studies reported significantly greater responsiveness in I/I subjects.	(72)
APOB (Ins/Del signal peptide)	231 unrelated subjects (146 women/ 85 men). BMI > 25	25% reduction in energy intake during 2.5 months	Del allele associated with higher baseline LDL-C levels but also with increased response to dietary intervention.	(55)

(*Continued*)

TABLE 1 *(Continued)*

Gene/polymorphism	Population	Dietary factors examined	Conclusions	Reference
Apolipoprotein C-III (APOC3)				
APOC3 (SstI, C1100T)	Systematic review	Various interventions	Variation at the apo C-III *Sst*I site influenced dietary responsiveness such that after the subjects changed from a low-fat diet to a high-MUFA diet, LDL-cholesterol concentrations increased in *S1/S1* subjects but decreased in *S1/S2* subjects. When the effect of this polymorphism with the APOA1–75G/A polymorphism was studied, it was found that total and LDL-cholesterol concentrations decreased most in subjects with the G/G-S1/S2 polymorphism and increased most in subjects with the G/A-S1/S1 polymorphism. The C1100T polymorphic site has not been associated with the magnitude of the lipid response.	(72)
APOC3 (SstI)	59 volunteers (18 smokers: 8 with the S1S1 genotype, 10 with the S2 allele; 41 nonsmokers: 29 with the S1S1 genotype, 12 with the S1S2 genotype)	Three different diets: a diet enriched in saturated fatty acids (SFA) (38% fat, 20% SFA) followed by a randomized, crossover period during which they ate a diet enriched in carbohydrates	S1S1 smokers were not influenced by any of the diets, but the atherogenic ratio decreased in S2 carriers when they changed from the diet rich in SFA to a diet rich in olive oil or carbohydrates. No significant difference was observed when the S2 nonsmokers changed from one diet to another, but there was a decrease in the LDL-C/HDL-C ratio when S1S1 subjects changed from the saturated diet to either of the other diets.	(92)

		(NCEP-1) (30% fat, 10% SFA, 55% carbohydrates) and a diet enriched in MUFA (8% fat, 22% MUFA).		
Apolipoprotein E (APOE)				
APOE (E2/E3/E4)		Various interventions	46 interventions involving altering the dietary fat content of the diet. Significantly different total and LDL-C responses between genotype groups were reported in 8 and 11 studies, respectively, with E4 subjects showing the greatest responses. However, subjects with the E2 allele had greatest responses to other diet interventions (i.e., wheat and oat bran, fiber)	(72)
APOE (E2/E3/E4)	65 normal males, mean age 37.5 years, BMI 29.2, recruited in the Quebec City area. Ethnic origin not indicated, most probably white.	High CHO versus high MUFA. Ad libitum, parallel design. Intervention lasting 6–7 weeks. Food was provided to the participants.	Variability in response to a high-CHO diet is primarily determined by APOE genotype, whereas the response to a high-MUFA is determined by waist circumference.	(27)
APOE (E2/E3/E4)	White women, mean age 60 (50–65 years), BMI approximately 32.4	10-week dietary intervention (Amer. Heart Assoc. Step I). Only advice was provided.	In response to the dietary advice to follow an AHA Step I diet, those with the E4 allele benefited the most, while the lipid profile could worsen in those without the E4 allele.	(79)

(Continued)

TABLE 1 *(Continued)*

Gene/polymorphism	Population	Dietary factors examined	Conclusions	Reference
APOE (E2/E3/E4)	104 patients with hyperlipidemia. Mean age about 54, BMI around 22.5. Presumably Japanese. Approximately 50% male.	Response to dietary therapy (not specified)	Plasma TC and TG levels were significantly lowered by the dietary treatment in patients with 3/3, 2/3, and 3/4 genotypes; but 2/4 subjects did not respond to the diet.	(112)
APOE (E2/E3/E4)	205 women (ages 49–65 years)	Double-blind, placebo-controlled trial of 43.5 mg red clover–derived isoflavones/d.	Interactions between apoE genotype and treatment tended to be significant for changes in total and LDL cholesterol ($P = 0.06$ and $P = 0.05$), and differences between treatments were significant in E2/E3 women.	(6)
APOE (E2/E3/E4)	84 healthy subjects	3 dietary periods, each lasting 4 weeks. The first was an SFA-enriched diet (38% fat, 20% SFA), which was followed by a carbohydrate (CHO)-rich diet (30% fat, <10% SFA, 55% carbohydrate) or a monounsaturated	LDL size was significantly higher in APOE3/4 subjects compared with APOE3/3 and APOE2/3 subjects in the basal state. LDL size was smaller after the CHO diet than after the MUFA or SFA diets. After the CHO diet, a significant increase in LDL size was noted with respect to the MUFA diet in APOE3/4 subjects, whereas a significant decrease was observed in the APOE3/3 individuals. Therefore, a diet high in MUFA increases LDL particle size compared with a CHO diet, and this effect is dependent of APOE genotypes.	(75)

		fatty acid (MUFA) olive oil–rich diet (38% fat, 22% MUFA) following a randomized crossover design.		
Cholesteryl ester transfer protein (CETP)				
CETP (Taq1B)	Systematic review	Various interventions	B1B1 subjects showed greater total and LDL-cholesterol responses to changes in the type of dietary fat than did subjects who were homozygous or heterozygous for the B2 allele in 1 of 3 studies.	(72)
CETP (I405V)	Subjects with moderate primary hypercholesterolemia (ages 20–60; 50 women, 10 men)	Margarine (20 g/d) without PSE (placebo) or with PSE (2.8 g/d = 1.68 g/d phytosterols) for four weeks each period, in a crossover, double-blind study	Percent reductions in TC with consumption of PSE for the II, IV, and VV phenotypes were 7.2, 4.2, and not significant, respectively, whereas for LDL-C significant reductions occurred only for II (9.5%). However, the CETP concentration diminished only in the II phenotype.	(68)
CETP (I405V and Taq1B) and APOE (E2/E3/E4)	60 subjects with moderate primary hypercholesterolemia (ages 20–60; 50 women; 10 men)	Margarine (20 g/d) without PSE (placebo) or with PSE for four weeks each period, in a crossover, double-blind study	In relation to the I405V CETP polymorphism, the % reductions in TC with consumption of PSE for the II, IV, and VV phenotypes were 7.2, 4.2, and not significant, respectively.	(68)

(*Continued*)

TABLE 1 (*Continued*)

Gene/polymorphism	Population	Dietary factors examined	Conclusions	Reference
Cholesterol 7-alpha-hydroxylase (CYP7A1)				
CYP7A1 (A278-C)	Systematic review	Various interventions	This SNP was not associated with dietary responsiveness in one study.	(72)
CYP7A1 (A278-C)	496 normolipidemic subjects (meta-analysis including 26 previously published dietary trials)	Increased intake in dietary cholesterol (742 mg/d), cafestol (57 mg/d), saturated fat [change of 8–9 energy percent/d (en%/d)] and trans fat (change of 10–11 en%/d) in 496 normolipidemic subjects	After adjustment for the apolipoprotein E genotype effect, AA subjects consuming a cholesterol-rich diet had a smaller increase in plasma HDL cholesterol than did CC subjects (0.00 ± 0.02 versus 0.17 ± 0.04 mmol/L; $P < 0.001$). Upon intake of cafestol, AA subjects had a smaller increase in plasma total cholesterol than did CC subjects (0.69 ± 0.10 versus 1.01 ± 0.10 mmol/L; $P = 0.028$). No effects of the polymorphism were found in the saturated and trans fat interventions. In conclusion, the CYP7A1 polymorphism has a small but significant effect on the increase in plasma HDL cholesterol and plasma total cholesterol after an increased intake of dietary cholesterol and cafestol.	(43)
Intestinal fatty acid–binding protein (FABP2)				
FABP2 A54T	Systematic review	Various interventions	One study showed that T54/T54 subjects had greater total and LDL cholesterol responses to a soluble-fiber diet than did the other two genotypes, and the heterozygotes had a significantly greater total cholesterol response to soluble fiber than did the A54/A54 homozygotes.	(72)

Low-density lipoprotein receptor (LDLR)				
LDLR (HincII, PvuII)	Systematic review	Various interventions	A significant interaction between diet and variation in the LDL receptor gene was shown in two studies. After wheat- or oat-bran supplementation, the total and LDL cholesterol reductions were significantly different among the HincII genotype groups, with 2/2 subjects showing the greatest reduction and 1/1 subjects showing the smallest reduction. In terms of the PvuII site, subjects lacking the cutting site were found to have greater HDL responses to low-fat diets.	(72)
Hepatic lipase (LIPC)				
LIPC (NlaIII, MspI)	Systematic review	Various interventions	These SNPs were not associated with the response to diet.	(72)
Endothelial lipase (EL)				
LIPG (Thr111Ile)	83 sedentary, healthy men and women ages 50–75	Subjects were weight-maintained on an Amer. Heart Assoc. Step 1 Diet and then studied before and after aerobic exercise training	The LIPG genotype was associated with interindividual variability in HDL-C and its subfractions and their response to exercise training.	(39)

(*Continued*)

TABLE 1 (*Continued*)

Gene/polymorphism	Population	Dietary factors examined	Conclusions	Reference
Lipoprotein lipase (LPL)				
LPL (HindIII, S447X, N291S)	Systematic review	Various interventions	The H-allele at the HindIII SNP was associated with greater cholesterol and TG responses. Subjects with the S447X polymorphism showed significantly greater decreases in LDL-C levels than did S/S subjects when PUFA replaced SFA in the diet. Subjects heterozygous for the N291S SNP showed greater responses in TG than did N/N subjects. No significant interactions were noted for the PvuII and the T-93G SNPs.	(72)
Paraoxonase 1 (PON1)				
PON1 (G192Arg)	37 healthy, nonsmoking women	A controlled, crossover dietary intervention of two 5-week periods was conducted. The two study diets were either low or high in vegetables, and thus in natural antioxidants, with some differences in fatty acid contents.	The reduction of PON1 activity due to the high-vegetable diet was greatest among the women with the PON1(192Arg) allele and PON1(55Leu/Leu) genotype.	(99)

Peroxisome proliferator-activated receptor gamma (PPARG)				
PPARG (Pro12Ala)	76 men and 74 women (age 49, BMI 26.5 kg/m^2	Subjects were randomly assigned to consume either fish oil supplements or placebo capsules containing olive oil for three months.	Carriers of the Ala12 allele presented a greater decrease in TG concentration in response to n-3 fatty acid supplementation than did subjects with the Pro12Pro genotype when the total dietary fat intake was below 37 E% or the intake of saturated fatty acids was below 10 E%.	(63)
Scavenger receptor class B, member 1 (SCARB1)				
SCARBI [exon 1 (G–>A)]	97 healthy volunteers with exon 1 polymorphism	Both groups consumed 3 diets (SFA-rich, CHO-rich, MUFA-rich diets) lasting 4 weeks each according to a randomized crossover design.	Carriers of the minor allele, 1/2, are more susceptible to the presence of SFA in the diet because of a greater increase in LDL cholesterol.	(94)

*Abbreviations: BMI, body mass index; CHO, carbohydrate; HDL, high-density lipoprotein; LDL, low-density lipoprotein; MUFA, monounsaturated fatty acid; PUFA, polyunsaturated fatty acid; PSE, plant sterol esters; SFA, saturated fatty acid; SNP, single nucleotide polymorphism.

systematic review as well as an enumeration of more recent reports (after 2002) (6, 27, 39, 43, 55, 63, 68, 72, 75, 79, 92, 94, 97, 99, 112, 120) examining gene-diet interactions in the fasting state. In addition to the above-mentioned reasons contributing to the lack of replication of these types of studies, it should be noted that the composition of the dietary intervention greatly varies between studies. It would be appropriate to standardize a minimum set of variables when considering the design of future intervention studies in order to fix certain conditions (e.g., patients characteristics, medications, and composition and length of the dietary treatment and sample size) and to allow better comparison among studies and even potentially to carry out meta analyses, something that it is impossible under the current experimental conditions.

RESULTS FROM OBSERVATIONAL STUDIES In observational studies, large numbers of subjects can be studied and long-term dietary habits can be estimated. However, the level of evidence of the results obtained from these studies traditionally has been considered to be lower than that of experimental studies. This level can be increased by taking into consideration the principle of Mendelian randomization that was discussed in the "Methodological Issues Assessing Gene-Diet Interaction" section above. Table 2 summarizes the findings of a number of observational studies involving gene-diet interactions on lipid metabolism in the fasting state (15–17, 23–25, 32, 34, 45, 66, 73, 84, 85, 89, 95, 103, 104, 110, 111, 115). In general, as pointed out for the intervention studies, replication of results is still very low. However, taking into account that larger sample sizes are required in observational studies as compared with intervention studies, one factor that has limited replication is the lack of published studies analyzing the same SNPs and dietary factors. In addition, these findings need an increased interface with nutrigenomic studies to acquire mechanistic knowledge for the reported statistical interactions.

GENE-DIET INTERACTIONS IN THE POSTPRANDIAL STATE Humans are typically in a nonfasting state. Postprandial lipemia, characterized by a rise in TRLs after eating, is a dynamic, nonsteady-state condition (49). Over 25 years ago, Zilversmit (125) proposed that atherogenesis was a postprandial phenomenon as postprandial lipoproteins and their remnants could deposit into the arterial wall and accumulate in atheromatous plaques. Several studies have investigated the potential interaction between some polymorphisms in candidate genes and diet on postprandial lipids. Table 3 summarizes the findings of these studies involving *APOA1, APOA5, APOC3, APOE, LPL, NPY,* and *SCARB1* gene variants (26, 54, 67, 70, 71, 74, 93, 102, 107, 125). In postprandial studies, subjects usually receive a fat-loading test meal in which composition varies depending on the nutrient(s) to be tested. After the test meal, blood samples are taken again to measure postprandial lipids. Meal absorption is a complex phenomenon, and because postprandial hyperlipidemia

TABLE 2 Summary of studies analyzing gene-diet interactions with plasma lipid outcomes in observational studies

Gene/polymorphism	Population	Dietary factors examined	Conclusions	Reference
Apolipoprotein A-I (APOA1)				
APOA1 (−75G/A)	755 men and 822 women from the Framingham Offspring Study	Semiquantitative FFQ	In women carriers of the A allele, higher PUFA intakes were associated with higher HDL-C concentrations, whereas the opposite effect was observed in G/G women.	(85)
Apolipoprotein A-IV (APOA4)				
APOA4 [G360H; 347(Thr→Ser)]	758 randomly selected subjects (mean age 36.7) from two Spanish regions differing in latitude and fat intake: Aragon and Comunidad Valenciana	Ecological data (3 household budget surveys, Natl. Inst. Statistics)	The magnitude of the effects associated with the APOA4 alleles was higher in subjects from Aragon compared with the Comunidad Valenciana, suggesting a possible influence of the higher fat intake in Aragon. In the combined association analysis, subjects with the 360Gln/347Ser pseudohaplotype had the highest LDL-C concentrations, supporting the antagonistic effect between the 360His and the 347Ser alleles on this trait.	(34)
APOA4 (G360H)	222 men and 236 from rural and urban Costa Rica	FFQ	Lifestyles associated with an urban environment, such as increased saturated fat intake, elicit a more adverse plasma lipoprotein profile among Costa Rican carriers of the APOA4-360H allele than in APOA41 homozygotes. Therefore, under the conditions studied, persons with the APOA4-360H allele may be more susceptible to CHD.	(17)

(*Continued*)

TABLE 2 (*Continued*)

Gene/polymorphism	Population	Dietary factors examined	Conclusions	Reference
Apolipoprotein C-III (APOC3)				
APOC3 (T-455C, T-625del & C3238G 3′ UTR)	336 randomly selected residents from Costa Rica	FFQ	Compared to a SAT-rich diet is associated with a beneficial lipoprotein profile only among homozygotes of the APOC3 promoter 455T-625T polymorphism.	(15)
Apolipoprotein E (APOE)				
APOE (E2/E3/E4)	132 free-living subjects participating in the EPIC study	FFQ	Elevated plasma cholesterol levels associated with high SAT fat intake can be expected, particularly in those individuals who combine a risky dietary behavior with the presence of the E4 allele.	(65)
APOE (E2/E3/E4)	420 randomly selected free-living Costa Ricans	FFQ	The APOE2 allele could modulate the effect of habitual saturated fat on VLDL-C and HDLC in a population with an average habitual total fat intake of less that 30%.	(16)
APOE (E2/E3/E4)	284 men and 130 women with CAD (mean age 61 years), participants in the EUROASPIRE Study	Four-day food record	CAD patients with the E2 allele will likely have a greater TG response to high dietary sucrose intakes than will patients with the E3 or E4 alleles.	(32)

APOE (E2/E3/E4)	Population control for a case-control Alzheimer's study, >60 years of age. 46 E4+ (30.4% male) and 171 E4− subjects (48.5% male). Ethnicity not indicated.	Dietary recall over two age periods (20–39 and 40–59 years)	The proportion of subjects with the E4 allele was higher in the lowest tertile of fat intake compared with subjects in the highest tertile, suggesting that older persons with the E4 allele who survived free of disease may be protected by a lifelong lower dietary fat intake.	(95)
APOE (E2/E3/E4)	396 men and 513 women aged 18 to 66 years from a Mediterranean Spanish population	Ecological data (three household budget surveys, National Institute of Statistics)	In women, an interaction between alcohol consumption and APOE in determining LDL-C concentrations was found. LDL-C concentrations in female drinkers with the E2 variant were significantly lower than in nondrinkers with the E2 variant. Likewise, in female drinkers with the E4 variant, LDL-C concentrations were significantly lower than in nondrinkers with E4. Moreover, in female drinkers, LDL-C concentrations did not differ between carriers of the E4 and the E3 variants, and in nondrinkers, LDL-C concentrations did not differ between carriers of the E2 and the E3 variants. We also found a statistically significant interaction effect between the APOE polymorphism and physical activity in determining HDL-C concentrations in men.	(23)
APOE (E2/E3/E4)	1014 men and 1133 women from the Framingham Offspring Study	FFQ	In men, the effects of alcohol intake on LDL cholesterol were modulated in part by variability at the APOE locus. Alcohol-related increases in LDL-C concentrations are noted for APOE4 males, whereas the opposite effect is seen in APOE2 males.	(25)

(*Continued*)

TABLE 2 *(Continued)*

Gene/polymorphism	Population	Dietary factors examined	Conclusions	Reference
APOE (E2/E3/E4) and CYP-7A1 (−204A→C)	131 males for whom dietary composition markedly changed and total cholesterol decreased (from 6.21 +/− 1.31 mmol/L in 1988 to 5.43 +/− 1.06 mmol/L in 1996) over an eight-year follow-up study	Changes in food intake according to food questionnaire during an 8-year period	APOE genotype influenced plasma total and LDL cholesterol, with carriers of the E4 having the highest and E2 carriers the lowest levels, this reached borderline significance for cholesterol in 1988 and strongly affected the 1996 levels of LDL-C. However, APOE did not influence the change in these measures over time. In contrast, the CYP-7A1 −204A→C polymorphism did not affect lipid measures per se but was strongly associated with a decrease in plasma total cholesterol over the eight-year time period.	(45)
Cholesteryl ester transfer protein (CETP)				
CETP (TaqIB and −629C > A)	1300 Chinese, 364 Malay and 282 Asian Indian men, and in 1558 Chinese, 397 Malay, and 306 Asian Indian women	FFQ	Dietary cholesterol showed a significant interaction with the TaqIB polymorphism in determining HDL-C concentrations in Indians and Malays, but not in Chinese.	(111)
Liver fatty acid–binding protein (FABP1)				
FABP1 T94A	623 French-Canadian men	FFQ	T94/T94 exhibit higher apoB levels, whereas carriers of the A94 allele seem to be protected against high apoB levels when consuming a high-fat and high-saturated-fat diet.	(104)

Hepatic lipase (LIPC)				
LIPC (−514C/T)	1020 men and 1110 women participating in the Framingham Offspring Study. Mostly from white ethnicity	Semiquantitative FFQ	Dietary fat intake modifies the effect of the −514(C/T) polymorphism on HDL-C concentrations and subclasses. TT subjects may have an impaired adaptation to higher animal fat diets that could result in higher CVD risk.	(84)
LIPC (−514C/T)	Singaporean men and women (1324 Chinese, 471 Malay, and 375 Asian Indian)	FFQ	There were differences in the association of −514C > T polymorphism with plasma lipids according to dietary intake and ethnic background. Specifically, the TT genotype is associated with a more atherogenic lipid profile when subjects consume diets with a fat content >30%.	(110)
Endothelial lipase (EL)				
LIPG (Thr111Ile)	281 white women and 216 white men, ages 17 to 76 years (mean age ~39 years), from the Quebec Family Study. BMI ranging from 16.8 to 64.9 (mean ~29.0).	Three-day dietary record	A gender-specific gene-diet interaction among women suggests that the T111I missense mutation may confer protection against the lowering effect of a high dietary PUFA intake on plasma apoA-I and HDL3-C levels.	(89)

(Continued)

TABLE 2 (*Continued*)

Gene/polymorphism	Population	Dietary factors examined	Conclusions	Reference
Lipoprotein lipase (LPL)				
LPL-HindIII, LPL-S447X, and APOC3-SstI APOE (E2/E3/E4)	Spanish population ($n = 1029$)	Ecological data (three household budget surveys, National Institute of Statistics)	There was a significant interaction between APOE and LPL variants and HDL-C levels in both genders ($P < 0.05$). The increases in HDL-C observed for the rare alleles were higher in epsilon4 than in epsilon3 subjects, and absent in epsilon2 individuals. This effect was modulated by smoking (interaction HindIII-APOE-smoking, $P = 0.019$), indicating that smoking abolished the increase in HDL-C levels observed in epsilon4/H(−) subjects.	(24)
Paraoxonase 1 (PON1)				
PON1-192	654 males, ages 25 to 74, randomly selected from the REGICOR Study	72-hour recall questionnaire	The beneficial effect of increasing oleic acid intake on HDL and PON1 activity at population level is especially observed in subjects carrying the R allele of the PON1-192 polymorphism.	(115)

Peroxisome proliferator-activated receptor alpha (PPARα)				
PPARα-L162V	Men with (n = 281) and without (n = 351) the metabolic syndrome	FFQ	The frequency of the V162 allele was higher in subjects with simultaneous abdominal obesity, hypertriglyceridemia, and low HDL-C levels. Carriers of the V162 were characterized by higher plasma apolipoprotein B and TG levels. In a model including the PPARalpha-L162V polymorphism, fat or saturated fat, the interaction term between the polymorphism and fat intake, and covariates (smoking habits and energy and alcohol intake), the interaction explained a significant percentage of the variance observed in waist circumference.	(103)
Peroxisome proliferator-activated receptor gamma (PPARG)				
PPARG (Pro12Ala)	Subjects (n = 2141) were controls selected for three case-control studies nested within the Nurses' Health Study	Semiquantitative FFQ	Among Pro/Pro individuals, those in the highest quintile of total fat intake had higher BMI compared with those in the lowest quintile, whereas among 12Ala variant allele carriers, no significant trend was observed between dietary fat intake and BMI. In contrast, intake of MUFA was not associated with BMI among homozygous wild-type women but was inversely associated with BMI among 12Ala variant allele carriers. The relationship between dietary fat intake and plasma lipids also differed according to PPARG genotype.	(73)

*Abbreviations: BMI, body mass index; CAD, coronary artery disease; CHD, coronary heart disease; CHO, carbohydrate; FFQ, food frequency questionnaire; HDL, high-density lipoprotein; LDL, low-density lipoprotein; MUFA, monounsaturated fatty acid; PUFA, polyunsaturated fatty acid; PSE, plant sterol esters; SFA, saturated fatty acid; SNP, single nucleotide polymorphism; TG, triglyceride.

TABLE 3 Summary of studies analyzing gene-diet interactions with plasma lipid outcomes in postprandial studies

Gene/polymorphism	Population	Phenotypes	Dietary factors examined	Conclusions	Reference
Apolipoprotein A-I (APOA1)					
APOA1 (−75G/A)	28 G/G and 23 G/A healthy males, homozygotes for the apo E3 allele	Postprandial lipids	Fat loading test	A greater postprandial response in large TRLs was observed in G/A than in G/G subjects.	(70)
Apolipoprotein A-V (APOA5)					
APOA5 (−1131T > C)	Healthy, nonobese subjects [n = 158; mean (± SEM) age: 33.8 ± 1.2 year; body mass index (in kg/m^2): 23.3 ± 0.3]	Measurements included fasting and postprandial lipid concentrations, lipid peroxidation, C-reactive protein concentrations, and DNA damage.	Fat loading test	After consumption of a mixed meal, carriers of the C allele had significantly greater increases in total chylomicron and VLDL TAG than did subjects with the TT genotype. Moreover, carriers of the C allele had higher dense LDL, serum C-reactive protein, and urinary 8-epi-prostaglandin F(2alpha) concentrations and more lymphocyte DNA damage.	(54)
APOA5 (S19W, −1131T > C; −12238T > C)	Healthy young men (n = 774) who had undergone both an OFTT and an OGTT. Participants in the EARSII Study.	Fasting and postprandial lipids and insulin	OFTT and OGTT	Results strongly support the role of APOA5 in determining plasma TG levels.	(71)

Apolipoprotein C-III (APOC3)					
(apo) CIII C3238G, C-482T, and T-455C	122 viscerally obese men (abdominal visceral AT area ≥130 cm^2)	Lipoproteins and response to a 75 g OGTT	OGTT	S1/S2 heterozygotes (n = 24) were characterized by increased fasting plasma TG concentrations compared with S1/S1 homozygotes. No association was found between the response to the OGTT and any of the apoC-III gene variants (SstI, T-455C, or C-482T) examined.	(26)
Apo CIII T2854G	Healthy and normolipidemic Korean men (n = 262)	Postprandial lipids	Fat loading test	The data show that the APOAC3 T2854G polymorphism is associated with elevated postprandial TAG concentrations in the study population of Korean men.	(124)
Apolipoprotein E (APOE)					
APOE (−219G/T)	51 healthy white APOE3/3 subjects. Average age ~23, BMI ~24.5	Postprandial lipids	Oral fat loading test	The −219G/T polymorphism influences postprandial lipid metabolism, prolonging postprandial lipemia in subjects with the TT genotype.	(74)
APOE (E2/E3/E4)	16 FCH parents (52 ± 9 years eld), 16 offspring (22 ± 5 years) and 12 healthy controls. Ethnic origin not indicated, but probably white	Postprandial lipids	Oral fat loading test	The six-hour postprandial TG values were correlated with fasting TG and were associated with the APOE4 allele.	(102)

(*Continued*)

TABLE 3 *(Continued)*

Gene/polymorphism	Population	Phenotypes	Dietary factors examined	Conclusions	Reference
Neuropeptide Y (NPY)					
NPY (Leu7Pro)	Seven middle-aged obese subjects with Leu7Pro genotype were matched with seven subjects with Leu7Leu genotype for gender, age, apolipoprotein E phenotype, and BMI	Postprandial lipemia, postheparin plasma LPL and HL	Oral eight-hour fat tolerance test	This study suggests compositional differences in lipoprotein particles might exist between the genotype groups that affect postprandial lipid metabolism.	(107)
Lipoprotein lipase (LPL)					
LPL HindIII (H1/H2) and Serine 447-Stop (S447X)	51 healthy male volunteers	Postprandial lipid levels	Fat loading test	Data revealed that subjects that are homozygous for the H2 allele (H2H2) showed a higher postprandial response for small TRL, RP, large TRL-RP, large TRL-B48, and small TRL-B48 levels. Furthermore, in the	(67)

				case of the S447X polymorphism, 447Ter carriers had a lower postprandial response for small TRL-RP, large TRL-B48, and small TRL-RP. Subjects with the LPL H2S447 genotype had higher plasmaTAG, larger TRL-TAG, larger TRL-RP, smaller TRL-RP, and larger TRL-B48 ($P < 0.037$) than did H1X447 subjects.	
Scavenger receptor class B, member 1 (SCARB1)					
SCARBI [exon 1 (G→A)]	47 normolipidemic volunteers who were homozygous for the E3 allele at the APOE gene	Postprandial lipid levels	Fat loading test	Postprandial responses for TAGs and RP in small TAG-rich lipoproteins were higher in 1/1 individuals than in 1/2 individuals.	(93)

*Abbreviations: BMI, body mass index; FCH, familial combined hyperlipidemia; HL, hepatic lipase; LPL, lipoprotein lipase; MUFA, monounsaturated fatty acid; PUFA, polyunsaturated fatty acid; RP, retinyl palmitate; PSE, plant sterol esters; SFA, saturated fatty acid; SNP, single nucleotide polymorphism; OFTT, oral fat tolerance test; OGTT, oral glucose tolerance test; TAG, triacylglycerols; TG, triglyceride; TRL-RP, dial triglyceride-rich lipoproteins-retinyl palmitate; VLDL, very-low-density lipoprotein.

and hyperglycemia are simultaneously present in the postabsorptive phase, particularly in diabetics and in subjects with impaired glucose tolerance, the distinct role of these two factors is a matter of debate (26). Consistency is still very low and, similar to the conclusions reached above for the other experimental approaches, replication is a major need for postprandial studies, where the number of subjects and the complexity of the designs may add even more bias than that of other experimental approaches.

FUTURE OPPORTUNITIES FOR PERSONALIZED NUTRITION: WHAT NEEDS TO BE DONE?

Although the current evidence from both experimental and observational nutrigenetics studies is not strong enough to start making specific personalized nutritional recommendations based on genetic information, we have many examples of common SNPs that modulate the individual response to diet as proof of concept of how gene-diet interactions can influence lipid metabolism. It is critical that these preliminary studies go through further replication in nutrigenetic designs. Overall, the evidence from intervention trials showing gene-diet interactions in lipid metabolism is weak. Many of the trials were short term, of poor experimental design for the stated purpose, and conducted on small sample sizes. To assess the modulation by specific SNPs of the effects of dietary interventions on lipid metabolism, there is a need for well-designed, adequately powered, randomized controlled studies, or studies that are of equivalent level, of greater duration, and in which careful consideration is given to which patients to include. Emphasis should be placed on carrying out appropriate studies to increase consistency. Moreover, nutrigenomic research should also investigate the potential mechanisms involved in the gene-diet interactions reported by nutrigenetic studies. In a few years, both nutrigenetics and nutrigenomics will increase the level of evidence of some of the observed interactions, and personalized nutrition will be both possible and potentially successful (119). One of the first applications of personalized nutrition seems to be centered in dislipidemic patients who require special intervention with dietary treatment. It is known that these individuals will display dramatic heterogeneity in response to the currently recommended therapeutic diets and that the recommendations will need to be adjusted individually. This process could be more efficient if the recommendations are carried out based on genetic and molecular knowledge. Moreover, compliance with dietary advice may increase when it is supported with information based on nutritional genomics and when the patient feels that the advice is personalized. However, a number of important changes in the provision of health care are needed in order to achieve the potential benefits associated with this concept, including a teamwork approach, with greater integration among physicians, dieticians, and genetic counselors. After more experience is gained from patients and/or individuals at high risk, these approaches could be applied toward primary prevention.

SUMMARY AND CONCLUSIONS

In summary, the current evidence supports the concept that gene-diet interactions modulate plasma lipid concentrations and, potentially, cardiovascular risk. However, the application of these findings to the clinical environment is not ready for prime time. Current and future findings need to be replicated using experimental approaches providing the highest level of scientific evidence. Moreover, most of the past and current studies are being conducted using the simplest scenarios, i.e., one single dietary component, one single SNP, and one single risk factor. We have to evolve toward more realistic situations involving interactions of multiple genes, dietary components, and risk factors. This will require large genetic epidemiological studies and intervention studies involving groups of individuals selected for specific genotype combinations and phenotypic characteristics. Another current major gap relates to the inaccuracies of the dietary instruments used in epidemiological studies and the databases used to translate foods into nutrients. These areas need further development to achieve more precision and consistency from nutrigenomic studies.

ACKNOWLEDGMENTS

The authors' study is supported by grants from the American Heart Association (0335432T), USDA/FAS/ICD/RSED/SCRP, and NIH/NHLBI (HL54776); contracts 53-K06-5-10 and 58-1950-9-001 from the U.S. Department of Agriculture Research Service; and grants G03/140 and PI02-1096 from the Instituto de Salud Carlos III, Spain.

The *Annual Review of Nutrition* is online at http://nutr.annualreviews.org

LITERATURE CITED

1. Altmann SW, Davis HR Jr, Zhu LJ, Yao X, Hoos LM, et al. 2004. Niemann-Pick C1 Like 1 protein is critical for intestinal cholesterol absorption. *Science* 303:1201–4
2. Antonarakis SE, Nomenclature Working Group. 1998. Recommendations for a nomenclature system for human gene mutations. *Hum. Mutat.* 11:1–3
3. Assmann G, Gotto AM Jr. 2004. HDL cholesterol and protective factors in atherosclerosis. *Circulation* 109 (23 Suppl. 1): III8–14
4. Assmann G, Nofer JR. 2003. Atheroprotective effects of high-density lipoproteins. *Annu. Rev. Med.* 54:321–41
5. Asztalos B, Lefevre M, Wong L, Foster TA, Tulley R, et al. 2000. Differential response to low-fat diet between low and normal HDL-cholesterol subjects. *J. Lipid Res.* 41:321–28
6. Atkinson C, Oosthuizen W, Scollen S, Loktionov A, Day NE, Bingham SA. 2004. Modest protective effects of isoflavones from a red clover–derived dietary supplement on cardiovascular disease risk factors in perimenopausal women, and evidence of an interaction with ApoE genotype in 49–65-year-old women. *J. Nutr.* 134:1759–64
7. Austin MA, Hutter CM, Zimmern RL, Humphries SE. 2004. Familial hypercholesterolemia and coronary heart

disease: a HuGE association review. *Am. J. Epidemiol.* 160:421–29

8. Austin MA, Hutter CM, Zimmern RL, Humphries SE. 2004. Genetic causes of monogenic heterozygous familial hypercholesterolemia: a HuGE prevalence review. *Am. J. Epidemiol.* 160:407–20
9. Beaty TH, Khoury MJ. 2000. Interface of genetics and epidemiology. *Epidemiol. Rev.* 22:120–25
10. Bertolini S, Cantafora A, Averna M, Cortese C, Motti C, et al. 2000. Clinical expression of familial hypercholesterolemia in clusters of mutations of the LDL receptor gene that cause a receptor-defective or receptor-negative phenotype. *Arterioscler. Thromb. Vasc. Biol.* 20:E41–52
11. Bertolini S, Pisciotta L, Di Scala L, Langheim S, Bellocchio A, et al. 2004. Genetic polymorphisms affecting the phenotypic expression of familial hypercholesterolemia. *Atherosclerosis* 174:57–65
12. Botto LD, Khoury MJ. 2001. Commentary: facing the challenge of gene-environment interaction: the two-by-four table and beyond. *Am. J. Epidemiol.* 153: 1016–20
13. Breslow JL. 2000. Genetics of lipoprotein abnormalities associated with coronary artery disease susceptibility. *Annu. Rev. Genet.* 34:233–54
14. Brown MS, Goldstein JL. 1976. Analysis of a mutant strain of human fibroblasts with a defect in the internalization of receptor-bound low density lipoprotein. *Cell* 9:663–74
15. Brown S, Ordovas JM, Campos H. 2003. Interaction between the APOC3 gene promoter polymorphisms, saturated fat intake and plasma lipoproteins. *Atherosclerosis* 170:307–13
16. Campos H, D'Agostino M, Ordovas JM. 2001. Gene-diet interactions and plasma lipoproteins: role of apolipoprotein E and habitual saturated fat intake. *Genet. Epidemiol.* 20:117–28
17. Campos H, Lopez-Miranda J, Rodriguez C, Albajar M, Schaefer EJ, Ordovas JM. 1997. Urbanization elicits a more atherogenic lipoprotein profile in carriers of the apolipoprotein A-IV-2 allele than in A-IV-1 homozygotes. *Arterioscler. Thromb. Vasc. Biol.* 17:1074–81
18. Cargill M, Altshuler D, Ireland J, Sklar P, Ardlie K, et al. 1999. Characterization of single-nucleotide polymorphisms in coding regions of human genes. *Nat. Genet.* 22:231–38
19. Cederbaum S. 2002. Phenylketonuria: an update. *Curr. Opin. Pediatr.* 14:702–6
20. Chahoud G, Aude YW, Mehta JL. 2004. Dietary recommendations in the prevention and treatment of coronary heart disease: Do we have the ideal diet yet? *Am. J. Cardiol.* 94:1260–67
21. Civeira F, Intl. Panel Manag. Familial Hypercholesterolemia. 2004. Guidelines for the diagnosis and management of heterozygous familial hypercholesterolemia. *Atherosclerosis* 173:55–68
22. Connelly MA, Williams DL. 2004. Scavenger receptor BI: a scavenger receptor with a mission to transport high density lipoprotein lipids. *Curr. Opin. Lipidol.* 15: 287–95
23. Corella D, Guillen M, Saiz C, Portoles O, Sabater A, et al. 2001. Environmental factors modulate the effect of the APOE genetic polymorphism on plasma lipid concentrations: ecogenetic studies in a Mediterranean Spanish population. *Metabolism* 50:936–44
24. Corella D, Guillen M, Saiz C, Portoles O, Sabater A, et al. 2002. Associations of LPL and APOC3 gene polymorphisms on plasma lipids in a Mediterranean population: interaction with tobacco smoking and the APOE locus. *J. Lipid Res.* 43:416–27
25. Corella D, Tucker K, Lahoz C, Coltell O, Cupples LA, et al. 2001. Alcohol drinking determines the effect of the APOE locus on LDL-cholesterol concentrations

in men: the Framingham Offspring Study. *Am. J. Clin. Nutr.* 73:736–45
26. Couillard C, Vohl MC, Engert JC, Lemieux I, Houde A, et al. 2003. Effect of apoC-III gene polymorphisms on the lipoprotein-lipid profile of viscerally obese men. *J. Lipid Res.* 44:986–93
27. Couture P, Archer WR, Lamarche B, Landry N, Deriaz O, et al. 2003. Influences of apolipoprotein E polymorphism on the response of plasma lipids to the ad libitum consumption of a high-carbohydrate diet compared with a high-monounsaturated fatty acid diet. *Metabolism* 52:1454–59
28. Davey Smith G, Ebrahim S. 2003. Mendelian randomization: Can genetic epidemiology contribute to understanding environmental determinants of disease? *Int. J. Epidemiol.* 32:1–22
29. Davis HR Jr, Zhu LJ, Hoos LM, Tetzloff G, Maguire M, et al. 2004. Niemann-Pick C1 Like 1 (NPC1L1) is the intestinal phytosterol and cholesterol transporter and a key modulator of whole-body cholesterol homeostasis. *J. Biol. Chem.* 279:33586–92
30. de Andrade M, Amos CI, Thiel TJ. 1999. Methods to estimate genetic components of variance for quantitative traits in family studies. *Genet. Epidemiol.* 17:64–76
31. Dedoussis GV, Schmidt H, Genschel J. 2004. LDL-receptor mutations in Europe. *Hum. Mutat.* 24:443–59
32. Erkkila AT, Sarkkinen ES, Lindi V, Lehto S, Laakso M, Uusitupa MI. 2001. APOE polymorphism and the hypertriglyceridemic effect of dietary sucrose. *Am. J. Clin. Nutr.* 73:746–52
33. Fujino T, Navaratnam N, Scott J. 1998. Human apolipoprotein B RNA editing deaminase gene (APOBEC1). *Genomics* 47:266–75
34. Ganan A, Corella D, Guillen M, Ordovas JM, Pocovi M. 2004. Frequencies of apolipoprotein A4 gene polymorphisms and association with serum lipid concentrations in two healthy Spanish populations. *Hum. Biol.* 76:253–66
35. Garcia-Closas M, Lubin JH. 1999. Power and sample size calculations in case-control studies of gene-environment interactions: comments on different approaches. *Am. J. Epidemiol.* 149:689–92
36. Gibbons GF, Wiggins D, Brown AM, Hebbachi AM. 2004. Synthesis and function of hepatic very-low-density lipoprotein. *Biochem. Soc. Trans.* 32(Pt. 1):59–64
37. Greenland S. 1993. Basic problems in interaction assessment. *Environ. Health Perspect.* 101(Suppl. 4):59–66
38. Hagberg JM, Wilund KR, Ferrell RE. 2000. APO E gene and gene-environment effects on plasma lipoprotein-lipid levels. *Physiol. Genomics* 4:101–8
39. Halverstadt A, Phares DA, Ferrell RE, Wilund KR, Goldberg AP, Hagberg JM. 2003. High-density lipoprotein-cholesterol, its subfractions, and responses to exercise training are dependent on endothelial lipase genotype. *Metabolism* 52:1505–11
40. Havel RJ, Kane JP. 1975. Quantification of triglyceride transport in blood plasma: a critical analysis. *Fed. Proc.* 34:2250–57
41. Hegele RA. 2002. Environmental modulation of atherosclerosis end points in familial hypercholesterolemia. *Atherosclerosis* 2(Suppl.):5–7
42. Heller DA, de Faire U, Pedersen NL, Dahlen G, McClearn GE. 1993. Genetic and environmental influences on serum lipid levels in twins. *N. Engl. J. Med.* 328:1150–56
43. Hofman MK, Weggemans RM, Zock PL, Schouten EG, Katan MB, Princen HM. 2004. CYP7A1 A-278C polymorphism affects the response of plasma lipids after dietary cholesterol or cafestol interventions in humans. *J. Nutr.* 134:2200–4
44. Holtzman NA. 1988. Genetic variation in nutritional requirements and susceptibility to disease: policy implications. *Am. J. Clin. Nutr.* 48:1510–16
45. Hubacek JA, Pitha J, Skodova Z, Poledne R, Lanska V, et al. 2003. Polymorphisms

in CYP-7A1, not APOE, influence the change in plasma lipids in response to population dietary change in an 8-year follow-up; results from the Czech MONICA study. *Clin. Biochem.* 36:263–67
46. Huff MW. 2003. Dietary cholesterol, cholesterol absorption, postprandial lipemia and atherosclerosis. *Can. J. Clin. Pharmacol.* 10(Suppl. A):26–32
47. Humphries SE, Montgomery HE, Talmud PJ. 2001. Predisposing genes, high-risk environments and coronary artery disease: LPL and fibrinogen as examples. *World Rev. Nutr. Diet.* 89:61–67
48. Humphries SE, Ridker PM, Talmud PJ. 2004. Genetic testing for cardiovascular disease susceptibility: a useful clinical management tool or possible misinformation? *Arterioscler. Thromb. Vasc. Biol.* 24:628–36
49. Hussain MM, Shi J, Dreizen P. 2003. Microsomal triglyceride transfer protein and its role in apoB-lipoprotein assembly. *J. Lipid Res.* 44:22–32
50. Hyson D, Rutledge JC, Berglund L. 2003. Postprandial lipemia and cardiovascular disease. *Curr. Atheroscler. Rep.* 5:437–44
51. Ioannidis JP, Ntzani EE, Trikalinos TA, Contopoulos-Ioannidis DG. 2001. Replication validity of genetic association studies. *Nat. Genet.* 29:306–9
52. Jacobs B, De Angelis-Schierbaum G, Egert S, Assmann G, Kratz M. 2004. Individual serum triglyceride responses to high-fat and low-fat diets differ in men with modest and severe hypertriglyceridemia. *J. Nutr.* 134:1400–5
53. Jacobs DR Jr, Anderson JT, Hannan P, Keys A, Blackburn H. 1983. Variability in individual serum cholesterol response to change in diet. *Arteriosclerosis* 3:349–56
54. Jang Y, Kim JY, Kim OY, Lee JE, Cho H, et al. 2004. The 1131T→C polymorphism in the apolipoprotein A5 gene is associated with postprandial hypertriacylglycerolemia; elevated small, dense LDL concentrations; and oxidative stress in nonobese Korean men. *Am. J. Clin. Nutr.* 80:832–40
55. Jemaa R, Mebazaa A, Fumeron F. 2004. Apolipoprotein B signal peptide polymorphism and plasma LDL-cholesterol response to low-calorie diet. *Int. J. Obes. Relat. Metab. Disord.* 28:902–5
56. Kardia SL. 2000. Context-dependent genetic effects in hypertension. *Curr. Hypertens. Rep.* 2:32–38
57. Katan MB, Beynen AC, De Vries JH, Nobels A. 1986. Existence of consistent hypo- and hyperresponders to dietary cholesterol in man. *Am. J. Epidemiol.* 123: 221–34
58. Katan MB, Grundy SM, Willett WC. 1997. Should a low-fat, high-carbohydrate diet be recommended for everyone? Beyond low-fat diets. *N. Engl. J. Med.* 337: 563–66
59. Krauss RM. 2001. Atherogenic lipoprotein phenotype and diet-gene interactions. *J. Nutr.* 131:340–43S
60. Krauss RM. 2001. Dietary and genetic effects on low-density lipoprotein heterogeneity. *Annu. Rev. Nutr.* 21:283–95
61. Krieger M. 2001. Scavenger receptor class B type I is a multiligand HDL receptor that influences diverse physiologic systems. *J. Clin. Invest.* 108:793–97
62. LeLorier J, Gregoire G, Benhaddad A, Lapierre J, Derderian F. 1997. Discrepancies between meta-analyses and subsequent large, randomized, controlled trials. *N. Engl. J. Med.* 337:536–42
63. Lindi V, Schwab U, Louheranta A, Laakso M, Vessby B, et al. 2003. Impact of the Pro12Ala polymorphism of the PPAR-gamma2 gene on serum triacylglycerol response to n-3 fatty acid supplementation. *Mol. Genet. Metab.* 79:52–60
64. Little J, Bradley L, Bray MS, Clyne M, Dorman J, et al. 2002. Reporting, appraising, and integrating data on genotype prevalence and gene-disease associations. *Am. J. Epidemiol.* 156:300–10
65. Loktionov A. 2003. Common gene polymorphisms and nutrition: emerging

links with pathogenesis of multifactorial chronic diseases. *J. Nutr. Biochem.* 14: 426–51

66. Loktionov A, Scollen S, McKeown N, Bingham SA. 2000. Gene-nutrient interactions: dietary behaviour associated with high coronary heart disease risk particularly affects serum LDL cholesterol in apolipoprotein E epsilon4-carrying free-living individuals. *Br. J. Nutr.* 84:885–90
67. Lopez-Miranda J, Cruz G, Gomez P, Marin C, Paz E, et al. 2004. The influence of lipoprotein lipase gene variation on postprandial lipoprotein metabolism. *J. Clin. Endocrinol. Metabolism* 89:4721–28
68. Lottenberg AM, Nunes VS, Nakandakare ER, Neves M, Bernik M, et al. 2003. The human cholesteryl ester transfer protein I405V polymorphism is associated with plasma cholesterol concentration and its reduction by dietary phytosterol esters. *J. Nutr.* 133:1800–5
69. Lusis AJ, Mar R, Pajukanta P. 2004. Genetics of atherosclerosis. *Annu. Rev. Genomics Hum. Genet.* 5:189–218
70. Marin C, Lopez-Miranda J, Gomez P, Paz E, Perez-Martinez P, et al. 2002. Effects of the human apolipoprotein A-I promoter G-A mutation on postprandial lipoprotein metabolism. *Am. J. Clin. Nutr.* 76:319–25
71. Martin S, Nicaud V, Humphries SE, Talmud PJ, EARS Group. 2003. Contribution of APOA5 gene variants to plasma triglyceride determination and to the response to both fat and glucose tolerance challenges. *Biochim. Biophys. Acta* 1637:217–25
72. Masson LF, McNeill G, Avenell A. 2003. Genetic variation and the lipid response to dietary intervention: a systematic review. *Am. J. Clin. Nutr.* 77:1098–111
73. Memisoglu A, Hu FB, Hankinson SE, Liu S, Meigs JB, et al. 2003. Prospective study of the association between the proline to alanine codon 12 polymorphism in the PPARgamma gene and type 2 diabetes. *Diabetes Care* 26:2915–17
74. Moreno JA, Lopez-Miranda J, Marin C, Gomez P, Perez-Martinez P, et al. 2003. The influence of the apolipoprotein E gene promoter (−219G/T) polymorphism on postprandial lipoprotein metabolism in young normolipemic males. *J. Lipid Res.* 44:2059–64
75. Moreno JA, Perez-Jimenez F, Marin C, Gomez P, Perez-Martinez P, et al. 2004. The effect of dietary fat on LDL size is influenced by apolipoprotein E genotype in healthy subjects. *J. Nutr.* 134:2517–22
76. Mu H, Hoy CE. 2004. The digestion of dietary triacylglycerols. *Prog. Lipid Res.* 43:105–33
77. Muller M, Kersten S. 2003. Nutrigenomics: goals and strategies. *Nat. Rev. Genet.* 4:315–22
78. Neale BM, Sham PC. 2004. The future of association studies: gene-based analysis and replication. *Am. J. Hum. Genet.* 75: 353–62
79. Nicklas BJ, Ferrell RE, Bunyard LB, Berman DM, Dennis KE, Goldberg AP. 2002. Effects of apolipoprotein E genotype on dietary-induced changes in high-density lipoprotein cholesterol in obese postmenopausal women. *Metabolism* 51:853–58
80. Ordovas JM. 2000. Genetic polymorphisms and activity of cholesterol ester transfer protein (CETP): Should we be measuring them? *Clin. Chem. Lab. Med.* 38:945–49
81. Ordovas JM. 2001. Genetics, postprandial lipemia and obesity. *Nutr. Metab. Cardiovasc. Dis.* 11:118–33
82. Ordovas JM. 2002. HDL genetics: candidate genes, genome wide scans and gene-environment interactions. *Cardiovasc. Drugs Ther.* 16:273–81
83. Ordovas JM, Corella D. 2004. Nutritional genomics. *Annu. Rev. Genomics Hum. Genet.* 5:71–118
84. Ordovas JM, Corella D, Demissie S, Cupples LA, Couture P, et al. 2002. Dietary fat intake determines the effect of a common polymorphism in the hepatic lipase

gene promoter on high-density lipoprotein metabolism: evidence of a strong dose effect in this gene-nutrient interaction in the Framingham Study. *Circulation* 106:2315–21
85. Ordovas JM, Corella D, Cupples LA, Demissie S, Kelleher A, et al. 2002. Polyunsaturated fatty acids modulate the effects of the APOA1 G-A polymorphism on HDL-cholesterol concentrations in a sex-specific manner: the Framingham Study. *Am. J. Clin. Nutr.* 75:38–46
86. Ordovas JM, Mooser V. 2002. The APOE locus and the pharmacogenetics of lipid response. *Curr. Opin. Lipidol.* 13:113–17
87. Ordovas JM, Tai ES. 2002. The babel of the ABCs: novel transporters involved in the regulation of sterol absorption and excretion. *Nutr. Rev.* 60:30–33
88. Ottman R. 1990. An epidemiological approach to gene-environment interaction. *Genet. Epidemiol.* 7:177–85
89. Paradis ME, Couture P, Bosse Y, Despres JP, Perusse L, et al. 2003. The T111I mutation in the EL gene modulates the impact of dietary fat on the HDL profile in women. *J. Lipid Res.* 44:1902–8
90. Parks EJ, Rutledge JC, Davis PA, Hyson DA, Schneeman BO, Kappagoda CT. 2001. Predictors of plasma triglyceride elevation in patients participating in a coronary atherosclerosis treatment program. *J. Cardiopulm. Rehabil.* 21:73–79
91. Pennacchio LA, Rubin EM. 2003. Apolipoprotein A5, a newly identified gene that affects plasma triglyceride levels in humans and mice. *Arterioscler. Thromb. Vasc. Biol.* 23:529–34
92. Perez-Martinez P, Gomez P, Paz E, Marin C, Gavilan Moral E, et al. 2001. Interaction between smoking and the Sstl polymorphism of the apo C-III gene determines plasma lipid response to diet. *Nutr. Metab. Cardiovasc. Dis.* 11:237–43
93. Perez-Martinez P, Lopez-Miranda J, Ordovas JM, Bellido C, Marin C, et al. 2004. Postprandial lipemia is modified by the presence of the polymorphism present in the exon 1 variant at the SR-BI gene locus. *J. Mol. Endocrinol.* 32:237–45
94. Perez-Martinez P, Ordovas JM, Lopez-Miranda J, Gomez P, Marin C, et al. 2003. Polymorphism exon 1 variant at the locus of the scavenger receptor class B type I gene: influence on plasma LDL cholesterol in healthy subjects during the consumption of diets with different fat contents. *Am. J. Clin. Nutr.* 77:809–13
95. Petot GJ, Traore F, Debanne SM, Lerner AJ, Smyth KA, Friedland RP. 2003. Interactions of apolipoprotein E genotype and dietary fat intake of healthy older persons during mid-adult life. *Metabolism* 52:279–81
96. Pimstone SN, Sun XM, du Souich C, Frohlich JJ, Hayden MR, Soutar AK. 1998. Phenotypic variation in heterozygous familial hypercholesterolemia: a comparison of Chinese patients with the same or similar mutations in the LDL receptor gene in China or Canada. *Arterioscler. Thromb. Vasc. Biol.* 18:309–15
97. Plat J, Mensink RP. 2002. Relationship of genetic variation in genes encoding apolipoprotein A-IV, scavenger receptor BI, HMG-CoA reductase, CETP and apolipoprotein E with cholesterol metabolism and the response to plant stanol ester consumption. *Eur. J. Clin. Invest.* 32:242–50
98. Poustie VJ, Rutherford P. 2001. Dietary treatment for familial hypercholesterolaemia. *Cochrane Database Syst. Rev.* 2:CD001918
98a. Rantala M, Rantala TT, Savolainen MJ, Friedlander Y, Kesaniemi YA. 2000. Apolipoprotein B gene polymorphisms and serum lipids: meta-analysis of the role of genetic variation in responsiveness to diet. *Am. J. Clin. Nutr.* 71(3):713–24
99. Rantala M, Silaste ML, Tuominen A, Kaikkonen J, Salonen JT, et al. 2002. Dietary modifications and gene polymorphisms alter serum paraoxonase activity in healthy women. *J. Nutr.* 132:3012–17
100. Rebbeck TR, Spitz M, Wu X. 2004.

Assessing the function of genetic variants in candidate gene association studies. *Nat. Rev. Genet.* 5:589–97
101. Redgrave TG. 2004. Chylomicron metabolism. *Biochem. Soc. Trans.* 32(Pt. 1):79–82
102. Reiber I, Mezo I, Kalina A, Palos G, Romics L, Csaszar A. 2003. Postprandial triglyceride levels in familial combined hyperlipidemia. The role of apolipoprotein E and lipoprotein lipase polymorphisms. *J. Nutr. Biochem.* 14:394–400
103. Robitaille J, Brouillette C, Houde A, Lemieux S, Perusse L, et al. 2004. Association between the PPARα-L162V polymorphism and components of the metabolic syndrome. *J. Hum. Genet.* 49: 482–89
104. Robitaille J, Brouillette C, Lemieux S, Perusse L, Gaudet D, Vohl MC. 2004. Plasma concentrations of apolipoprotein B are modulated by a gene-diet interaction effect between the LFABP T94A polymorphism and dietary fat intake in French-Canadian men. *Mol. Genet. Metab.* 82:296–303
105. Rothman KJ, Greenland S, Walker AM. 1980. Concepts of interaction. *Am. J. Epidemiol.* 112:467–70
106. Schaefer EJ, Lamon-Fava S, Ausman LM, Ordovas JM, Clevidence BA, et al. 1997. Individual variability in lipoprotein cholesterol response to National Cholesterol Education Program Step 2 diets. *Am. J. Clin. Nutr.* 65:823–30
107. Schwab US, Agren JJ, Valve R, Hallikainen MA, Sarkkinen ES, et al. 2002. The impact of the leucine 7 to proline 7 polymorphism of the neuropeptide Y gene on postprandial lipemia and on the response of serum total and lipoprotein lipids to a reduced fat diet. *Eur. J. Clin. Nutr.* 56:149–56
108. Sijbrands EJ, Westendorp RG, Defesche JC, de Meier PH, Smelt AH, Kastelein JJ. 2001. Mortality over two centuries in large pedigree with familial hypercholesterolaemia: family tree mortality study. *BMJ* 322:1019–23
109. Sun XM, Patel DD, Webb JC, Knight BL, Fan LM, et al. 1994. Familial hypercholesterolemia in China. Identification of mutations in the LDL-receptor gene that result in a receptor-negative phenotype. *Arterioscler. Thromb.* 14:85–94
110. Tai ES, Corella D, Deurenberg-Yap M, Cutter J, Chew SK, et al. 2003. Dietary fat interacts with the $-514C > T$ polymorphism in the hepatic lipase gene promoter on plasma lipid profiles in a multiethnic Asian population: the 1998 Singapore National Health Survey. *J. Nutr.* 133:3399–408
111. Tai ES, Ordovas JM, Corella D, Deurenberg-Yap M, Chan E, et al. 2003. The TaqIB and $-629C > A$ polymorphisms at the cholesteryl ester transfer protein locus: associations with lipid levels in a multiethnic population. The 1998 Singapore National Health Survey. *Clin. Genet.* 63:19–30
112. Tamasawa N, Murakami H, Yamato K, Matsui J, Tanabe J, Suda T. 2003. Influence of apolipoprotein E genotype on the response to caloric restriction in type 2 diabetic patients with hyperlipidaemia. *Diabetes Obes. Metab.* 5:345–48
113. Tiret L. 2002. Gene-environment interaction: a central concept in multifactorial diseases. *Proc. Nutr. Soc.* 61:457–63
114. Tobin MD, Minelli C, Burton PR, Thompson JR. 2004. Development of Mendelian randomization: from hypothesis test to "Mendelian deconfounding". *Int. J. Epidemiol.* 33:26–29
115. Tomas M, Senti M, Elosua R, Vila J, Sala J, et al. 2001. Interaction between the Gln-Arg 192 variants of the paraoxonase gene and oleic acid intake as a determinant of high-density lipoprotein cholesterol and paraoxonase activity. *Eur. J. Pharmacol.* 432:121–28
116. Trayhurn P. 2003. Nutritional genomics—"Nutrigenomics". *Br. J. Nutr.* 89:1–2
117. Umans-Eckenhausen MA, Defesche JC,

Sijbrands EJ, Scheerder RL, Kastelein JJ. 2001. Review of first 5 years of screening for familial hypercholesterolaemia in the Netherlands. *Lancet* 357:165–68

118. van Dijk KW, Rensen PC, Voshol PJ, Havekes LM. 2004. The role and mode of action of apolipoproteins CIII and AV: synergistic actors in triglyceride metabolism? *Curr. Opin. Lipidol.* 15:239–46
119. van Ommen B, Stierum R. 2002. Nutrigenomics: exploiting systems biology in the nutrition and health arena. *Curr. Opin. Biotechnol.* 13:517–21
120. Vincent S, Planells R, Defoort C, Bernard MC, Gerber M, et al. 2002. Genetic polymorphisms and lipoprotein responses to diets. *Proc. Nutr. Soc.* 61:427–34
121. Vuorio AF, Gylling H, Turtola H, Kontula K, Ketonen P, Miettinen TA. 2000. Stanol ester margarine alone and with simvastatin lowers serum cholesterol in families with familial hypercholesterolemia caused by the FH-North Karelia mutation. *Arterioscler. Thromb. Vasc. Biol.* 20:500–6
122. Wiegman A, Hutten BA, de Groot E, Rodenburg J, Bakker HD, et al. 2004. Efficacy and safety of statin therapy in children with familial hypercholesterolemia: a randomized controlled trial. *JAMA* 292:331–37
123. Williams RR, Hasstedt SJ, Wilson DE, Ash KO, Yanowitz FF. 1986. Evidence that men with familial hypercholesterolemia can avoid early coronary death. An analysis of 77 gene carriers in four Utah pedigrees. *JAMA* 255:219–24
124. Woo SK, Kang HS. 2003. The apolipoprotein CIII T2854G variants are associated with postprandial triacylglycerol concentrations in normolipidemic Korean men. *J. Hum. Genet.* 48:551–55
125. Zilversmit DB. 1979. Atherogenesis: a postprandial phenomenon. *Circulation* 60:473–85

Annu. Rev. Nutr. 2005. 25:391–406
doi: 10.1146/annurev.nutr.24.012003.132155

First published online as a Review in Advance on February 11, 2005

THE INSULIN RESISTANCE SYNDROME: Definition and Dietary Approaches to Treatment

Gerald M. Reaven
Division of Cardiovascular Medicine, Department of Medicine, Stanford University School of Medicine, Stanford, California 94305; email: greaven@cvmed.stanford.edu

Key Words hyperinsulinemia, cardiovascular disease, dietary carbohydrate, dietary fat, weight loss

■ **Abstract** The ability of insulin to stimulate glucose disposal varies at least sixfold in apparently healthy individuals, and approximately one-third of the population that is most resistant to this action of insulin is at greatly increased risk to develop a number of adverse clinical outcomes. Type 2 diabetes occurs when insulin resistant individuals are unable to secrete enough insulin to compensate for the defect in insulin action, and this was the first clinical syndrome identified as being related to insulin resistance. Although the majority of insulin-resistant individuals are able to maintain the level of compensatory hyperinsulinemia needed to prevent the development of a significant degree of hyperglycemia, the combination of insulin resistance and hyperinsulinemia greatly increases the likelihood of developing a cluster of closely related abnormalities and the resultant clinical diagnoses that can be considered to make up the insulin resistance syndrome (IRS). Since being overweight/obese and sedentary decreases insulin sensitivity, it is not surprising that the prevalence of the manifestations of the IRS is increasing at a rapid rate. From a dietary standpoint, there are two approaches to attenuating the manifestations of the IRS: (*a*) weight loss to enhance insulin sensitivity in those overweight/obese individuals who are insulin resistant/hyperinsulinemic; and (*b*) changes in macronutrient content of diets to avoid the adverse effects of the compensatory hyperinsulinemia. This chapter will focus on defining the abnormalities and clinical syndromes that compose the IRS and evaluating the dietary changes that can ameliorate its adverse consequences.

CONTENTS

INTRODUCTION

The aim of this chapter is to consider the role that changes in the amount and kind of calories consumed can play in attenuating the manifestations of the insulin resistance syndrome (IRS). Prevalence of the adverse clinical consequences of the IRS is growing rapidly in parallel with worldwide increases in body weight, and successful weight loss in overweight/obese individuals can moderate the abnormalities and clinical syndromes associated with insulin resistance (9, 26, 30, 35, 37, 42, 45, 56, 58). However, weight loss is difficult to achieve, and not all overweight/obese individuals are insulin resistant (1, 35, 37, 39). Thus, a major goal of this review is to define the relationship between excess adiposity, insulin resistance, and the IRS, as well as to offer suggestions to help identify those overweight/obese individuals who will benefit the most from weight loss.

Although weight loss of 5%–10% of initial body weight can enhance insulin sensitivity in overweight/obese individuals who are insulin resistant, not all of the abnormalities in these individuals return to the levels seen in insulin-sensitive individuals (35, 37). Furthermore, normal-weight individuals are not all insulin sensitive, nor are they spared from developing manifestations of the IRS (1, 39). Fortunately, the therapeutic benefits of dietary intervention in insulin-resistant persons are not limited to decreasing total caloric intake, and evidence is reviewed showing that clinically useful changes can also occur in insulin-resistant individuals by changing the macronutrient composition of isocaloric diets. In contrast to weight loss, which both enhances insulin sensitivity and lowers plasma insulin concentrations, variations in the relative proportion of macronutrients in the diet have little, or no, effect on insulin-mediated glucose disposal. However, by modifying the level of circulating insulin required to maintain glucose homeostasis in insulin-resistant individuals, variations in diet composition have the ability to either accentuate, or attenuate, the manifestations of the IRS.

Based on the general considerations outlined above, the remainder of this chapter (*a*) describes the abnormalities and clinical syndromes associated with insulin resistance (the IRS); (*b*) defines the relationship between excess adiposity and insulin resistance, and outlines approaches to identify those overweight/obese individuals who will benefit the most from weight loss; and (*c*) explains why the usual recommended "prudent" diet based on replacing saturated fat (SF) with carbohydrate (CHO) will have adverse consequences in individuals with the IRS. Although implicit in the discussion to this point, it should be explicitly stated that only experimental results obtained in human beings are considered in addressing the issues outlined above.

DEFINITION OF THE INSULIN RESISTANCE SYNDROME (IRS)

Differentiation from the Metabolic Syndrome

Sensitivity to insulin-mediated glucose disposal varies widely in the population at large (61). When insulin-resistant individuals cannot maintain the degree of hyperinsulinemia needed to overcome the defect in insulin action, type 2 diabetes develops (46). Although the vast majority of individuals can sustain the level of compensatory hyperinsulinemia needed to maintain normal or near-normal glucose tolerance, this philanthropic effort on the part of the pancreatic beta cell is a mixed blessing. The combination of insulin resistance and compensatory hyperinsulinemia prevents the development of frank hyperglycemia, but greatly increases the risk of having some degree of glucose intolerance, a high plasma triglyceride (TG) and low high-density lipoprotein cholesterol (HDL-C) concentration, and essential hypertension (46). In 1988, it was proposed that individuals displaying this cluster of abnormalities associated with insulin resistance/compensatory hyperinsulinemia were at significantly increased risk of cardiovascular disease (CVD) (46). Because the importance of insulin resistance and associated abnormalities as CVD risk factors was not widely appreciated at that time, the cluster of associated abnormalities was subsumed under the rubric of syndrome X.

Since the introduction of the concept of syndrome X, considerable information has evolved relevant to the role of insulin resistance in human diseases. This has resulted in two somewhat disparate approaches to thinking about the clinical implications of insulin resistance and its consequences. One view recognizes that the abnormalities related to insulin resistance have broadened considerably, and the adverse clinical outcomes extend beyond type 2 diabetes and CVD. Because CVD is recognized to be just one of the multiple clinical syndromes associated with insulin resistance, it seems appropriate to replace the term syndrome X with one that more aptly deals with this new information. In this context, the IRS seems to be a logical choice to provide a pathophysiological construct with which to view the different abnormalities and clinical syndromes that occur more commonly in insulin-resistant individuals.

During a period when the number of abnormalities and clinical syndromes related to insulin resistance was expanding rapidly, the cardiological community acknowledged the importance of this defect in insulin action as increasing CVD risk with the report of the Adult Treatment Panel III (ATP III) of the National Cholesterol Education Program (12). The ATP III recognized the importance of CVD risk factors of what they referred to as a "constellation of lipid and nonlipid risk factors of metabolic origin," designated this cluster as the metabolic syndrome,

TABLE 1 ATP III[a] criteria for diagnosing the metabolic syndrome[b]

Abdominal obesity	
Men: waist circumference >40 inches	
Women: waist circumference >35 inches	
Fasting glucose ≥110, <126 mg/dl	
Blood pressure ≥130/80 mm Hg	
Triglycerides ≥150 mg/dl	
High-density lipoprotein cholesterol	
Men <40 mg/dl	
Women <50 mg/dl	

[a]Adult Treatment Panel III of the National Cholesterol Education Program.

[b]The metabolic syndrome is present when three or more of the five criteria are met.

and stated, "This syndrome is closely related to insulin resistance." Table 1 lists the five criteria selected by the ATP III with which to diagnose the metabolic syndrome. Other than the inclusion of abdominal obesity, the abnormalities selected by the ATP III are those initially proposed to comprise syndrome X, and these choices reflect their view that insulin resistance is at the root of the problem. On the other hand, the stated purpose of the ATP III is to provide criteria to make a clinical diagnosis of the metabolic syndrome, not to provide a physiological construct to explain why insulin resistant/hyperinsulinemic individuals are at increased CVD risk.

Put more explicitly; in contrast to the physiological construct underlying the IRS, the metabolic syndrome is aimed at providing the means to make a clinical diagnosis. Whether or not this effort will prove to be of clinical benefit remains to be seen, but because of its broader construct, the focus of this chapter is on the IRS.

Abnormalities and Clinical Syndromes Associated with Insulin Resistance

Insulin resistance is not a disease unto itself, but a physiological abnormality that increases the likelihood that one or more of the abnormalities listed in Table 2 will be present. Furthermore, because these abnormalities occur more commonly in insulin-resistant individuals, these individuals are at increased risk to develop the clinical syndromes listed in Table 3. However, the relationship between insulin resistance and the changes listed in Tables 2 and 3 is complicated, and the abnormalities and clinical syndromes can occur in the absence of insulin resistance. It must also be emphasized that insulin-resistant individuals do not necessarily develop any of the clinical syndromes listed in Table 3.

TABLE 2 Abnormalities associated with insulin resistance/ compensatory hyperinsulinemia

- Some degree of glucose intolerance
  - Impaired fasting glucose
  - Impaired glucose tolerance
- Dyslipidemia
  - ↑ Triglycerides
  - ↓ HDL-C
  - ↓ LDL-particle diameter (small, dense LDL particles)
  - ↑ Postprandial accumulation of triglyceride-rich lipoproteins
- Endothelial dysfunction
  - ↑ Mononuclear cell adhesion
  - ↑ Plasma concentration of cellular adhesion molecules
  - ↑ Plasma concentration of asymmetric dimethylarginine
  - ↓ Endothelial-dependent vasodilatation
- Procoagulant factors
  - ↑ Plasminogen activator inhibitor-1
  - ↑ Fibrinogen
- Hemodynamic changes
  - ↑ Sympathetic nervous system activity
  - ↑ Renal sodium retention
- Markers of inflammation
  - ↑ C-reactive protein, white blood cell count, etc.
- Abnormal uric acid metabolism
  - ↑ Plasma uric acid concentration
  - ↓ Renal uric acid clearance
- Increased testosterone secretion (ovary)
- Sleep-disordered breathing

HDL-C, high-density lipoprotein cholesterol; LDL, low-density lipoprotein.

TABLE 3 Clinical syndromes associated with insulin resistance

- Type 2 diabetes
- Cardiovascular disease
- Essential hypertension
- Polycystic ovary syndrome
- Nonalcoholic fatty liver disease
- Certain forms of cancer
- Sleep apnea

The focus of this chapter does not permit an extensive discussion of the complex relationship between insulin resistance, compensatory hyperinsulinemia, and the abnormalities and clinical syndromes that make up the IRS, but an extensive review of these issues has recently been published (51). However, it is important to briefly address the question of differential tissue insulin sensitivity, for if this phenomenon did not exist, there would be no IRS. The ability of insulin to stimulate muscle glucose uptake and inhibit free fatty acid (FFA) release from the adipose tissue is highly correlated (3), and the similar degree of insulin resistance in these two tissues initiates the series of events that leads to the abnormalities and clinical syndromes listed in Tables 2 and 3. There are many instances of this phenomenon, but the following three should suffice to make the point. Perhaps the most important example is the relationship between muscle, adipose tissue, and liver. Daylong increases in plasma insulin (muscle insulin resistance) and FFA (adipose tissue insulin resistance) concentrations act upon a liver that is insulin sensitive to stimulate hepatic TG synthesis (44, 53). One consequence of these events will be an increase in hepatic very-low-density lipoprotein (VLDL)-TG synthesis and secretion, leading to hypertriglyceridemia, while at the same time there will be a tendency for the fat content of the liver to increase, and nonalcoholic fatty liver disease to develop. The kidney is another example of an organ that retains normal insulin sensitivity in the presence of muscle and adipose tissue insulin resistance (48), and the compensatory hyperinsulinemia increases renal sodium retention and decreases uric acid clearance, thus contributing to the increased prevalence of essential hypertension and higher plasma uric acid concentrations in individuals with the IRS. The third example is polycystic ovary syndrome, in which the hyperinsulinemia in insulin-resistant women acts on an ovary, which may even be hypersensitive to the ability of insulin to increase testosterone secretion (11). Indeed, the compensatory hyperinsulinemia that prevents the development of type 2 diabetes in insulin-resistant individuals is responsible for most, if not all, of the abnormalities and clinical syndromes that constitute the IRS.

IMPROVING INSULIN SENSITIVITY WITH WEIGHT LOSS

Consideration of dietary approaches to attenuate the abnormalities and clinical syndromes related to the IRS should differentiate between efforts to enhance insulin sensitivity and changes aimed at minimizing its adverse consequences. In this context, there is substantial evidence that insulin sensitivity can be enhanced, and manifestations of the IRS improve when insulin-resistant individuals lose weight (9, 26, 30, 35, 37, 42, 45, 49, 50, 56, 58). In contrast, variations in macronutrient content of isocaloric diets have little, if any, impact on insulin sensitivity (5, 17, 20), and their benefits are limited primarily, if not entirely, to decreasing the adverse metabolic consequences of insulin resistance/hyperinsulinemia (49, 50). Thus, in this section, attention is focused on the ability of weight loss to improve insulin sensitivity, and thereby to attenuate the abnormalities associated with the IRS.

Weight Loss Can Improve Insulin Sensitivity

The results of the Third National Health and Nutrition Examination Survey (28) indicated that more than 50% of those surveyed between 1988 and 1994 were overweight/obese, and the magnitude of this problem continues to increase. Although the gravity of the obesity epidemic is well appreciated, efforts to deal with it effectively are compromised by widespread pessimism concerning the ability to achieve sustained weight loss in overweight/obese individuals. The problem is further confounded by continuing controversies concerning the relative superiority of weight-loss diets that vary widely in their macronutrient content. In the absence of compelling evidence that compliance is greater with any specific macronutrient combination, other than the necessity that the individuals are willing and able to follow a diet containing less energy than they use, it does not seem possible to propose the "best" diet to help overweight/obese individuals with the IRS lose weight.

On the other hand, it is possible to address the fact that not all overweight/obese individuals are insulin resistant and at increased risk of developing the adverse consequences associated with the defect in insulin action. Prospective studies from our research group have indicated that the upper one-third of an apparently healthy population is sufficiently insulin resistant to develop the adverse clinical syndromes of the IRS, whereas those in the lower one-third of the population are at much less risk (13, 62). Although approximately 75% of individuals in the most insulin-resistant tertile are overweight/obese, 30% of those in the most insulin-sensitive tertile are also overweight/obese, and at low risk of the IRS (39). Thus, it seems sensible that the most intensive efforts at weight loss be initiated in those overweight/obese individuals who will benefit the most if the intervention is successful. Obviously, the first step in accomplishing that goal would be the ability to identify such individuals, and it appears that there is a relatively simple way to accomplish that task (36).

How to Identify Overweight/Obese Individuals Who Will Benefit the Most from Weight Loss

Because there is no simple clinical way to quantify insulin resistance, the alternative is to either initiate similar effort at weight loss in all overweight/obese persons, or to use surrogate estimates of insulin resistance to identify those who will benefit the most from weight loss. Health care professionals electing the second course usually rely on measurements of fasting plasma insulin (FPI) concentrations, or various formulae involving the use of both fasting plasma glucose (FPG) and insulin concentrations (HOMA-IR, QUICKI, FPG $\times$ FPI, etc.) to identify insulin-resistant persons. FPI concentrations are reasonably predictive of direct measures of insulin resistance in nondiabetic individuals, but the relationship (r-value $\sim$0.6) only accounts for $\sim$36% of the variability in insulin action, and the use of the more complicated surrogate estimates of insulin action does not substantially increase the magnitude of the relationship (25, 61). More importantly, plasma insulin measurements are not standardized, and it is not possible to interpret the clinical significance of values from one laboratory to another. We have shown in overweight/obese individuals that the plasma TG/HDL-C concentration ratio is as good a surrogate marker of insulin resistance as is FPI concentration; in addition, it can be used to identify individuals who have the atherogenic profile that characterizes the IRS and thereby are at increased risk of CVD (36). Based upon the results of these studies, we have suggested that an overweight/obese person with a TG/HDL-C concentration ratio (mg/dl) $\geq$3.0 is highly likely to be both insulin resistant and at increased CVD risk; the higher the value, the less sensitive and the more specific the ratio, whereas values $<$3.0 increase sensitivity and lose specificity. This approach is certainly not perfect, but it does provide a way to decrease the number of overweight/obese individuals who meet the criteria for intensive weight loss efforts and to identify those who will benefit the most if weight loss can be accomplished.

Insulin-Resistant Individuals Can Lose Weight

Although there appears to be a perception that insulin-resistant/hyperinsulinemic individuals cannot lose weight, several studies, performed in different ethnic groups, have indicated that insulin-resistant individuals, using either insulin concentrations as a surrogate measure of insulin resistance or direct measures of insulin-mediated glucose disposal, either gain the same weight, or less weight, over time (18, 23, 55, 57, 59, 63). Furthermore, the ability to lose weight in response to calorie-restricted diets does not vary as a function of differences in either insulin resistance or insulin secretion (35, 37, 38). Consequently, although it is very difficult to carry out successful weight loss programs, the impediment is not because the individual may be insulin resistant /hyperinsulinemic.

Benefits of Weight Loss in Insulin-Resistant Overweight/Obese Individuals

Studies published 30 years ago demonstrated that insulin sensitivity improved when nondiabetic overweight/obese individuals lost weight, which was associated with a decrease in the plasma insulin response to oral glucose and lower plasma TG concentrations (45). Similar improvements in insulin sensitivity have been demonstrated in several subsequent studies, and we have also shown that following moderate weight loss the slightly elevated daylong plasma glucose and FFA concentrations seen in nondiabetic, insulin-resistant, overweight individuals return to the values of equally overweight, insulin-sensitive person (35, 37, 38). However, although the daylong hyperinsulinemia that characterizes nondiabetic, overweight, insulin-resistant individuals also declines with weight loss, it does not fall to the level seen in insulin-sensitive, equally obese individuals (35, 37, 38). Similarly, C-reactive protein concentrations are higher in insulin-resistant than in insulin-sensitive individuals matched for adiposity, and although concentrations fall in association with weight loss in the insulin-resistant persons, they do not reach the level seen in the insulin-sensitive subjects (37). Thus, a moderate amount of weight loss in insulin-resistant, overweight/obese individuals improves insulin sensitivity, resulting in changes in carbohydrate and lipid metabolism and a marker of vascular inflammation that would decrease the risk of type 2 diabetes, CVD, and other clinical syndromes associated with the IRS.

EFFECT OF VARIATIONS IN MACRONUTRIENT CONTENT ON THE MANIFESTATIONS OF THE INSULIN-RESISTANCE SYNDROME

In contrast to the lack of compelling evidence showing that variations in macronutrient content affect the ability to lose weight, data concerning the metabolic effects of such manipulations in weight-maintenance diets are more consistent. In this section, the ability of changes in relative amounts and kinds of dietary CHO and fat to modify the abnormalities and clinical syndromes associated with the IRS is discussed.

Variations in Amount of Fat and Carbohydrate

Until relatively recently, the prudent diet recommended for all Americans contained (as percentages of total calories) approximately 15% protein, 25%–30% fat, and 55%–60% CHO; this approach was aimed at decreasing SF intake. The rationale for this recommendation was that it would help decrease CVD risk by maintaining the lowest possible plasma low-density lipoprotein cholesterol (LDL-C) concentration (15, 41).

Replacing SF with CHO in isocaloric diets requires that more insulin be secreted to maintain glucose homeostasis, and the more insulin resistant the individual, the greater will be the requisite degree of compensatory hyperinsulinemia. The additional CHO does not require a substantial increase in insulin secretion in order for insulin-sensitive persons to maintain glucose homeostasis, and low-fat/high-CHO diets will help maintain low LDL-C concentration in these individuals without adverse metabolic consequences. Although the beneficial effects of low-fat/high-CHO diets on LDL-C concentrations are not lost in insulin-resistant individuals, this dietary modification will have one of two effects in these persons, neither of which is desirable. If they are unable to respond to the need to secrete even more insulin, their ability to maintain normal glucose tolerance will be compromised. Alternatively, if they are capable of further increasing their degree of compensatory hyperinsulinemia, the abnormalities associated with the IRS (Table 1) will be accentuated, and the likelihood of developing one of the clinical syndromes listed in Table 2 will increase.

It is not possible within the context of this review to discuss all of the adverse consequences of low-fat/high-CHO diets in insulin-resistant/hyperinsulinemic individuals. However, the relationship between CVD risk and the dyslipidemic changes of the IRS are well established, and there is considerable evidence of the metabolic effects of low-fat/high-CHO diets on lipoprotein metabolism in insulin-resistant individuals. Thus, a brief summary of these issues will hopefully serve the useful purpose of pointing out the dangers of replacing SF with CHO in the approximately one-third (13, 62) of the U.S. population that is sufficiently insulin resistant to be at increased risk of all of the adverse manifestations of the IRS.

TRIGLYCERIDE-RICH LIPOPROTEINS The fact that low-fat/high-CHO diets increase fasting plasma TG concentrations has been repeatedly confirmed since the pioneering studies by Ahrens and associates (4). Fasting hypertriglyceridemia is perhaps the most characteristic metabolic abnormality in insulin-resistant/hyperinsulinemic individuals, and the ingestion of low-fat/high-CHO diets increases hepatic VLDL-TG synthesis and secretion, resulting in higher fasting TG concentrations in both nondiabetic individuals and in patients with type 2 diabetes (2, 14, 16, 40, 47, 53).

The original suggestion by Zilversmit (64) that atherogenesis is a postprandial phenomenon continues to gain support (31), and there is evidence that degree of postprandial lipemia is accentuated in insulin resistant/hyperinsulinemic individuals (22, 24, 32, 33). Not surprisingly, there is also evidence that increasing dietary intake of CHO accentuates the postprandial accumulation of TG-rich lipoproteins (2, 7, 8, 24). Thus, the predictable effect of low fat-high CHO diets in insulin resistant and hyperinsulinemic individuals will be to both increase fasting plasma TG concentration, and accentuate the daylong accumulation of TG-rich remnant lipoproteins.

HIGH-DENSITY LIPOPROTEIN CHOLESTEROL CONCENTRATION In light of evidence that there is an independent relationship between insulin resistance/hyperinsulinemia and HDL-C concentration (29), the conclusion from two meta-analyses (15, 41) that low-fat/high-CHO diets result in lower HDL-C concentrations is not unexpected. More controversial is whether the kind of fat affects HDL-C concentration. Thus, Mattson & Grundy (34) suggested some time ago that there was an accentuated decline in HDL-C concentrations when SF was replaced with polyunsaturated fat (PUF), as compared with substitution of SF with monounsaturated fat (MUF), whereas Howard and associates (19) were unable to confirm this observation. If the data from the meta-analyses (15, 41) are considered, it appears that the effect on HDL-C concentration is reasonably similar when either MUF or PUF replaces SF.

LOW-DENSITY LIPOPROTEIN CHOLESTEROL PARTICLE DIAMETER A study in 100 healthy volunteers (52) demonstrated that a highly significant inverse relationship exists between degree of insulin resistance and LDL particle diameter. The study also demonstrated that individuals with small, dense LDL (pattern B) are relatively insulin resistant, glucose intolerant, hyperinsulinemic, with higher TG and lower HDL-C concentrations, and elevated levels of blood pressure as compared with individuals with a preponderance of larger LDL particles (pattern A). Given evidence that the appearance of small, dense LDL particles is one of the abnormalities that occurs more commonly in patients with the IRS, it is not surprising that the prevalence of pattern A is more common in patients on diets relatively high in fat, whereas conversion to pattern B is seen when the switch is made to a diet relatively high in CHO (10, 27, 60).

LOW-DENSITY LIPOPROTEIN CHOLESTEROL CONCENTRATION There is abundant evidence that LDL-C concentrations will fall when SF is replaced with PUF or MUF (15, 41), and because differences in insulin resistance and/or hyperinsulinemia do not modulate LDL-C concentration, this effect will be similar in insulin-resistant individuals. Furthermore, it has been shown (43) that the effect on LDL-C concentrations of diets containing ~20% versus ~40% of total fat was similar, as long as the ratios of polyunsaturated to saturated fat (P:S) were identical (1.0), as well as the n-3:n-6 ratio and the ratio of MUF to total fat. In other words, it appears that there may be little or no increase in LDL-C levels in response to the ingestion of more fat, as long as the fat is unsaturated. These data are congruent with the results of two large meta-analyses (15, 41), and seem to apply equally well to patients with type 2 diabetes (16, 17).

Variations in the Kind of Carbohydrate

Replacement of SF with MUF and/or PUF, rather than CHO, will lower LDL-C concentrations and will not lead to a significant increase in ambient plasma insulin concentrations and the manifestations of the IRS, thus providing a simple and useful dietary approach for patients with pure hypercholesterolemia, the IRS, or combined dyslipidemia. On the other hand, other dietary modifications have been suggested in order to limit the untoward metabolic consequences of the conventional low-fat/high-CHO diets.

For example, one suggestion aimed at avoiding the untoward effects of low-fat/high-CHO diets in patients with type 2 diabetes has been to vary the glycemic index of the CHO ingested, rather than to simply replace SF with unsaturated fat (UF) and reduce the CHO intake (21, 54). Alternatively, it has been suggested that the untoward effects of low-fat/high-CHO diets in patients with type 2 diabetes can be avoided by doubling the recommended fiber intake to 50 g/d (6). Even if it is assumed that patients would be willing to consume diets made up almost entirely of oranges (300 g/d), green peas (110 g/d), zucchini (195 g/d), papaya (250 g/d), peaches (300 g/d), fruit cocktail (200 g/d), and cherries (100 g/d), it did not appear that the improvement in daylong plasma glucose and insulin concentrations and fasting plasma lipid concentrations in this study (6) was as great as when a low-fat/high-CHO diet was compared with a diet in which MUF was increased and CHO decreased (16). Similarly, in a study in which the glycemic index was varied in low-fat/high-CHO diets (21), the improvements in daylong plasma glucose and insulin concentrations were also of lesser magnitude than the study in which the

CHO intake was reduced and the MUF intake increased (16). It is worth noting that the results of these two studies, in which either the fiber intake (6) or the glycemic index (21) was varied, indicated that estimates of insulin sensitivity and several aspects of lipoprotein metabolism improved on *both* the control and experimental diets, without any significant differences between them for many of the experimental variables measured. A more recent study (54) compared the metabolic effects of two diets that seemed to be approximately equal in fat and CHO intake, but differed in glycemic index. It was concluded that four weeks of the lower glycemic index diet led to a variety of benefits, including lower postprandial glucose and insulin concentrations and enhanced insulin sensitivity. Unfortunately, these values were also significantly lower at baseline when the lower glycemic diet was used, and measurements of diet-associated changes in insulin secretion and sensitivity did not show any consistent diet effect.

It is not clear from the available data whether the clinical utility of increasing the fiber content or decreasing the glycemic index of low-fat/high-CHO diets is preferable to simply replacing SF with UF and decreasing CHO intake. In order to resolve this question it is necessary to initiate studies in which these alternatives can be directly compared. In the absence of such information, it is argued that it is simpler, and at least as beneficial, to simply replace SF with UF, not CHO, and thereby avoid the adverse effects of low-fat/high-CHO intake.

SUMMARY

The most dramatic improvements in manifestations of IRS occur in overweight, insulin-resistant/hyperinsulinemic individuals when they lose weight. However, as long as the energy content is kept constant, there appears to be little, or no, evidence that low fat-/high CHO diets will directly improve insulin sensitivity. On the other hand, there is considerable evidence that isocaloric diets, low in fat and enriched in CHO, will accentuate the manifestations of the IRS. The more insulin resistant an individual, the greater is the amount of insulin that must be secreted in response to a CHO-enriched diet in order to maintain glucose homeostasis. Thus, the inevitable, and consistently replicated, effect of replacing SF with CHO in insulin-resistant individuals is to increase daylong concentration of glucose or insulin, or both. In addition, this dietary approach has consistently been shown to stimulate hepatic VLDL-TG synthesis and secretion, leading to an increase in concentration of TG-rich lipoproteins, both in the fasting and postprandial states. The increase in the ambient TG-rich lipoproteins seen following low-fat/high-CHO diets has previously been shown to be associated with a decrease in HDL-C concentration, and it appears that such diets will change the LDL subclass pattern to B in 36 of 87 individuals (41%) who had either pattern A or an intermediate pattern at the outset (27).

Given the evidence that low-fat/high-CHO diets do not modify the basic defect in the IRS (insulin resistance) and accentuate all of its metabolic manifestations, there seems to be little rationale for substituting SF with CHO. This is particularly true in light of the multiple observations that replacing SF with MUF or PUF, or both, will lead to the same fall in LDL-C concentrations, without any of the adverse metabolic effects seen with low-fat/high-CHO diets (15, 41).

Finally, the prevalence of the manifestations of the IRS is increasing rapidly as the world becomes heavier and less fit. There is considerable evidence that dietary manipulations can play a powerful role in modulating the manifestations of the IRS, as well as reasonably good understanding of interventions that either can be helpful or actually make the situation worse. Thus, inability of nutritional means to prevent and/or treat the manifestations of the IRS will result from a failure of implementation, not from a lack of clinically relevant information.

The *Annual Review of Nutrition* is online at http://nutr.annualreviews.org

LITERATURE CITED

1. Abbasi F, Brown BWB, Lamendola C, McLaughlin T, Reaven GM. 2002. Relationship between obesity, insulin resistance, and coronary heart disease risk. *J. Am. Coll. Card.* 40:937–43
2. Abbasi F, McLaughlin T, Lamendola C, Kim HS, Tanaka A, et al. 2000. High carbohydrate diets, triglyceride-rich lipoproteins, and coronary heart disease risk. *Am. J. Cardiol.* 85:45–48
3. Abbasi F, McLaughlin T, Lamendola C, Reaven GM. 2000. The relationship between glucose disposal in response to physiological hyperinsulinemia and basal glucose and free fatty acid concentrations in healthy volunteers. *J. Clin. Endocrinol. Metab.* 85:1251–54
4. Ahrens EH, Hirsch J, Oette K, Farquahar JW, Stein Y. 1961. Carbohydrate-induced and fat-induced lipemia. *Trans. Assoc. Am. Phys.* 74:134–36
5. Borkman M, Campbell LV, Chisholm DJ, Storlien LH. 1991. High-carbohydrate low-fat diets do not enhance insulin sensitivity in normal subjects. *J. Clin. Endocrinol. Metab.* 72:432–37
6. Chandalia M, Garg A, Lutjohann D, von Bergmann K, Grundy SM, Brinkley L. 2002. Beneficial effects of high dietary fiber intake in patients with type 2 diabetes mellitus. *N. Engl. J. Med.* 342:1392–98
7. Chen YD-I, Coulston AM, Zhou M-Y, Hollenbeck CB, Reaven GM. 1995. Why do low-fat high-carbohydrate diets accentuate postprandial lipemia in patients with NIDDM? *Diabetes Care* 18:10–16
8. Chen YD-I, Swami S, Skowronski R, Coulston AM, Reaven GM. 1993. Effect of variations in dietary fat and carbohydrate intake on postprandial lipemia in patients with noninsulin dependent diabetes mellitus. *J. Clin. Endocrinol. Metab.* 76:347–51
9. Dixon JB, Bhathal PS, Hughes NR, O'Brien PE. 2004. Nonalcoholic fatty liver disease. Improvement in liver histological analysis with weight loss. *Hepatology* 39:1647–54
10. Dreon DM, Fernstrom HA, Miller B, Krauss RM. 1995. Apolipoprotein E isoform phenotype and LDL subclass response to a reduced-fat diet. *Arterioscler. Thromb. Vasc. Biol.* 15:105–11
11. Dunaif A, Segal KR, Futterweit W, Dobrjansky A. 1989. Profound peripheral insulin resistance, independent of obesity, in the polycystic ovary syndrome. *Diabetes* 38:1165–74

12. Executive summary of the third report of the National Cholesterol Education Program (NCEP) expert panel on detection, evaluation, and treatment of high blood cholesterol in adults (adult treatment panel III). 2002. *JAMA* 285:2846–97
13. Facchini FS, Hua N, Abbasi F, Reaven GM. 2001. Insulin resistance as a predictor of age-related diseases. *J. Clin. Endocrinol. Metab.* 86:3574–78
14. Farquhar JW, Frank A, Gross RC, Reaven GM. 1966. Glucose, insulin, and triglyceride responses to high and low carbohydrate diets in man. *J. Clin. Invest.* 45:1648–56
15. Gardner CD, Kraemer HC. 1995. Monounsaturated versus polyunsaturated dietary fat and serum lipids—a meta-analysis. *Arterioscler. Thromb. Vasc. Biol.* 15:1917–27
16. Garg A, Bantle JP, Henry RR, Coulston AM, Griver KA, et al. 1994. Effects of varying carbohydrate content of diet in patients with non-insulin dependent diabetes mellitus. *JAMA* 271:1421–28
17. Garg A, Grundy SM, Unger RH. 1992. Comparison of effects of high and low carbohydrate diets on plasma lipoproteins and insulin sensitivity in patients with mild NIDDM. *Diabetes* 41:1278–85
18. Hoag S, Marshall JA, Jones RH, Hamman RF. 1995. High fasting insulin levels associated with lower rates of weight gain in persons with normal glucose tolerance: the San Luis Valley Diabetes Study. *Int. J. Obes.* 19:175–80
19. Howard BV, Hannah JS, Heiser CC, Jablonski KA, Paidi MC, et al. 1995. Polyunsaturated fatty acids result in greater cholesterol lowering and less triacylglycerol elevation than do monounsaturated fatty acids in a dose-response comparison in a multiracial study group. *Am. J. Clin. Nutr.* 62:392–402
20. Hughes VA, Fiatarone MA, Fielding RA, Ferrara CM, Elahi D, Evans WJ. 1995. Long-term effects of a high-carbohydrate diet and exercise on insulin action in older subjects with impaired glucose tolerance. *Am. J. Clin. Nutr.* 62:426–33
21. Jarvi AE, Karlstrom BE, Granfeldt YE, Bjorck IE, Asp N-GL, Vessby BOH. 1999. Improved glycemic control and lipid profile and normalized fibrinolytic activity on a low-glycemic index diet in type 2 diabetic patients. *Diabetes Care* 22:10–18
22. Jeppesen J, Hollenbeck CB, Zhou M-Y, Coulston AM, Jones C, et al. 1995. Relation between insulin resistance, hyperinsulinemia, postheparin plasma lipoprotein lipase activity, and postprandial lipemia. *Arterioscler. Thromb. Vasc. Biol.* 15:320–24
23. Jones CNO, Abbasi F, Carantoni M, Polonsky KS, Reaven GM. 2000. Roles of insulin resistance and obesity in regulation of plasma insulin concentrations. *Am. J. Physiol.* 278:E504–8
24. Kim H-S, Abbasi F, Lamendola C, McLaughlin T, Reaven GM. 2001. Effect of insulin resistance on postprandial elevations of remnant lipoprotein concentrations in postmenopausal women. *Am. J. Clin. Nutr.* 74:592–95
25. Kim SH, Abbasi F, Reaven GM. 2004. Impact of degree of obesity on surrogate estimates of insulin resistance. *Diabetes Care* 27:1998–2002
26. Knowler WC, Barrett-Connor E, Fowler SE, Hamman RF, Lachin JL, et al. 2002. Reduction in the incidence of type 2 diabetes with lifestyle intervention or metformin. *N. Engl. J. Med.* 346:393–403
27. Krauss RM, Dreon DM. 1995. Low-density lipoprotein subclasses and responses to a low-fat diet in healthy man. *Am. J. Clin. Nutr.* 62:478S–487S
28. Kuczmarski RJ, Carroll MD, Flegal KM, Troiano RP. 1997. Varying body mass index cutoff points to describe overweight prevalence among U.S. adults: NHANES III (1988 to 1994). *Obes. Res.* 5(6): 542–48
29. Laws A, Reaven GM. 1992. Evidence for an independent relationship between insulin resistance and fasting plasma

HDL-cholesterol, triglyceride and insulin concentrations. *J. Int. Med.* 231:25–30

30. Liu GC, Coulston AM, Lardinois CK, Hollenbeck CB, Moore JG, Reaven G. 1985. Moderate weight loss and sulfonylurea treatment of non-insulin-dependent diabetes mellitus. *Arch. Intern. Med.* 145:665–69
31. Mamo JCL. 1995. Atherosclerosis as a post-prandial disease. *Endocrinol. Metab.* 2:229–44
32. Masumi A, Tanaka A, Ogita K, Sekine M, Numano F, et al. 2000. Relationship between hyperinsulinemia and remnant lipoprotein concentrations in patients with impaired glucose tolerance. *J. Clin. Endocrinol. Metab.* 85:3557–60
33. Masumi A, Tanaka A, Ogita K, Sekine M, Numano F, et al. 2001. Relationship between plasma insulin concentration and plasma remnant lipoprotein response to an oral fat load in patients with type 2 diabetes. *J. Am. Coll. Cardiol.* 38:1628–32
34. Mattson FH, Grundy SM. 1985. Comparison of effects of dietary saturated, monounsaturated, and polyunsaturated fatty acids on plasma lipids and lipoproteins in man. *J. Lipid. Res.* 26:194–202
35. McLaughlin T, Abbasi F, Carantoni M, Schaaf P, Reaven GM. 1999. Differences in insulin resistance do not predict weight loss in response to hypocaloric diets in healthy obese women. *J. Clin. Endocrinol. Metab.* 84:578–81
36. McLaughlin T, Abbasi F, Cheal K, Chu J, Lamendola C, Reaven G. 2003. Use of metabolic markers to identify overweight individuals who are insulin resistant. *Ann. Intern. Med.* 139:802–9
37. McLaughlin T, Abbasi F, Lamendola C, Liang L, Reaven G, et al. 2002. Differentiation between obesity and insulin resistance in the association with C-reactive protein. *Circulation* 106:2908–12
38. McLaughlin T, Abbasi F, Lamendola C, Kim H-S, Reaven GM. 2001. Metabolic changes following sibutramine-assisted weight loss in obese individuals: role of plasma free fatty acids in the insulin resistance of obesity. *Metabolism* 50:819–82
39. McLaughlin T, Allison G, Abbasi F, Lamendola C, Reaven G. 2004. Prevalence of insulin resistance and associated cardiovascular disease risk factors among normal weight, overweight, and obese individuals. *Metabolism* 53:495–99
40. McLaughlin T, Abbasi F, Lamendola C, Yeni-Komshian H, Reaven G. 2000. Carbohydrate-induced hypertriglyceridemia: an insight into the link between plasma insulin and triglyceride concentrations. *J. Clin. Endocrinol. Metab.* 85:3085–88
41. Mensink RP, Katan MB. 1992. Effect of dietary fatty acids on serum lipids and lipoproteins. *Arterioscler. Thromb.* 12: 911–19
42. Moran LJ, Noakes M, Clifton PM, Tomlinson L, Galletly C, Norman RJ. 2003. Dietary composition in restoring reproductive and metabolic physiology in overweight women with polycystic ovary syndrome. *J. Clin. Endocrinol. Metab.* 88:812–19
43. Nelson GJ, Schmidt PC, Kelley DS. 1995. Low-fat diets do not lower plasma cholesterol levels in healthy men compared to high-fat diets with similar fatty acid composition at constant caloric intake. *Lipids* 30:969–76
44. Olefsky JM, Farquhar JW, Reaven GM. 1974. Reappraisal of the role of insulin in hypertriglyceridemia. *Am. J. Med.* 57:551–60
45. Olefsky JM, Reaven GM, Farquhar JW. 1974. Effects of weight reduction on obesity: studies of carbohydrate and lipid metabolism. *J. Clin. Invest.* 53:64–76
46. Reaven GM. 1988. Role of insulin resistance in human disease. *Diabetes* 37:1595–607
47. Reaven GM. 1996. Hypertriglyceridemia: the central feature of syndrome X. *Cardiovasc. Risk Factors* 6:29–35
48. Reaven GM. 1997. The kidney: an unwilling accomplice in syndrome X. *Am. J. Kidney Dis.* 30:928–31

49. Reaven GM. 1997. Do high carbohydrate diets prevent the development or attenuate the manifestations (or both) of syndrome X? A viewpoint strongly against. *Curr. Opin. Lipidol.* 8:23–27
50. Reaven GM. 2000. Diet and syndrome X. *Curr. Atheroscler. Rep.* 2:503–7
51. Reaven GM. 2004. The metabolic syndrome or the insulin resistance syndrome? Different names, different concepts, and different goals. *Endocrinol. Metab. Clin. N. Am.* 33:283–303
52. Reaven GM, Chen Y-DI, Jeppesen J, Maheux P, Krauss RM. 1993. Insulin resistance and hyperinsulinemia in individuals with small dense, low density lipoprotein particles. *J. Clin. Invest.* 92:141–46
53. Reaven GM, Lerner R, Stern M, Farquhar JW. 1967. Role of insulin in endogenous hypertriglyceridemia. *J. Clin. Invest.* 46:1756–67
54. Ruzkalla SW, Taghrid L, Laromiguiere M, Hueit D, Boillot J, et al. 2004. Improved plasma glucose control, whole-body glucose utilization, and lipid profile on a low-glycemic index diet in type 2 diabetic men. *Diabetes Care* 27:1866–72
55. Schwartz MW, Boyko EJ, Kahn SE, et al. 1995. Reduced insulin secretion: an independent predictor of body weight gain. *J. Clin. Endocrinol. Metab.* 80:1571–76
56. Su H-Y, Sheu WH-H, Chin H-ML, Jeng C-Y, Chen Y-DI, Reaven GM. 1995. Effect of weight loss on blood pressure and insulin resistance in normotensive and hypertensive obese individuals. *Am. J. Hypertens.* 8:1067–71
57. Swinburn BA, Nyomba BL, Saad MF, Zurlo F, Raz I, Knowler WC. 1991. Insulin resistance associated with lower rates of weight gain in Pima Indians. *J. Clin. Invest.* 88:168–73
58. Tuomilehto J, Lindstrom J, Eriksson JG, Valle TT, Hamalainen H, et al. 2001. Prevention of type 2 diabetes by changes in lifestyle among subjects with impaired glucose tolerance. *N. Engl. J. Med.* 344:1343–50
59. Valdez R, Mitchell BD, Haffner SM, Hazuda HP, Morales PA, et al. 1994. Predictors of weight change in a bi-ethnic population. The San Antonio Heart Study. *Int. J. Obes.* 18:85–91
60. Williams PT, Dreon DM, Krauss RM. 1995. Effects of dietary fat on high-density lipoprotein subclasses are influenced by both apolipoprotein E isoforms and low-density lipoprotein subclass patterns. *Am. J. Clin. Nutr.* 61:1234–40
61. Yeni-Komshian H, Carantoni M, Abbasi F, Reaven GM. 2000. Relationship between several surrogate estimates of insulin resistance and quantification of insulin-mediated glucose disposal in 490 healthy, nondiabetic volunteers. *Diabetes Care* 23: 171–75
62. Yip J, Facchini FS, Reaven GM. 1998. Resistance to insulin-mediated glucose disposal as a predictor of cardiovascular disease. *J. Clin. Endocrinol. Metab.* 83:2773–76
63. Zavaroni I, Zuccarelli A, Gasparini P, Massironi P, Barilli A, Reaven GM. 1998. Can weight gain in healthy, nonobese volunteers be predicted by differences in baseline plasma insulin concentrations? *J. Clin. Endocrinol. Metab.* 83:3498–500
64. Zilversmit DB. 1979. Atherogenesis: a postprandial phenomenon. *Circulation* 60: 473–85

Annu. Rev. Nutr. 2005. 25:407–34
doi: 10.1146/annurev.nutr.25.050304.092538

First published online as a Review in Advance on May 4, 2005

DEVELOPMENTAL DETERMINANTS OF BLOOD PRESSURE IN ADULTS

Linda Adair and Darren Dahly
Department of Nutrition, Schools of Public Health and Medicine, University of North Carolina at Chapel Hill, North Carolina 27599-8120; email: Linda_adair@unc.edu, dahly@email.unc.edu

Key Words hypertension, birth weight, fetal programming

■ **Abstract** Over the past 20 years a large and varied body of research has attempted to make the case for the developmental origins of elevated adult blood pressure (BP). Experimental animal research has identified plausible biological mechanisms through which fetal nutritional insufficiency may affect adult BP. The majority of human epidemiologic studies demonstrate an inverse association of birth weight (the most commonly used marker of fetal nutrition) with adult BP and higher risk of hypertension among individuals with lower weight at birth. The most adverse BP outcomes occur among individuals who were small at birth but relatively large as adults, a finding that suggests a role for postnatal growth. We critically review the literature on proposed mechanisms and epidemiologic evidence for developmental origins of adult BP and hypertension, considering associations with birth weight, maternal nutrition during pregnancy, child growth patterns, and infant feeding.

CONTENTS

INTRODUCTION

Hypertension represents a major public health challenge worldwide owing to its high prevalence, worsening trends, and importance as a risk factor for cardiovascular disease mortality. Based on the most recent U.S. National Health and Nutrition Examination Survey (1999–2000), age-adjusted prevalence of hypertension among adults was 28.4%, and this represents a 30% increase since the prior (1988–1994) survey (34). A selection of age-adjusted prevalence rates from other countries is presented in Table 1 (61). These data provide impressive evidence of the magnitude of this worldwide problem.

Although a great deal is known about modifiable risk factors for hypertension, including obesity, smoking, alcohol consumption, diet, and physical activity, these factors do not fully explain differences in its occurrence. A newer and still controversial area of research draws our attention to the developmental origins of elevated blood pressure (BP) and other noncommunicable diseases. The main tenet of the developmental origins of adult health and disease (DOHaD) hypothesis is that nutritional insufficiency in early life programs disease risk through persistent effects on structure and metabolic function of organ systems. Early life responses to nutritional insufficiency may enhance survival in the short run, but may be maladaptive in later life when the organism no longer is faced with insufficiency (40).

BP is the most studied outcome in tests of the DOHaD hypothesis, largely because of its ease of measurement and known association with cardiovascular disease mortality. A vast literature on this topic has developed over the past two decades. Extensive reviews and meta-analyses of the animal and epidemiologic literature have been published. In addition, the *Annual Review of Nutrition* recently published a review (106) of the effects of maternal nutrition in pregnancy on long-term health outcomes in offspring. Here, we provide a broad overview of the developmental origins of BP and cite recent reviews for readers to consult for further details. We begin by discussing mechanisms through which nutritional

TABLE 1 Age-adjusted prevalence of hypertension in selection populations, based on national survey data (except for India)

	Year	Age range	% Male	% Female
United States	1999–2000	18+	38.3	28.7
Germany	1997–1999	18–79	55.4	56.6
Mexico	1992–1993	20–69	38.6	30.1
China	2000–2001	35–74	28.8	26.6
India*	2002	35+	47.5	48.4
South Africa	1998	15–65	22.9	23.4

*Based on survey of urban adults in Mumbai; n = 88,653.

Data from (61).

factors in early life may influence BP, with an emphasis on kidney development and the role of glucocorticoids. We then review the epidemiologic literature, examining how BP relates to birth weight, maternal nutrition during pregnancy, child growth patterns, and infant feeding. Limitations of human studies are discussed and linked with suggestions for future research.

BLOOD PRESSURE REGULATION: WHAT IS "PROGRAMMABLE" AND WHAT ARE THE MECHANISMS?

BP is regulated through complex physiological mechanisms, involving the kidneys, factors that affect endothelial function and arterial compliance, the sympathetic nervous system, the hypothalamic pituitary adrenal (HPA) axis, and the renin-angiotensin system. Prenatal influences on these systems have been explored as potential mechanisms through which fetal nutritional insufficiency affects long-term BP. The biological plausibility of the DOHaD hypothesis is generally well established by experimental research in animals. Nutritional insufficiency is thought to be the primary programming stimulus (45), although other stressors also play a role. Strong evidence from animal studies shows that fetal growth restriction secondary to maternal dietary restriction (11, 68, 127, 136), manipulation of uterine blood supply (3), or administration of corticosteroids during pregnancy (26, 27) elevates offspring BP. Animal models typically induce fetal nutritional insufficiency by restricting maternal intake of food or specific nutrients. Administration of glucocorticoids during pregnancy mimics the effects of dietary restriction on fetal growth, and this method has been used often in animal models of fetal programming.

Potential Mechanisms

FETAL EXPOSURE TO EXCESS GLUCOCORTICOIDS Glucocorticoid exposure is an attractive explanation for fetal programming of BP because it is a common underlying factor for many structural and physiological changes related to BP regulation. Extensive reviews on the HPA axis and glucocorticoids have been published (e.g., 13, 35, 65, 91, 114). Briefly, fetal exposure to glucocorticoids is normally limited until late in gestation because of low fetal endogenous production, and protection from maternal cortisol through the action of 11ß-hydroxysteroid dehydrogenase type 2 (11ßHSD-2), which converts active cortisol to its inactive form in the placenta. When maternal cortisol levels are elevated or placental expression of 11ßHSD-2 is low (either of which can follow maternal nutritional insufficiency), the fetus can be exposed to excess cortisol. High fetal exposure can reset the fetal HPA axis, resulting in chronic elevation of cortisol levels and altered response to stimuli, with consequences for development of hypertension (13, 104). Cortisol also affects organ growth and differentiation, and can produce permanent deficits such as reduced nephron number (see below). High cortisol may also affect the mother's ability to properly nourish offspring during lactation (131).

ALTERATIONS IN KIDNEY STRUCTURE AND FUNCTION The hypothesis linking fewer nephrons at birth with increased hypertension risk in adulthood followed the observation that BP is elevated when renal mass is surgically reduced (15, 81, 82). The role of nephrogenesis in fetal programming of adult BP has been reviewed extensively (67, 85). Animal models show that maternal dietary protein restriction or glucocorticoid administration during pregnancy impairs nephrogenesis and results in offspring with smaller kidneys with fewer nephrons (136, 137). Structural deficits have also been observed in the kidneys of growth-retarded human infants (53, 118).

Nephrogenesis may be impaired by alterations in the activity of the renin-angiotensin system [reviewed by Rasch and colleagues (105)], possibly through lower renal expression of the angiotensin II type 2 receptor (93). Although protein restriction has been the main animal model, there is also evidence that maternal vitamin A (16) and iron deficiency (77) result in reduced nephron number. When nephron number is reduced, the glomerular filtration rate is increased, resulting in further nephron loss, an increase in BP to sustain hemodynamic function, and a progressive worsening of kidney damage that leads to elevated BP. Altered gene expression in nephron-deficient kidneys (12, 84) may also affect the capacity of nephrons to retain salt and water.

THE VASCULAR SYSTEM In growth-restricted fetuses, elastin in the walls of the aorta and large arteries is deficient, and this defect could eventually lead to arterial stiffness and elevated BP (89, 90). Inconsistent results from humans reflect differences in methods used to measure arterial stiffness, site of measurement, and degree of control for confounding. There is evidence of lower arterial compliance (often measured by pulse wave velocity) in adults who were small at birth (88). Other studies found no relationship of birth weight to pulse wave velocity [e.g., among adults in India (63), Wales (95), and the Netherlands (101)]. A study in Ireland (96) found opposite effects in men and women, whereas a Dutch study (126) found a positive association of birth weight with carotid arterial compliance, but a weaker relationship with brachial and femoral arterial compliance that attenuated when adjusted for height.

Brawley and colleagues (14) reviewed mechanisms through which maternal dietary restriction affects peripheral arterial function, and suggested reduced sensitivity to nitric oxide and reduced endothelium-dependent relaxation as fetal responses with long-term implications for elevated BP. IJzerman and colleagues (58) found a significant association of low birth weight with impaired microvascular function, leading to their suggestion that impaired capillary recruitment is a potential mechanism for fetal programming of BP.

EPIGENETIC MECHANISMS Researchers have suggested alterations in telomere length as a potential mechanism through which hypertension is programmed (7,

25). Briefly, telomeres are noncoding nucleotide sequences found at the ends of chromosomes. During each cycle of DNA replication, a few nucleotides at the ends of chromosomes are invariably lost, thus the telomeres act as a buffer to protect the coding portions of the chromosomes. Telomere attrition eventually prohibits further cell division and results in cellular senescence. As telomeres erode over time, they can be relengthened by the action of the enzyme telomerase, thus preventing the telomeres from becoming too short for cell division.

The potential role for telomere length as a mechanism to explain the developmental origins of adult disease is derived from the following points: Telomere length is largely determined before birth, through genetics and environmental factors (99); short telomeres are associated with elevated pulse pressure and hypertension in adults (5, 25, 115); telomerase activity is high in many fetal tissues, in association with rapid growth in this period (7); and telomerase activity can be regulated by estrogen and possibly other steroid hormones active in utero (5, 6, 25). If telomerase activity were somehow reduced, then the tissues affected, which could include the kidneys, heart, or vasculature, would suffer from abnormally reduced telomeres, which could in turn lead to earlier deterioration of these tissues in adulthood and the resulting hypertension. There is little evidence yet to support this hypothesis, but in recent experiments, fetal growth retardation followed by rapid catch-up growth resulted in elevated telomere attrition in rodent kidneys (5, 25).

Other epigenetic mechanisms have also been proposed. There is evidence that fetal DNA methylation (an important regulator of gene transcription) in utero can be altered through restricting the supply of nutrients to the fetus (83). Folic acid intake has also been suggested as an important factor in fetal DNA methylation (92). For example, feeding pregnant agouti (Avy/a) mice a methyl-supplemented diet (that included folate) altered the offspring's expression of the *agouti* (*Avy*) gene (135), which is associated with obesity and hyperinsulinemia. It has also been recently demonstrated in rats that uteroplacental insufficiency alters gene methylation in the fetal rat kidney (39, 103).

It is also possible, but not well investigated, that clonal selection among rapidly dividing cells during development could select cell lines that are adapted to an abnormal intrauterine environment but that cause chronic disease later in life (132). Metabolic differentiation of cells could have similar effects (132).

OTHER PROPOSED MECHANISMS Fowden & Forhead (35) reviewed endocrine mechanisms of intrauterine programming, with a focus on insulin, thyroid hormones, growth hormone and insulin-like growth factors (IGFs), and glucocorticoids. IGFs are of interest because they are highly responsive to maternal nutritional insufficiency (41), play an important role in prenatal growth, and are related to adult cardiovascular function [see review by Holt (51)]. IGF-I may affect BP through its role in growth of vascular smooth muscle cells and control of regional blood flow by nitric oxide–mediated vasodilation [reviewed by Green (43)].

Hattersley & Tooke (48) proposed that genetically determined insulin resistance underlies both restricted fetal growth and adult insulin resistance and cardiovascular disease. This hypothesis is supported by a study showing that allele differences in an insulin gene are associated with size at birth (29). Complicating the fetal insulin hypothesis, however, is the possibility of intergenerational programming effects that could be a nongenetic mechanism of inheritance of low birth weight and elevated adult BP. These potential effects are summarized by Drake & Walker (28).

THE ROLE OF BODY COMPOSITION Adult body mass index (BMI) is often considered as a potential confounder of the relationship of birth size to later BP. If variation in body composition is the result of fetal programming, indicators of body composition should be considered as potential mediators rather than confounders. Rogers (109), Oken & Gillman (98), and Martorell et al. (87) recently reviewed evidence for fetal origins of obesity. Most studies report a positive association of birth weight to BMI later in life, although a J-shaped association has also been observed (24). The attenuation of this relationship with adjustment for maternal BMI suggests a role for genetic or behavioral factors that contribute to both enhanced fetal growth and postnatal development of obesity. There is stronger, though not entirely consistent, evidence for fetal programming of fat patterning, with lower birth weight associated with central adiposity after adjustment for BMI. Early postnatal catch-up growth following intrauterine growth restriction may also relate to increased central fat (100).

Vickers and colleagues (128, 129) offer intriguing evidence that maternal undernutrition in pregnancy produces offspring that are less physically active and hyperphagic throughout their postnatal life, particularly in response to a high-calorie diet. This combination of high energy intake and low activity leads to higher levels of body fat and significantly elevated BP.

There is also evidence of prenatal effects on lean body mass. Singhal and colleagues (122) show that higher birth weight is associated with an increase in fat-free mass, but not fat mass, in adolescents. Similarly, a Guatemalan study found lower fat-free mass in individuals with a history of growth retardation (76). Yajnik describes the "thin-fat" Indian baby who, in response to maternal nutritional insufficiency, is born with a deficit of skeletal muscle but not fat. This pattern persists into adulthood, and is associated with insulin resistance and cardiovascular disease (138).

HUMAN EPIDEMIOLOGIC STUDIES

Although plausible mechanisms have been identified in animal studies, human epidemiologic studies are mostly observational and are ill suited to allow causal inferences about the consequences of early life exposures. Given the recent focus on DOHaD, there are currently no adult studies designed specifically to test the hypothesis. Data used to explore developmental origins of adult BP typically derive from prospective cohort studies or data sources established for other purposes (e.g., registries), or from studies that measure current BP and related factors and obtain birth information retrospectively. These studies often lack sufficient data on early exposures and are therefore not ideally suited to test fully the DOHaD hypothesis. Furthermore, the literature is dominated by European studies, where more data are available, particularly from large cohorts, but where poor maternal and fetal nutrition is less prevalent.

The majority of studies use birth weight as an indicator of fetal nutritional status. Studies from the 1980s to mid 1990s typically presented correlation coefficients or beta coefficients from models in which BP is regressed on birth weight. Criticism of birth weight as an indicator of fetal nutritional sufficiency led to studies that considered other birth outcomes (gestational age, length, and body proportions at birth) and maternal diet and nutritional status during pregnancy. The observation that an inverse relation of size at birth to later BP is amplified or seen only when adult size is taken into account led to a new emphasis on the role of postnatal growth (8) and a broadening of emphasis to include "developmental" rather than just fetal origins of adult disease. The human literature is now characterized by a greater focus on potential mechanisms, with measurement of factors that influence BP, such as cortisol levels, arterial compliance, or sympathetic nervous system activity.

Relationship of Birth Weight to Adult Blood Pressure

A substantial body of literature documents an association of birth weight with later BP. The first studies were published in the 1980s: In a large national U.K. cohort, Wadsworth et al. (130) found an inverse relation of birth weight to systolic BP at age 36. Gennser and colleagues (37) found a significantly higher risk of having elevated diastolic BP among Swedish army conscripts who had been growth retarded at birth compared with those whose birth weight was appropriate for gestational age (OR 3.63; 95% CI 1.14 to 12.57).

There have been many subsequent studies, and those published through 1996, with quantitative assessment of the relationship of birth weight to later BP, were reviewed by Leon & Koupilova (73) and Law & Shiell (70). Huxley et al. (57) updated the latter review with 1996–2000 publications. In addition, Huxley et al. (54) more formally reviewed studies that reported regression coefficients of systolic BP on birth weight. In all but 3 of 55 reports (for which the total sample size was 382,514), these regressions, adjusted for current body size, produced a negative coefficient on birth weight, with effects in adults ranging from −0.35 to −5.9 mm Hg per kg. However, many of the estimates have wide confidence intervals, and the 95% CI excluded zero in only about half of the studies. In a formal meta-analysis of systolic BP adjusted for sample sizes, the pooled estimate of the effect of birth weight was −1.38 mm Hg per kg in children and adults combined (113). There was substantial heterogeneity, with smaller studies having larger negative regression coefficients. Huxley et al. (54) point out that of 48 studies that did not report a regression coefficient but included a direction of effect, only 25 found it to be inverse, suggesting publication bias.

Table 2 summarizes adult studies published since 2000, identified by a Pub Med search using key words "blood pressure or hypertension" and "birth weight or fetal growth retardation or fetal programming." This was not intended as an exhaustive search for a formal review or meta-analysis, but to provide a sense of the range of study types and new findings.

The recent studies remain consistent with earlier ones in finding a modest inverse relation of birth weight to adult systolic BP, or a significantly increased risk of hypertension with lower birth weight. Given the controversy about adjustment for current body size, many of the studies report unadjusted values, or values both adjusted and unadjusted for size in adulthood. Details of several of the larger studies are presented to illustrate typical methods and results.

The largest studies take advantage of data collected during physical examinations for military conscription and linked with birth records. For example, in a sample of 165,136 Swedish conscripts, Leon et al. (74) reported a 0.6 (95% CI 0.5–0.7) mm Hg decrease in systolic BP per kg increase in birth weight unadjusted, and a 1.47 (1.37–1.57) mm Hg decrease adjusted for adult height and weight. Lundgren et al. (80), in an even larger sample (276,033) of Swedish 17- to 24-year-old conscripts, reported that risk of having systolic BP above the 90th height-standardized percentile increased by 15% (17% when adjusted for birth length, gestational age, adult height, and BMI) for each 1-standard deviation increase in birth weight. A strength shared by these studies is their very large, representative samples of young adult males. Estimates of effect tend to be precise and highly significant, even when coefficients are small. However, as noted by Leon (74), measurement of BP at conscription may be subject to more error than measurement using more standardized protocols, leading to a possible underestimation of effects.

Among 7876 participants in the Vasterbotten Intervention Program in Sweden, Mogren et al. (94) found that low birth weight (LBW; less than 2.5 kg) significantly elevated risk of hypertension (based on standard cut points and measured BP) in adult men and women, ages 29–41 years. Adjustment for current BMI slightly increased the odds ratios and effects were stronger in women than in men: LBW was associated with a seven times higher likelihood of having adult systolic BP > 160, while the odds ratio in men was 2.16.

In an ongoing prospective Iceland Heart Association study, Gunnarsdottir and colleagues (44) found that increased hypertension risk (defined using cut points of 140 mm Hg for systolic and 90 mm Hg for diastolic BP, or taking medication to lower BP) was associated with lower birth weight in women, but not men. Further analysis of the large Helsinki University Central Hospital 1924–1944 birth cohorts in Finland also show lower odds (9) and a lower cumulative incidence of hypertension (defined as a record of having taken medication to lower BP) with increasing birth weight (10, 30, 31).

The inverse association of birth weight with adult BP in these populations with low mortality, little nutritional insufficiency, and high mean birth weights underscores the need to consider failure to reach growth potential rather than small birth size as a measure of fetal nutritional insufficiency. More studies from

TABLE 2 Summary of papers (published since 2000) relating birth weight to adult blood pressure or hypertension*

Location of study	Reference	Sample and study type	n	Age	Result (regression coefficient units are mm Hg per kg BW, 95% CI in parentheses unless otherwise noted)
United Kingdom	(56)	Offspring of participants in Oxford Nutrition Survey of wartime dietary rations in pregnant women	137	50	No association of BW to BP in 110 adults not taking medication for HTN, adjusted (age, gender, BMI, social class, smoking) or unadjusted
United Kingdom	(47)	1946 birth cohort, MRC NSHD	3,157	43	SBP: −2.3 (0.8, 3.5) (men) SBP: −1.8 (0.1, 3.5) (women) Similar when adjusted for adult BMI
United Kingdom	(46)	1946 birth cohort, MRC NSHD	3,534	36–53	See (40). No amplification of effect with age
United Kingdom	(71)	Brompton Study Cohort	346	22	SBP: −2.7 (−0.4, −5.0) unadjusted DBP: −1.6 (−0.1, −3.2) unadjusted
Scotland	(59)	Follow-up of LBW infants and controls born in Edinburgh hospital	61	24	BW < 2 kg predicted higher mean SBP (122 +/− 12 versus 115 +/− 9 in controls, ($P < 0.05$). No effect of BW on DBP
Netherlands	(126)	Amsterdam Growth and Health Longitudinal Study Cohort	281	36	SBP: −3.3 (−5.75, −0.88) unadjusted DBP: −1.8 (−3.49, −0.21) unadjusted SBP: −3.05 (−5.51, −0.60) adjusted (height and weight) DBP: −1.55 (−3.19, 0.08) adjusted
Sweden	(60)	Twins born 1973–1979 Birth/conscription record link	886 male	17–19	Within-twin pairs: SBP: MZ −1.30 (−4.14, 1.54), DZ 0.14 (−3.49, 3.76). Between pairs −2.68 (−4.95, −0.42) MZ, 0.28 (−2.35, 2.91) DZ, adjusted (age, where examined, GA, current height, weight)

(*Continued*)

TABLE 2 (*Continued*)

Location of study	Reference	Sample and study type	n	Age	Result (regression coefficient units are mm Hg per kg BW, 95% CI in parentheses unless otherwise noted)
Sweden	(74)	Conscripts born 1973–1976 linked to birth registry	165,136	18	SBP: −0.60 (−0.7,−0.5) unadjusted SBP: −1.47 (−1.57,−1.37) adjusted (height and weight)
Finland	(33)	FinnDiane study, Finnish diabetic nephropathy	1,543 type I diabetics	33	SBP: −0.96 (−2.54, 0.63) adjusted (age, sex) unchanged by control for BMI, social class, medication. Among full term SBP: −1.90 (−3.71, −0.09) unadjusted SBP 2.37 (−4.08, −0.65) adjusted (medication use, GFR, glycemic control, urinary albumin excretion rate) effects stronger in females, ns in males No effects on DBP SBP: −6.4 (1.0, 11.9) in the 213 people previously diagnosed as having hypertension
Finland	(139)	Subgroup of cohort from Helsinki University Central Hospital 1924–1944 births	500	70	
Denmark	(112)	Obese and nonobese identified at draft board exam	327 obese, 285 nonobese	19.8, 38.8 47.9	SBP: −2.0 (−3.8, 2.2) unadjusted (estimated per kg: at age 38 from reported values for 1-SD BW) SBP: −2.7 (−5.2, 0) adjusted (BMI, age)
Belgium	(78)	Twins	418 twin pairs	18–36	Women: SBP: −4.27 (unadjusted, $p < 0.001$) SBP: −4.20 (adjusted, $p < 0.01$) GA, BMI, age DPB: −2.18 (unadjusted, $p = 0.02$) DBP: −1.23 (adjusted, ns)

					Men: SBP: 0.46 (unadjusted, ns) SBP: −0.89 (adjusted, ns) DBP: 0.90 (crude, ns) DBP: −0.80 (adjusted, ns)
New Zealand	(133)	Dunnedin Multidisciplinary Health and Development Study cohort	891 with 1+ obs.	26 (repeat measures up to age 26)	SBP: −0.55 (−.32, 1.46) adjusted (age, sex, age*sex) SBP: −1.84 (−2.65, 1.02) adjusted (age, sex, height, weight)
Hong Kong	(18)	Follow-up of 1967 Hong Kong hospital birth cohort	122	30	SBP: −6.0 (−10.6, −1.3) adjusted (sex, BMI, mother's education and health during pregnancy) DBP: −3.2 (−6.8, 0.5)
South Africa	(75)	Case control: UGA versus AGA at birth	73 UGA 64 AGA	20	SBP mean = 126 (13.3 SD) versus 122 (11.7) in underweight versus adequate birthweight for GA DBP mean = 73.2 (8.4) versus 69.5 (8.7)
Guatemala	(124)	Follow-up of nutrition intervention study	385	20–29	Women: BW positively associated with SBP ($P < 0.001$) and DBP ($P < 0.05$): no regression analysis Men: no association of BW with BP
Japan	(125)	Medical students	299	23	No correlation of BW with SBP or DBP
Korea	(19)	Students	22 males	20	Significant inverse correlation of BW with DBP (−0.47)
Sweden	(94)	Vasterbotten Intervention Program	7,876	29–41	Males: SBP > 160 OR for LBW = 2.16 (0.51, 9.19) unadjusted, 2.45 (0.57–10.48) adjusted (BMI) SBP > 140 OR for LBW = 1.22 (0.72, 2.06) unadjusted, 1.31 (0.77, 2.22) adjusted DBP > 95 OR for LBW = 2.46 (1.11, 5.44) unadjusted, 3.05 (1.35, 6.89) adjusted DBP > 90 OR for LBW = 1.36 (0.73, 2.51) unadjusted, 1.52 (0.81, 2.82) adjusted

(*Continued*)

TABLE 2 (*Continued*)

Location of study	Reference	Sample and study type	n	Age	Result (regression coefficient units are mm Hg per kg BW, 95% CI in parentheses unless otherwise noted)
					Females: SBP > 160: OR for LBW = 7.59 (2.74, 21.01) unadjusted, 7.70 (2.76, 21.47) adjusted SBP > 140: OR for LBW = 2.29 (1.26, 4.140) unadjusted, 2.32 (1.27, 4.23) adjusted DBP > 95: OR for LBW = 1.58 (1.48, 5.16) unadjusted, 1.59 (0.48, 5.19) adjusted DBP > 90: OR for LBW = 1.10 (0.47, 2.54) unadjusted, 1.10 (0.47, 2.56) adjusted
Sweden	(80)	Conscript-birth registry link	276,033 males	17–24	High SBP (>90th percentile, height standardized) OR for BW < −2 SD = 1.15 (1.07–1.23) crude, 1.17 (1.08,1.27) adjusted (birth length, GA, adult height, BMI) OR for high SBP if light for GA = 1.33 (1.20, 1.46) adjusted
Sweden	(4)	Subgroup of population-based study of births in 1908, 1914, 1918, 1922, and 1930 Goteborg	438 women	50, 60	BW significantly predicts risk of HTN[a] at age 60 but not at 50 OR for HTN = 0.96 (0.92, 0.99) per 100 g increase in BW unchanged by adjustment for BMI
Sweden	(32)	1913 birth cohort from Gothenburg	478 men	50	SBP: −2.7 (−5.8, 0.4) unadjusted SBP: −3.7 (−6.7, −0.8) adjusted (current weight, GA, place of birth, parity, maternal diabetes, smoking) RR for HTN[b] 0.73 (0.54–0.98) per kg BW unadjusted 0.68 (0.50–0.93) adjusted
Iceland	(44)	Subgroup from Reykjavik study, 1914–1935 birth cohort	4601	50	Referent BW category = 3.75–4.0 kg In women: odds of HTN[c] if BW < 3.45 kg = 1.4 (1.1–1.8)

					No effect in men: OR = 1.0 (0.8–1.3) SBP: −1.2 (p = 0.110 in men, 0.093 in women) adjusted (age) SBP: −1.7 men (p = 0.01) 1.6 women (p = 0.023), adjusted (age, BMI) no association of BW with DBP
Finland	(9)	Helsinki University Hospital 1924–1944 births	13,517	57–77	OR for HTN[b] 0.77 (0.71–0.84) per kg BW, unadjusted
Finland	(10)	Helsinki University Central Hospital births 1934–1944	8,760		Cumulative incidence of HTN[b] related to BW: 20.2% (18.3, 22.1) in BW < 3.0 kg versus 12.3% (10.1, 14.6) in >4.0 kg, unadjusted
Finland	(30)	Helsinki University Central Hospital	7,086	Born 1924–1933	Cumulative incidence of HTN[b] declines with increasing BW in men and women (28.9% in BW ≤ 2.5 kg, 23.8% in BW > 4.0 kg)
Shanghai	(140)	Shanghai Women's Health Study	13,467 women	40–70	Inverse relationship of BW to HTN[d], p for trend = 0.07 BW > 2.5 kg associated with 20%–30% reduction in risk of HTN versus BW < 2.5 kg, unadjusted
Australia	(119)	Community study among Aborigines	767	7–43	SBP: −2.9 (−0.3, −5.5) in adults, adjusted (age, sex, weight) Women: SBP: −4.7 (−0.5, B8.6) Men: SBP: −1.4 (−1.7, B5.0) OR for HTN[e] if LBW = 2.3 (1.3, 3.5)

[a]HTN medication, BP cutpoints SBP > 160, DBP > 95.

[b]HTN medication record.

[c]BP cutpoints SBP > 140, DBP > 90 or medication.

[d]Self report of HTN medication use.

[e]BP cutpoints, SBP > 130, DBP > 85.

*Abbreviations: AGA, adequate weight for gestational age; BMI, body mass index; BP, blood pressure; BW, birthweight; DBP, diastolic blood pressure; GA, gestational age; HTN, hypertension; LBW, low birth weight; MRC NSHD, Medical Research Council National Survey of Health and Development; obs, observation; OR, odds ratio; RR, relative risk; SBP, systolic blood pressure; UGA, underweight for gestational age.

developing and transitional populations with a higher prevalence of poor nutrition are needed to broaden the range of exposures under study. Transitional populations are also more likely to experience changing (in many cases improving) nutritional conditions during childhood and young adulthood. The mismatch of pre- and postnatal environment is precisely the combination of exposures under which we would expect the strongest manifestation of DOHaD (40).

Unfortunately, few studies have been conducted in non-Western populations. Among participants in the Shanghai Women's Health Study (140), LBW was associated with a 20%–30% increase in the risk of hypertension (defined as use of medication) compared with birth weight >2.5 kg. Those who were LBW but were heavier than average as adults were four times more likely to have early-onset (age 20–40) hypertension. Unfortunately, this study relies solely on self-reports, and the sample able to report birth weight represents only about 18% of all study participants, thus raising concerns about recall and selection bias.

In a community of Australian Aborigines, birth weight was inversely associated with systolic BP, and odds of hypertension were elevated with history of LBW, with effects stronger in women than in men (adjusted for current weight) (119). One of the few developing-country studies that do not show an inverse association of birth weight with adult BP is a follow-up of a nutrition intervention study in Guatemala (113). In women whose mothers had received energy or protein supplements during pregnancy, birth weight was *positively* associated with systolic and diastolic BP, but no association was found in men.

Because differences in the association of birth weight with BP have been reported for males and females, Lawlor et al. (72) conducted a meta-regression analysis of 59 observational studies to assess sex differences. Of studies among adults that included males and females and reported linear regression coefficients, 9 presented sex-specific results and 11 presented results for males and females combined. Regression coefficients did not differ by sex: −2.21 (−3.56, −0.86) mm Hg per kg birth weight in males and −2.33 (−3.55, −1.10) in females. Pooled regression coefficients were about one unit larger in studies with males and females combined, which led the authors to suggest that separate results for males and females were more likely to be reported when overall results were weak.

Given the limitations of birth weight, some studies examined the effects of gestational age, birth length, or relative weight (ponderal index or BMI) [see (57) for a review]. For example, a study in 30-year-old Hong Kong adults shows a negative association of birth length and ponderal index with systolic BP and a negative association of length but not weight with diastolic BP (18). Leon et al. (74) compared the separate effects of weight, length, and gestational age on BP in 18-year-old Swedish conscripts. They concluded that the rate of accretion of fetal mass, independent of gestational age, matters most for later BP. Other studies have found associations with both weight and length, but typically considered their separate effects (4).

The clinical relevance of prenatal factors has been questioned based on the small size of birth weight coefficients (generally −1 to −4 mm Hg per kg birth weight). Although such differences may seem small in relation to effects associated with adult lifestyle risk factors and weight status, even small reductions in a population's mean BP can reduce the number of individuals at risk for hypertension. Although studies typically find weak or no associations of birth weight with diastolic BP, the clinical relevance of effects of systolic BP is greater because high systolic BP, at least in persons older than 50 years, is a much more important cardiovascular disease risk factor than is diastolic BP.

Studies of hypertension risk typically show strong effects of early nutrition and provide perspective on the potential importance of early interventions. For example, young adult males had a 33% increased odds of having high systolic BP if they were born light for gestational age (80). LBW was associated with more than double the risk of systolic BP > 160 mm Hg in 29- to 41-year-old males, and a greater than sevenfold increase in risk among females (94). When estimates are adjusted for adult BMI, coefficients represent the average effect of birth weight on BP at all levels of BMI. However, the most frequent finding is that risk is concentrated in those who were small at birth but large as adults. Judgments about the importance of fetal nutrition should also consider this important combination and potential synergism of risk factors.

In sum, the literature over the past two decades is consistent in showing an inverse association of birth weight with adult systolic BP or an increased risk of hypertension in adults with lower weight at birth.

Maternal Nutrition During Pregnancy and Later Blood Pressure

Fetal growth restriction and metabolic adaptations associated with programming later disease risk are assumed to be the result of fetal *nutritional* insufficiency (45). In most cases, this is secondary to poor maternal nutrition, but may also reflect adequate maternal nutrition along with placental insufficiency or other factors that reduce nutrient availability to the fetus. The ability to study inadequate maternal nutrition is limited by a scarcity of data since, unlike birth weight, maternal nutrition data aside from weight gain are not routinely recorded in clinical records. Animal models provide strong evidence of long-term effects of maternal dietary restriction on offspring BP, but the role of maternal diet and nutritional status during pregnancy has been directly assessed in relatively few human studies.

Several studies used the "natural experiments" of the Dutch Famine and Leningrad Siege, when women were exposed to severe rationing during pregnancy. Offspring exposed to famine in utero did not have significantly elevated BP as adults (110, 111, 123), although their insulin resistance was altered (107). Unfortunately, individual maternal dietary intake data are not available from these studies, so it is difficult to draw conclusions on the effects of maternal dietary restriction. Some studies with individual dietary data show effects of macronutrient imbalance during pregnancy on offspring BP. For example, Sheill et al. (116, 117) found higher BP, and Herrick et al. (50) found higher adult cortisol levels in offspring of mothers who reported high intakes of meat and fish in the second half of pregnancy. Roseboom et al. (111) found a positive association of maternal dietary protein to carbohydrate ratio with offspring BP, and Campbell et al. (17) found differing effects of carbohydrate, depending on the level of protein intake. In contrast, Huxley & Neil (56) found no relationship of maternal blood levels (more precise indicators of diet) during pregnancy to adult BP in a small sample from the United Kingdom.

Few studies used anthropometric indicators of nutrition status during pregnancy, and most involved youths rather than adults. Maternal prepregnancy BMI and weight gain during pregnancy were unrelated to offspring BP in a study of 17-year-old Israeli military conscripts (69), but other studies in children find elevated offspring BP if the mother had lower skinfold thickness in pregnancy or poor maternal weight gain. For example, in offspring of British women with below-median triceps skinfold thickness, weight gain from 18 to 28 weeks gestation was inversely related to BP at age 11 (22). Godfrey et al. (42) found an inverse relation between maternal skinfold thickness during pregnancy and offspring BP in Jamaican children. In addition, a prospective study of Filipino youths shows that maternal nutritional status during pregnancy is inversely associated with adolescent offspring BP, independent of birth weight (2).

The Role of Postnatal Growth

The relationship of birth size to later BP is often enhanced or present only when current size, typically represented as adult BMI, is taken into account. Studies typically find the highest mean BP or highest risk of hypertension in people who were relatively small at birth but relatively large as adults. This has been interpreted as evidence for an effect of postnatal growth (79); in order to start out small but end up large relative to the population distribution, one must have grown faster in height and/or weight at some time between birth and adulthood. An expanded research focus on postnatal growth has led to a refinement of the fetal origins hypothesis to include postnatal influences (10, 108). Catch-up or more rapid postnatal growth is a hypothesized risk factor for elevated BP in later life, and it has been suggested that coronary heart disease is a disorder of growth (108).

The newer focus on postnatal growth is plagued by some of the same problems of interpretation posed by the use of birth weight to represent fetal nutritional sufficiency. First, postnatal growth is the product of complex interactions among genetic and environmental variables. Like birth weight, it is a sensitive but non-specific indicator of nutritional sufficiency. Faster growth typically leads to larger body size, which is positively associated with BP, raising questions about the importance of growth versus its "end product." Growth entails increases in both lean tissue and fat, each of which has different consequences for chronic disease risk. Second, growth in any given interval is not independent of size at the beginning of the interval. Pre- and postnatal growth are part of a continuum, linked by common underlying determinants and because postnatal growth may represent a response to prenatal growth restriction. Thus, evaluation of the separate effects of fetal and postnatal factors is challenging.

Although an effect of growth has sometimes been inferred in the absence of longitudinal growth data, a full understanding of how postnatal growth relates to adult BP requires analysis of serial data from birth to adulthood. Critical questions relate to the timing of effects (e.g., is there a difference in risk associated with more rapid growth in infancy versus childhood?) and to whether rapid linear growth and rapid weight gain are associated with similar risks. See Huxley et al. (57) for a review of studies (published up to 2000) that examine the role of skeletal and nonskeletal growth in predicting systolic BP.

Studies with serial growth data have been conducted primarily in Europe, where childhood school health records can be linked with birth records or where earlier child growth studies were conducted. The different methods used to evaluate the effects of growth are illustrated by the studies described below.

Several analyses that strongly influenced thought about the role of growth are based on a follow-up of cohorts born in the Helsinki University Central Hospital. Eriksson et al. (30) calculated child height, weight, and BMI Z-scores for the large birth cohorts, then plotted mean Z-scores of those with hypertension as adults. Different growth trajectories are demonstrated when Z-scores of those with hypertension deviate from zero. Men from the 1922–1933 birth cohort with hypertension had lower weight at birth, but had caught up in weight by age 7 and had higher weight and BMI Z-scores from age 7 to 15. The Z-scores of those with hypertension increasingly deviated from zero with age, but the differences were small (0.08 SD units at age 15 in males, which is equivalent to about 0.6 kg above the mean in weight), a statistically significant effect because of the large sample. In a similar study of the 1933–1944 cohort, men and women who later developed hypertension were smaller at birth but had BMI and weight Z-scores above zero (0.1–0.15 SD) by age 12. The effects of lower birth weight and higher BMI were found to be additive rather than interactive.

Law and colleagues (71) compared the effects of birth weight, growth in infancy, and growth in early childhood (age 1–5 years) using a method that accounted for their intercorrelation. More rapid early childhood, but not infancy growth, was associated with increased BP in this sample of young adults in the United Kingdom. The highest mean systolic BP was in those who were light at birth but had the most rapid childhood weight gains. However, the effects of growth were substantially attenuated and no longer significant when adult BMI was taken into account. This suggests that more rapid child growth is simply a predictor of greater adult size, a known risk factor for elevated BP. In contrast, Hardy et al. (47) found independent associations of BMI at ages 2, 4, 7, and 15 years with systolic BP at age 43. The associations were negative prior to age 15 in women and up to age 43 in men, but not fully explained by adult BMI in women.

Another approach to the analysis of the relationship of child growth to adult BP was developed by Cole (23) and applied to data from Brazil (52) and Cebu, Philippines (1, 23) to assess the relative importance of growth velocity at different ages. Although these were studies of adolescents rather than adults, they are important in demonstrating the method. When BP is regressed on Z-scores of weight at different ages in the same model, each coefficient is an age-specific measure of the association between weight and BP. A positive coefficient indicates that faster growth during that interval predicts higher BP. In the Brazil sample, there was a similar effect of weight gain at all ages, whereas in Filipino males, increased risk of elevated BP was associated primarily with mid-childhood to adolescence weight gain. The effects of rapid weight gain on risk of having high BP at age 16 were confined to males who were relatively thin at birth, but had accelerated gain from mid-childhood to adolescence (1).

The question of whether the effects of rapid growth are age-specific has generated considerable controversy. Evidence suggests that small size at birth followed by rapid early postnatal weight gain adversely programs later risk of insulin resistance and hypertension (71, 120). This finding has raised questions about the wisdom of promoting rapid infant growth among those with fetal growth restriction (121). However, not all studies find increased risk associated with infant growth; in fact, a protective effect of more rapid infant growth is suggested by the results from Cebu, Philippines (1). Similarly, in Hong Kong adults, change in ponderal index from 6–18 months of age was inversely associated with BP, that is, becoming relatively fatter in early life reduced systolic BP in adulthood (18).

Few studies directly compare linear growth with growth in weight. Faster height gain is positively associated with BP in some studies (30, 49, 62, 134), but Lundgren and colleagues (80) found that males born small for gestational age have an increased risk of high systolic BP, especially if they are short as adults. More evidence supports a role for accelerated weight gain, which may represent the accumulation of body fat.

In sum, the cumulative evidence suggests that childhood growth trajectories, particularly among those with a history of fetal growth restriction, affect risk of elevated BP in adulthood. It is still not clear whether risks differ depending on the age when more rapid growth occurs or whether the effects of growth are independent of attained size or body composition in adulthood. The inference of growth effects from the observation that risk is highest among those who were small at birth but large as adults does not provide sufficient insight into the nature of the risk that may be related to excess growth. More studies need to span the full growth period, with serial measurements of height, weight, and body composition as well as exposures that influence growth. More rapid growth may itself be programmed: Metabolic adaptations may alter the response to diet and activity of those with a history of nutritional insufficiency in utero (40), facilitating their more rapid growth. A more promising line of research may involve examination of differential growth responses to environmental factors in those with and without a history of fetal nutritional insufficiency.

Other Postnatal Factors

Adult BP may be influenced by early diet. In a recent systematic review (102), data were compiled to examine how BP relates to infant feeding. Exclusive breastfeeding was compared with formula feeding, with adjustment for current age, sex, height, and BMI using data from 26 estimates of systolic BP and 24 estimates of diastolic BP. On average, breast-feeding was associated with modestly lower average systolic BP (−1.10 mm Hg) compared with formula feeding, with no marked differences by age. The effect was larger in small studies than in large studies, suggesting publication bias. No effects of feeding on diastolic BP were found. Differences in composition of breast milk versus formula, in particular in their fat and sodium content, are thought to be the relevant determinants of long-term effects of infant feeding on BP. This hypothesis is supported by data from a randomized trial to study the effect of a low- or normal-sodium diet (average daily consumption of 0.89 ± 0.26 mol and 2.50 ± 0.95 mol, respectively, over a 25-week intervention period) in Dutch infants ($n = 476$) (36). At age 15 years ($n = 167$) systolic and diastolic BP were lower (−3.6 mm Hg and −2.2 mm Hg, respectively) in the low-sodium group.

Further evidence of early diet composition effects comes from a follow-up study of mothers and offspring randomly assigned to receive a dried milk supplement. In young adulthood (age 23–27 years), BP was higher among those who consumed more supplement at 3 months of age [+1.07 mm HG systolic BP per quartile of milk consumption ($\leq$682, 710–795, 824–909, $\geq$937 ml)], independent of birth weight and adult BMI, a finding that suggests an effect of diet composition independent of growth (86).

Summary of Study Limitations and Directions for Future Research

Taken as a whole, animal and human studies provide strong evidence that adult BP has developmental origins. However, the human epidemiologic literature is characterized by weaknesses that have led to continued skepticism about the importance of developmental versus adult lifestyle factors (38, 55). Below, we consider some of these weaknesses and suggest directions for future research to address them.

THE NEED FOR BETTER CHARACTERIZATION OF NUTRITIONAL EXPOSURES Although it is convenient, birth weight is an inadequate marker of fetal nutritional insufficiency. This is underscored by a lack of strong evidence that maternal diet affects birth weight, and by the fact that maternal diet in pregnancy can affect offspring BP independent of size at birth (2, 66). There has been inadequate research on maternal nutrition during pregnancy with careful quantification of maternal dietary intakes and nutritional stores. A promising new approach is the use of a maternal supply–fetal demand model (64) to better characterize fetal nutritional sufficiency. Better characterization of fetal growth patterns, and in particular growth of specific organs through serial fetal ultrasound, may also improve our ability to identify the key programming influences.

INCONSISTENT MEASUREMENT AND DEFINITION OF BP OUTCOMES For practical reasons, most studies use casual or single-occasion rather than ambulatory BP measurements. Few studies compare effects of birth weight on BP using both methods. One such study found similar coefficients estimated using casual versus ambulatory BP measurement in elderly adults (139), one found stronger effects with casual measurements in young adults (78), and one found stronger effects of ambulatory measurements in adolescent girls (97). In addition, hypertension has not been consistently defined across studies. Records or self-report of using medications to lower BP may bias estimates toward the null since many cases of hypertension are not diagnosed and treated. Studies that use different BP cutpoints to define hypertension make it difficult to compare results across studies. Ideally, studies should use standardized measurement and definition of outcomes.

INADEQUATE CONSIDERATION OF POSTNATAL EXPOSURES, INCLUDING LACK OF LONGITUDINAL DATA ON POSTNATAL GROWTH, AND FACTORS SUCH AS DIET AND PHYSICAL ACTIVITY THAT INFLUENCE GROWTH There is no research testing whether responsiveness to environmental factors is altered by early nutrition. The observation that fetal growth restriction in rats results in lower levels of physical activity (128) and overeating, particularly in response to a high-fat diet (117), provides the biological rationale for asking whether there may be similar effects in humans.

INAPPROPRIATE STATISTICAL MODELING There is controversy about interpretation of results when models adjust for current body size in assessing early life predictors of adult BP (38). Typically, variables such as adult BMI are considered as potential confounders of the relationship. However, growth and adult body size may *mediate* the relationship of early life factors and adult BP and their inclusion in the model may bias estimates. When adult size is included in models, the effects of early size can be interpreted only in the context of adult size. Lucas and colleagues (79) therefore recommend assessing and reporting results from three regression models, illustrated here with birth weight and adult BMI as the exposures. The "early" model includes birth weight alone, the "combined" model includes birth weight and adult BMI, and the "interaction" model includes a birth weight × adult BMI interaction term. The early origins hypothesis would be supported when there is a negative coefficient on birth weight in the early model, and a negative coefficient of birth weight and the interaction term in the interaction model. The most important aspect of developmental factors may be their ability to potentiate the effects of adverse lifestyle factors in adulthood; thus, future research should focus on explorations of interactions of early and later life risk factors.

LACK OF CLARITY ABOUT THE ROLE OF GROWTH AND INADEQUATE INFORMATION ABOUT THE IMPORTANCE OF TIMING OF EXPOSURES The expansion of the fetal origins hypothesis to include postnatal developmental factors is important but not sufficient. Future research should focus on the identification of precisely what aspect of growth matters. Is it simply a predictor of adult body composition, which, in turn, affects risk of elevated BP? Or does rapid growth pose other challenges, for example, to kidney function compromised by prenatally impaired nephrogenesis? To inform appropriate interventions, we need to determine whether more rapid growth has different long-term consequences depending on when it occurs and whether there are differential effects of rapid growth of lean versus fat mass.

THE ROLE OF GENETICS The design of most epidemiologic studies does not allow for testing hypotheses about the role of genetics. If common genetic factors relate to both poor fetal growth and elevated BP in adults, we may mistakenly infer a casual affect of fetal retardation. Moreover, maternal BP may be an important confounder of the association between fetal growth retardation and adult hypertension since it is both inversely associated with infant birth weight and the offspring's adult BP (21). Twin studies show that controlling for genetic factors may attenuate, but not fully explain, the observed inverse association of birth weight with adult BP (20, 78).

CONCLUSION

Substantial evidence from animal and human studies supports a role for long-term effects of early nutritional exposures in the development of elevated BP and hypertension. Although developmental factors may not be among the strongest risk factors for hypertension, their importance should be recognized and used to bolster early life prevention efforts, including optimization of maternal nutrition during pregnancy and prevention of excess weight gain. Developmental factors may play a greater role in developing and transitional country settings, where populations of adults among whom low birth weight was common are now exposed to rapid changes in diet and activity that are conducive to the development of cardiovascular diseases. An appreciation of the potential for greater susceptibility of such individuals offers further opportunities for targeted intervention in adulthood.

The *Annual Review of Nutrition* is online at http://nutr.annualreviews.org

LITERATURE CITED

1. Adair LS, Cole TJ. 2003. Rapid child growth raises blood pressure in adolescent boys who were thin at birth. *Hypertension* 41:451–56
2. Adair LS, Kuzawa C, Borja JR. 2001. Maternal energy stores and diet composition during pregnancy program adolescent blood pressure. *Circulation* 104:1034–39
3. Alexander BT. 2003. Placental insufficiency leads to development of hypertension in growth-restricted offspring. *Hypertension* 41:457–62
4. Andersson SW, Lapidus L, Niklasson A, Hallberg L, Bengtsson C, Hulthen L. 2000. Blood pressure and hypertension in middle-aged women in relation to weight and length at birth: a follow-up study. *J. Hypertens.* 18:1753–61
5. Aviv A. 2001. Hypothesis: pulse pressure and human longevity. *Hypertension* 37:1060–66
6. Aviv A. 2002. Chronology versus biology: telomeres, essential hypertension, and vascular aging. *Hypertension* 40:229–32

7. Aviv A, Aviv H. 1997. Reflections on telomeres, growth, aging, and essential hypertension. *Hypertension* 29:1067–72
8. Barker DJ. 2003. Coronary heart disease: a disorder of growth. *Horm. Res.* 59(Suppl. 1):35–41
9. Barker DJ, Eriksson JG, Forsen T, Osmond C. 2002. Fetal origins of adult disease: strength of effects and biological basis. *Int. J. Epidemiol.* 31:1235–39
10. Barker DJ, Forsen T, Eriksson JG, Osmond C. 2002. Growth and living conditions in childhood and hypertension in adult life: a longitudinal study. *J. Hypertens.* 20:1951–56
11. Battista MC, Oligny LL, St-Louis J, Brochu M. 2002. Intrauterine growth restriction in rats is associated with hypertension and renal dysfunction in adulthood. *Am. J. Physiol. Endocrinol. Metab.* 283:E124–31
12. Bertram C, Trowern AR, Copin N, Jackson AA, Whorwood CB. 2001. The maternal diet during pregnancy programs altered expression of the glucocorticoid receptor and type 2 11ß-hydroxysteroid dehydrogenase: potential molecular mechanisms underlying the programming of hypertension in utero. *Endocrinology* 142:2841–53
13. Bertram CE, Hanson MA. 2002. Prenatal programming of postnatal endocrine responses by glucocorticoids. *Reproduction* 124:459–67
14. Brawley L, Poston L, Hanson MA. 2003. Mechanisms underlying the programming of small artery dysfunction: review of the model using low-protein diet in pregnancy in the rat. *Arch. Physiol. Biochem.* 111:23–35
15. Brenner BM, Garcia DL, Anderson S. 1988. Glomeruli and blood pressure. Less of one, more the other? *Am. J. Hypertens.* 1:335–47
16. Burrow CR. 2000. Retinoids and renal development. *Exp. Nephrol.* 8:219–25
17. Campbell DM, Hall MH, Barker DJ, Cross J, Shiell AW, Godfrey KM. 1996. Diet in pregnancy and the offspring's blood pressure 40 years later. *Br. J. Obstet. Gynaecol.* 103:273–80
18. Cheung YB, Low L, Osmond C, Barker D, Karlberg J. 2000. Fetal growth and early postnatal growth are related to blood pressure in adults. *Hypertension* 36:795–800
19. Choi CS, Kim C, Lee WJ, Park JY, Hong SK, et al. 2000. Association between birth weight and insulin sensitivity in healthy young men in Korea: role of visceral adiposity. *Diabetes Res. Clin. Pract.* 49:53–59
20. Christensen K, Stovring H, McGue M. 2001. Do genetic factors contribute to the association between birth weight and blood pressure? *J. Epidemiol. Community Health* 55:583–87
21. Churchill D, Perry IJ, Beevers DG. 1997. Ambulatory blood pressure in pregnancy and fetal growth. *Lancet* 349:7–10
22. Clark PM, Atton C, Law CM, Shiell A, Godfrey K, Barker DJ. 1998. Weight gain in pregnancy, triceps skinfold thickness, and blood pressure in offspring. *Obstet. Gynecol.* 91:103–7
23. Cole T. 2003. Modelling post-natal exposures and their interactions with birth size. *J. Nutr.* 134:201–4
24. Curhan GC, Chertow GM, Willett WC, Spiegelman D, Colditz GA, et al. 1996. Birth weight and adult hypertension and obesity in women. *Circulation* 94:1310–15
25. Demerath EW, Cameron N, Gillman MW, Towne B, Siervogel RM. 2004. Telomeres and telomerase in the fetal origins of cardiovascular disease: a review. *Hum. Biol.* 76:127–46
26. Dodic M, Hantzis V, Duncan J, Rees S, Koukoulas I, et al. 2002. Programming effects of short prenatal exposure to cortisol. *FASEB J.* 16:1017–26
27. Dodic M, Moritz K, Koukoulas I, Wintour EM. 2002. Programmed hypertension: kidney, brain or both? *Trends Endocrinol. Metab.* 13:403–8

28. Drake AJ, Walker BR. 2004. The intergenerational effects of fetal programming: non-genomic mechanisms for the inheritance of low birth weight and cardiovascular risk. *J. Endocrinol.* 180:1–16
29. Dunger DB, Ong KK, Huxtable SJ, Sherriff A, Woods KA, et al. 1998. Association of the INS VNTR with size at birth. ALSPAC Study Team. Avon Longitudinal Study of Pregnancy and Childhood. *Nat. Genet.* 19:98–100
30. Eriksson J, Forsen T, Tuomilehto J, Osmond C, Barker D. 2000. Fetal and childhood growth and hypertension in adult life. *Hypertension* 36:790–94
31. Eriksson JG, Forsen T. 2002. Unravelling the fetal origins hypothesis. *Lancet* 360:2072
32. Eriksson M, Wallander MA, Krakau I, Wedel H, Svardsudd K. 2004. Birth weight and cardiovascular risk factors in a cohort followed until 80 years of age: the study of men born in 1913. *J. Intern. Med.* 255:236–46
33. Fagerudd J, Forsblom C, Pettersson-Fernholm K, Saraheimo M, Waden J, et al. 2004. Birth weight is inversely correlated to adult systolic blood pressure and pulse pressure in type 1 diabetes. *Hypertension* 44:1–6
34. Fields LE, Burt VL, Cutler JA, Hughes J, Roccella EJ, Sorlie P. 2004. The burden of adult hypertension in the United States 1999 to 2000: a rising tide. *Hypertension* 44:398–404
35. Fowden AL, Forhead AJ. 2004. Endocrine mechanisms of intrauterine programming. *Reproduction* 127:515–26
36. Geleijnse JM, Hofman A, Witteman JC, Hazebroek AA, Valkenburg HA, Grobbee DE. 1997. Long-term effects of neonatal sodium restriction on blood pressure. *Hypertension* 29:913–17
37. Gennser G, Rymark P, Isberg PE. 1988. Low birth weight and risk of high blood pressure in adulthood. *Br. Med. J. (Clin. Res. Ed.)* 296:1498–500
38. Gillman MW. 2002. Epidemiological challenges in studying the fetal origins of adult chronic disease. *Int. J. Epidemiol.* 31:294–99
39. Gluckman PD, Hanson MA. 2004. The developmental origins of the metabolic syndrome. *Trends Endocrinol. Metab.* 15:183–87
40. Gluckman PD, Hanson MA. 2004. Living with the past: evolution, development, and patterns of disease. *Science* 305:1733–36
41. Gluckman PD, Pinal CS. 2002. Maternal-placental-fetal interactions in the endocrine regulation of fetal growth: role of somatotrophic axes. *Endocrine* 19:81–89
42. Godfrey KM, Forrester T, Barker DJ, Jackson AA, Landman JP, et al. 1994. Maternal nutritional status in pregnancy and blood pressure in childhood. *Br. J. Obstet. Gynaecol.* 101:398–403
43. Green LR. 2001. Programming of endocrine mechanisms of cardiovascular control and growth. *J. Soc. Gynecol. Investig.* 8:57–68
44. Gunnarsdottir I, Birgisdottir BE, Benediktsson R, Gudnason V, Thorsdottir I. 2002. Relationship between size at birth and hypertension in a genetically homogeneous population of high birth weight. *J. Hypertens.* 20:623–28
45. Harding JE. 2001. The nutritional basis of the fetal origins of adult disease. *Int. J. Epidemiol.* 30:15–23
46. Hardy R, Kuh D, Langenberg C, Wadsworth ME. 2003. Birthweight, childhood social class, and change in adult blood pressure in the 1946 British birth cohort. *Lancet* 362:1178–83
47. Hardy R, Wadsworth ME, Langenberg C, Kuh D. 2004. Birthweight, childhood growth, and blood pressure at 43 years in a British birth cohort. *Int. J. Epidemiol.* 33:121–9
48. Hattersley AT, Tooke JE. 1999. The fetal insulin hypothesis: an alternative explanation of the association of low birthweight with diabetes and vascular disease. *Lancet* 353:1789–92

49. Hennessy E, Alberman E. 1997. The effects of own fetal growth on reported hypertension in parous women aged 33. *Int. J. Epidemiol.* 26:562–70
50. Herrick K, Phillips DI, Haselden S, Shiell AW, Campbell-Brown M, Godfrey KM. 2003. Maternal consumption of a high-meat, low-carbohydrate diet in late pregnancy: relation to adult cortisol concentrations in the offspring. *J. Clin. Endocrinol. Metab.* 88:3554–60
51. Holt RI. 2002. Fetal programming of the growth hormone–insulin-like growth factor axis. *Trends Endocrinol. Metab.* 13:392–97
52. Horta BL, Barros FC, Victora CG, Cole TJ. 2003. Early and late growth and blood pressure in adolescence. *J. Epidemiol. Community Health* 57:226–30
53. Hughson M, Farris AB 3rd, Douglas-Denton R, Hoy WE, Bertram JF. 2003. Glomerular number and size in autopsy kidneys: the relationship to birth weight. *Kidney Int.* 63:2113–22
54. Huxley R, Neil A, Collins R. 2002. Unravelling the fetal origins hypothesis: Is there really an inverse association between birthweight and subsequent blood pressure? *Lancet* 360:659–65
55. Deleted in proof
56. Huxley RR, Neil HA. 2004. Does maternal nutrition in pregnancy and birth weight influence levels of CHD risk factors in adult life? *Br. J. Nutr.* 91:459–68
57. Huxley RR, Shiell AW, Law CM. 2000. The role of size at birth and postnatal catch-up growth in determining systolic blood pressure: a systematic review of the literature. *J. Hypertens.* 18:815–31
58. IJzerman RG, van Weissenbruch MM, Voordouw JJ, Yudkin JS, Serne EH, et al. 2002. The association between birth weight and capillary recruitment is independent of blood pressure and insulin sensitivity: a study in prepubertal children. *J. Hypertens.* 20:1957–63
59. Irving RJ, Shore AC, Belton NR, Elton RA, Webb DJ, Walker BR. 2004. Low birth weight predicts higher blood pressure but not dermal capillary density in two populations. *Hypertension* 43:610–13
60. Johansson-Kark M, Rasmussen F, DeStavola B, Leon DA. 2002. Fetal growth and systolic blood pressure in young adulthood: the Swedish Young Male Twins Study. *Paediatr. Perinat. Epidemiol.* 16:200–9
61. Kearney PM, Whelton M, Reynolds K, Whelton PK, He J. 2004. Worldwide prevalence of hypertension: a systematic review. *J. Hypertens.* 22:11–19
62. Koupilova I, Leon DA, Lithell HO, Berglund L. 1997. Size at birth and hypertension in longitudinally followed 50–70-year- old men. *Blood Press.* 6:223–28
63. Kumaran K, Fall CH, Martyn CN, Vijayakumar M, Stein C, Shier R. 2000. Blood pressure, arterial compliance, and left ventricular mass: no relation to small size at birth in south Indian adults. *Heart* 83:272–77
64. Kuzawa CW. 2004. Modeling fetal adaptation to nutrient restriction: testing the fetal origins hypothesis with a supply-demand model. *J. Nutr.* 134:194–200
65. Langley-Evans SC. 2001. Fetal programming of cardiovascular function through exposure to maternal undernutrition. *Proc. Nutr. Soc.* 60:505–13
66. Langley-Evans SC, Gardner DS, Jackson AA. 1996. Association of disproportionate growth of fetal rats in late gestation with raised systolic blood pressure in later life. *J. Reprod. Fertil.* 106:307–12
67. Langley-Evans SC, Langley-Evans AJ, Marchand MC. 2003. Nutritional programming of blood pressure and renal morphology. *Arch. Physiol. Biochem.* 111:8–16
68. Langley-Evans SC, Welham SJ, Jackson AA. 1999. Fetal exposure to a maternal protein diet impairs nephrogenesis and promotes hypertension in the rat. *Life Sci.* 64:965–74
69. Laor A, Stevenson D, Shemer J, Gale R,

Seidman D. 1997. Size at birth, maternal nutritional status in pregnancy, and blood pressure at age 17: population-based analysis. *BMJ* 315:449–53
70. Law CM, Shiell AW. 1996. Is blood pressure inversely related to birth weight? The strength of evidence from a systematic review of the literature. *J. Hypertens.* 14:935–41
71. Law CM, Shiell AW, Newsome CA, Syddall HE, Shinebourne EA, et al. 2002. Fetal, infant, and childhood growth and adult blood pressure: a longitudinal study from birth to 22 years of age. *Circulation* 105:1088–92
72. Lawlor DA, Ebrahim S, Davey Smith G. 2002. Is there a sex difference in the association between birth weight and systolic blood pressure in later life? Findings from a meta-regression analysis. *Am. J. Epidemiol.* 156:1100–4
73. Leon D, Koupilova I. 1999. Birthweight, blood pressure and hypertension: epidemiologic studies. In *Fetal Origins of Cardiovascular and Lung Disease*, ed. DJP Barker, pp. 23–48. New York: Marcel Dekker
74. Leon DA, Johansson M, Rasmussen F. 2000. Gestational age and growth rate of fetal mass are inversely associated with systolic blood pressure in young adults: an epidemiologic study of 165,136 Swedish men aged 18 years. *Am. J. Epidemiol.* 152:597–604
75. Levitt NS, Lambert EV, Woods D, Hales CN, Andrew R, Seckl JR. 2000. Impaired glucose tolerance and elevated blood pressure in low birth weight, nonobese, young South African adults: early programming of cortisol axis. *J. Clin. Endocrinol. Metab.* 85:4611–18
76. Li H, Stein AD, Barnhart HX, Ramakrishnan U, Martorell R. 2003. Associations between prenatal and postnatal growth and adult body size and composition. *Am. J. Clin. Nutr.* 77:1498–505
77. Lisle SJ, Lewis RM, Petry CJ, Ozanne SE, Hales CN, Forhead AJ. 2003. Effect of maternal iron restriction during pregnancy on renal morphology in the adult rat offspring. *Br. J. Nutr.* 90:33–39
78. Loos RJ, Fagard R, Beunen G, Derom C, Vlietinck R. 2001. Birth weight and blood pressure in young adults: a prospective twin study. *Circulation* 104:1633–38
79. Lucas A, Fewtrell MS, Cole TJ. 1999. Fetal origins of adult disease—the hypothesis revisited. *BMJ* 319:245–49
80. Lundgren EM, Cnattingius HM, Jonsson GB, Tuvemo TH. 2001. Linear catch-up growth does not increase the risk of elevated blood pressure and reduces the risk of overweight in males. *J. Hypertens.* 19:1533–38
81. Mackenzie HS, Brenner BM. 1995. Fewer nephrons at birth: a missing link in the etiology of essential hypertension? *Am. J. Kidney Dis.* 26:91–98
82. Mackenzie HS, Lawler EV, Brenner BM. 1996. Congenital oligonephropathy: the fetal flaw in essential hypertension? *Kidney Int.* (Suppl.)55:S30–34
83. MacLennan NK, James SJ, Melnyk S, Piroozi A, Jernigan S, et al. 2004. Uteroplacental insufficiency alters DNA methylation, one-carbon metabolism, and histone acetylation in IUGR rats. *Physiol. Genomics* 18:43–50
84. Manning J, Beutler K, Knepper MA, Vehaskari VM. 2002. Upregulation of renal BSC1 and TSC in prenatally programmed hypertension. *Am. J. Physiol. Renal. Physiol.* 283:F202–6
85. Marchand MC, Langley-Evans SC. 2001. Intrauterine programming of nephron number: the fetal flaw revisited. *J. Nephrol.* 14:327–31
86. Martin RM, McCarthy A, Smith GD, Davies DP, Ben-Shlomo Y. 2003. Infant nutrition and blood pressure in early adulthood: the Barry Caerphilly Growth study. *Am. J. Clin. Nutr.* 77:1489–97
87. Martorell R, Stein AD, Schroeder DG. 2001. Early nutrition and later adiposity. *J. Nutr.* 131:874–80S

88. Martyn CN, Barker DJ, Jespersen S, Greenwald S, Osmond C, Berry C. 1995. Growth in utero, adult blood pressure, and arterial compliance. *Br. Heart J.* 73:116–21
89. Martyn CN, Greenwald SE. 1997. Impaired synthesis of elastin in walls of aorta and large conduit arteries during early development as an initiating event in pathogenesis of systemic hypertension. *Lancet* 350:953–55
90. Martyn CN, Greenwald SE. 2001. A hypothesis about a mechanism for the programming of blood pressure and vascular disease in early life. *Clin. Exp. Pharmacol. Physiol.* 28:948–51
91. Matthews SG. 2002. Early programming of the hypothalamo-pituitary-adrenal axis. *Trends Endocrinol. Metab.* 13:373–80
92. McKay JA, Williams EA, Mathers JC. 2004. Folate and DNA methylation during in utero development and aging. *Biochem. Soc. Trans.* 32:1006–7
93. McMullen S, Gardner DS, Langley-Evans SC. 2004. Prenatal programming of angiotensin II type 2 receptor expression in the rat. *Br. J. Nutr.* 91:133–40
94. Mogren I, Hogberg U, Stegmayr B, Lindahl B, Stenlund H. 2001. Fetal exposure, heredity and risk indicators for cardiovascular disease in a Swedish welfare cohort. *Int. J. Epidemiol.* 30:853–62
95. Montgomery AA, Ben-Shlomo Y, McCarthy A, Davies D, Elwood P, Smith GD. 2000. Birth size and arterial compliance in young adults. *Lancet* 355:2136–37
96. Murray LJ, Gallagher AM, Boreham CA, Savage M, Smith GD. 2001. Sex-specific difference in the relation between birth weight and arterial compliance in young adults: the Young Hearts Project. *J. Epidemiol. Community Health* 55:665–66
97. O'Sullivan J, Wright C, Pearce MS, Parker L. 2002. The influence of age and gender on the relationship between birth weight and blood pressure in childhood: a study using 24-hour and casual blood pressure. *Eur. J. Pediatr.* 161:423–27
98. Oken E, Gillman MW. 2003. Fetal origins of obesity. *Obes. Res.* 11:496–506
99. Okuda K, Bardeguez A, Gardner JP, Rodriguez P, Ganesh V, et al. 2002 Telomere length in the newborn. *Pediatr. Res.* 52:377–81
100. Ong KK, Ahmed ML, Emmett PM, Preece MA, Dunger DB. 2000. Association between postnatal catch-up growth and obesity in childhood: prospective cohort study. 320:967–71
101. Oren A, Vos LE, Bos WJ, Safar ME, Uiterwaal CS, et al. 2003. Gestational age and birth weight in relation to aortic stiffness in healthy young adults: two separate mechanisms? *Am. J. Hypertens.* 16:76–79
102. Owen CG, Whincup PH, Gilg JA, Cook DG. 2003. Effect of breast feeding in infancy on blood pressure in later life: systematic review and meta-analysis. *BMJ* 327:1189–95
103. Pham TD, MacLennan NK, Chiu CT, Laksana GS, Hsu JL, Lane RH. 2003. Uteroplacental insufficiency increases apoptosis and alters p53 gene methylation in the full-term IUGR rat kidney. *Am. J. Physiol. Regul. Integr. Comp. Physiol.* 285:R962–70
104. Phillips DI, Walker BR, Reynolds RM, Flanagan DE, Wood PJ, et al. 2000. Low birth weight predicts elevated plasma cortisol concentrations in adults from 3 populations. *Hypertension* 35:1301–6
105. Rasch R, Skriver E, Woods LL. 2004. The role of the RAS in programming of adult hypertension. *Acta Physiol. Scand.* 181:537–42
106. Rasmussen KM. 2001. The "fetal origins" hypothesis: challenges and opportunities for maternal and child nutrition. *Annu. Rev. Nutr.* 21:73–95
107. Ravelli AC, van der Meulen JH, Michels RP, Osmond C, Barker DJ, et al. 1998. Glucose tolerance in adults after prenatal exposure to famine. *Lancet* 351:173–77

108. Robinson SM, Barker DJ. 2002. Coronary heart disease: a disorder of growth. *Proc. Nutr. Soc.* 61:537–42
109. Rogers I. 2003. The influence of birthweight and intrauterine environment on adiposity and fat distribution in later life. *Int. J. Obes. Relat. Metab. Disord.* 27:755–77
110. Roseboom TJ, van der Meulen JH, Ravelli AC, van Montfrans GA, Osmond C, et al. 1999. Blood pressure in adults after prenatal exposure to famine. *J. Hypertens.* 17:325–30
111. Roseboom TJ, van der Meulen JH, van Montfrans GA, Ravelli AC, Osmond C, et al. 2001. Maternal nutrition during gestation and blood pressure in later life. *J. Hypertens.* 19:29–34
112. Schack-Nielsen L, Holst C, Sorensen TI. 2002. Blood pressure in relation to relative weight at birth through childhood and youth in obese and non-obese adult men. *Int. J. Obes. Relat. Metab. Disord.* 26:1539–46
113. Schluchter MD. 2003. Publication bias and heterogeneity in the relationship between systolic blood pressure, birth weight, and catch-up growth—a meta analysis. *J. Hypertens.* 21:273–79
114. Seckl JR. 2001. Glucocorticoid programming of the fetus: adult phenotypes and molecular mechanisms. *Mol. Cell. Endocrinol.* 185:61–71
115. Serrano AL, Andres V. 2004. Telomeres and cardiovascular disease: Does size matter? *Circ. Res.* 94:575–84
116. Shiell AW, Campbell-Brown M, Haselden S, Robinson S, Godfrey KM, Barker DJ. 2001. High-meat, low-carbohydrate diet in pregnancy: relation to adult blood pressure in the offspring. *Hypertension* 38:1282–88
117. Shiell AW, Campbell DM, Hall MH, Barker DJ. 2000. Diet in late pregnancy and glucose-insulin metabolism of the offspring 40 years later. *BJOG* 107:890–95
118. Silver LE, Decamps PJ, Korst LM, Platt LD, Castro LC. 2003. Intrauterine growth restriction is accompanied by decreased renal volume in the human fetus. *Am. J. Obstet. Gynecol.* 188:1320–25
119. Singh GR, Hoy WE. 2003. The association between birthweight and current blood pressure: a cross-sectional study in an Australian Aboriginal community. *Med. J. Aust.* 179:532–35
120. Singhal A, Fewtrell M, Cole TJ, Lucas A. 2003. Low nutrient intake and early growth for later insulin resistance in adolescents born preterm. *Lancet* 361:1089–97
121. Singhal A, Lucas A. 2004. Early origins of cardiovascular disease: Is there a unifying hypothesis? *Lancet* 363:1642–45
122. Singhal A, Wells J, Cole TJ, Fewtrell M, Lucas A. 2003. Programming of lean body mass: a link between birth weight, obesity, and cardiovascular disease? *Am. J. Clin. Nutr.* 77:726–30
123. Stanner SA, Bulmer K, Andres C, Lantseva OE, Borodina V, et al. 1997. Does malnutrition in utero determine diabetes and coronary heart disease in adulthood? Results from the Leningrad siege study, a cross sectional study. *BMJ* 315:1342–48
124. Stein AD, Conlisk A, Torun B, Schroeder DG, Grajeda R, Martorell R. 2002. Cardiovascular disease risk factors are related to adult adiposity but not birth weight in young Guatemalan adults. *J. Nutr.* 132:2208–14
125. Suzuki T, Minami J, Ohrui M, Ishimitsu T, Matsuoka H. 2000. Relationship between birth weight and cardiovascular risk factors in Japanese young adults. *Am. J. Hypertens.* 13:907–13
126. te Velde SJ, Ferreira I, Twisk JW, Stehouwer CD, van Mechelen W, Kemper HC. 2004. Birthweight and arterial stiffness and blood pressure in adulthood—results from the Amsterdam Growth and Health Longitudinal Study. *Int. J. Epidemiol.* 33:154–61
127. Vehaskari VM, Aviles DH, Manning J. 2001. Prenatal programming of adult

hypertension in the rat. *Kidney Int.* 59: 238–45
128. Vickers MH, Breier BH, Cutfield WS, Hofman PL, Gluckman PD. 2000. Fetal origins of hyperphagia, obesity, and hypertension and postnatal amplification by hypercaloric nutrition. *Am. J. Physiol. Endocrinol. Metab.* 279:E83–87
129. Vickers MH, Breier BH, McCarthy D, Gluckman PD. 2003. Sedentary behavior during postnatal life is determined by the prenatal environment and exacerbated by postnatal hypercaloric nutrition. *Am. J. Physiol. Regul. Integr. Comp. Physiol.* 285:R271–73
130. Wadsworth ME, Cripps HA, Midwinter RE, Colley JR. 1985. Blood pressure in a national birth cohort at the age of 36 related to social and familial factors, smoking, and body mass. *Br. Med. J. (Clin. Res. Ed.)* 291:1534–38
131. Ward JW, Wooding FB, Fowden AL. 2002. The effects of cortisol on the binucleate cell population in the ovine placenta during late gestation. *Placenta* 23:451–58
132. Waterland RA, Garza C. 1999. Potential mechanisms of metabolic imprinting that lead to chronic disease. *Am. J. Clin. Nutr.* 69:179–97
133. Williams S, Poulton R. 2002. Birth size, growth, and blood pressure between the ages of 7 and 26 years: failure to support the fetal origins hypothesis. *Am. J. Epidemiol.* 155:849–52
134. Williams S, St George IM, Silva PA. 1992. Intrauterine growth retardation and blood pressure at age seven and eighteen. *J. Clin. Epidemiol.* 45:1257–63
135. Wolff GL, Kodell RL, Moore SR, Cooney CA. 1998. Maternal epigenetics and methyl supplements affect *agouti* gene expression in A^{vy}/a mice. *FASEB J.* 12:949–57
136. Woods LL, Ingelfinger JR, Nyengaard JR, Rasch R. 2001. Maternal protein restriction suppresses the newborn renin-angiotensin system and programs adult hypertension in rats. *Pediatr. Res.* 49:460–67
137. Woods LL, Weeks DA, Rasch R. 2004. Programming of adult blood pressure by maternal protein restriction: role of nephrogenesis. *Kidney Int.* 65:1339–48
138. Yajnik CS. 2004. Obesity epidemic in India: intrauterine origins? *Proc. Nutr. Soc.* 63:387–96
139. Yliharsila H, Eriksson JG, Forsen T, Kajantie E, Osmond C, Barker DJ. 2003. Self-perpetuating effects of birth size on blood pressure levels in elderly people. *Hypertension* 41:446–50
140. Zhao M, Shu XO, Jin F, Yang G, Li HL, et al. 2002. Birthweight, childhood growth and hypertension in adulthood. *Int. J. Epidemiol.* 31:1043–51

Annu. Rev. Nutr. 2005. 25:435–68
doi: 10.1146/annurev.nutr.25.050304.092625

First published online as a Review in Advance on April 15, 2005

PEDIATRIC OBESITY AND INSULIN RESISTANCE: Chronic Disease Risk and Implications for Treatment and Prevention Beyond Body Weight Modification

M.L. Cruz,[1] G.Q. Shaibi,[2] M.J. Weigensberg,[3]
D. Spruijt-Metz,[4] G.D.C. Ball,[5] and M.I. Goran[6]
[1,4,6]Department of Preventive Medicine, [2]Department of Biokinesiology and Physical Therapy, [3]Department of Pediatrics, University of Southern California, Los Angeles, California 90033; [5]Department of Pediatrics, University of Alberta, Edmonton, Alberta 2C3 WMC Canada; email: marthacr@usc.edu, shaibi@usc.edu, weigensb@usc.edu, dmetz@usc.edu, gdball@pop.srv.ualberta.ca, goran@usc.edu

Key Words children, adiposity, insulin sensitivity

■ **Abstract** The study of childhood obesity has continued to grow exponentially in the past decade. This has been driven in part by the increasing prevalence of this problem and the widespread potential effects of increased obesity in childhood on lifelong chronic disease risk. The focus of this review is on recent findings regarding the link between obesity and disease risk during childhood and adolescence. We describe recent reports relating to type 2 diabetes in youth (2), prediabetes (69, 166), metabolic syndrome (33, 35), polycystic ovarian syndrome (77), and nonalcoholic fatty liver disease (58, 146), and the mediating role of insulin resistance in these conditions. In addition, we review the implications of this research for the design of more effective treatment and prevention strategies that focus more on the improvement of obesity-related metabolic abnormalities and chronic disease risk reduction than on the conventional energy balance approach that focuses on weight management.

CONTENTS

0199-9885/05/0714-0435$20.00

CONSEQUENCES OF OBESITY IN CHILDREN AND ADOLESCENTS

Type 2 Diabetes and Prediabetes

The incidence of type 2 diabetes has increased among children worldwide (49, 132, 140, 154), and this is thought to be a consequence of the pediatric obesity epidemic (87, 135). Estimates suggest a 20-fold increase in the incidence of type 2 diabetes in children and adolescents in the past two decades. However, because these estimates are based almost entirely on clinical observations of the number of diagnosed cases of type 1 versus type 2 diabetes, they should be interpreted with caution. Several small studies have examined the prevalence of type 2 diabetes as well as prediabetes in high-risk populations, and these are summarized in Table 1. Among these studies, relatively small numbers of children have been diagnosed with type 2 diabetes (Table 1). In addition, the documentation of type 2 diabetes in pediatric obesity is not a new phenomenon. For example, one study from 1968 found 6% of obese multiethnic children had diabetes, presumably type 2 (139).

Unfortunately, the current overall prevalence of type 2 diabetes in childhood remains unknown. One study in U.S. adolescents aged 12–19 who participated in National Health and Nutrition Examination Survey (NHANES) III (1988–1994) reported a 0.41% prevalence for all forms of diabetes, approximately one third of which were considered to represent type 2 (49) (Table 1). However, the sample size in this study was too small to provide a stable estimate of diabetes prevalence. In addition, these data preceded more recent reports regarding the rise in obesity (135) in adolescents, and therefore may underestimate the true prevalence of type 2 diabetes in the general pediatric population.

Youth diagnosed with type 2 diabetes are almost always obese, have usually reached puberty, and have a family history of type 2 diabetes (2). In the United States, the increase in type 2 diabetes appears particularly noteworthy among minority populations such as African Americans, Latinos, and Native Americans (37, 50, 65), groups that also have the highest prevalence of obesity among North American youth (87, 135). Prevalence estimates of type 2 diabetes in higher risk Native American adolescent populations in Canada and the United States approach 3%–5% (37, 50, 65). Thus, obesity in childhood seems to be a primary risk factor for type 2 diabetes (2), as it is in adults (55, 129), particularly among high-risk

TABLE 1 Prevalence of prediabetes (impaired fasting glucose and impaired glucose tolerance) and type 2 diabetes in pediatric populations*

Reference	Population	Age (years)	Test	Impaired fasting glucose	Impaired glucose tolerance	Type 2 diabetes
(139)	66 multiethnic obese children	4–16	OGTT	Not reported	17%	6%
(49)	U.S. general adolescent population, oversampling of African American and Mexican American; n = 2867	12–19	Fasting glucose (n = 1083), random glucose (n = 1784)	1.76%[a]	Not assessed	0.14%
(165)	U.S. obese children; BMI = 30–32; mixed ethnicity (62% non-Hispanic white); n = 55	4–10	OGTT	Not reported	25.4%	0%
	U.S. obese adolescents; BMI = 37–41; mixed ethnicity (56% non-Hispanic white) n = 112	11–18			20.5%	3.6%
(69)	Overweight, Latino children; BMI percentile = 94%–96%; positive family history type 2 diabetes; n = 150	8–13	OGTT	0%[a] 12.3%[b]	28%	0%

(Continued)

TABLE 1 *(Continued)*

Reference	Population	Age (years)	Test	Impaired fasting glucose	Impaired glucose tolerance	Type 2 diabetes
(189a)	Obese; BMI-SDS 2.6–3.0; European, mixed ethnicity (89% Caucasian); n = 102	7–18	OGTT	11.8%[a]	36.3%	5.9%
(182a)	Obese; BMI-SDS 1.9–4.7; European, Caucasian; n = 520	8.9–20.3	OGTT	3.7%[c]	2.1%	1.5%[d]
(188)	Moderate to severe obesity; BMI-SDS 2.3–2.8; U.S. mixed ethnicity (40% white; 30% black; 27% Hispanic); n = 439	10.9–13.1	OGTT	Not reported	14.4%–19.9%	0%

[a]Impaired fasting glucose defined as fasting plasma glucose ≥110 and <126.

[b]Impaired fasting glucose defined as fasting plasma glucose ≥100 and <126 in extended study cohort (n = 211) (186).

[c]Impaired fasting glucose defined as fasting plasma glucose 100–109.

[d]Diabetes defined as fasting plasma glucose ≥110 (misclassified), or two-hour OGTT glucose ≥200.

*Abbreviations: BMI, body mass index; OGTT, oral glucose tolerance test; SDS, standard deviation score.

ethnic groups. In adults, the progression from normal glucose tolerance to overt type 2 diabetes involves an intermediate stage of hyperglycemia, characterized by impaired fasting glucose and/or impaired glucose tolerance, now known as prediabetes (3). Recent reports have documented a high prevalence of prediabetes among obese children and adolescents (summarized in Table 1).

In a clinic-based population, Caprio and colleagues (166) detected impaired glucose tolerance in 25% of obese children (4–10 years of age) and in 21% of obese adolescents (11–18 years of age); type 2 diabetes was identified in 4% of the obese adolescents. Similarly, we found that 28% of obese Hispanic children with a positive family history for type 2 had impaired glucose tolerance, but found no cases of type 2 diabetes (69). An unexpected finding was that the prevalence of children with impaired glucose tolerance was unaffected by overweight severity (69). These studies have also revealed another interesting common feature in that prediabetes in children and youth is more frequently characterized by impaired glucose tolerance, whereas the prevalence of impaired fasting glucose (glucose $\geq$110 mg/dl $<$125 mg/dl) is typically low (69, 166).

The findings from these studies have important clinical implication for the screening of high-risk children for prediabetes based on a fasting blood sample, as is recommended by the American Diabetes Association (2). In other words, the use of a fasting blood sample, as opposed to an oral glucose tolerance test, may miss the diagnosis of a significant number of children who have prediabetes. The recent lowering of the cut point for diagnosis of impaired fasting glucose from 110 mg/dl to 100 mg/dl by the American Diabetes Association may increase the likelihood of detecting adverse changes in glucose homeostasis. We found that when a fasting glucose threshold of 100 mg/dl was used in a cohort of overweight Hispanic children in Los Angeles, 12% of children were identified as having impaired fasting glucose, compared with less than 1% when the 110 mg/dl cut point was used (186). However, the relative risk of developing type 2 diabetes if a child has impaired fasting glucose, impaired glucose tolerance, or both remains to be determined through ongoing longitudinal studies. Although studies in adults suggest that both states of glucose dysregulation increase the risk of progression to overt type 2 diabetes (3), this remains to be shown in children.

The Metabolic Syndrome

The metabolic syndrome was first described by Reaven in 1988 (148), but it wasn't until recently that both the World Health Organization (136) and the Adult Treatment Panel (ATP) III of the National Cholesterol Education Program proposed clinical definitions (48). The availability of a clinical definition prompted numerous reports on the prevalence of the metabolic syndrome and provided evidence that the metabolic syndrome is an entity that places individuals at risk of type 2 diabetes (86, 110) and cardiovascular disease that is associated with increased cardiovascular disease mortality (93, 112).

Although a clinical definition of the metabolic syndrome in children does not currently exist, several large population studies have attempted to establish the prevalence of the metabolic syndrome during childhood. Despite differences in definitions and cut points (26, 27, 33, 109, 144), these studies suggest that the prevalence of the metabolic syndrome in children and adolescents is relatively low (3%–4%) when compared with rates in the adult population. For instance, the age-adjusted prevalence of the metabolic syndrome in U.S. adults, based on the ATP III definition, was 23.7%, whereas in adults aged 20–29 years it was 6.7% (59). The overall prevalence of the metabolic syndrome in U.S. adolescents was 4.2% (33). In this study, the authors chose to use a definition similar to that proposed in ATP III. Adolescents were classified as having the metabolic syndrome if they had three or more of the following: triglycerides $\geq$110 mg/dl, high-density lipoprotein-cholesterol (HDL-C) $\leq$40 mg/dl; waist circumference >90th percentile (for age and gender), fasting glucose >110 mg/dl, and blood pressure $\geq$90th percentile (for age, gender, and height) (33).

Although the above studies suggest that overall prevalence rates of the metabolic syndrome in youth are low, the perspective is very different in overweight adolescents (33, 188). In NHANES III, the prevalence of the metabolic syndrome was 28.7% in overweight adolescents (BMI $\geq$ 95th percentile) compared with 6.1% in adolescents at risk for overweight (BMI $\geq$ 85th but lower than 95th percentile), and 0.1% in those with a BMI below the 85th percentile (33). Eighty-nine percent of overweight adolescents had at least one abnormality of the metabolic syndrome and more than half (56%) had two abnormalities (33). The individual prevalence of abdominal obesity, high triglycerides, low HDL-C, and high blood pressure in overweight adolescents was 74.5%, 51.8%, 50%, and 11.2%, respectively. Impaired fasting glucose was only present in 2.6% of overweight adolescents. Similarly, several other studies have found a high prevalence of the metabolic syndrome among severely overweight children and adolescents. For example, Cruz et al. (35) described a prevalence of 30% in Hispanic children >85th percentile for BMI, and Weiss et al. (188) saw a prevalence of 39% and 49.7% in obese adolescents above the 97th and 99th percentile, respectively, for BMI. Thus, the prevalence of the metabolic syndrome is clearly related to increasing severity of obesity.

Nonalcoholic Fatty Liver Disease

Nonalcoholic fatty liver disease (NAFLD) encompasses the entire spectrum of liver disease, which includes simple hepatic steatosis without inflammation (which may not lead to progressive liver injury), nonalcoholic steatohepatitis (NASH), and the resulting cirrhosis (which may be devoid of steatosis). NAFLD is thought to be the most common liver disease in the United States and obesity is probably the single most important risk factor (30). The disorder is increasingly recognized in the pediatric population (11, 146, 153, 175), especially in children who are obese or with type 2 diabetes (11, 159, 175). In one study, 83% of patients diagnosed with NASH were obese, 30% had elevated serum triglycerides, and 19% had elevated serum cholesterol (146). Collectively, these studies have brought to light the magnitude of the problem of NAFLD in overweight children as well as the potential for the future burden of liver disease in affected subjects (146, 153).

The early development of NASH in childhood may lead to chronic end-stage liver disease later in life, most significantly cirrhosis (20, 125). In fact, a recent case study report documented the development of cirrhosis from NASH in two overweight boys aged 10 and 14 (125).

Polycystic Ovarian Syndrome

Polycystic ovarian syndrome (PCOS) is a common comorbidity of obesity in adolescent girls (77). PCOS is defined as ovulatory dysfunction with evidence of hyperandrogenism not due to other causes (115). Most girls with PCOS demonstrate reduced sex hormone–binding globulin (163) and elevated free testosterone (7, 77, 116, 163); elevations in total testosterone, androstenedione, and DHEA-sulfate may also be seen (115, 163). Insulin resistance is generally present and may be higher than in BMI-matched controls (116). About half of adult women with PCOS are obese (18, 61, 66), and there is a predisposition to central obesity (88). Comparable percentages among adolescents are not known, but PCOS can be seen in both obese and nonobese adolescents (163). Women with PCOS have increased incidence of other comorbidities including prediabetes, type 2 diabetes, hypertension, and dyslipidemia (46, 190). With respect to comorbidities in adolescents, Palmert (138) showed that 33% of overweight predominantly Caucasian adolescents with PCOS had either impaired glucose tolerance or undiagnosed type 2 diabetes. The prevalence of impaired glucose tolerance in adolescents with PCOS may approach 50% in some populations (7).

WHY IS FAT BAD? RELATIONSHIP BETWEEN INCREASED ADIPOSITY AND HEALTH RISK IN CHILDREN

Location of Body Fat

For children as well as adults, there are several hypotheses that might explain the link between increased body fat and health risk (62). The following sections review these hypotheses and the evidence for them in pediatric studies.

One of the earlier theories, termed the "portal theory," links visceral adipose tissue to insulin resistance and is based on the direct effects of free fatty acids on the liver (62). Numerous studies support a link between body fat, visceral fat, and metabolic risk factors in children (23, 63, 80, 114). Earlier studies showed the presence of visceral fat in children at an early age (72), although to a highly variable degree (73), and the gradual expansion of this fat compartment during growth and development (90). Due to the high colinearity between visceral fat, subcutaneous abdominal fat, and total body fat, it is challenging to obtain a representative indication of the unique contribution of each of these fat compartments to health risk.

More recently, the "ectopic fat" theory has been proposed (147). This approach suggests that fat deposition outside of adipose tissue (e.g., in muscle or liver) contributes to insulin resistance. Intramyocellular lipid (IMCL), for example, has been shown to be a major determinant of insulin resistance in adults (101), as well as obese individuals (60) including adolescents (9, 165). In addition to IMCL, fat deposition in the liver has also been associated with insulin resistance and hyperinsulinemia in both nonobese normal subjects (122, 133, 161) and in obese subjects with type 2 diabetes (102, 122), and this association seems to be independent of total body adiposity. Liver fat may also be a significant factor in children, although there are no studies in this area. In support of both the portal theory and ectopic fat theory, a recent study in adults showed that removal of subcutaneous abdominal fat by liposuction had no metabolic benefits, a finding that suggests other fat depots may be more clinically relevant (104). Thus, the location of body fat deposition seems to be an important factor in explaining the link between adiposity and health risk, though more direct evidence of this concept is needed.

Fat as Endocrine Organ

Since the discovery of leptin in 1994 (191), it has become evident that adipose tissue is not an inert tissue but instead is a critical tissue involved with metabolic regulation (103). Adipocytes produce and secrete several important mediators related to insulin resistance, cardiovascular disease, and type 2 diabetes. These mediators, collectively termed "adipocytokines," exhibit diverse actions at various central (e.g., hypothalamus) and peripheral (e.g., skeletal muscle) sites and may provide insight into the underlying mechanisms linking adiposity with disease risk. Although the number of identified adipocytokines has grown exponentially in recent years, the current section focuses on leptin, tumor necrosis factor alpha (TNF-alpha), interleukin-6 (IL-6), and adiponectin and their respective relations to metabolic and cardiovascular health in children.

The majority of mechanistic evidence in relation to adipocytokine action is derived from animal models of obesity, whereas the data from pediatric populations has primarily looked at associations between adipocytokines and markers of health. In general, the findings from pediatric studies are similar to those from studies of adults, showing significant positive correlations between adipocytokines and measures of adiposity (130), with the exception of adiponectin, which appears to have insulin-sensitizing properties and is inversely related to measures of obesity (10). Although it remains unclear whether adipocytokines in children are simply markers of degree of adiposity, several recent reports have established significant relations between adipocytokines and insulin resistance that are independent of body composition (10, 172).

LEPTIN Leptin was the first characterized adipocytokine, and has its primary mechanism of action in the hypothalamus, where it is thought to regulate energy intake and expenditure by suppressing food intake and stimulating energy expenditure (191). Leptin is directly related to adiposity and insulin resistance in children (84, 128), which suggests that overweight children, like adults, exhibit resistance to the antiobesity effects of leptin (111). Recent research further extends adipose-related leptin resistance in overweight children to include the associated metabolic complications. Chu and colleagues (29) observed significant positive associations between leptin levels and both insulin resistance as well as metabolic syndrome scores that were independent of body composition in children. Because leptin has been shown in animal models to stimulate both lipid and glucose metabolism, it is not altogether surprising that leptin resistance in youth extends beyond the dysregulation of body composition (98). For example, baseline leptin levels predict the development of diabetes in Japanese men (but not women), and this effect was independent of baseline body fat and insulin resistance (124). We are not aware of similar studies in children and adolescents.

TNF-ALPHA AND INTERLEUKIN-6 (IL-6) These two adipocytokines are proinflammatory mediators with detrimental effects on insulin sensitivity and atherosclerosis in adults (176). Similar to leptin, TNF-alpha and IL-6 are positively correlated with measures of adiposity in children (16, 130), but unlike leptin, TNF-alpha and IL-6 have been shown to impair glucose homeostasis in rodent models (160, 181). Plasma levels of TNF-alpha and IL-6 increase in response to acute and chronic inflammatory events in children (157). Obesity and the metabolic syndrome are considered disorders related to chronic inflammation (56), and TNF-alpha and IL-6 presumably act as inflammatory mediators of adiposity-associated metabolic disturbances in children. To date, very little work has established relations between metabolic dysregulation independent of body composition and TNF-alpha or IL-6.

ADIPONECTIN In contrast to other adipocytokines, adiponectin is inversely related to total adiposity in children (130). Weight loss in children is associated with an increase in adiponectin and an improvement in insulin resistance (149, 150). These observations have led to studies of the potential role of adiponectin as a protective adipocytokine against insulin resistance and early cardiovascular disease in youth. Weiss and colleagues (187) evaluated adiponectin, insulin sensitivity, abdominal fat distribution, and IMCL levels in 8 nonobese and 14 obese adolescents. Significantly lower adiponectin levels were observed in obese compared with nonobese children. Additionally, they found a strong inverse correlation between adiponectin and IMCL ($r = 0.73$, $P < 0.001$) that was independent of both total and abdominal fat. However, when groups were analyzed separately, the inverse association was only significant in the obese children, a finding that suggests a potential adiposity-related threshold effect between adiponectin and IMCL levels. Adiponectin was also found to correlate positively with insulin sensitivity ($r = 0.52$, $P < 0.02$) and negatively with plasma triglyceride ($r = -0.80$, $P < 0.001$), and these relations persisted after controlling for percent body fat.

Bacha et al. (10) observed similar differences in adiponectin levels between lean and obese youth. However, in contrast to Weiss et al. (187), Bacha and colleagues found a significant relationship between adiponectin and abdominal adiposity whereby obese adolescents with higher visceral fat had lower levels of adiponectin compared with those with lower visceral fat. These relations were not reported in the lean children. Significant associations between adiponectin and several features of the metabolic syndrome were also established in that systolic and diastolic blood pressure and triglycerides were inversely associated with adiponectin, whereas HDL-C was directly associated. After controlling for adiposity, however, adiponectin levels were significantly correlated only with HDL-C. Collectively, these observations suggest that adiponectin is more than a biomarker of adiposity in youth and may prove to be an important mediator of adiposity-related metabolic dysregulation. Changes in adiponectin levels track closely with changes in body fat and precede changes in insulin sensitivity (169). Adiponectin levels predict the development of diabetes (low levels = increased risk) in Pima Indians (118), but not changes in body weight (182).

SUMMARY Undoubtedly, the number of cytokines produced and secreted by adipose tissue will expand, as will the diverse mechanisms by which these proteins regulate adiposity-related pathophysiology. Very little is known regarding how the pattern of secreted cytokines changes during growth and development or of the role these factors play in regulating the growth process. As a better understanding of these complex and interconnected relations is elucidated, researchers and clinicians may be better able to develop meaningful interventions to help delay or prevent the comorbidities associated with childhood obesity.

The Role of Insulin Resistance

Perhaps the most accepted hypothesis linking adiposity to increased chronic disease risk, and one supported by prospective studies, relates to insulin resistance (40, 148). The following sections review the pediatric evidence relating to the role of insulin resistance in various chronic diseases associated with obesity as depicted in Figure 1.

TYPE 2 DIABETES Insulin resistance is one of two primary features in the pathogenesis of type 2 diabetes; the other feature is impairment of insulin secretion. Prospective longitudinal studies demonstrate that both insulin resistance and diminished insulin secretion are independent predictors of the development of type 2 diabetes in obese adult Mexican American and Pima Indian populations (83, 189). Insulin resistance places increased secretory demand on the pancreatic B cell, resulting in increased compensatory insulin secretion and hyperinsulinemia (39). Although normoglycemia is maintained as long as compensatory insulin secretion is adequate, a relative failure to compensate for insulin resistance with adequate insulin secretion appears to develop in some individuals over time, leading to impairment in glucose homeostasis (19, 39). The cause of beta cell failure in the face of insulin resistance remains unknown, although it may relate to genetic factors or to physiologic events such as the accumulation of amyloid polypeptide in the pancreatic islets (91).

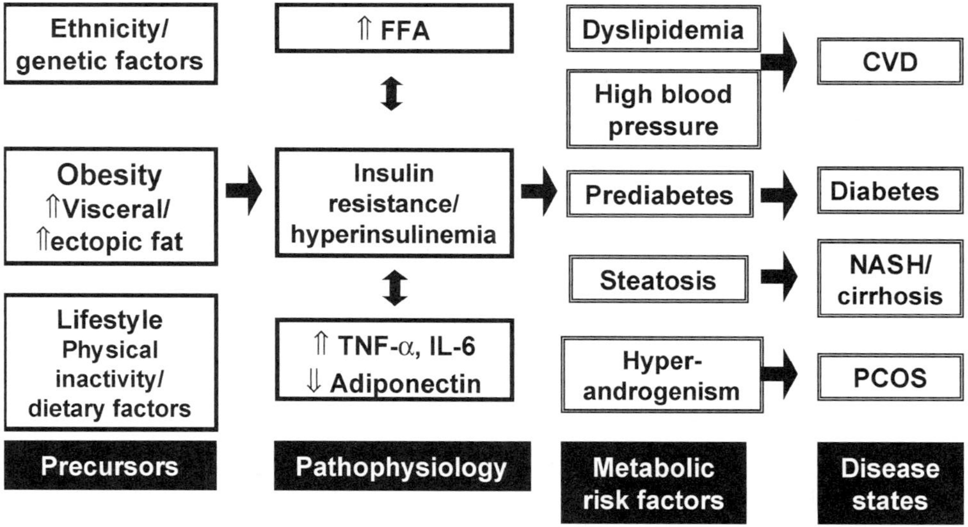

Figure 1 The central role of insulin resistance is highlighted in the proposed relationship between obesity and associated disease outcomes in children.

Early evidence indicates that the pathogenesis of type 2 diabetes in youth is likely to be quite similar to that in adults, albeit with an expression over a more accelerated time course. Studies in children have suggested that both insulin resistance and poor beta cell function may be responsible for dysregulation of glucose homeostasis (69, 166). In a multiethnic clinic-based study of obese children and adolescents, Caprio and colleagues found that insulin sensitivity measured indirectly via the homeostatic model was decreased in children with impaired fasting glucose compared with children with normal glucose tolerance (166). In contrast, among overweight Hispanic children, there were no differences in insulin sensitivity (measured via the frequently sampled intravenous glucose tolerance test and minimal modeling) between impaired glucose- and normal glucose-tolerant obese Hispanic children, but impaired glucose tolerance (69, 166) and impaired fasting glucose (186) were associated with deteriorating beta cell function. Ongoing longitudinal studies of such childhood cohorts should elucidate the relative risk of future development of type 2 diabetes in overweight children with prediabetes.

METABOLIC SYNDROME The role of obesity and insulin resistance in the etiology of the metabolic syndrome has been recently explored in children through cross-sectional and prospective studies (35, 145, 168). The Cardiovascular Risk in Young Finns Study was one of the analyses of the childhood predictors of the metabolic syndrome. To explore this, fasting insulin at baseline was related to the development of the metabolic syndrome [defined as having the three following conditions: high triglycerides and high blood pressure (>75th percentile) and low HDL-C (<25th percentile)] after six years of follow up in 1865 children and adolescents (aged 6–18 years) (145). The results from this study showed that baseline insulin concentration was higher in children who subsequently developed the metabolic syndrome, lending support to the view that insulin resistance precedes the development of the metabolic syndrome in childhood (144). Since obesity in childhood is closely associated with insulin resistance, it would have been important to establish if children and adolescents who developed the metabolic syndrome after a six-year follow-up period were also more overweight.

More recently, data from the Bogalusa Heart Study (a biracial community-based longitudinal cohort) was used to disentangle the relative contribution of childhood obesity (measured via BMI) versus insulin resistance (measured via fasting insulin) to the adulthood risk of developing the metabolic syndrome (168). In this study, 718 children aged 8–17 years at baseline were followed for an average of 11.6 years. The metabolic syndrome was defined as comprising the following four factors: BMI, fasting insulin, systolic (or mean arterial) blood pressure, and triglyceride/HDL ratio in the highest quartile for age, gender, ethnicity, and study year (168). Significant positive trends were seen between childhood BMI as well as insulin quartiles and the incidence of clustering in adulthood. Children in the top quartile of BMI and insulin versus those in the bottom quartile were 11.7 and 3.6 times more likely to develop clustering, respectively, as adults. A high childhood BMI was significantly associated with the incidence of clustering in adulthood even after adjustment for childhood insulin levels. However, in this study, adjustment for childhood BMI eliminated the influence of insulin on the incidence of clustering in adulthood. Thus, in this biethnic, community-based study, childhood obesity (measured via BMI) was more closely associated with the presence of the metabolic syndrome in adulthood than was fasting insulin (168). These findings suggest that obesity in childhood precedes the development of the metabolic syndrome in adulthood.

Although obesity in childhood may be more closely associated than insulin resistance with the development of the metabolic syndrome, the question remains as to why some obese children develop the metabolic syndrome and others do not. The recent NHANES III data on the prevalence of the metabolic syndrome among U.S. adolescents found that approximately 30% of overweight children (BMI > 95th percentile) had the metabolic syndrome, whereas the remaining 70% did not (33). We recently addressed this issue in a cohort ($n = 126$) of overweight Hispanic adolescents (mean BMI percentile 97 ± 2.9; aged 8–13 years) with a family history for type 2 diabetes (35). We hypothesized that in overweight Hispanic children, insulin resistance would be more closely associated than overall adiposity with the metabolic syndrome. In this study, insulin sensitivity was measured via the frequently sampled intravenous glucose tolerance test and minimal modeling, and overall adiposity was measured via dual energy X-ray absorptiometry. We found that insulin sensitivity (after adjustment for differences in adiposity) was 62% lower in overweight youth with the metabolic syndrome (defined as having three or more of the following: hypertriglyceridemia, low HDL-C, high blood pressure, high waist circumference, or impaired glucose tolerance) compared with overweight youth without the metabolic syndrome. Furthermore, in multivariate regression analysis, insulin sensitivity, but not fat mass, was independently and negatively related to triglycerides and blood pressure and positively related to HDL-C. These results suggest that the effect of adiposity on lipids and blood pressure control is mediated via insulin resistance.

These findings in overweight Hispanic youth are in agreement with previous results in which directly measured insulin sensitivity has been shown to be independently associated with the separate components of the metabolic syndrome (34, 95, 164). Collectively, these findings in pediatric studies suggest that obesity coupled with insulin resistance may contribute to the development of the metabolic syndrome in childhood.

NONALCOHOLIC FATTY LIVER DISEASE In adults, insulin resistance is regarded as an essential factor for the development of NAFLD, and in turn, NAFLD is considered a feature of the metabolic syndrome (102, 122). Peripheral insulin resistance may lead to steatosis through increased adipose tissue lipolysis and delivery of fatty acids to the liver (156). In turn, excess delivery of free fatty acids to the liver may lead to hepatic insulin resistance, as has been observed in adults with NAFLD (102, 122). Supporting a central role of insulin resistance in NASH is a recent report that treatment with the insulin sensitizer pioglitazone was associated with improvements in biochemical and histological features of NASH (143). In children, NAFLD has been shown to occur most commonly in conditions associated with insulin resistance, including obesity and type 2 diabetes (11, 146, 159, 175). A recent retrospective study found that children with biopsy-proven NAFLD were almost exclusively obese and had fasting hyperinsulinemia (159). These data suggest that NAFLD in childhood is also associated with an insulin-resistant state and may be a further metabolic abnormality associated with the metabolic syndrome.

POLYCYSTIC OVARIAN SYNDROME The majority of both obese and nonobese women with PCOS are insulin resistant, and the insulin resistance tends to be greater in obese women (41). Obese adolescents with PCOS show greater insulin resistance than those without PCOS matched for total body and abdominal adiposity (116). The relationship of obesity and insulin resistance to the pathogenesis of PCOS is still incompletely understood. The prevailing hypothesis is that insulin resistance resulting in increased compensatory insulin secretion and hyperinsulinemia leads to the hyperandrogenism seen in PCOS through multiple complex mechanisms. Insulin increases the pituitary gonadotrope sensitivity to gonadotropin-releasing hormone, which results in greater luteinizing hormone secretion (1); increases insulin-like growth factor-I binding to the ovary (142), which amplifies the effect of luteinizing hormone on androgen production in the ovary (25); directly stimulates ovarian androgen production via either the insulin receptor or the insulin-like growth factor-I receptor (13); activates ovarian enzymes involved in androgen synthesis (45); and decreases hepatic sex hormone–binding globulin production, resulting in higher free androgen levels (131).

INFLUENCE OF ETHNICITY ON INSULIN RESISTANCE Detailed studies comparing ethnic differences in metabolic risk factors have been helpful in understanding why certain subgroups of the population may be at increased disease risk. Studies in children are of increased significance because they allow examination of potentially underlying biological differences across subgroups of the population in the absence of potential confounding factors such as smoking, alcohol, aging, and menopausal status. Data from the Bogalusa Heart Study were the first to show evidence of increased insulin resistance in African American compared with Caucasian children based on measures of fasting insulin (63). Subsequently, other studies have demonstrated greater insulin resistance and a greater acute insulin response in African American than in Caucasian children (6, 76), and these differences were independent of body fat, visceral fat, dietary factors, and physical activity. Previous studies have shown that African American children have a higher than expected acute insulin response to glucose than do Caucasian children (68); the higher insulin levels in African Americans are partly attributable to increased secretion and a lower hepatic extraction (75, 180) and may have a genetic basis (74).

Studies of obesity, insulin resistance, insulin secretion, and the beta cell response in the Hispanic population are limited, even in adults. The limited studies show that Hispanic adults have greater fasting and postchallenge insulin (82), greater insulin resistance (83, 85), and a higher second-phase insulin response (28) compared with Caucasians. We recently showed that Hispanic and African American children are equally more insulin resistant than are Caucasian children (70). Interestingly, the compensatory response to the same degree of insulin resistance was different in Hispanic compared with African American children. African American children compensated with a higher acute insulin response to glucose, and this effect was in part due to a reduction in hepatic insulin extraction. Hispanic children compensated to the same degree of insulin resistance with greater second-phase insulin secretion (70). This difference may be the basis that could explain ethnic differences in disease risk profile.

The well-documented ethnic differences in insulin action and secretion could be explained by either genetic or environmental factors. We have been unable to explain the lower insulin sensitivity and higher acute insulin response in African American compared with Caucasian children by factors such as diet, physical activity, and socioeconomic status (108, 117). We have shown that greater African American genetic admixture was independently related to lower insulin sensitivity ($P < 0.001$) and higher fasting insulin ($P < 0.01$) (74). This analysis provides initial evidence that these ethnic differences may have a genetic basis.

In summary, distinct biological differences exist between high-risk ethnic groups, and we have only begun to scratch the surface of this concept. One clear finding is that minority children are more insulin resistant, and this seems to be independent of adiposity and other biological and behavioral factors and could have a genetic basis. From the limited available evidence, it seems that the pathophysiology of obesity-related metabolic conditions, and in particular the compensatory responses to insulin resistance, may be different across the various ethnic groups. These differences are likely to have implications for the development of effective intervention strategies that may need to be focused on ethnic-specific and/or target-specific metabolic factors.

THE INFLUENCE OF PUBERTY ON INSULIN RESISTANCE Puberty is associated with rapid and dynamic changes in various metabolic systems, including hormonal regulation, changes in body fat and fat distribution, as well as transient changes in insulin resistance. Several studies have demonstrated that insulin sensitivity decreases at the onset of puberty and recovers by the end of the maturation process (4, 32, 71, 126). In Caucasian children, decreased insulin sensitivity during puberty is accompanied by increased insulin secretion that normalizes as insulin resistance improves near the end of puberty (24). In a large cross-sectional study (164), insulin sensitivity (measured using the euglycemic-hyperinsulinemic clamp) was highest in Tanner stage I and lowest in Tanner stage III (~20% lower than stage I) and near prepubertal levels in Tanner stage V. Using a longitudinal design, we have previously observed (71) that the pubertal transition from Tanner stage I to III was associated with a 32% reduction in insulin sensitivity (measured by the intravenous glucose tolerance test) in Caucasian and African Americans, and this change was consistent across a range of body fatness.

PUTTING IT ALL TOGETHER: THE ADDITIVE EFFECTS In the prior sections, we have reviewed the multiple factors that influence insulin resistance (including ethnicity, puberty, and greater body fat, especially muscle, liver, and visceral fat). These factors seem to have additive and independent effects on insulin resistance. To understand the physiological impact of insulin resistance, Kahn et al. proposed the disposition index that characterizes the hyperbolic relationship between insulin resistance and insulin secretion (Figure 2). Thus, as insulin sensitivity of tissues decreases (i.e., greater insulin resistance), beta cells in the pancreas have to work harder to secrete more insulin. This relationship is characterized by a hyperbola. Figure 2 demonstrates hypothetical examples in the pediatric population at various degrees of insulin resistance. At the tail end of the hyperbola, very large decreases in insulin sensitivity are associated with very small requisite increases in insulin secretion. At the other end of the extreme, the same relative reduction in insulin sensitivity requires a huge increase in insulin secretion. Thus, overweight minority children are operating in the zone of the hyperbola where periods of exposure to insulin resistance (e.g., due to more weight gain or due to puberty) will have a significant impact on insulin secretion. These requisite increases in insulin secretion are hypothesized to lead to beta cell exhaustion over time in predisposed individuals.

Figure 2 also demonstrates that a key feature of effective interventions to improve metabolic health is based on a focus to decrease insulin resistance to move individuals into the "safe zone" of the hyperbola. In the sections that follow, we review various strategies to accomplish this aim that move beyond traditional energy balance/weight loss strategies.

PREVENTION AND TREATMENT OF THE METABOLIC CONSEQUENCES OF OBESITY IN CHILDREN AND ADOLESCENTS

The increased prevalence and incidence of pediatric overweight over the past 15 to 20 years has prompted health organizations and scientific associations to advocate for increased attention, resources, and research to address this emerging health crisis through prevention and treatment initiatives. Numerous reviews have been published, highlighting promising research and underscoring the need for additional study of pediatric overweight prevention and treatment strategies. However, there are very few examples of intervention studies designed specifically to address the underlying metabolic abnormalities. Most typical "weight management" programs for youth have been based on the traditional "energy balance" model and used restrictive diets, behavior modification techniques, physical activity, and/or drugs, but these approaches have generally not been successful and don't necessarily address insulin resistance and the underlying risks beyond weight loss. In addition, a recent study shows that dieting approaches are generally ineffective in children and adolescents and may actually promote weight gain (57). Thus, as was

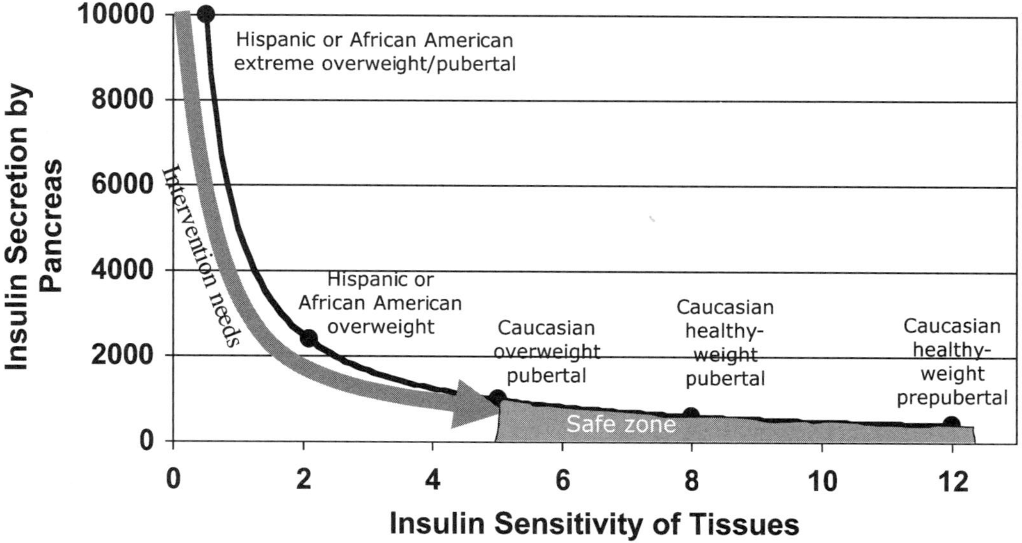

Figure 2 Hyperbolic relationship between insulin sensitivity and insulin secretion. This figure demonstrates examples at various degrees of insulin resistance and the focus of interventions to improve insulin resistance and secretion.

concluded in a recent *Cochran* review, conventional approaches targeting weight management in children have not been effective (173). The purpose of the discussion that follows is to review intervention studies that have addressed metabolic abnormalities related to obesity and aimed to reduce chronic disease risk beyond weight reduction.

Studies Using Physical Activity

In adults, regular physical activity and high levels of physical fitness are associated with reduced chronic disease risk (67, 92, 100, 105, 106), but much less research has examined this issue in children and adolescents; a summary of findings is presented below with a focus on effects on reducing chronic disease risk.

Cross-sectional studies in pediatrics have shown a positive influence of activity/fitness on disease risk (107, 158), whereas others show no effect (12, 81). Unfortunately, few intervention studies have been conducted in youth to examine the effects of physical activity/exercise on chronic disease risk reduction. Ferguson et al. (54) reported that four months of intensive aerobic-type exercise training without dietary intervention (five days/week for four months; 40-minute training sessions at a heart rate >150 beats per minute) in obese boys and girls (n = 79) resulted in significant decreases in percentage body fat as well as fasting insulin and triglyceride levels in comparison with control children. Although the authors were unable to determine whether reductions in insulin and triglyceride levels were a result of parallel decreases in body fat, these findings support the notion that increases in physical activity can lead to improvements of metabolic risk profile in overweight children. However, in another study from the same group, a comparison of 10-week programs for 7- to 11-year-old obese African American girls (79), neither aerobic training (n = 12) nor lifestyle education (n = 10) led to improvements in fasting insulin levels. Although some other investigations (99, 185) in youth provide evidence that increased physical activity can lead to improvements in the metabolic and cardiovascular risk of overweight children, the mechanisms of these improvements remain largely unclear. Furthermore, it has yet to be determined whether improvements in risk profile lead to decreases in future diabetes and/or cardiovascular disease outcomes.

Although most studies in pediatrics have implemented aerobic training as a modality of exercise, evidence from adults (21, 22, 155, 178) suggests that incorporation of strength training (resistance training) may be important for improving insulin sensitivity, body composition (increased muscle mass and decreased fat mass), and fat redistribution (reduced visceral fat and IMCL). Resistance training has also been shown to improve insulin sensitivity and glucose regulation in adults with impaired glucose tolerance or type 2 diabetes (36, 42, 167). However, further studies are needed to identify whether these effects are mediated through changes in body composition or through other mechanisms. One previous study (141), for example, showed that improvement in insulin sensitivity after resistance training disappeared once the data were normalized for fat-free mass, a finding that suggests the increased glucose disposal rate was due to a mass effect rather than an alteration in the intrinsic properties of the skeletal muscle.

Resistance training therefore may be an important exercise modality for overweight youth. Several organizations, including the American Academy of Pediatrics, have recently endorsed resistance training (with appropriate supervision and instruction) as a safe activity for children and adolescents as a means of improving strength and decreasing risk of sports-related injuries (51). However, to date, most studies of resistance training in younger populations have focused on issues related to safety, strength improvements, and musculature changes (53, 52). One prior study examined a six-week program that combined a dietary intervention (low energy, 20%–25% calories from fat, high in complex carbohydrate) with strength training in obese children (174). This study focused on lipid profile, which improved after the intervention (6% reduction in total cholesterol). We previously conducted a resistance training trial with 12 overweight Caucasian girls (178, 179). This study showed that resistance training (20-minute sessions, three days/week for five months) led to increased strength and improvement in visceral fat. Small improvements in glucose tolerance and insulin levels (determined using an oral glucose tolerance test) were noted, but these changes did not achieve statistical significance. In one other study recently completed (162), 16 weeks of twice-per-week progressive resistance training in Hispanic males (15.2 ± 1.7 years, Tanner stage 3–5, BMI percentile $= 97.7 \pm 2.8$) led to a significant increase in insulin sensitivity in the training group by $45.1 \pm 24.2\%$ versus no change in the control group ($-0.8 \pm 40.7\%$). The between-group difference in change score was highly significant ($p < 0.001$).

Given the increasing prevalence rates of pediatric obesity and diabetes in this population and the potential for resistance training to improve parameters related to glucose homeostasis, further studies using this approach seem warranted. Moreover, resistance training may be a practical form of exercise, especially for very overweight children who may be extremely challenged by the difficulty in performing typical aerobic exercise interventions. In contrast, it seems very likely that overweight children who participate in resistance training will experience success and quick results that will encourage them to continue in an intervention.

In summary, current research suggests that physical activity interventions in overweight youth are efficacious for improving overall body composition (113), and perhaps more importantly, may improve the disease risk profile of overweight children (54, 78, 99, 177, 184). Further research is warranted to address the many questions that remain regarding the optimal frequency, intensity, duration, and mode of activity necessary to invoke risk profile improvement.

Dietary Approaches

The most successful long-term studies of obesity reduction in children have been reported by Epstein et al. (47). The dietary components of these family-based behavioral interventions have used what is called the "Traffic Light Diet, Food Guide Pyramid," which differentiates food choices primarily based on fat content.

Other expert dietary recommendations for children have been nonspecific and have promoted well-balanced, healthy meals based on the food pyramid (15), nutritionally balanced meals to support growth (31), and a general emphasis on reduction in dietary fat intake rather than on types of fat or carbohydrate in the diet. Current clinical treatment guidelines therefore are generally based on empirical evidence and expert opinion (14).

Remarkably few studies have examined nutritional approaches for reducing obesity and chronic disease risk factors in children. Most studies have focused on diet and weight loss and have been conducted in Caucasian children. In terms of risk reduction, most previous studies have examined dietary intervention for lipid improvement in children. The Dietary Intervention Study in Children (DISC) examined the effects of nutrition education on lipid profiles in 663 children, mostly Caucasian, over three years (134). There was a small but significant 8% reduction in LDL-cholesterol, which was sustained two years after the intervention ended. However, a general trend of increasing triglyceride levels was identified in both the control and intervention groups, which indicates that other dietary combinations may be needed to obtain beneficial effects on multiple risk factors. Another large trial (Child and Adolescent Trial for Cardiovascular Health, or CATCH) sought to improve diet and physical activity in a national study involving 5000 children from approximately 100 schools. Despite improvements in diet and physical activity in schools, CATCH had very limited effects on overall dietary intake and physical activity and no significant changes were acheived in obesity measures, blood pressure, or cholesterol (121).

Based on our review of the literature we conclude that more specific, targeted, and individualized dietary approaches are needed for risk reduction in overweight children. Specifically, good evidence suggests that modification of the types and quality of carbohydrates in the diet may be effective for improving insulin sensitivity and reducing insulin secretion and may contribute to weight loss. This dietary strategy may be more effective than previous interventions to reduce calories and/or proportion of calories from carbohydrate in the diet (89). In particular, diets enriched with whole-grain carbohydrates, foods that elicit a lower glucose response, and foods higher in fiber have been shown to have beneficial effects. In a cross-sectional study in adolescents, whole-grain intake was associated with a lower body mass index as well as improved insulin sensitivity (170). In addition, epidemiological studies show that intake of whole grains is associated with protection from type 2 diabetes (127) as well as coronary artery disease (171). Dietary fiber, especially soluble fiber (e.g., psyllium), has beneficial effects on blood glucose control and blood lipids (38, 94, 119). Fiber intake also has beneficial effects on regulating food intake (by inducing satiation and satiety) and can improve glycemic control and reduce lipids (120).

These carbohydrate effects may work through improvement in the glycemic load (a measure of how much glucose is released into the blood after ingestion of a particular food). Foods with a low glycemic value have been hypothesized to be beneficial for reducing risk for type 2 diabetes because they reduce the demand for high levels of insulin secretion (89). In both short-term (44) and long-term (43) studies in obese children, a low glycemic index has been shown to reduce plasma glucose and improve insulin resistance. An additional benefit is that voluntary food intake tends to be lower after consumption of foods with a low glycemic index (152). A recent 12-month intervention in obese children showed that promotion of a diet with a low glycemic index led to greater weight loss and improvement in insulin resistance than promotion of a typical low-fat diet (43). Another study in children has shown that a low-glycemic-index breakfast meal led to a reduced calorie intake in lunch (183). Previous studies that have modified the glycemic index of foods while retaining a Hispanic-style diet have been successful in improving glucose control and lipids in Hispanic patients with type 2 diabetes (96, 97). The low-glycemic-index approach also tackles the issue of soda and juice intake. Replacement of sugary drinks with water or lower-sugar versions may also result in improved glucose control. In fact, a recent school-based intervention that promoted water intake and reduced consumption of sugared beverages led to significant improvements in fasting glucose and insulin response (151).

Pharmacological Approaches

Although no medications are currently approved for the management of pediatric overweight (because of safety concerns), pharmacotherapy may be appropriate in overweight youth with comorbidities (e.g., prediabetes, sleep apnea) that increase health risk.

As with dietary and physical activity interventions in overweight youth, most interventions using pharmacotherapy have targeted weight loss. In a randomized and controlled study (137), Orlistat (a gastrointestinal lipase inhibitor) decreased BMI in obese adolescents to a greater degree in the experimental group than in the control group (-4.09 ± 2.9 kg/m^2 versus $+0.11 \pm 2.49$ kg/m^2, respectively; $p < 0.001$). In another trial (123) of 20 adolescents (mean age 14.6 years, mean BMI 44), orlistat (120 mg) was administered three times daily with a multivitamin and a behavioral program (this was not a randomized study). Gastrointestinal side effects similar to those in adults were observed, and these decreased with time. The main outcomes were also similar to those of adults (4% weight loss and 21 mg/dl reduction in cholesterol, 17 mg/dl reduction in LDL-C, 14 uU/ml reduction in fasting insulin, and 15 mg/dl reduction in fasting glucose). In the concluding words of the authors, "Short-term treatment with orlistat, in the context of a behavioral program, is well-tolerated and has a side-effect profile similar to that observed in adults, but its true benefit versus conventional therapy remains to be determined in placebo-controlled trials."

The other FDA-approved drug for obesity, sibutramine, has also been tested in adolescents in a randomized double-blind study (N = 82; 13–17 years of age). This study compared a 6-month behavior intervention with placebo versus behavior intervention with sibutramine (17). There was significantly greater weight loss with the drug (8% versus 4%), but medication had to be reduced or discontinued in 33 patients to manage increases in blood pressure or other symptoms. The authors concluded, "Until more extensive safety and efficacy data are available, medications for weight loss should be used only on an experimental basis in adolescents and children." Thus, the studies show that the general responses to these drugs in terms of safety and efficacy are similar in children and adults, and more additional longer-term safety/efficacy data are needed.

Few pharmacological studies have targeted the underlying insulin resistance associated with obesity. In one study, metformin, an insulin-sensitizing drug used for the treatment of type 2 diabetes in both adults and children, was used to treat overweight youth with a family history of type 2 diabetes and hyperinsulinemia. In a double-blind controlled trial in 29 obese adolescents (64), metformin (500 mg twice/day, administered for six months) resulted in significant improvements in body mass index and fasting insulin but not in insulin sensitivity. In another study, metformin was shown to improve insulin sensitivity and lower plasma total and free testosterone in obese adolescent girls with PCOS (8). Other agents that may prove beneficial in the treatment of insulin resistance in high-risk youth are the thiazolidinediones, which are much more potent insulin sensitizers than metformin. Thiazolidinediones have been shown to improve insulin sensitivity, glucose tolerance, and cardiovascular risk factors in nondiabetic obese subjects with impaired glucose tolerance (5).

In summary, pharmacotherapy may be indicated in children with comorbidities and in cases in which attempts to improve risk through lifestyle interventions have failed. Well-designed randomized controlled studies of the safety and efficacy of pharmacological agents in pediatrics are needed.

SUMMARY AND IMPLICATIONS: CONCEPT OF MULTIPLE TARGETS FOR TREATMENT AND PREVENTION

Most prior interventions for treating and preventing obesity in children have traditionally targeted body weight/body mass index through conventional approaches based on the energy balance model. Several arguments against this approach can be made. For example, it may take generations to reverse the population BMI trend, short-term weight loss may be effective but is not usually sustainable, and weight loss per se does not necessarily address health and metabolic risk factors. Finally, evidence suggests that a focus on body weight in children and adolescents is not effective. In a large cohort study, children who reported more dieting attempts were more likely to gain weight over a three-year period (57). Thus, the risks of a focus on weight loss in children and adolescents include greater weight gain, lower self-esteem (due to repeated failures), and body image and eating disorders.

Interventions designed to target specific metabolic factors/health outcomes may be more effective, especially in high-risk groups with elevated metabolic risk factors. One approach based on the centrally mediating role of insulin resistance, for example, is to identify interventions for improving insulin sensitivity and reducing insulin secretion. Improvement in insulin resistance may be an efficient intervention strategy because this addresses multiple risk factors, targeted through one common mechanism. It remains to be tested, for example, whether improvement of insulin resistance can lead to reduced risk of type 2 diabetes and cardiovascular disease over and above any effects on risk reduction through weight loss.

Alternative diet and exercise strategies can be designed around this concept. For example, traditional dietary approaches (e.g., reduced calorie, low fat, and low carbohydrate) generally have been designed to lead to weight loss and have failed to recognize the data suggesting that the quality and type of fats and carbohydrates are more important than the amount in affecting metabolic outcomes and thereby potentially improving risk factors associated with obesity. For fat, replacing foods high in saturated fat and trans fats with foods rich in plant-based fat sources (MUFAs and PUFAs; nuts, fish, soy) may be effective. For carbohydrate, data are beginning to show that replacing sugary foods based on simple/processed carbohydrates with foods high in whole grain/unprocessed carbohydrates, fiber, and low glycemic index value may be effective not only for weight loss but also for disease risk reduction.

The purpose of this review was to summarize the negative health outcomes associated with obesity during childhood and to review the case for insulin resistance as a potentially mediating factor in this relationship. We presented existing data showing the efficacy of intervention strategies that also address risk factor reduction, beyond weight loss. Our general premise does not exclude any focus on body weight, but suggests a focus on multiple targets. Indeed, the emphasis on risk reduction (rather than weight reduction) may be more effective in the long run because it may take the patient's focus off body weight, a focus for which self-efficacy and outcome expectancy may not be optimal.

The *Annual Review of Nutrition* is online at http://nutr.annualreviews.org

LITERATURE CITED

1. Adashi EY, Hsueh AJ, Yen SS. 1981. Insulin enhancement of luteinizing hormone and follicle-stimulating hormone release by cultured pituitary cells. *Endocrinology* 108:1441–49
1a. Alberti KGMM, Zimmet PZ, for the WHO Consultation. 1998. Definition, diagnosis and classification of diabetes mellitus and its complications. Part 1: diagnosis and classification of diabetes mellitus. Provisional report of a WHO consultation. *Diabetic Med.* 15:539–53
2. Am. Diabetes Assoc. 2000. Type 2 diabetes in children and adolescents. *Pediatrics* 105:671–80
3. Am. Diabetes Assoc. 2004. Expert Committee on the Diagnosis and Classification of Diabetes. *Diabetes Care* 27:S5–10
4. Amiel SA, Sherwin RS, Simonson DC, Lauritano AA, Tamborlane WV. 1986. Impaired insulin action in puberty: a contributing factor to poor glycemic control in adolescents with diabetes. *N. Engl. J. Med.* 315:215–19
5. Antonucci T, Whitcomb R, McLain R,

Lockwood D, Norris RM. 1997. Impaired glucose tolerance is normalized by treatment with the thiazolidinedione troglitazone. *Diabetes Care* 20:188–93
6. Arslanian S, Suprasongsin C, Janosky JE. 1997. Insulin secretion and sensitivity in black versus white prepubertal healthy children. *J. Clin. Endocrinol. Metab.* 82:1923–27
7. Arslanian SA, Lewy VD, Danadian K. 2001. Glucose intolerance in obese adolescents with polycystic ovary syndrome: roles of insulin resistance and beta-cell dysfunction and risk of cardiovascular disease. *J. Clin. Endocrinol. Metab.* 86:66–71
8. Arslanian SA, Lewy V, Danadian K, Saad R. 2002. Metformin therapy in obese adolescents with polycystic ovary syndrome and impaired glucose tolerance: amelioration of exaggerated adrenal response to adrenocorticotropin with reduction of insulinemia/insulin resistance. 87:1555–59
9. Ashley MA, Buckley AJ, Criss AL, Ward JA, Kemp A, et al. 2002. Familial, anthropometric and metabolic associations of intromyocellular lipid levels in prepubertal males. *Pediatr. Res.* 51:81–86
10. Bacha F, Saad R, Gungor N, Arslanian SA. 2004. Adiponectin in youth: relationship to visceral adiposity, insulin sensitivity, and beta-cell function. *Diabetes Care* 27:547–52
11. Baldridge AD, Perez-Atayde AR, Graeme-Cook F, Higgins L, Lavine JE. 1995. Idiopathic steatohepatitis in childhood: a multicenter retrospective study. *J. Pediatr.* 127:700–4
12. Ball GD, Shaibi GQ, Cruz ML, Watkins MP, Weigensberg MJ, Goran MI. 2004. Insulin sensitivity, cardiorespiratory fitness, and physical activity in overweight Hispanic youth. *Obes. Res.* 12:77–85
13. Barbieri RL, Makris A, Ryan KJ. 1983. Effects of insulin on steroidogenesis in cultured porcine ovarian theca. *Fertil. Steril.* 40:237–41
14. Barlow SE, Dietz WH. 1998. Obesity evaluation and treatment: Expert Committee recommendations. The Maternal and Child Health Bureau, Health Resources and Services Administration and the Department of Health and Human Services. 102:E29
15. Barlow SE, Dietz WH. 2002. Management of child and adolescent obesity: summary and recommendations based on reports from pediatricians, pediatric nurse practitioners, and registered dietitians. *Pediatrics* 110:236–38
16. Berberoglu M. 2001. Evaluation of the correlation between serum tumor necrosis factor-alpha and relative body mass index (RBMI) in childhood. *J. Pediatr. Endocrinol. Metab.* 14:543–47
17. Berkowitz RI, Wadden TA, Tershakovec AM, Cronquist JL. 2003. Behavior therapy and sibutramine for the treatment of adolescent obesity: a randomized controlled trial. *JAMA* 289:1805–12
18. Bringer J, Lefebvre P, Boulet F, Grigorescu F, Renard E, et al. 1993. Body composition and regional fat distribution in polycystic ovarian syndrome. Relationship to hormonal and metabolic profiles. *Ann. NY Acad. Sci.* 687:115–23
19. Buchanan TA. 2003. Pancreatic beta-cell loss and preservation in type 2 diabetes. *Clin. Ther.* 25(Suppl. B):B32–46
20. Bugianesi E, Leone N, Vanni E, Marchesini G, Brunello F, et al. 2002. Expanding the natural history of nonalcoholic steatohepatitis: from cryptogenic cirrhosis to hepatocellular carcinoma. *Gastroenterology* 123:134–40
21. Campbell WW, Crim MC, Young VR, Evans WJ. 1994. Increased energy requirements and changes in body composition with resistance training in older adults. *Am. J. Clin. Nutr.* 60(2):167–75
22. Campbell WW, Crim MC, Young VR, Joseph LJ, Evans WJ. 1995. Effects of resistance training and dietary protein intake on protein metabolism in

older adults. *Am. J. Physiol. Endocrinol. Metabol.* 268:E1143–53
23. Caprio S, Hyman LD, Limb C, McCarthy S, Lange R, et al. 1995. Central adiposity and its metabolic correlates in obese adolescent girls. *Am. J. Physiol. Endocrinol. Metabol.* 269:E118–26
24. Caprio S, Plewe G, Diamond MP, Simonson DC, Boulware SD, et al. 1989. Increased insulin secretion in puberty: a compensatory response to reductions in insulin sensitivity. *J. Pediatr.* 114:963–67
25. Cara JF, Rosenfield RL. 1988. Insulin-like growth factor I and insulin potentiate luteinizing hormone-induced androgen synthesis by rat ovarian thecal-interstitial cells. *Endocrinology* 123: 733–39
26. Chen W, Bao W, Begum S, Elkasabany A, Srinivasan SR, Berenson GS. 2000. Age-related patterns of the clustering of cardiovascular risk variables of syndrome X from childhood to young adulthood in a population made up of black and white subjects: the Bogalusa Heart Study. *Diabetes* 49:1042–48
27. Chen W, Srinivasan SR, Elkasabany A, Berenson GS. 1999. Cardiovascular risk factors clustering features of insulin resistance syndrome (syndrome X) in a biracial (black-white) population of children, adolescents, and young adults: the Bogalusa Heart Study. *Am. J. Epidemiol.* 150:667–74
28. Chiu KC, Cohan P, Lee NP, Chuang LM. 2000. Insulin sensitivity differs among ethnic groups with a compensatory response in B-cell function. *Diabetes Care* 23:1353–58
29. Chu NF, Wang D-J, Shieh S-M, Rimm EB. 2000. Plasma leptin concentrations and obesity in relation to insulin resistance syndrome components among school children in Taiwan: the Taipei Children Heart Study. *Int. J. Obes.* 24: 1265–71
30. Clark JM, Brancati FL, Diehl AM. 2002. Nonalcoholic fatty liver disease. *Gastroenterology* 122:1649–57
31. Committee Nutr., Am. Acad. Pediatr. 1998. *Obesity in Children*. Oak Grove, IL: Am. Acad. Pediatr.
32. Cook JS, Hoffman RP, Stene MA, Hansen JR. 1993. Effects of maturational stage on insulin sensitivity during puberty. *J. Clin. Endocrinol. Metab.* 77: 725–30
33. Cook S, Weitzman M, Auinger P, Nguyen M, Dietz WH. 2003. Prevalence of a metabolic syndrome phenotype in adolescents: findings from the third National Health and Nutrition Examination Survey, 1988–1994. *Arch. Pediatr. Adolesc. Med.* 157:821–27
34. Cruz ML, Huang TTK, Johnson MS, Gower BA, Goran MI. 2002. Insulin sensitivity and blood pressure in black and white children. *Hypertension* 40:18–22
35. Cruz ML, Weigensberg MJ, Huang T, Ball GDC, Shaibi GQ, Goran MI. 2004. The metabolic syndrome in overweight Hispanic youth and the role of insulin sensitivity. *J. Clin. Endocrinol. Metab.* 89:108–13
36. Cuff DJ, Meneilly GS, Martin A, Ignaszewski A, Tildesley HD, Frohlich JJ. 2003. Effective exercise modality to reduce insulin resistance in women with type 2 diabetes. *Diabetes Care* 26:2977–82
37. Dabelea D, Pettitt DJ, Jones KL, Arslanian SA. 1999. Type 2 diabetes mellitus in minority children and adolescents. An emerging problem. *Endocrinol. Metab. Clin. North Am.* 28:709–29
38. Davidson MH, Maki KC, Kong JC, Dugan LD, Torri SA, et al. 1998. Long-term effects of consuming foods containing psyllium seed husk on serum lipids in subjects with hypercholesterolemia. *Am. J. Clin. Nutr.* 67:367–76
39. DeFronzo RA, Bonadonna RC, Ferrannini E. 1992. Pathogenesis of NIDDM. A balanced overview. *Diabetes Care* 15: 318–68

40. DeFronzo RA, Ferrannini E. 1991. Insulin resistance. A multifaceted syndrome responsible for NIDDM, obesity, hypertension, dyslipidemia, and atherosclerotic cardiovascular disease. *Diabetes Care* 14:173–94
41. Dunaif A, Graf M, Mandeli J, Laumas V, Dobrjansky A. 1987. Characterization of groups of hyperandrogenic women with acanthosis nigricans, impaired glucose tolerance, and/or hyperinsulinemia. *J. Clin. Endocrinol. Metab.* 65:499–507
42. Dunstan DW, Daly RM, Owen N, Jolley D, De Courten M, et al. 2002. High-intensity resistance training improves glycemic control in older patients with type 2 diabetes. *Diabetes Care* 25:1729–36
43. Ebbeling CB, Leidig MM, Sinclair KB, Hangen JP, Ludwig DS. 2003. A reduced-glycemic load diet in the treatment of adolescent obesity. *Arch. Pediatr. Adolesc. Med.* 157:773–79
44. Ebbeling CB, Ludwig DS. 2001. Treating obesity in youth: Should dietary glycemic load be a consideration? *Adv. Pediatr.* 48:179–212
45. Ehrmann DA, Barnes RB, Rosenfield RL. 1995. Polycystic ovary syndrome as a form of functional ovarian hyperandrogenism due to dysregulation of androgen secretion. *Endocr. Rev.* 16:322–53
46. Ehrmann DA, Barnes RB, Rosenfield RL, Cavaghan MK, Imperial J. 1999. Prevalence of impaired glucose tolerance and diabetes in women with polycystic ovary syndrome. *Diabetes Care* 22:141–46
47. Epstein LH, Roemmich JN, Raynor HA. 2001. Behavioral therapy in the treatment of pediatric obesity. *Pediatr. Clin. North Am.* 48:981–93
48. Expert Panel Detection, Eval., Treat., High Blood Cholesterol in Adults. 2001. Executive Summary of the Third Report of the National Cholesterol Education Program (NCEP) Expert Panel on Detection, Evaluation, and Treatment of High Blood Cholesterol in Adults (Adult Treatment Panel III). *JAMA* 285:2486–97
49. Fagot-Campagna A, Flegal KM, Saaddine JB, Beckles GLA. 2001. Diabetes, impaired fasting glucose, and elevated HbA1c in U.S. adolescents: the Third National Health and Nutrition Examination Survey. *Diabetes Care* 5: 834–37
50. Fagot-Campagna A, Pettitt DJ, Engelgau MM, Burrows NR, Geiss LS, et al. 2000. Type 2 diabetes among North American children and adolescents: an epidemiologic review and a public health perspective. *J. Pediatr.* 136:664–72
51. Faigenbaum AD. 2003. *Youth strength training*. http://www.afpafitness.com/articles/YouthTrain.htm
52. Faigenbaum AD, Loud RL, O'Connell J, Glover S, O'Connell J, Westcott WL. 2001. Effects of different resistance training protocols on upper-body strength and endurance development in children. *J. Strength Cond. Res.* 15:459–65
53. Faigenbaum AD, Westcott W, Loud R, Long C. 1999. The effects of different resistance training protocols on muscular strength and endurance development in children. *Pediatrics* 104(1):e5
54. Ferguson MA, Gutin B, Le NA, Karp W, Litaker M, et al. 1999. Effects of exercise training and its cessation on components of the insulin resistance syndrome in obese children. *Int. J. Obes. Relat. Metab. Disord.* 23:889–95
55. Ferrannini E, Camastra S. 1998. Relationship between impaired glucose tolerance, non-insulin-dependent diabetes mellitus and obesity. *Eur. J. Clin. Invest.* 28(Suppl. 2):3–6
56. Festa A, D'Agostino R Jr, Howard G, Mykkanen L, Tracy RP, Haffner SM. 2000. Chronic subclinical inflammation as part of the insulin resistance syndrome: the Insulin Resistance

Atherosclerosis Study (IRAS). *Circulation* 102:42–47
57. Field AE, Austin SB, Taylor CB, Malspeis S, Rosner B, et al. 2003. Relation between dieting and weight change among preadolescents and adolescents. *Pediatrics* 112:900–6
58. Fishbein MH, Miner M, Mogren C, Chalekson J. 2003. The spectrum of fatty liver in obese children and the relationship of serum aminotransferases to severity of steatosis. *J. Pediatr. Gastroenterol. Nutr.* 36:54–61
59. Ford ES, Giles WH, Dietz WH. 2002. Prevalence of the metabolic syndrome among U.S. adults: findings from the Third National Health and Nutrition Examination Survey. *JAMA* 287:356–59
60. Forouhi N, Jekinson G, Thomas E, Mullick S, Mierisova S, et al. 1999. Relation of triglyceride stores in skeletal muscle cells to central obesity and insulin sensitivity in European and South Asian men. *Diabetologia* 42:932–35
61. Franks S. 1995. Polycystic ovary syndrome. *N. Engl. J. Med.* 333:853–61
62. Frayn KN. 2000. Visceral fat and insulin resistance—causative or correlative? *Br. J. Nutr.* 83:S71–77
63. Freedman DS, Srinivasan SR, Burke GL, Shear CL, Smoak CG, et al. 1987. Relation of body fat distribution to hyperinsulinemia in children and adolescents: the Bogalusa Heart Study. *Am. J. Clin. Nutr.* 46:403–10
64. Freemark M, Bursey D. 2001. The effects of metformin on body mass index and glucose tolerance in obese adolescents with fasting hyperinsulinemia and a family history of type 2 diabetes. *Pediatrics* 107:1–7
65. Gahagan S, Silverstein J. 2003. Prevention and treatment of type 2 diabetes mellitus in children, with special emphasis on American Indian and Alaska Native children. American Academy of Pediatrics Committee on Native American Child Health. *Pediatrics* 112:e328
66. Gambineri A, Pelusi C, Vicennati V, Pagotto U, Pasquali R. 2002. Obesity and the polycystic ovary syndrome. *Int. J. Obes. Relat. Metab. Disord.* 26:883–96
67. Goodpaster BH, Katsiaras A, Kelley DE. 2003. Enhanced fat oxidation through physical activity is associated with improvements in insulin sensitivity in obesity. *Diabetes* 52:2191–97
68. Goran MI. 1997. Energy expenditure, body composition, and disease risk in children and adolescents. *Proc. Nutr. Soc.* 56:195–209
69. Goran MI, Bergman RN, Avila Q, Watkins M, Ball GDC, et al. 2004. Impaired glucose tolerance and reduced beta-cell function in overweight Latino children with a positive family history for type 2 diabetes. *J. Clin. Endocrinol. Metab.* 89:207–12
70. Goran MI, Cruz ML, Bergman RN, Watanabe RM. 2002. Insulin resistance and the associated compensatory response in Caucasian, African American and Hispanic children. *Diabetes Care* 25:2184–90
71. Goran MI, Gower BA. 2001. Longitudinal study of pubertal insulin resistance. *Diabetes* 50:2444–50
72. Goran MI, Kaskoun MC, Shuman WP. 1995. Intra-abdominal adipose tissue in young children. *Int. J. Obes.* 19:279–83
73. Goran MI, Nagy TR, Treuth MT, Trowbridge C, Dezenberg C, et al. 1997. Visceral fat in Caucasian and African-American pre-pubertal children. *Am. J. Clin. Nutr.* 65:1703–9
74. Gower BA, Fernandez JR, Beasley TM, Shriver MD, Goran MI. 2003. Using genetic admixture to explain racial differences in insulin-related phenotypes. *Diabetes* 52:1047–51
75. Gower BA, Granger WM, Franklin F, Shewchuk RM, Goran MI. 2002. Contribution of insulin secretion and clearance to the greater acute insulin response

to glucose in African-American versus Caucasian children and adolescents. *J. Clin. Endocrinol. Metab.* 87:2218–24
76. Gower BA, Nagy TR, Goran MI. 1999. Visceral fat, insulin sensitivity, and lipids in prepubertal children. *Diabetes* 48: 1515–21
77. Gulekli B, Turhan NO, Senoz S, Kukner S, Oral H, Gokmen O. 1993. Endocrinological, ultrasonographic and clinical findings in adolescent and adult polycystic ovary patients: a comparative study. *Gynecol. Endocrinol.* 7:273–77
78. Gutin B, Barbeau P, Owens S, Lemmon CR, Bauman M, et al. 2002. Effects of exercise intensity on cardiovascular fitness, total body composition, and visceral adiposity of obese adolescents. *Am. J. Clin. Nutr.* 75:818–26
79. Gutin B, Cucuzzo N, Islam S, Smith C, Stachura ME. 1995. Physical training, lifestyle education and coronary risk factors in obese girls. *Med. Sci. Sports Exerc.* 28:19–23
80. Gutin B, Islam S, Manos T, Cucuzzo N, Smith C, Stachura ME. 1994. Relation of percentage of body fat and maximal aerobic capacity to risk factors for atherosclerosis and diabetes in black and white seven- to eleven-year-old children. *J. Pediatr.* 125:847–52
81. Gutin B, Owens S, Treiber F, Islam S, Karp W, Slavens G. 1997. Weight-independent cardiovascular fitness and coronary risk factors. *Arch. Pediatr. Adolesc. Med.* 151:462–65
82. Haffner SM, D'Agostino R, Saad MF, Rewers M, Mykkanen L, et al. 1996. Increased insulin resistance and insulin secretion in nondiabetic African-Americans and Hispanics compared with non-Hispanic whites. The Insulin Resistance Atherosclerosis Study. *Diabetes* 45:742–48
83. Haffner SM, Miettinen H, Gaskill SP, Stern MP. 1995. Decreased insulin secretion and increased insulin resistance are independently related to the 7-year risk of NIDDM in Mexican-Americans. *Diabetes* 44:1386–91
84. Haffner SM, Mykkanen L, Rainwater DL, Karhapaa P, Laakso M. 1999. Is leptin concentration associated with the insulin resistance syndrome in nondiabetic men? *Obes. Res.* 7:164–69
85. Haffner SM, Stern MP, Hazuda HP, Mitchell BD, Patterson JK. 1990. Cardiovascular risk factors in confirmed prediabetic individuals. Does the clock for coronary heart disease start ticking before the onset of clinical diabetes? *JAMA* 263:2893–98
86. Hanson RL, Imperatore G, Bennett PH, Knowler WC. 2002. Components of the "metabolic syndrome" and incidence of type 2 diabetes. *Diabetes* 51:3120–27
87. Hedley AA, Ogden CL, Johnson CL, Carroll MD, Curtin LR, Flegal KM. 2004. Prevalence of overweight and obesity among U.S. children, adolescents, and adults, 1999–2002. *JAMA* 291: 2847–50
88. Hoeger K. 2001. Obesity and weight loss in polycystic ovary syndrome. *Obstet. Gynecol. Clin. North Am.* 28:85–97
89. Hu FB, van Dam RM, Liu S. 2001. Diet and risk of Type II diabetes: the role of types of fat and carbohydrate. *Diabetologia* 44:805–17
90. Huang T-K, Johnson MS, Figueroa-Colon R, Dwyer JH, Goran MI. 2001. Growth of visceral fat, subcutaneous abdominal fat and total body fat in children. *Obes. Res.* 9:283–89
91. Hull RL, Westermark GT, Westermark P, Kahn SE. 2004. Islet amyloid: a critical entity in the pathogenesis of type 2 diabetes. *J. Clin. Endocrinol. Metab.* 89: 3629–43
92. Irwin ML, Mayer-Davis EJ, Addy CL, Pate RR, Durstine JL, et al. 2000. Moderate-intensity physical activity and fasting insulin levels in women: the Cross-Cultural Activity Participation Study. *Diabetes Care* 23:449–54
93. Isomaa B, Almgren P, Tuomi T, Forsen

B, Lahti K, et al. 2001. Cardiovascular morbidity and mortality associated with the metabolic syndrome. *Diabetes Care* 24:683–89

94. Jenkins DJ, Kendall CW, Vuksan V, Vidgen E, Parker T, et al. 2002. Soluble fiber intake at a dose approved by the U.S. Food and Drug Administration for a claim of health benefits: serum lipid risk factors for cardiovascular disease assessed in a randomized controlled crossover trial. *Am. J. Clin. Nutr.* 75: 834–39
95. Jiang X, Srinivasan SR, Webber LS, Wattigney WA, Berenson GS. 1995. Association of fasting insulin level with serum lipid and lipoprotein levels in children, adolescents, and young adults: the Bogalusa Heart Study. *Arch. Intern. Med.* 155:190–96
96. Jimenez-Cruz A, Bacardi-Gascon M, Turnbull WH, Rosales-Garay P, Severino-Lugo I. 2003. A flexible, low-glycemic index Mexican-style diet in overweight and obese subjects with type 2 diabetes improves metabolic parameters during a 6-week treatment period. *Diabetes Care* 26:1967–70
97. Jimenez-Cruz A, Turnbull WH, Bacardi-Gascon M, Rosales-Garay P. 2004. A high-fiber, moderate glycemic index, Mexican-style diet improves dyslipidemia in individuals with type 2 diabetes. *Nutr. Res.* 24:19–27

97a. Kahn SE, Prigeon RL, McCulloch DK, Boyko EJ, Bergman RN, et al. 1993. Quantification of the relationship between insulin sensitivity and beta-cell function in human subjects. Evidence for a hyperbolic function. *Diabetes* 42(11): 1663–72

98. Kamohara S, Burcelin R, Halaas JL, Friedman JM, Charron MJ. 1997. Acute stimulation of glucose metabolism in mice by leptin treatment. *Nature* 389: 374–77
99. Kang HS, Gutin B, Barbeau P, Owens S, Lemmon CR, et al. 2002. Physical training improves insulin resistance syndrome markers in obese adolescents. *Med. Sci. Sports Exerc.* 34:1920–27
100. Kelley DE, Goodpaster BH. 2001. Effects of physical activity on insulin action and glucose tolerance in obesity. *Med. Sci. Sports Exerc.* 31:S619–23
101. Kelley DE, Goodpaster BH. 2001. Skeletal muscle triglyceride an aspect of regional adiposity and insulin resistance. *Diabetes Care* 24:933–41
102. Kelley DE, McKolanis TM, Hegazi R, Kuller L, Kalhan S. 2003. Fatty liver in type 2 diabetes mellitus: relation to regional adiposity, fatty acids, and insulin resistance. *Am. J. Physiol.* 285:E906–16
103. Kershaw EE, Flier JS. 2004. Adipose tissue as an endocrine organ. *J. Clin. Endocrinol. Metab.* 89:2548–56
104. Klein S, Fontana L, Young VL, Coggan AR, Kilo C, et al. 2004. Absence of an effect of liposuction on insulin action and risk factors for coronary heart disease. *N. Engl. J. Med.* 350:2549–57
105. Kriska AM, Hanley AJ, Harris SB, Zinman B. 2001. Physical activity, physical fitness, and insulin and glucose concentrations in an isolated Native Canadian population experiencing rapid lifestyle change. *Diabetes Care* 24:1787–92
106. Kriska AM, Pereira MA, Hanson RL, de Courten MP, Zimmet PZ, et al. 2001. Association of physical activity and serum insulin concentrations in two populations at high risk for type 2 diabetes but differing by BMI. *Diabetes Care* 24: 1175–80
107. Ku CY, Gower BA, Hunter GR, Goran MI. 2000. Racial differences in insulin secretion and sensitivity in prepubertal children: role of physical fitness and physical activity. *Obes. Res.* 8:506–15
108. Deleted in proof
109. Laaksonen DE, Lakka HM, Lynch J, Lakka TA, Niskanen L, et al. 2003. Cardiorespiratory fitness and vigorous leisure-time physical activity modify the association of small size at birth with

the metabolic syndrome. *Diabetes Care* 26:2156–64

110. Laaksonen DE, Lakka HM, Niskanen LK, Kaplan GA, Salonen JT, Lakka TA. 2002. Metabolic syndrome and development of diabetes mellitus: application and validation of recently suggested definitions of the metabolic syndrome in a prospective cohort study. *Am. J. Epidemiol.* 156:1070–77
111. Lahlou N, Landais P, Boissiey D, Bougneres P. 1997. Circulating leptin in normal children and during the dynamic phase of juvenile obesity. *Diabetes* 46: 989–93
112. Lakka HM, Laaksonen DE, Lakka TA, Niskanen LK, Kumpusalo E, et al. 2002. The metabolic syndrome and total and cardiovascular disease mortality in middle-aged men. *JAMA* 288:2709–16
113. LeMura LM, Maziekas MT. 2002. Factors that alter body fat, body mass, and fat-free mass in pediatric obesity. *Med. Sci. Sports Exerc.* 34:487–96
114. Le Stunff C, Bougnäres P. 1994. Early changes in postprandial insulin secretion, not in insulin sensitivity, characterize juvenile obesity. *Diabetes* 43:696–702
115. Lewis V. 2001. Polycystic ovary syndrome. A diagnostic challenge. *Obstet. Gynecol. Clin. North Am.* 28:1–20
116. Lewy VD, Danadian K, Witchel SF, Arslanian S. 2001. Early metabolic abnormalities in adolescent girls with polycystic ovarian syndrome. *J. Pediatr.* 138: 38–44
117. Lindquist CH, Gower BA, Goran MI. 2000. Role of dietary factors in ethnic differences in early risk of cardiovascular disease and type 2 diabetes. *Am. J. Clin. Nutr.* 71:725–32
118. Lindsay RS, Funahashi T, Hanson RL, Matsuzawa Y, Tanaka S, et al. 2002. Adiponectin and development of type 2 diabetes in the Pima Indian population. *Lancet* 360:57–58
119. Ludwig DS. 2002. The glycemic index: physiological mechanisms relating to obesity, diabetes, and cardiovascular disease. *JAMA* 287:2414–23
120. Ludwig DS, Pereira M, Kroenke C, Hilner JE, Van Horn L, et al. 1999. Dietary fiber, weight gain, and cardiovascular disease risk factors in young adults. *JAMA* 282:1539–46
121. Luepker RV, Perry CL, McKinlay SM, Nader PR, Parcel GS, et al. 1996. Outcomes of a field trial to improve children's dietary patterns and physical activity: the Child and Adolescent Trial for Cardiovascular Health (CATCH). *JAMA* 275:768–76
122. Marchesini G, Brizi M, Bianchi G, Tomassetti S, Bugianesi E, et al. 2001. Nonalcoholic fatty liver disease: a feature of the metabolic syndrome. *Diabetes* 50:1844–50
123. McDuffie JR, Calis KA, Uwaifo GI, Sebring NG, Fallon EM, et al. 2002. Three-month tolerability of orlistat in adolescents with obesity-related comorbid conditions. *Obes. Res.* 10:642–50
124. McNeely MJ, Boyko EJ, Weigle DS, Shofer JB, Chessler SD, et al. 1999. Association between baseline plasma leptin levels and subsequent development of diabetes in Japanese Americans. *Diabetes Care* 22:65–70
125. Molleston JP, White F, Teckman J, Fitzgerald JF. 2002. Obese children with steatohepatitis can develop cirrhosis in childhood. *Am. J. Gastroenterol.* 97: 2460–62
126. Moran A, Jacobs DRJ, Steinberger J, Hong C-P, Prineas R, et al. 1999. Insulin resistance during puberty: result from clamp studies in 357 children. *Diabetes* 48:2039–44
127. Murtaugh MA, Jacobs DR Jr, Jacob B, Steffen LM, Marquart L. 2003. Epidemiological support for the protection of whole grains against diabetes. *Proc. Nutr. Soc.* 62:143–49
128. Nagy TR, Gower BA, Trowbridge CA, Dezenberg C, Shewchuk RM, Goran

MI. 1997. Effects of gender, ethnicity, body composition, and fat distribution on serum leptin concentrartions in children. *J. Clin. Endocrinol. Metab.* 82:2148

129. Neel JV, Weder AB, Julius S. 1998. Type II diabetes, essential hypertension, and obesity as "syndromes of impaired genetic homeostasis": the "thrifty genotype" hypothesis enters the 21st century. *Perspect. Biol. Med.* 42:44–74
130. Nemet D, Wang P, Funahashi T, Matsuzawa Y, Tanaka S, et al. 2003. Adipocytokines, body composition, and fitness in children. *Pediatr. Res.* 53:148–52
131. Nestler JE, Jakubowicz DJ, Reamer P, Gunn RD, Allan G. 1999. Ovulatory and metabolic effects of D-chiro-inositol in the polycystic ovary syndrome. *New Engl. J. Med.* 340:1314–20
132. Neufeld ND, Raffel LJ, Landon C, Chen Y-D, Vadheim CM. 1998. Early presentation of type 2 diabetes in Mexican-American youth. *Diabetes Care* 21:80–86
133. Nguyen-Duy TB, Nichaman MZ, Church TS, Blair SN, Ross R. 2003. Visceral fat and liver fat are independent predictors of metabolic risk factors in men. *Am. J. Physiol.* 284:E1065–71
134. Obarzanek E, Kimm S, Barton BA, VanHorn L, Kwiterovich JPO, et al. 2001. Long-term safety and efficacy of a cholesterol-lowering diet in children with elevated low-density lipoprotein cholesterol: seven-year results of the dietary intervention study in children (DISC). *Pediatrics* 107:256–64
135. Ogden CL, Flegal KM, Carroll MD, Johnson CL. 2002. Prevalence and trends in overweight among U.S. children and adolescents, 1999–2000. *JAMA* 288:1728–32
136. Deleted in proof
137. Ozkan B, Bereket A, Turan S, Keskin S. 2004. Addition of orlistat to conventional treatment in adolescents with severe obesity. *Eur. J. Pediatr.* 163(12):738–41
138. Palmert MR, Gordon CM, Kartashov AI, Legro RS, Emans SJ, Dunaif A. 2002. Screening for abnormal glucose tolerance in adolescents with polycystic ovary syndrome. *J. Clin. Endocrinol. Metab.* 87:1017–23
139. Paulsen EP, Richenderfer L, Ginsberg-Fellner F. 1968. Plasma glucose, free fatty acids and immunoreactive insulin in sixty-six obese children. *Diabetes* 17:261–69
140. Pinhas-Hamiel O, Dolan LM, Daniels SR, Standiford D, Khoury PR, Zeitler P. 1996. Increased incidence of non-insulin-dependent diabetes mellitus among adolescents. *J. Pediatr.* 128:608–15
141. Poehlman ET, Dvorak R, DeNino W, Brochu M, Ades PA. 2000. Effects of resistance training and endurance training on isulin sensitivity in nonobese, young women: a controlled randomized trial. *J. Clin. Endrocrinol. Metab.* 85:2463–68
142. Poretsky L, Glover B, Laumas V, Kalin M, Dunaif A. 1988. The effects of experimental hyperinsulinemia on steroid secretion, ovarian [125I]insulin binding, and ovarian [125I]insulin-like growth-factor I binding in the rat. *Endocrinology* 122:581–85
143. Promrat K, Lutchman G, Uwaifo GI, Freedman RJ, Soza A, et al. 2004. A pilot study of pioglitazone treatment for nonalcoholic steatohepatitis. *Hepatology* 39:188–96
144. Raitakari OT, Porkka KV, Ronnemaa T, Knip M, Uhari M, et al. 1995. The role of insulin in clustering of serum lipids and blood pressure in children and adolescents. The Cardiovascular Risk in Young Finns Study. *Diabetologia* 38:1042–50
145. Deleted in proof
146. Rashid M, Roberts EA. 2000. Nonalcoholic steatohepatitis in children. *J. Pediatr. Gastroenterol. Nutr.* 30:48–53
147. Ravussin E, Smith SR. 2002. Increased fat intake, impaired fat oxidation, and failure of fat cell proliferation result in ectopic fat storage, insulin resistance,

and type 2 diabetes mellitus. *Ann. NY Acad. Sci.* 967:363–78
148. Reaven GM. 1988. Role on insulin resistance in human disease. *Diabetes* 37: 1595–607
149. Reinehr T, Kiess W, Kapellen T, Andler W. 2004. Insulin sensitivity among obese children and adolescents, according to degree of weight loss. *Pediatrics* 114:1569–73
150. Reinehr T, Roth C, Menke T, Andler W. 2004. Adiponectin before and after weight loss in obese children. *J. Clin. Endocrinol. Metab.* 89:3790–94
151. Ritenbaugh C, Teufel-Shone NI, Aickin MG, Joe JR, Poirier S, et al. 2003. A lifestyle intervention improves plasma insulin levels among Native American high school youth. *Prev. Med.* 36:309–19
152. Robers SB. 2000. High-glycemic index foods, hunger and obesity: Is there a connection? *Nutr. Rev.* 58:163–69
153. Roberts EA. 2003. Nonalcoholic steatohepatitis in children. *Curr. Gastroenterol. Rep.* 5:253–59
154. Rosenbloom AL, Joe JR, Young RS, Winter WE. 1999. Emerging epidemic of type 2 diabetes in youth. *Diabetes Care* 22:345–54
155. Ryan AS, Pratley RE, Elahi D, Goldberg AP. 1995. Resistive training increases fat-free mass and maintains RMR despite weight loss in postmenopausal women. *J. Appl. Physiol.* 79:818–23
156. Sanyal AJ, Campbell-Sargent C, Mirshahi F, Rizzo WB, Contos MJ, et al. 2001. Nonalcoholic steatohepatitis: association of insulin resistance and mitochondrial abnormalities. *Gastroenterology* 120:1183–92
157. Scheett TP, Nemet D, Stoppani J, Maresh CM, Newcomb R, Cooper DM. 2002. The effect of endurance-type exercise training on growth mediators and inflammatory cytokines in pre-pubertal and early pubertal males. *Pediatr. Res.* 52:491–97
158. Schmitz KH, Jacobs DR Jr, Hong CP, Steinberger J, Moran A, Sinaiko AR. 2002. Association of physical activity with insulin sensitivity in children. 26: 1310–16
159. Schwimmer JB, Deutsch R, Rauch JB, Behling C, Newbury R, Lavine JE. 2003. Obesity, insulin resistance, and other clinicopathological correlates of pediatric nonalcoholic fatty liver disease. *J. Pediatr.* 143:500–5
160. Senn JJ, Klover PJ, Nowak IA, Mooney RA. 2002. Interleukin-6 induces cellular insulin resistance in hepatocytes. *Diabetes* 51:3391–99
161. Seppala-Lindroos A, Vehkavaara S, Hakkinen AM, Goto T, Westerbacka J, et al. 2002. Fat accumulation in the liver is associated with defects in insulin suppression of glucose production and serum free fatty acids independent of obesity in normal men. *J. Clin. Endocrinol. Metab.* 87:3023–28
162. Shaibi GQ, Ball G, Salem G, Cruz ML, Weigensberg MJ, et al. 2004. Resistance training significantly improves insulin sensitivity in overweight Hispanic adolescent males. *Obes. Res.* 12:A65 (Abstr.)
163. Silfen ME, Denburg MR, Manibo AM, Lobo RA, Jaffe R, et al. 2003. Early endocrine, metabolic, and sonographic characteristics of polycystic ovary syndrome (PCOS): comparison between nonobese and obese adolescents. *J. Clin. Endocrinol. Metab.* 88:4682–88
164. Sinaiko AR, Jacobs DR Jr, Steinberger J, Moran A, Luepker R, et al. 2001. Insulin resistance syndrome in childhood: associations of the euglycemic insulin clamp and fasting insulin with fatness and other risk factors. *J. Pediatr.* 139:700–7
165. Sinha R, Dufour S, Petersen KF, Lebon V, Enoksson S, et al. 2002. Assessment of skeletal muscle triglyceride content by (1)H nuclear magnetic resonance spectroscopy in lean and obese adolescents: relationships to insulin sensitivity, total

body fat, and central adiposity. *Diabetes* 51:1022–27

166. Sinha R, Fisch G, Teague B, Tamborlane WV, Banyas B, et al. 2002. Prevalence of impaired glucose tolerance among children and adolescents with marked obesity. *New Engl. J. Med.* 346:802–10
167. Smutok MA, Kokkinos PF, Farmer C, Dawson P, Shulman R, et al. 1993. Aerobic versus strength training for risk factor intervention in middle-aged men at high risk for coronary heart disease. *Metabolism* 42(2):177–84
168. Srinivasan SR, Myers L, Berenson GS. 2002. Predictability of childhood adiposity and insulin for developing insulin resistance syndrome (syndrome X) in young adulthood: the Bogalusa Heart Study. *Diabetes* 51:204–9
169. Stefan N, Vozarova B, Funahashi T, Matsuzawa Y, Weyer C, et al. 2002. Plasma adiponectin concentration is associated with skeletal muscle insulin receptor tyrosine phosphorylation, and low plasma concentration precedes a decrease in whole-body insulin sensitivity in humans. *Diabetes* 51:1884–88
170. Steffen LM, Jacobs DR Jr, Murtaugh MA, Moran A, Steinberger J, et al. 2003. Whole grain intake is associated with lower body mass and greater insulin sensitivity among adolescents. *Am. J. Epidemiol.* 158:243–50
171. Steffen LM, Jacobs DR Jr, Stevens J, Shahar E, Carithers T, Folsom AR. 2003. Associations of whole-grain, refined grain, and fruit and vegetable consumption with risks of all-cause mortality and incident coronary artery disease and ischemic stroke: the Atherosclerosis Risk in Communities (ARIC) Study. *Am. J. Clin. Nutr.* 78:383–90
172. Steinberger J, Steffen L, Jacobs DR Jr, Moran A, Hong CP, Sinaiko AR. 2003. Relation of leptin to insulin resistance syndrome in children. *Obes. Res.* 11:1124–30
173. Summerbell C, Ashton V, Campbell K, Edmunds L, Kelly S, Waters E. 2003. Interventions for treating obesity in children. *Cochrane Database Syst. Rev.* 3:CD001872
174. Sung RY, Yu CW, Chang SK, Mo SW, Woo KS, Lam CW. 2002. Effects of dietary intervention and strength training on blood lipid level in obese children. *Arch. Dis. Child.* 86:407–10
175. Tominaga K, Kurata JH, Chen YK, Fujimoto E, Miyagawa S, et al. 1995. Prevalence of fatty liver in Japanese children and relationship to obesity. An epidemiological ultrasonographic survey. *Dig. Dis. Sci.* 40:2002–9
176. Trayhurn P, Beattie JH. 2001. Physiological role of adipose tissue: white adipose tissue as an endocrine and secretory organ. *Proc. Nutr. Soc.* 60:329–39
177. Treuth MS, Hunter GR, Figueroa-Colon R, Goran MI. 1998. Effects of strength training on intra-abdominal adipose tissue in obese prepubertal girls. *Med. Sci. Sports Exerc.* 30:1738–43
178. Treuth MS, Hunter GR, Kekes-Szabo T, Weinsier RL, Goran MI, Berland L. 1995. Strength training reduces intra-abdominal adipose tissue in older women. *J. Appl. Physiol.* 78:1425–31
179. Treuth MS, Ryan RE, Pratley RE, Rubin MA, Miller JP, et al. 1994. Effects of strength training on total and regional body composition in older men. *J. Appl. Physiol.* 77:614–20
180. Uwaifo GI, Nguyen TT, Keil MF, Russell DL, Nicholson JC, et al. 2002. Differences in insulin secretion and sensitivity of Caucasian and African American prepubertal children. *J. Pediatr.* 140: 673–80
181. Uysal KT, Wiesbrock SM, Marino MW, Hotamisligil GS. 1997. Protection from obesity-induced insulin resistance in mice lacking TNF-alpha function. *Nature* 389:610–14
182. Vozarova B, Stefan N, Lindsay RS, Krakoff J, Knowler WC, et al. 2002. Low plasma adiponectin concentrations

do not predict weight gain in humans. *Diabetes* 51:2964–67

182a. Wabitsch M, Hauner H, Hertrampf M, Muche R, Hay B, et al. 2004. Type II diabetes mellitus and impaired glucose regulation in Caucasian children and adolescents with obesity living in Germany. *Int. J. Obes. Relat. Metab. Disord.* 28:307–13

183. Warren JM, Henry CJ, Simonite V. 2003. Low glycemic index breakfasts and reduced food intake in preadolescent children. *Pediatrics* 112:e414–19

184. Watts K, Beye P, Siafarikas A, Davis EA, Jones TW, et al. 2004. Exercise training normalizes vascular dysfunction and improves central adiposity in obese adolescents. *J. Am. Coll. Cardiol.* 43:1823–27

185. Watts K, Beye P, Siafarikas A, O'Driscoll G, Jones TW, et al. 2004. Effects of exercise training on vascular function in obese children. *J. Pediatr.* 144: 620–25

186. Weigensberg MJ, Ball G, Shaibi GQ, Cruz ML, Goran MI. 2004. Overweight Latino children meeting new diagnostic criteria for impaired fasting glucose (IFG) have decreased beta-cell function. *Obes. Res.* 12:A120;467-P (Abstr.)

187. Weiss R, Dufour S, Groszmann A, Petersen K, Dziura J, et al. 2003. Low adiponectin levels in adolescent obesity: a marker of increased intramyocellular lipid accumulation. *J. Clin. Endocrinol. Metab.* 88:2014–18

188. Weiss R, Dziura J, Burgert TS, Tamborlane WV, Taksali SE, et al. 2004. Obesity and the metabolic syndrome in children and adolescents. *N. Engl. J. Med.* 350:2362–74

189. Weyer C, Bogardus C, Mott DM, Pratley RE. 1999. The natural history of insulin secretory dysfunction and insulin resistance in the pathogenesis of type 2 diabetes mellitus. *J. Clin. Invest.* 104:787–94

189a. Wiegand S, Maikowski U, Blankenstein O, Biebermann H, Tarnow P, Gruters A. 2004. Type 2 diabetes and impaired glucose tolerance in European children and adolescents with obesity—a problem that is no longer restricted to minority groups. *Eur. J. Endocrinol.* 151:199–206

190. Wild S, Pierpoint T, McKeigue P, Jacobs H. 2000. Cardiovascular disease in women with polycystic ovary syndrome at long-term follow-up: a retrospective cohort study. *Clin. Endocrinol. (Oxf.)* 52:595–600

191. Zhang Y, Proenca R, Maffel M, Barone M, Leopold L, Friedman JM. 1994. Position cloning of the mouse obese gene and its human homologue. *Nature* 372:425–32

Annu. Rev. Nutr. 2005. 25:469–97
doi: 10.1146/annurev.nutr.25.050304.092514

First published online as a Review in Advance on May 4, 2005

ANNUAL LIPID CYCLES IN HIBERNATORS: Integration of Physiology and Behavior

John Dark
Department of Psychology, University of California, Berkeley, California 94720-1650; email: johndark@berkeley.edu

Key Words white adipose tissue, brown adipose tissue, energy balance, thermoregulation, circannual rhythms

■ **Abstract** Mammalian hibernation is a temporary suspension of euthermia allowing endotherms to undergo reversible hypothermia and generate a marked savings in energy expenditure. In most fat-storing hibernator species, seasonal changes in food intake, triacylglycerol deposition, metabolism, and reproductive development are controlled by a circannual clock. In ground-dwelling sciurid rodents (ground squirrels and marmots), for example, energy intake increases during a summer body mass gain phase, and toward the end of this phase metabolic rate also begins to decrease, resulting in a profound increase in lipid deposition as fat. Increased activity of lipogenic hormones and enzymes correspond with this increase. The hibernation mass loss phase begins after the body mass peak in the fall and ends in spring. During this phase, stored lipids are slowly utilized in a programmed manner by undergoing deep torpor or hibernation during which the hypothalamic setpoint for body temperature is typically reduced to just above 0°C. Throughout the hibernation season, bouts of deep torpor are punctuated by periodic arousals in which brown adipose tissue thermogenesis plays a critical role. Lipid oxidation nearly exclusively fuels deep torpor and most of the rewarming process. The fatty acid composition of stored lipids can affect the depth and duration of deep torpor, and saturated fatty acids may be preferentially used during hibernation, whereas polyunsaturated fatty acids may be preferentially retained. Female and underweight male hibernators terminate hibernation in spring when aboveground food becomes available; in contrast, heavier males with sufficient lipid reserves spontaneously terminate hibernation several weeks before females and independent of food availability. Mating occurs shortly after emergence from hibernation, and the lipid cycle begins again with the completion of reproduction. Lipid deposition and mobilization, temperature regulation, reproduction, and circannual timing are intimately interdependent. The unique manner in which they are controlled during the annual cycle, especially lipid reserves, makes hibernators valuable and promising models for research into the mechanisms underlying these processes in all mammals.

CONTENTS

INTRODUCTION

> It was the best of times, it was the worst of times . . . it was the season of Light, it was the season of Darkness, it was the spring of hope, it was the winter of despair, we had everything before us, we had nothing before us. . . .
>
> (Charles Dickens, *A Tale of Two Cities*)

These familiar lines at the beginning of the Dickens classic could just as well be the first lines of a text on environmental physiology entitled *A Tale of Two Seasons*. For animals living in temperate or more extreme latitudes, summer is a period of plenty, with moderate temperatures and a bounty of food. Winter, on the other hand, can be bitter, with reduced temperatures and decreased food availability and/or quality. Organisms living in such an environment are faced with the challenge of how to take advantage of a summer of abundance yet survive or, better still, avoid the harsh demands of winter.

BACKGROUND

Definition of Hibernation

Most mammalian species are homeothermic, i.e., they more or less always remain euthermic (i.e., body temperature = 35°C–37°C). Hibernating mammals periodically abandon homeothermy in favor of heterothermy, in which body temperature (T_b) may be reduced to nearly 0°C, then returned to euthermia without ill effect—a degree of hypothermia lethal to most mammals, including humans. T_b decreases to close to T_a, typically as low as 2°C–3°C in ground squirrels and marmots (107, but see 11). T_b, heart rate, breathing, and metabolic rate (MR) are all profoundly reduced during hibernation (30, 69, 107). Fat-storing hibernators generally remain in their burrows or dens throughout winter, and hibernation has been estimated to provide a savings of ~85% over the energetic cost of remaining euthermic during the entire hibernation season (see, e.g., 3).

Reversible hypothermia most likely evolved independently in several mammalian groups (see, e.g., 21, 69) as a de novo adaptation and represents an extension of temperature regulation around a new low T_b setpoint, possibly an extension of the circadian decrease in T_b during deep, slow-wave sleep (for a review, see 82). The apparent central regulation of T_b during hibernation suggests that mammalian hibernation is not the re-emergence of a more primitive or reptilian form of thermoregulation (105).

Most fat-storing hibernators continue to undergo cycles in body mass, food consumption, and reproduction despite being housed in the laboratory under constant conditions of light, temperature, etc. (reviewed in 151). The annual changes persist, but their timing only approximates a year; the duration or period of each animal's circannual rhythm (e.g., days from peak body mass to peak body mass) is unique. One animal may have a period of 320 days, and the animal in the adjacent cage a 370-day cycle. After two years in the laboratory, the circannual cycles of these two hibernators will be ~100 days, or more than three months, out of phase. The fact that 20 animals in the same room express circannual cycles with 20 different periods implies generation by an endogenous circannual clock. The evidence for an endogenous circannual clock is overwhelming; nevertheless, its neural substrate has yet to be identified (see 151). Although the rhythm persists in constant conditions, its period is adjusted to ~365 days by the natural progression of daylight duration in the spring and summer after constant darkness during winter (103).

Scope

This review focuses primarily on annual lipid cycles in fat-storing ground squirrels and marmots because of my own bias and their prominence in the literature (for a recent review on food-storing hibernators, see 90).

ANNUAL CYCLES IN FOOD INGESTION, FAT STORAGE, HIBERNATION, AND REPRODUCTION

It is practically impossible to discuss one of these four functions without considering its interaction with the others. The annual cycle of a typical hibernator, such as the golden-mantled ground squirrel (*Spermophilus lateralis*), has several characteristic phases: (*a*) a body mass gain phase typically is initiated during the spring or summer after reproductive activity is completed; (*b*) a body mass loss phase begins in late summer or fall, depending on latitude or altitude, and is characterized by the animals' immergence into burrows and onset of hibernation; and (*c*) a reproductive phase, which generally produces a single litter each year, begins with emergence from hibernation in the spring. Hibernation invariably is accompanied by body mass loss.

BODY MASS GAIN PHASE

Body Mass Gain is not Simply a Consequence of Increased Food Intake

A neural mechanism appears to control or regulate the deposition and mobilization of lipid stores in white adipose tissue (WAT) around a preferred level (see 38, 108, 122). This in turn presumes the availability of a feedback signal from WAT to the brain sufficiently accurate to reflect total body fat reserves. Regulation of WAT mass has been a point of contention in research on obesity and ingestive behavior, as well as hibernation, for decades. Some of the most convincing evidence for centrally mediated body fat regulation comes from heterothermic species in which WAT mass progressively changes over the course of the annual cycle (see 109).

The increases in fat stores during the body mass gain phase can be quite remarkable. Golden-mantled ground squirrels double their body mass and triple their fat mass (97). Despite its larger size, the arctic ground squirrel also doubles body mass and in a much shorter active season (four months active, eight months hibernating) (67). Plasma lipids mimic the changes in fat reserves during the body mass gain phase (88). Plasma lipids in both males and females are decreasing at emergence from hibernation and continue to decrease until fattening begins. Males start fattening after mating and plasma lipids and fatty acid (FA) synthesis coincidently increase (20, 88). Although female body mass increases during pregnancy and lactation, FA synthesis and plasma lipids continue to decrease until the young are weaned and fat deposition commences, up to seven weeks later than males (88).

Annual Changes in Lipids of Hibernators are Generally Circannual

Peak body mass of juvenile ground squirrels is only two-thirds that of adults (91), exemplifying the challenge for young to both grow and lay down adequate fat reserves. Although their body mass is lower than that of adults before the initial hibernation season, linear or skeletal growth is completed during the first body mass gain phase (32, 94). The initial body mass peak is significantly lower than the second peak, even under presumably optimal laboratory conditions (43). Increased second-year body mass represents a programmed increase in fat deposition (12%) and fat-free dry mass (15%) (43). During the second mass gain phase, neither total subcutaneous WAT mass nor subcutaneous adipocyte number increases. Both WAT mass and fat cell number increase in abdominal fat from the first to second body mass peak. Perhaps because of its insulative value in low T_as, subcutaneous WAT achieves its full mass and cellularity during the first mass gain phase, whereas final maturity of abdominal WAT depots is delayed one year.

Circannual Interaction of Food Intake and Metabolic Rate

Peak body and fat mass and peak food intake do not occur concomitantly, as is also the case for minimum body and fat mass and food intake (see 35). Food consumption peaks and begins to decrease well before body mass maxima are achieved. This counterintuitive outcome derives from the systematic decreases in metabolic rate during the body mass gain phase. Over the course of the year, the oxygen (O_2) consumption, food intake, and body mass cycles are slightly out of phase (5, 145). In spring, O_2 consumption increases before the spring increase in food intake, accounting for continued decreases in body mass after food intake begins to increase. Similarly, MR begins decreasing by midsummer, several weeks before food intake declines, thereby enhancing late lipid deposition by shifting the energy balance equation toward energy surfeit. Although all three processes are ultimately controlled by the endogenous circannual clock, body fat mass control is the critical function and the other two are likely subservient to its maintenance at a prescribed level.

Metabolic rate of European hedgehogs housed at constant T_a progressively decreases from June to October, but respiratory quotient (RQ) remains steady at a value indicative of the mixed oxidation of carbohydrate and FAs (132). Similarly, from midwinter to spring, hedgehogs housed at a low T_a increase their minimum MR during deep torpor; again RQ remains constant but at 0.72, a value indicating nearly 100% FA oxidation. Marmots and ground squirrels undergo a comparable decrease in euthermic MR during mass gain, decreasing MR by nearly half at the end of the weight-gain phase (8, 135); insectivorous bats even undergo daily torpor to enhance fat deposition before the hibernation season (131). Circannual changes in MR explain the discrepancies between circannual changes in food intake and body mass, and reduced MR at the end of mass gain may function to exaggerate the critical deposition of stored lipids for hibernation.

Changes in Lipogenic Factors During Body Mass Gain

Male ground squirrels emerge from hibernation with residual fat stores that are lost during the first few weeks of aboveground activity, whereas females emerge at their body mass nadir (see, e.g., 22, 93). In the field, maximum mass occurs in both sexes in late summer–early fall, when male plasma insulin concentrations also peak (22). Female insulin concentrations peak during pregnancy and lactation and remain elevated until peak body mass is achieved. Adequate glucocorticoids provide a necessary permissive anabolic effect for insulin's lipogenic actions (see 22); adrenal glucocorticoids also increase over the mass gain phase, peaking with body mass. In the laboratory, plasma insulin concentrations in fasted yellow-bellied marmots (*Marmota flaviventris*) change little during the annual cycle except during the final weeks of mass gain, when fasting plasma insulin concentrations nearly double (56). Insulin responsiveness to exogenous dextrose, on the other hand, progressively increases throughout the mass gain phase, peaking as body mass peaks; dextrose-induced insulin release remains consistently low during mass loss (56, 137). Interestingly, when insulin concentrations are highest at peak mass, glucose absorption is lowest, indicating adipocyte insensitivity to insulin at the body mass maximum. Insulin concentrations and insulin responsiveness progressively increase during lipid deposition in hibernators and correspond to a shift toward lipogenesis until peak WAT lipid stores are attained and adipocytes become insulin resistant.

Whether adipocytes are lipogenic or lipolytic is a product of shifts in the balance between those factors that promote fat storage (e.g., insulin) versus those that promote energy liberation (e.g., norepinephrine). This balance is then reflected in the ratio of lipogenic enzymes [e.g., lipoprotein lipase (LPL)] to lipolytic enzymes [e.g., hormone-sensitive lipase (HSL)]. A shift to a preponderance of lipogenic factors generally occurs when energy intake exceeds energy expenditure and lipolytic factors usually prevail during negative energy balance. During mass gain in marmots, the ratio of HSL mRNA concentrations (and presumably HSL activity) to LPL mRNA concentrations favors lipogenesis, coinciding with profound fat deposition (147). Fatty acid synthase (FAS), and presumably FA synthesis, increases in WAT, brown adipose tissue (BAT), and liver during body mass gain, peaking at peak mass; FAS activity was highest in liver, moderate in WAT, and lowest in BAT (118, 144). WAT fatty acid CoA ligase, representing the first step in triacylglycerol (TG) synthesis from FA, and another enzyme in TG synthesis, diacylglycerol acetyltransferase (DGAT), follow the same pattern as FAS, increasing in WAT from minimal values in hibernation to maximal values during mass gain. Although hepatic and BAT CoA ligase are moderately high during mass gain, they are much higher during hibernation (see below) (118), possibly reflecting reconversion into TG of the excess FAs liberated by the marked sympathetic activity during arousal from hibernation (see below). When fat deposition is at its greatest, factors for hepatic and WAT FA synthesis and TG synthesis markedly increase.

Although marmot monoacylglycerol acetyltransferase (MGAT) activity—another enzyme involved in TG synthesis—is comparatively low in WAT and BAT relative to liver, it increases significantly during mass gain (118). MGAT activity was 80 times higher in liver than in WAT or BAT and evidenced no annual variation. Because of MGAT's unique properties that specifically retain polyunsaturated fatty acids in TGs, this enzyme is discussed in detail in the "Hibernation" section below.

Programmed Changes in Lipid Mass

The prodigious fat deposition during the mass gain phase is not simply the product of hyperphagia and/or decreased MR, but rather represents a programmed change in the preferred level of WAT lipid reserves. Several lines of evidence support this contention. Temporary restricted access to food does not prevent projected increases in body mass. Ground squirrels food-deprived for 2–3 days overeat when food is returned and accumulate weight at a more rapid rate than previously until they catch up to the body mass extrapolated from their previous rate of increase (15). Trapping ground squirrels in the field regularly and holding them for part of each day (without food) limits their foraging time and they lose body mass (7). This mass loss represents a decrease in lean mass, but fat mass remains unchanged from that of unrestricted squirrels. In the laboratory, ground squirrels fed a daily ration of food comparable to their daily intake at their spring nadir (which produces marked mass loss at one time of year) undergo a significant mass gain phase even though peak mass is less than that of freely feeding squirrels (35, 38). Although peak body mass is reduced, total abdominal WAT mass is not different from that of freely feeding squirrels. In other words, caloric intake that results in negative energy balance and mass loss during one phase is sufficient for positive energy balance and fat deposition comparable to controls during another phase. Presumably, MR is sufficiently changed to compensate for reduced caloric intake. Circannual increases in preferred WAT mass level appear paramount and circannual changes in ingestion and metabolism more labile.

Although brain lesions that produce obesity in laboratory rats also substantially increase body mass in hibernators, circannual changes in body mass persist. For example, ablation of the ventromedial nucleus of the hypothalamus (VMH) produces a significant increase in peak body mass; however, trough body mass is essentially unaffected (15, 119, 120). VMH ablation shifts body fat mass at its peak upward without otherwise affecting its programmed circannual changes. Ablation of the paraventricular nucleus of the hypothalamus, which can also produce obesity, altered neither peak body mass nor circannual body mass changes (44).

Direct manipulation of WAT mass also supports the concept of programmed changes in preferred WAT mass. Surgical excision of a substantial quantity of WAT (~30 g) from the inguinal subcutaneous depot and retroperitoneal and gonadal abdominal fat depots during mass gain (or mass loss) is quickly recovered (37). Regardless of whether WAT is ablated during mass gain or loss, body mass is quickly restored to a value appropriate to that extrapolated from its previous pattern of mass change. Peak body mass was unaffected when as much inguinal, retroperitoneal, and gonadal fat as feasible was extirpated four months earlier (36). Total lipid mass was identical to that of intact squirrels and was restored without compensatory increases in food intake. Ablated gonadal fat was not recovered; gonadal WAT mass was only ~15% that of normal and total gonadal adipocyte number was reduced by ~85%. Retroperitoneal WAT, on the other hand, differed in neither mass, adipocyte number, nor adipocyte size between treatments; presumably, excised adipocytes completely regenerated and matured in this depot. Total subcutaneous fat (measures of individual subcutaneous depots are not feasible at peak mass because all subcutaneous fat becomes contiguous) was significantly heavier in lipectomized squirrels. Although total subcutaneous fat cell number was comparable in lipectomized and intact animals, fat cell size from the inguinal WAT region was 25% greater and from the dorsal WAT region was 19% greater than corresponding adipocytes of intact squirrels (36). Ground squirrels quickly recover WAT mass after lipectomy, without increasing food intake, by complete regeneration of retroperitoneal adipocytes and a mix of adipocyte hyperplasia and hypertrophy in subcutaneous WAT (cf. 36, 38). It appears that the programmed peak lipid mass is still achieved after lipectomy despite lack of recovery in gonadal WAT, presumably by compensatory changes in MR and regionally specific changes in adipocyte cellularity.

Leptin and Hibernators

A requirement for regulating WAT mass, especially at an annually changing level, is a feedback signal accurately reflecting total body lipid stores. A sufficiently accurate feedback signal(s) from WAT to the CNS allowing subtle changes in energy balance (food intake and/or MR) to appropriately maintain WAT mass has not yet been identified in hibernators; however, the peptide, leptin, may provide such feedback. Chronic leptin levels provide an accurate WAT feedback signal to the CNS in a number of species (for reviews, see 1, 127, 142). Exogenous leptin decreases food intake and body mass in ground squirrels (23, 124) as in laboratory animals. The few studies of leptin concentrations and lipid mass have yielded contradictory results. During prehibernatory body mass gain of the little brown bat, the usual relation between increased WAT mass and increased leptin does not appear to hold. Circulating leptin levels increase before body mass and decrease as body mass increases to its peak (100). Leptin may be dissociated from WAT mass during hibernation because leptin increases energy expenditure; therefore, leptin may be dissociated to permit decreased MR during maximum fat deposition and, subsequently, deep torpor (100). Indeed, high leptin titers inhibit shallow, daily torpor expression in several species (64, 74). Leptin concentrations, on the other hand, closely follow circannual changes in body mass in woodchucks held at a room temperature (20°C–23°C) that prevents hibernation (34). The relation between leptin and the annual lipid cycle and hibernation remains an open question.

BODY MASS LOSS PHASE

Because the annual mass loss phase is coincident with hibernation, programmed changes in lipid metabolism are discussed primarily with relation to hibernation.

Little is known of the programmed progression of WAT changes during mass loss in the field because the animals are inaccessible after immergence into their burrows. Nevertheless, mass loss is apparent upon emergence in the spring. For example, golden-mantled ground squirrels appear aboveground with little or no fat reserves in males and females (see, e.g., 24, 93), whereas in the larger Belding's ground squirrel both males and females emerge with considerable lipid reserves (88, 116). Larger hibernators emerge from hibernation with more substantial fat reserves, presumably their reduced rate of conductance and heat loss resulting from their decreased surface-to-volume ratio also reduces their rate of mass loss (see, e.g., 67, 118). Typically, food consumption in nonhibernating animals during body mass loss phase progressively decreases, reaching minimum intake 2–4 weeks before trough body mass (5, 35, 145); i.e., body and lipid mass continue decreasing even after food intake begins to increase. During body mass loss under optimal conditions of food availability and a T_a of ~23°C, nearly all loss represents decreased lipid mass (~85%); neither water, protein, nor ash mass decrease during mass loss (43). The mass of individual fat depots successively decrease at the same rate, and these decreases in lipid mass are entirely mirrored in proportional decreases in adipocyte size (43). Hibernators do not have access to water in their hibernacula throughout winter; for the arctic ground squirrel, at least, lipid catabolism liberates sufficient water to maintain proper hydration (67).

Changes in Lipolytic Factors During Body Mass Loss

Pancreatic content of the lipolytic hormone glucagon, unlike insulin, does not decrease during hibernation (18), possibly reflecting glucagon's lipolytic function during periodic arousals from hibernation. During the body mass loss phase, it is presumed that lipolytic enzyme activity increases, shifting the balance between lipolytic and lipogenic enzymes toward lipolysis. Indeed, marmots increase the ratio of HSL mRNA to LPL mRNA concentrations during mass loss (147). Sensitivity of marmot adipocytes to norepinephrine, a norepinephrine agonist, and glucagon, however, were comparable during mass gain and hibernation (33).

Evidence for Programmed Decreases in Body Mass

Body mass forced below its programmed level by food deprivation or by preventing deep torpor rapidly recovers when animals are allowed to eat. Recovery is not to previous levels but instead to a mass appropriate to the stage of the cycle (15, 81, 121). Although time spent torpid was not measured during recovery, it is likely that either food intake or time spent torpid increased, but not both, because digestion is precluded at low T_bs (see 30). Alternatively, a highly palatable diet resets maintained body mass upward slightly, and body mass increases somewhat before resuming its previous loss rate (15). Similarly, obesity-producing VMH lesions during the loss phase produce an immediate small increase in body mass before returning to the same pattern of loss (119). Both treatments shift preferred body mass upward without otherwise affecting programmed circannual changes in body mass.

HIBERNATION

Hibernators Markedly Reduce Metabolic Rate

The reduction in MR during deep torpor is remarkable. O_2 consumption at T_bs approaching 0°C is typically ~5% of euthermic values but can be as low as ~1% (e.g., 30, 69). Hibernation generally provides an energy savings of 80%–85% over expenditures if remaining euthermic (see, e.g., 3, 6, 69). A recent review (69) thoroughly described the several mechanisms proposed to underlie the decrease in metabolism and its energy-saving function. Hibernation is an active process and its initiation is under neuroendocrine control. Because euthermia isolates mammals from thermal effects on cellular metabolism, any mechanism eliciting hibernation must begin with the CNS lowering hypothalamic setpoint for T_b and eliminating thermoregulatory heat production. The primary evidence for the CNS's role in hibernation expression is that T_b is regulated during hibernation but at a very low setpoint (see, e.g., 26, 53, 79, 80, 107); nevertheless, CNS involvement in the initiation, maintenance, and termination of hibernation consistently receives little attention.

A rapid decrease in hypothalamic setpoint for T_b initiates two mechanisms that suppress MR during hibernation: (*a*) a neuroendocrine mechanism inhibiting thermoregulatory thermogenesis and (*b*) a separate mechanism, most likely also under neuroendocrine control, that suppresses cellular metabolism. Hibernation onset occurs during sleep and its concomitant decrease in T_b; however, T_b continues to progressively decrease, rapidly reaching a new lowered setpoint (53, 79, 80), often near 0°C (11, 26, 70, 72). The primacy of the change in hypothalamic setpoint is evident from the decrease in MR prior to any observable decrease in T_b (3, 69, 104, 125).

The sympathetic branch of the autonomic nervous system activates the organism. Increasing sympathetic activity enhances heart rate, respiration, blood flow, etc., which are counterproductive to hibernation; it was proposed to be an important function in hibernation nearly 30 years ago (140). Sympathetic neural activity also is the primary mediator of BAT nonshivering thermogenesis (NST) as well as WAT lipolysis (e.g., 9, 16, 29). Sympathetic activity suppression remains an important step in hibernation onset, especially as a means for "turning off" thermogenic heat production.

Lipid is the Primary Metabolic Fuel During Deep Torpor

Plasma metabolic fuel concentrations provide circumstantial evidence as to which fuel(s) may be the source of cellular oxidation during hibernation, reduced as it may be. Glucose is a major source of cellular energy in nonfasted animals; however, in the absence of food intake, the only sources of glucose are liver and muscle glycogen stores and glucose produced via gluconeogenesis. Because glycogen stores are very limited and gluconeogenesis from glycerol is inefficient, the required gluconeogenesis from amino acids would result in overwhelming muscle wasting if glucose were the primary metabolic fuel. Although capacity for gluconeogenesis from amino acids is increased during hibernation (28), there is little evidence of muscle wasting during hibernation (see, e.g., 107). It is likely, therefore, that non-carbohydrate fuels comprise most of the energy utilized during hibernation. Plasma glucose concentrations in ground squirrels and marmots remain remarkably stable at unchanged or elevated levels throughout a hibernation bout (55, 99, 123, 134, 139). In hibernating hedgehogs and dormice, glucose concentrations also are stable but at somewhat reduced levels (31, 98). Radiolabeled glucose incorporation into CO_2 is markedly suppressed during hibernation (134), and plasma lactate concentrations are correspondingly decreased during deep torpor (123, 150); both are indications of reduced glucose oxidation. Glycogen reserves may actually increase during deep torpor, which suggests that they may be preserved during deep torpor for a possibly critical role during arousal (107, 150). Additionally, a number of enzymes critical for glycolytic activity (e.g., pyruvate dehydrogenase and pyruvate phosphofructokinase) appear to be actively suppressed during hibernation (25, 27), a finding that supports this contention. Although glycolysis may be actively inhibited, this effect is reversible because carbohydrate oxidation can increase during deep torpor if an animal is energetically challenged (26). In addition, ketone bodies (β–hydroxybutyrate and acetoacetate) are a byproduct of hepatic oxidation of FA and can be utilized as metabolic fuel in several organs, especially the brain, during energetic challenge. Ketone concentrations are substantially elevated during deep torpor (99, 123, 126) and appear to contribute to glucose sparing during deep torpor by inhibiting glucose uptake by muscle (99). Ketones also may be actively preserved during hibernation.

The fact that most hibernators deposit considerable quantities of fat during the summer mass-gain phase and that this fat is subsequently lost during the hibernation phase is a priori evidence that stored lipids are the primary fuel during hibernation. Nevertheless, this is not evident from plasma FA concentrations during hibernation, which in ground squirrels do not appear to differ from euthermic values (99, 123), but are reduced during hibernation in hedgehogs (98). Triacylglycerol concentrations, in contrast, markedly decrease during deep torpor (123). Measures of metabolite concentrations during hibernation support the conclusion that lipids are the primary fuel.

RQ values calculated from measurements of O_2 consumption and CO_2 production during hibernation provide convincing evidence that FA oxidation nearly exclusively fuels deep torpor. RQ values vary from 0.7, representing nearly 100% FA oxidation, to 1.0, representing nearly 100% carbohydrate oxidation. Invariably, RQ during deep torpor is $\sim$0.7, indicative of nearly pure FA oxidation (see, e.g., 106, 114, 130, 133). The limited cellular metabolism during deep torpor, therefore, is fueled by FA oxidation.

T_b is regulated during deep torpor, and if T_a is reduced sufficiently below the T_b setpoint, MR must increase to maintain T_b. Increased MR at T_as $< \sim 0°C$ increases RQ from 0.7, indicating an increase in carbohydrate (i.e., glucose) utilization (26). There may be a limit on FA availability for oxidation at low temperatures such that increased O_2 consumption necessitates carbohydrate oxidation. If there are limits to FA availability at low temperatures, then FAs may not be mobilized by lipolysis during deep torpor. The enzyme pancreatic triacylglycerol lipase, found in pancreas of nonhibernators, is also expressed in heart and WAT of hibernating ground squirrels (17, 132). This enzyme may be able to mediate lipolysis during hibernation because it appears to continue functioning at very low temperatures without hormonal control. In this case, pancreatic triacylglycerol lipase–mediated lipolysis may be a slow source of FAs during deep torpor. This would seem to suggest that FAs can be mobilized during hibernation, but it does not address whether FAs actually are mobilized or whether their rate of mobilization is limited during hibernation.

There is little or no unstimulated glycerol release from hibernating jerboa or ground squirrel WAT incubated in vitro at 5°C–7°C, indicating that unstimulated lipolysis at T_bs characteristic of deep torpor is markedly suppressed (40, 115). Norepinephrine-stimulated glycerol release from WAT adipocytes in vitro also is nearly nonexistent at low tissue temperatures. Glycerol release from WAT continues to be suppressed until temperature exceeds ~15°C, then increases as temperature increases (40, 115). In addition, norepinephrine-stimulated glycerol release from BAT tissue of hibernating ground squirrels in vitro is nearly nil at 5°C (40). Although this suggests that BAT lipolysis may be suppressed at low temperatures, it has no bearing on the efficacy of norepinephrine to induce BAT NST, which presumably is unaffected at these same temperatures. Epinephrine-stimulated glycerol release of WAT in situ, as measured by microdialysis, also is markedly reduced during hibernation (52). It appears that spontaneous as well as neuroendocrine-stimulated lipolysis is inhibited at low temperatures characteristic of hibernation. A mechanism may exist capable of mediating lipolysis in WAT at very low temperatures, but any lipolysis that occurs at these T_bs is minimal because at $T_a <$ 0°C the increased MR necessary to maintain T_b is supported by an increase in carbohydrate, not lipid, oxidation (26).

Lipid Composition Affects Hibernation

Metabolic energy during hibernation is derived primarily from lipid stored in WAT in the form of TGs, which are composed of a single glycerol molecule and three FA molecules. The nature of the FAs comprising TG in WAT is variable and somewhat dependent upon diet. Although mammals can synthesize saturated fatty acids (SFAs) and monounsaturated (MUFAs) fatty acids de novo, they cannot synthesize polyunsaturated fatty acids (PUFAs). Many plants synthesize PUFAs, thus providing a readily available source of essential fatty acids, i.e., PUFAs that are necessary but not synthesized in the body. The presence of PUFAs in the WAT TG of hibernating ground-dwelling squirrels must come through dietary intake of plants containing PUFAs (57, 59). The most prevalent PUFA in plants consumed by hibernating ground-dwelling squirrels is linoleic fatty acid (see, e.g., 57, 60). Because T_bs during deep torpor are frequently as low as 1°C–3°C, or 20°C–25°C below the melting point of typical mammalian lipids, the relation between low T_bs and loss of lipid fluidity in WAT, as well as cellular membranes, is a long-standing issue (see 2, 68, 107). Lipid fluidity depends on degree of saturation of its composite FAs, therefore TG's melting point decreases as PUFA content increases (68). Increasing PUFA content of WAT in ground squirrels and marmots typically reduces WAT's melting point to 0°C to −5°C (63). Cell membranes are known to undergo structural changes prior to hibernation, presumably to maintain fluidity (see, e.g., 2, 107), but WAT TGs also would have to retain fluidity or lipolysis and mobilization of energy from stored lipids would be negatively affected at low T_bs (see, e.g., 63, 68), even if lipolysis is restricted to T_bs > 15°C.

Experiments on hibernating yellow pine chipmunks illustrate pronounced effects of lipid PUFA content on deep torpor (68, 71, 75). Diets supplemented with sunflower seed oil (high in PUFAs) consistently increase chipmunk hibernation bout duration over a range of low T_as (and T_bs), especially relative to those fed a diet supplemented with sheep fat (high in SFAs). On all measures, hibernation bouts of chipmunks fed the standard diet were at intermediate values at each T_a. The SFA diet increased O_2 consumption nearly twofold over that of PUFA-fed chipmunks; decreased metabolism was a consequence of the lower T_b in high-PUFA-fed animals. Slowly lowering T_a to determine minimum T_b ($T_{b\ min}$) before animals require increased MR to maintain T_b results in a $T_{b\ min}$ of SFA-fed chipmunks nearly fourfold higher than that of PUFA-fed chipmunks. PUFAs, in other words, lower T_b setpoint during hibernation, which decreases MR, thereby increasing torpor bout duration and ultimately reducing total energy expenditure.

In both the field and laboratory, three FAs comprise ~95% of the FAs found in ground-dwelling squirrel diets and their WAT lipids: palmitic, oleic, and linoleic FAs—an SFA, an MUFA, and a PUFA, respectively (see, e.g., 57, 60). MUFA and PUFA contents in WAT are comparable and proportionally greater than SFA content. PUFA intake occurs primarily in the final month prior to hibernation (see, e.g., 61). Diets high in PUFAs similarly affect hibernation in golden-mantled ground squirrels, yellow-bellied marmots, and black- and white-tailed prairie dogs (54, 59–61, 63, 73, 77). The most prevalent PUFA in plants available to hibernators is linoleic acid, and a diet increased in only linoleic acid content is sufficient to generate increases in torpor bout duration and reduced T_b (59). When offered diets varying in PUFA content, ground squirrels choose diets higher in PUFA content. Dietary preference for PUFAs, however, is controlled. Hibernators prefer a diet moderately high in PUFAs nearly threefold to one very high in PUFAs; if offered two diets, one very high in PUFAs and one very low in PUFA content, they consume approximately equal quantities of each. Total PUFA intake was equivalent in the two experiments and nearly comparable to PUFA content of animals in the field (62).

In contrast to diets reduced in PUFAs or higher in SFAs, diets higher in PUFAs enhance deep torpor. Surprisingly, hibernators fed a diet lacking PUFAs continue to hibernate, although $T_{b\ min}$ is increased and consequently torpor duration is nearly halved (54, 135). MR during deep torpor was significantly increased in PUFA-deficient animals, concomitantly increasing total energy expenditure during hibernation. Shortened torpor durations in PUFA-deficient animals negatively affect fat reserves, causing an accelerated rate of mass loss during the hibernation season. In other words, a hibernator whose diet is deficient in PUFAs during mass gain may maintain T_b only somewhat higher than normal animals, but will arouse from deep torpor nearly twice as often. Periodic arousals consume ~85%–90% of energy expended during the hibernation season; therefore, doubling the number of arousals is costly, increasing total energy utilization and jeopardizing overwinter survival, especially in males (see below).

Unlimited increases in WAT PUFA content do not necessarily translate into increases in depth and duration of torpor. Excessive dietary PUFA content contrarily increases $T_{b\ min}$ and decreases hibernation bout duration in the same manner as insufficient PUFAs (63). There appears to be an optimal level of dietary PUFAs, and animals will modify their dietary PUFA intake to achieve it. When offered diets varying in PUFA content, ground squirrels proportionally consume the diets such that total PUFA intake is within an optimal window (see 62). In addition, a rose may still be a rose, but a PUFA is not necessarily a PUFA. The predominant PUFA obtained from plants is linoleic acid (a diene, 18:2); however, hibernators in the field also typically possess measurable quantities of linolenic acid (a triene, 18:3). Supplementing diet with linseed oil, which increases WAT linolenic acid and concomitantly decreases WAT linoleic acid content, eliminates hibernation (83). Marmots remain euthermic and continue to feed throughout winter. Presumably, increased linolenic acids, and not reduced linoleic acid, somehow prevent hibernation because PUFA-deficient diets do not eliminate hibernation.

Increased linoleic acid content may be sufficient to improve hibernation parameters, but it may not be necessary. Increasing dietary MUFA content, for example, produces improvements in torpor duration and $T_{b\ min}$ comparable to a diet increased in linoleic acid content (75). Unsaturation of fatty acids is the key to lowering lipid melting point; thus, MUFA as well as PUFA content may affect hypothalamic setpoint for T_b, lowering $T_{b\ min}$s and improving chances for overwinter survival and successful reproduction. In fact, some propose that MUFAs sustain most of the improved hibernation characteristics; PUFAs only provide minor improvements (see, e.g., 51). Utilization of PUFAs during deep torpor has a downside, which would seem to jibe with this proposal. PUFAs have a greater propensity for peroxidation (auto-oxidation) than do either SFAs or MUFAs, and increasing PUFA content increases peroxidation rate. Additionally, deep torpor increases the rate of peroxidation, and the peroxides formed by this self-sustaining process are cellular toxins (see, e.g., 62). Although hibernators appear to markedly increase cellular antioxidants (e.g., ascorbate) during hibernation (48, 136), hibernators increase PUFA intake in a limited fashion, presumably in a trade-off of its beneficial versus detrimental consequences during hibernation (see 62). Peroxidation also may explain the reduced torpor bout duration after animals ingest diets containing excessive PUFAs, especially those with high linolenic acid content.

Hibernators appear to retain PUFAs specifically, preferentially oxidizing SFAs and MUFAs during hibernation. WAT composition changes across the hibernation season based upon FA saturation: The proportion of SFAs decreases, the proportion of MUFAs remains constant, and most interestingly, the proportion of PUFAs increases (54, 57). Venous blood exiting gonadal WAT contains proportionally more SFAs than found in gonadal WAT at that time, and proportionally less linoleic acid is in gonadal venous blood than is found in gonadal WAT (57). There is a primary utilization of SFAs, secondary utilization of MUFAs, and specific retention of PUFAs. Whether this occurs to retain the hibernation-enhancing effects of PUFAs or to exclude the negative effects of PUFA peroxidation is unknown. Animals undergoing exclusive FA oxidation (e.g., neonatal rats, chick embryos, and hibernators) evidence a secondary pathway for TG synthesis involving monoacylglycerol acetyltransferase (MGAT) primarily in the liver (118, 149). Hepatic MGAT concentrations in marmots, for example, are 80-fold greater than concentrations found in either WAT or BAT. MGAT acylates and accumulates monoacylglycerols containing PUFAs, specifically resulting in the retention of PUFAs in TG. MGAT therefore serves to retain PUFAs selectively in the face of increased lipolytic activity over prolonged periods. Regardless of the mechanism responsible for its original development, in hibernators this pathway retains PUFAs for their hibernation-facilitating effect while simultaneously reducing PUFA availability for possible toxic peroxide formation.

Arousal from Hibernation

One minimum requirement for successful hibernation is that the animal must be able to return to euthermia (i.e., rewarm). Mammalian hibernators arouse not just in spring as ectothermic hibernators do, but also periodically throughout the hibernation season. The occurrence of these periodic rewarmings probably represents the public's most common misunderstanding about hibernation. This erroneous concept evidences itself frequently in popular entertainment, everything from the spectacular *2001: A Space Odyssey* to the campy *Planet of the Apes.* In a favorite moment from the original *Star Trek* television series, Captain Kirk awakens a naughty Ricardo Montalban from centuries of continuous deep hibernation only to have him raise hell everywhere. This example is whimsical; nevertheless, it raises several relevant questions. For instance, if we ever can place humans into deep torpor for space travel or, more likely, for medical reasons (e.g., while they await a suitable organ for transplant), will they need to periodically arouse?

The duration of hibernation before a spontaneous arousal varies regularly from several days to several weeks (70), and the duration of the period of euthermia in fat-storing species is consistent and fairly short, typically $<$24 hours (see 30, 69, 107). Periodic arousals are energetically expensive; $\sim$85%–90% of a hibernator's energy budget during the hibernation season is used to fuel these periodic rewarmings to euthermia (see, e.g., 92, 143). Because it is so energetically costly to rewarm, frequent periodic arousals from hibernation appear contradictory and suggest that their occurrence is mandatory. Presumably, critical processes or functions that must be periodically restored at euthermic temperatures for the organism's survival necessitate spontaneous arousals. Functions that have been proposed to underlie spontaneous rewarming include renal function, restorative sleep, and most recently, neural memory functions (see 90 for a review). In light of the myriad critical processes that are suppressed at T_bs < ~15°C, including immune responsiveness, transcription, translation, renal function, and even norepinephrine-induced lipolysis, it is more than likely that no single cause is responsible for spontaneous arousals during the hibernation season (see, e.g., 90). There is a long-standing relation, nonetheless, that suggests that the lower the T_a and T_b (up to a point), the longer the hibernation bout (see, e.g., 70, 72, 138, 141). The proposed advantage from consuming adequate dietary PUFAs most likely is the basis for this relation. The resulting reduced $T_{b\ min}$ decreases MR and increases torpor bout duration, and this energy savings is compounded over the course of the hibernation season.

Metabolic fuel utilization during deep torpor represents almost 100% oxidation of FAs as indicated by its characteristic RQ of 0.7. Interestingly, O_2 consumption and CO_2 production during the earliest stage of arousal reveal a shift in RQ and a dramatic shift in metabolic fuel usage. During the initial stage of arousal until T_b increases to ~12°C–16°C, RQ is increased to ~1.0, indicating that carbohydrates comprise the primary fuel for cellular oxidation (see, e.g., 114, 130). At this point, RQ returns to ~0.7 and oxidation primarily of fat for the remainder of arousal. Although some of this most likely represents glycolysis of muscle and liver glycogen reserves, glucose oxidation increases as well. From T_b = 6°C to T_b = 15°C, disappearance of radiolabeled glucose and appearance of labeled CO_2 increase 15-fold over hibernation values, suggesting a marked increase in glucose oxidation (134). Concomitantly, lactate production that was suppressed during hibernation increases eightfold during arousal, also indicating increased glucose oxidation (123). Anti-insulin treatment at the initiation of rewarming produces marked hyperglycemia, signifying that endogenous insulin normally is facilitating glucose uptake and utilization (85). BAT's thermogenic contribution to rewarming is proposed to be paramount during initiation of arousal (see below) and to be dependent on increased insulin concentrations (45, 84, 89, 101). Because norepinephrine-stimulated lipolysis is suppressed at these T_bs (40), insulin-stimulated glucose oxidation may be critical for BAT NST. Indeed, glucose and acetate oxidation in BAT are markedly increased until T_b exceeds ~15°C (95).

Although protein loss is not programmed during the mass loss phase (43), there is some protein loss during hibernation (see, e.g., 67). Plasma free amino acids are not increased during hibernation, but do increase considerably during the later stages of arousal, possibly supporting increased gluconeogenesis for restoration of plasma glucose and muscle and hepatic glycogen reserves utilized during arousal (96, 146). Plasma ketones increase during hibernation (19, 99, 123) and subsequently decrease during arousal (99, 123), especially from T_b = 6°C to T_b = 15°C (19). A few tissues can utilize ketones as metabolic fuel, the most notable being the brain, which may rely on ketones as a substitute fuel during the energy demanding process of rewarming to euthermia. Glucose (including glycogen) and ketone oxidation may markedly increase during torpor initiation; nevertheless, the bulk of arousal remains dependent upon FA oxidation (see, e.g., 130). For example, despite glycerol concentrations increasing nearly fivefold during arousal, ground squirrel plasma FA concentrations actually decrease by 20%, demonstrating both increased lipolysis and increased fatty acid utilization (123). Rewarming to euthermia appears to utilize, if not require, combined glucose, ketone, and fatty acid oxidation.

Neither disruption of glucose oxidation with a low dose of nonmetabolizable glucose analogue, 2-deoxy-D-glucose (2DG), nor interference with FA oxidation by a low dose of mercaptoacetate (MA) affects time to rewarm (41). Injecting the same doses of 2DG and MA simultaneously, on the other hand, increases time required to reach euthermia; a minimum level of total metabolic fuel appears necessary for arousal to proceed at its normal pace. A large dose of MA at torpor initiation does not slow rewarming, but it reduces T_b during subsequent euthermia and often inordinately lengthens periodic arousal (39). If glucose metabolism is critical for the earliest stage of arousal, as appears to be the case, then disrupting glucose oxidation at this time should have a profound effect on the initiation of rewarming. This, indeed, is the case. A large dose of 2DG injected at the time of torpor initiation increases the time required to raise T_b to 15°C by >200% (39).

Time spent torpid throughout the hibernation season was increased by reducing ground squirrel lipid reserves by food restriction at hibernation outset (58). Increased time spent in deep torpor reduced rate of body mass loss and resulted in a total lipid mass in spring comparable to that of unrestricted animals. Surgically reducing total lipid mass by WAT lipectomy resulted in equivocal changes in torpor that were intermediate to that displayed by the food-restricted and normal-mass animals (58). Although lipectomy somewhat increased time in hibernation, body mass decreased at the same rate as that of normal squirrels and total lipid mass in spring was only ~50% of control values. Food restriction reduces lipid mass by decreasing adipocyte size, whereas lipectomy decreases adipocyte number. At room temperatures, lipid mass recovers following lipectomy by pronounced adipocyte hyperplasia in several WAT depots (36); T_bs characteristic of deep torpor preclude cellular proliferation (see 30), presumably including adipocyte hyperplasia and recovery after lipectomy. Increasing lipid mass of juvenile ground squirrels above its regulated level before the hibernation season by access to a high-fat diet produces no compensatory change in time spent torpid between high-fat-fed and chow-fed squirrels; thus, body mass and lipid mass of high-fat-fed juveniles remain elevated in spring (42). The ability of hibernators to undergo compensatory increases (or decreases) in time spent torpid to accommodate energetic challenges detrimental to programmed WAT mass remains little understood.

At some point, a hibernator rewarms from deep torpor and fails to re-enter hibernation. This defines the terminal arousal and the return to homeothermy. Although PUFAs are specifically retained throughout hibernation, resumption of continuous euthermy renders them superfluous and they are mobilized upon terminal arousal (57). The terminal arousal in the spring is followed by resumption of reproduction.

Timing of terminal arousal is shaped by sex and fat reserves, a topic that is discussed below.

Brown Adipose Tissue and Hibernation

Because of its pronounced development in hibernators, there has been a longstanding belief that BAT must be important during hibernation (e.g., 107, 129). In fact, BAT was often referred to as the "hibernating gland." Its importance for hibernation was not realized, however, until BAT's thermogenic mechanism and function as a major heat-producing organ were identified. There are numerous thorough reviews of the thermogenic mechanism underlying NST in BAT (see 29, 97). Briefly, BAT mitochondria have the unique ability to dissociate fuel oxidation from ATP production via uncoupling protein (UCP 1), resulting solely in the generation of heat. UCP 1 concentrations reflect BAT's thermogenic capacity; however, thermogenic activity is more accurately represented by guanosine 5′-diphosphate (GDP) binding in BAT. Surprisingly, UCP 1 content is constant across seasons in ground squirrel BAT; however, both BAT mass and BAT mitochondrial concentration increase during the hibernation season (113). During a deep torpor bout, UCP 1 levels remain elevated but GDP binding is markedly reduced (86, 113, 123). Because UCP 1 concentrations do not differ between deep torpor and arousal, the marked increase in GDP binding during arousal represents an unmasking of binding sites with the onset of arousal (113, 123).

Hibernation appears dependent upon a pronounced suppression of autonomic activity (see 140), and rewarming is characterized by exaggerated sympathetic activity, especially to BAT. BAT's influence during the initial stage of rewarming (until T_b exceeds ~15°C–16°C) is evident from the primacy of increases in BAT temperature over increases in T_b. During initiation of rewarming, BAT temperature increases markedly before T_b increases; in fact, BAT temperature exceeds 30°C before T_b reaches 15°C (87). Although shivering thermogenesis contributes significantly to rewarming from hibernation, shivering is not initiated until T_b exceeds 15°C–16°C (see, e.g., 78, 109, 129). What is not clear is whether neural input to skeletal muscle increases before T_b is > ~15°C and muscle is nonresponsive, or whether neural input to muscle is delayed until T_b exceeds this temperature. Even in the absence of muscle contractions, an increased rate of depolarizations at the neuromuscular junction would likely increase cellular metabolism (see, e.g., 49). BAT NST is critical for the initial stage of rewarming until T_b reaches ~15°C, when shivering and other functions that are suppressed during deep torpor resume. Preventing sympathetic activation (and BAT NST) during torpor initiation with a noradrenergic receptor blocker prevents rewarming (50), whereas preventing shivering thermogenesis with curare slows but does not prevent rewarming (129). Similarly, after surgically removing ~50% of BAT, hedgehogs cannot rewarm from hibernation (129). The juxtaposition of BAT near major blood vessels (see 129) suggests BAT heats circulating blood, thereby serving as a central heating system and indirectly rewarming peripheral tissues, specifically muscle, until they escape suppressive low temperatures.

HIBERNATION, FAT RESERVES, AND REPRODUCTION

Fat-storing hibernators are making a physiological bet with their lives in the balance. They are wagering that they have sufficient energy stored as lipids to survive within their burrows until aboveground conditions allow emergence and access to food resources. There are numerous reports of the dire consequences visited by late-season storms that delay emergence from hibernation (see, e.g., 4, 117, 128). Similarly, reduced food availability in the summer reduces fat deposition, which in turn increases overwinter mortality during hibernation (see, e.g., 47, 128).

Terminal arousal in fat-storing hibernators generally falls into two categories: (*a*) facultative terminators of hibernation that terminate dormancy when aboveground conditions (e.g., food availability) improve, and (*b*) obligate terminators of hibernation in which an endogenous circannual clock induces the terminal arousal, regardless of aboveground conditions.

Female Hibernators Facultatively Terminate Hibernation

Females typically emerge from hibernation several weeks later than males (see, e.g., 20, 24, 46, 65, 88, 91, 112, 116). For example, male Richardson's ground squirrels typically emerge in March, females emerge several weeks later, and by April 90% of females are pregnant (20). Female hibernators opportunistically terminate hibernation when the burrow mouth is free of snow and food availability returns. Providing hibernating females with food near the end of the hibernation phase induces terminal arousal, and delaying food availability prolongs hibernation (see, e.g., 65). Both pregnancy and lactation require marked increases in energy intake; intake is often doubled during lactation. Because of limits on energy intake and assimilation, the primary challenge for females is to be impregnated as soon as possible. The reproductive female must bear and wean her litter before she can begin to lay down sufficient WAT stores for the subsequent hibernation season. Similarly, the time that young of the year have to grow as well as deposit adequate adipose tissue for winter survival also is limited by the timing of weaning. Terminal arousal in females, therefore, appears to be opportunistic and keyed to the availability of adequate food resources.

Adult Male Hibernators Typically are Obligate Terminators of Hibernation

Male hibernators participating in reproduction terminate hibernation early, prior to reproductive females (20, 24, 46, 65, 88, 91, 112, 116). Often males will emerge from hibernation when snow is present and food is either unavailable or remains very limited (see, e.g., 46). Commitment to normothermy and subsequent testicular development occur before the possibility of emergence because testes are full grown, spermatogenesis is complete, and testosterone is maximal at first appearance aboveground (24, 93, 110, 111). As a result, only heavy males terminate hibernation early and possess large testes (see, e.g., 10, 42, 65, 93) because males committing to reproduction must rely on lipids remaining in adipose tissue reserves. Males spend less time torpid than females over the hibernation season, but this is mostly due to the male's early terminal arousal before emergence is possible (see, e.g., 112). The male ground squirrel's early termination of hibernation has serious ramifications; remaining euthermic for up to four weeks without food is costly, often equaling the entire cost of the preceding hibernation season (cf. 12).

Because testicular recrudescence and spermatogenesis require prolonged euthermia, a fascinating interplay takes place between energy reserves, the circannual clock, and the hypothalamic-pituitary-gonadal axis when males possess sufficient WAT reserves. Testis mass of golden-mantled ground squirrels increases from ~500 mg at hibernation outset to ~1100 mg at terminal arousal, but there is no spermatogenic development (12). The circannual clock increases hypothalamic sensitivity to gonadal steroid feedback such that very low testosterone titers are sufficient to inhibit gonadotropin release throughout most of the year (152). As the reproductive season approaches, the circannual clock markedly decreases hypothalamic sensitivity in normal weight males, resulting in increased gonadotropin release despite increasing plasma testosterone concentrations (112). Testosterone release and spermatogenesis require euthermic tissue temperatures because testicular tissue is unresponsive to the stimulatory effects of luteinizing hormone (LH) at T_bs characteristic of hibernation. Testosterone release from testicular tissue in vitro is nonexistent at 5° and 9°C, and testosterone release at 20°C is only 25% of the maximal value at 32°C (14). Plasma testosterone, LH, and follicle-stimulating hormone values remain at basal concentrations throughout the hibernation season, until approximately three weeks before terminal arousal, when testosterone and LH concentrations begin to rise, but only during periodic arousals, not during deep torpor (13). Hormone concentrations reach maximum values after approximately six hours of euthermia, then decrease to basal levels before deep torpor resumes. Maximal testosterone release during successive periodic arousals progressively increases, and during the rewarming that becomes the terminal arousal, testosterone and LH increase as before but this time remain elevated (cf. 13). Presumably, hypothalamic sensitivity to steroid feedback has decreased to the extent that testosterone concentrations rise sufficiently within six hours to prevent resumption of deep torpor. A negative relation between testosterone and hibernation has been presumed for some time, based on the inference that reproduction and hibernation are incompatible (see 148); exogenous testosterone treatment prevents hibernation (76, 102).

Only males with normal body mass generally terminate hibernation early in the field (see, e.g., 24, 65, 66, 116) because commitment to reproduction in males is dependent on adequate energy reserves. Ground squirrels fail to terminate hibernation spontaneously when starting hibernation underweight, whereas heavier males terminate hibernation early (see, e.g., 65). Both fasting- and lipectomy-induced WAT reduction immediately before the onset of hibernation inhibit male reproductive development in spring; testicular and accessory sex organ development are positively correlated with body mass (58). Although fasted squirrels spend more time hibernating than do either control or lipectomized animals, and thereby reduce the rate of body mass loss, reproductive development remains inhibited. It is not clear whether decreased hypothalamic sensitivity to testosterone feedback and terminal arousal in spring are dependent upon adequate fat reserves at hibernation outset in fall or on those present at the time of the terminal arousal in spring. Chronic leptin concentrations would provide an ideal feedback signal reflecting total body lipid stores; however, elevated leptin concentrations appear incompatible with reversible hypothermia (cf. 64, 74) and most likely leptin release may have to be suppressed during the hibernation phase to permit deep torpor (see 100). In this case, commitment to early terminal arousal would have to occur near peak body mass, when leptin concentrations may more accurately reflect total lipid mass. The relation between WAT mass, feedback from WAT (e.g., leptin), and reproductive development in male ground squirrels obviously is an area rife for future research.

Juvenile Male Hibernators Generally are Facultative Terminators of Hibernation

In the majority of fat-storing hibernators, juvenile males do not undergo an obligate terminal arousal, but await food availability in spring before terminating hibernation in the same manner as females (see 65). Although many juvenile female ground squirrels reproduce at the end of their first hibernation season, juvenile males generally are reproductively quiescent. In the limited time from weaning to winter's outset, juvenile energy intake must supply the requirements for growth as well as fat deposition. Insufficient lipid reserves in juvenile males somehow negate the circannual decrease in hypothalamic sensitivity to gonadal steroid feedback, which results in persistently low testosterone levels and a facultative termination of hibernation. Juvenile males initiating hibernation with lipid stores comparable to those of normal mass adults spontaneously terminate hibernation in spring (42, 65). Adult and juvenile male ground squirrels were provided either standard laboratory chow or a high-fat diet during the body mass gain phase before hibernating without food available. All adult males, regardless of diet, and 90% of high-fat-fed juvenile males spontaneously terminated hibernation (42). Body mass, lipid mass, testis mass, and testosterone concentrations of high-fat juveniles were greater than were those of chow-fed juveniles, but not different from values in adult males, regardless of diet. Lack of an obligate terminal arousal and accelerated reproductive development in juvenile ground squirrels is not a function of age, but a direct consequence of insufficient WAT mass.

SUMMARY

Hibernating mammals undergo remarkable annual cycles in body lipid content. During the summer and early fall, circannual changes in food intake, energy expenditure, and lipogenic factors combine to assure deposition of large reserves of white adipose tissue before the onset of winter. Attainment of a peak body mass precedes immergence and the onset of a body mass loss/hibernation phase. Profound metabolic suppression during deep torpor allows a slow utilization of stored lipids over winter and avoidance of the harsh climatic conditions aboveground. Not surprisingly, lipid oxidation nearly exclusively fuels deep torpor and the major portion of the brief periodic arousals to euthermia that regularly interrupt hibernation. T_b during deep torpor affects duration of hibernation bouts, and the degree of saturation of fatty acids comprising stored lipids affects T_b during deep torpor. Thus, a diet higher in unsaturated fatty acids during fattening decreases frequency of periodic arousals and may increase likelihood of overwinter survival. Females and juvenile males terminate hibernation in the spring when aboveground food becomes available. Males with sufficient WAT reserves, however, terminate hibernation early, before aboveground food is available, relying solely on WAT stores to complete reproductive development before emergence in spring. Mating occurs immediately upon emergence of females, and completion of reproductive duties marks the beginning of the next lipid deposition cycle.

ACKNOWLEDGMENTS

I am most grateful to Kimberly Pelz and Roberto Balmant dos Santos for all their help in preparing this manuscript, and I am especially indebted to Irving Zucker for his insightful and indispensable comments on the manuscript. Preparation of this manuscript was supported by National Institutes of Health Grant NS-30816.

The *Annual Review of Nutrition* is online at http://nutr.annualreviews.org

LITERATURE CITED

1. Ahima RS, Flier JS. 2000. Leptin. *Annu. Rev. Physiol.* 62:413–37
2. Aloia RC, Raison JK. 1989. Membrane function in mammalian hibernation. *Biochim. Biophys. Acta* 988:123–46
3. Armitage KB, Blumstein DT, Woods BC. 2003. Energetics of hibernating yellow-bellied marmots (*Marmota flaviventris*). *Compar. Biochem. Physiol.* 134A:101–14
4. Armitage KB, Downhower JF. 1974. Demography of yellow-bellied marmot populations. *Ecology* 55:1233–45
5. Armitage KB, Schulenberger E. 1972. Evidence of a circannual metabolic cycle in *Citellus tridecemlineatus*, a hibernator. *Comp. Biochem. Physiol.* 42A:667–88
6. Armitage KB, Woods BC. 2003. Group hibernation does not reduce energetic costs of young yellow-bellied marmots. *Physiol. Biochem. Zool.* 76:888–98
7. Bachman GC. 1994. Food restriction effects on the body composition of free-living ground squirrels, *Spermophilus beldingi*. *Physiol. Zool.* 67:756–70
8. Bailey ED. 1965. Seasonal changes in metabolic activity of non-hibernating woodchucks. *Can. J. Zool.* 43:905–9
9. Bamshad M, Song CK, Bartness TJ. 1999. CNS origins of the sympathetic nervous system outflow to brown adipose tissue. *Am. J. Physiol. Regul. Integr. Comp. Physiol.* 276:R1569–78
10. Barnes BM. 1984. Influence of energy stores on activation of reproduction function in male golden-mantled ground squirrels. *J. Comp. Physiol.* 154:425–31
11. Barnes BM. 1989. Freeze avoidance in a

mammal: body temperatures below 0°C in an Arctic hibernator. *Science* 244:1593–95

12. Barnes BM, Kretzmann M, Pelz K, Licht P, Zucker I. 1986. Influence of hibernation on testis growth and spermatogenesis in the golden-mantled ground squirrel, *Spermophilus lateralis*. *Biol. Reprod.* 35:1287–97
13. Barnes BM, Kretzmann M, Zucker I, Licht P. 1988. Plasma androgen and gonadotropin-levels during hibernation and testis maturation in golden-mantled ground squirrels. *Biol. Reprod.* 38:616–22
14. Barnes BM, Licht P, Zucker I. 1987. Temperature dependence of in vitro androgen production in testes from hibernating ground squirrels, *Spermophilus lateralis*. *Can. J. Zool.* 65:3020–23
15. Barnes DS, Mrosovsky N. 1974. Body weight regulation in ground squirrels and hypothalamically lesioned rats: slow and sudden set-point changes. *Physiol. Behav.* 12:251–58
16. Bartness TJ, Bamshad M. 1998. Innervation of mammalian white adipose tissue: implications for the regulation of total body fat. *Am. J. Physiol. Regul. Integr. Comp. Physiol.* 275:R1399–41
17. Bauer VW, Squire TL, Lowe ME, Andrews MT. 2001. Expression of a chimeric retroviral-lipase mRNA confers enhanced lipolysis in a hibernating mammal. *Am. J. Physiol. Regul. Integr. Comp. Physiol.* 281:R1186–92
18. Bauman WA, Meryn S, Florant GL. 1987. Pancreatic hormones in the nonhìbernating and hibernating golden mantled ground squirrel. *Comp. Biochem. Physiol.* 86A:241–44
19. Baumber J, South F, Farren L, Zatzman ML. 1971. A possible basis for periodic arousals during hibernation: accumulation of ketone bodies. *Life Sci.* 10:463–67
20. Bintz GL. 1988. Lipid synthesis and deposition by adult Richardson's ground squirrels in the natural environment. *J. Comp. Physiol. B* 158:199–204
21. Bligh J. 1973. Hibernation. Temperature regulation in mammals and other vertebrates. In *Frontiers of Biology*, ed. A Neuberger, EL Tatum, 30:1–436. Amsterdam: N. Holland Publ.
22. Boswell T, Woods SC, Kenagy GJ. 1994. Seasonal changes in body mass, insulin, and glucocorticoids of free-living golden-mantled ground squirrels. *Gen. Comp. Endocrinol.* 96:339–46
23. Boyer BB, Ormseth OA, Buck L, Nicolson M, Pelleymounter MA, Barnes BM. 1997. Leptin prevents posthibernation weight gain but does not reduce energy expenditure in arctic ground squirrels. *Comp. Biochem. Physiol.* 118C:405–12
24. Bronson MT. 1979. Altitudinal variation in the life history of the golden-mantled ground squirrel (*Spermophilus lateralis*). *Ecology* 60:272–79
25. Brooks SPJ, Storey KB. 1992. Mechanisms of glycolytic control during hibernation in the ground squirrel *Spermophilus lateralis*. *J. Comp. Physiol. B* 162:23–28
26. Buck CL, Barnes BM. 2000. Effects of ambient temperature on metabolic rate, respiratory quotient, and torpor in an arctic hibernator. *Am. J. Physiol. Regul. Integr. Comp. Physiol.* 279:R255–62
27. Buck ML, Squire TL, Andrews MT. 2002. Coordinate expression of the PDK4 gene: a means of regulating fuel selection in a hibernating mammal. *Physiol. Genom.* 8:5–13
28. Burlington RF, Klain GJ. 1967. Gluconeogenesis during hibernation and arousal from hibernation. *Comp. Biochem. Physiol.* 22:701–8
29. Cannon B, Nedergaard J. 2004. Brown adipose tissue: function and physiological significance. *Physiol. Rev.* 84:274–359
30. Carey HV, Andrews MT, Martin SL. 2003. Mammalian hibernation: cellular and molecular responses to depressed

metabolism and low temperature. *Physiol. Rev.* 83:1153–81
31. Castex C, Tahri A, Hoo-Paris R, Sutter BC. 1984. Insulin secretion in the hibernating edible dormouse (*Glis glis*): in vivo and in vitro studies. *Comp. Biochem. Physiol.* 79A:179–83
32. Clark TW, Skryja DD. 1969. Postnatal growth and development of the golden-mantled ground squirrel, *Spermophilus lateralis*. *J. Mammal.* 50:627–29
33. Cochet N, Meister R, Florant GL, Barré H. 1999. Regional variation of the white adipocyte lipolysis during the annual cycle of the alpine marmot. *Comp. Biochem. Physiol. C* 123:225–32
34. Concannon P, Levac K, Rawson R, Tennant B, Bensadoun A. 2001. Seasonal changes in serum leptin, food intake, and body weight in photoentrained woodchucks. *Am. J. Physiol. Regul. Integr. Comp. Physiol.* 281:R951–59
35. Dark J. 1984. Seasonal weight gain is attenuated in food-restricted ground squirrels with lesions of the suprachiasmatic nuclei. *Behav. Neurosci.* 98:830–35
36. Dark J, Forger NG, Stern JS, Zucker I. 1985. Recovery of lipid mass after lipectomy in ground squirrels. *Am. J. Physiol. Regul. Integr. Comp. Physiol.* 249:R73–78
37. Dark J, Forger NG, Zucker I. 1984. Complete and rapid recovery of body mass after surgical removal of adipose tissue in ground squirrels. *Proc. Natl. Acad. Sci. USA* 81:2270–72
38. Dark J, Forger NG, Zucker I. 1986. Regulation and function of lipid mass during the annual cycle of the golden-mantled ground squirrel. In *Living in the Cold: Physiological and Biochemical Adaptations*, ed. HC Heller, XJ Musacchia, LCH Wang, pp. 445–51. New York: Elsevier
39. Dark J, Miller DR. 1998. Metabolic fuel privation in hibernating and awake ground squirrels. *Physiol. Behav.* 63:59–65
40. Dark J, Miller DR, Lewis DA, Fried SK, Bunkin D. 2003. Norepinephrine-induced white adipose tissue lipolysis is suppressed at hibernation temperatures in ground squirrels. *J. Neuroendocrinol.* 15:451–58
41. Dark J, Ruby NF. 1993. Metabolic fuel utilization during hibernation. In *Life in the Cold: Ecological, Physiological, and Molecular Mechanisms*, ed. C Carey, GL Florant, BA Wunder, B Horwitz, pp. 167–74. Boulder, CO: Westview
42. Dark J, Ruby NF, Wade GN, Licht P, Zucker I. 1992. Accelerated reproductive development in juvenile male ground squirrels fed a high-fat diet. *Am. J. Physiol. Regul. Integr. Comp. Physiol.* 262:R644–50
43. Dark J, Stern JS, Zucker I. 1989. White adipose tissue cellularity dynamics during cyclic weight loss and weight gain of the golden-mantled ground squirrel. *Am. J. Physiol. Regul. Integr. Comp. Physiol.* 256:R1286–92
44. Dark J, Zucker I. 1986. Circannual rhythms of ground squirrels: role of the hypothalamic paraventricular nucleus. *J. Biol. Rhythms* 1:17–23
45. Daudova GM, Soliternova IB. 1972. Influence of insulin on the absorption of glucose by adipose tissue of the ground squirrel (*Citellus suslicus*) during hibernation and arousal. *J. Evol. Biochem. Physiol.* 8:399–401 [Transl. from *Zh. Evol. Biokhim. Fiziol.* 8:449–51]
46. Davis DE. 1976. Hibernation and circannual rhythms of food consumption in marmots and ground squirrels. *Q. Rev. Biol.* 51:477–514
47. Davis DE, Ludwig J. 1981. Mechanism for decline in a woodchuck population. *J. Wildl. Manag.* 45:658–68
48. Drew KL, Tøien A, Rivera PM, Smith MA, Perry G, Rice ME. 2002. Role of the antioxidant ascorbate in hibernation and warming from hibernation. *Comp. Biochem. Physiol. C* 133:483–92
49. Else PL, Hulbert AJ. 1987. Evolution of mammalian endothermic metabolism:

"leaky" membranes as a source of heat. *Am. J. Physiol. Regul. Integr. Comp. Physiol.* 253:R1–7
50. Feist DD. 1970. Blockade of arousal from hibernation by inhibition of norepinephrine synthesis in the golden hamster. *Life Sci.* 9:1117–25
51. Fietz J, Tataruch F, Dausmann KH, Ganzhorn JU. 2003. White adipose tissue composition in the free-ranging fat-tailed dwarf lemur (*Cheirogaleus medius*; primates), a tropical hibernator. *J. Comp. Physiol. B* 173:1–10
52. Flechtner-Mors M, Ditschuneit HH, Yip I, Alt A, Torres-Schow RM, et al. 1999. Reduced epinephrine-stimulated lipolytic activity in male golden-mantled ground squirrel during hibernation: an in situ microdialysis study. *Comp. Biochem. Physiol. B* 123:281–84
53. Florant GL, Heller HC. 1977. CNS regulation of body temperature in euthermic and hibernating marmots (*Marmota flaviventris*). *Am. J. Physiol. Regul. Integr. Comp. Physiol.* 232:R203–8
54. Florant GL, Hester L, Ameenuddin S, Rintoul DA. 1993. The effect of a low essential fatty acid diet on hibernation in marmots. *Am. J. Physiol. Regul. Integr. Comp. Physiol.* 264:R747–53
55. Florant GL, Hoo-Paris R, Castex C, Bauman WA, Sutter BC. 1986. Pancreatic A and B cell stimulation in euthermic and hibernating marmots (*Marmota flaviventris*): effects of glucose and arginine administration. *J. Comp. Physiol. B* 156:309–14
56. Florant GL, Lawrence AK, Williams K, Bauman WA. 1985. Seasonal changes in pancreatic B-cell function in euthermic yellow-bellied marmots. *Am. J. Physiol. Regul. Integr. Comp. Physiol.* 249:R159–65
57. Florant GL, Nuttle LC, Mullinex DE, Rintoul DA. 1990. Plasma and white adipose tissue lipid composition in marmots. *Am. J. Physiol. Regul. Integr. Comp. Physiol.* 258:R1123–31
58. Forger NG, Dark J, Barnes BM, Zucker I. 1986. Fat ablation and food restriction influence reproductive development and hibernation in ground squirrels. *Biol. Reprod.* 34:831–40
59. Frank CL. 1992. The influence of dietary fatty acids on hibernation by golden-mantled ground squirrels (*Spermophilus lateralis*). *Physiol. Zool.* 65:906–20
60. Frank CL. 1994. Polyunsaturate content and diet selection by ground squirrels (*Spermophilus lateralis*). *Ecology* 75: 458–63
61. Frank CL. 2002. Short-term variations in diet fatty acid composition and torpor by ground squirrels. *J. Mamm.* 83:1013–19
62. Frank CL, Dierenfeld ES, Storey KB. 1998. The relationship between lipid peroxidation, hibernation, and food selection in mammals. *Am. Zool.* 38:341–49
63. Frank CL, Storey KB. 1995. The optimal depot fat composition for hibernation by golden-mantled ground squirrels (*Spermophilus lateralis*). *J. Comp. Physiol. B* 164:536–42
64. Freeman DA, Lewis DA, Kauffman AS, Blum RM, Dark J. 2004. Reduced leptin concentrations are permissive for display of torpor in Siberian hamsters. *Am. J. Physiol. Regul. Integr. Comp. Physiol.* 287:R97–103
65. French AR. 1982. Intraspecific differences in the pattern of hibernation in the ground squirrel, *Spermophilus beldingi*. *J. Comp. Physiol.* 148:83–89
66. French AR. 1990. Age-class differences in the pattern of hibernation in yellow-bellied marmots, *Marmota flaviventris*. *Oecologia* 82:93–96
67. Galster WA, Morrison PR. 1976. Seasonal changes in body composition of the arctic ground squirrel, *Citellus undulatus*. *Can. J. Zool.* 54:740–78
68. Geiser F. 1990. Influence of polyunsaturated and saturated dietary lipids on adipose tissue, brain and mitochondrial membrane fatty acid composition

of hibernator. *Biochim. Biophys. Acta* 1046:159–66
69. Geiser F. 2004. Metabolic rate and body temperature reduction during hibernation and daily torpor. *Annu. Rev. Physiol.* 66: 239–74
70. Geiser F, Hiebert S, Kenagy GJ. 1990. Torpor bout duration during the hibernation season of 2 sciurid rodents—interrelations with temperature and metabolism. *Physiol. Zool.* 63:489–503
71. Geiser F, Kenagy GJ. 1987. Polyunsaturated lipid diet lengthens torpor and reduces body temperature in a hibernator. *Am. J. Physiol. Regul. Integr. Comp. Physiol.* 252:R897–901
72. Geiser F, Kenagy GJ. 1988. Torpor duration in relation to temperature and metabolism in hibernating ground squirrels. *Physiol. Zool.* 61:442–49
73. Geiser F, Kenagy GJ. 1993. Dietary fats and torpor patterns in hibernating ground squirrels. *Can. J. Zool.* 71:1182–86
74. Geiser F, Körtner G, Schmidt I. 1998. Leptin increases energy expenditure of a marsupial by inhibition of daily torpor. *Am. J. Physiol. Regul. Integr. Comp. Physiol.* 275:R1627–32
75. Geiser F, McAllan BM, Kenagy GJ. 1994. The degree of dietary fatty-acid unsaturation affects torpor patterns and lipid-composition in a hibernator. *J. Comp. Physiol. B* 164:299–305
76. Hall V, Goldman B. 1980. Effects of gonadal steroid hormones on hibernation in the Turkish hamster (*Mesocricetus brandti*). *J. Comp. Physiol. B* 135:107–14
77. Harlow HJ, Frank CL. 2001. The role of dietary fatty acids in the evolution of spontaneous and facultative hibernation patterns in prairie dogs. *J. Comp. Physiol. B* 171:77–84
78. Hashimoto M, Gao B, Kikuchi-Utsumi K, Ohinata H, Osborne PG. 2002. Arousal from hibernation and BAT thermogenesis against cold: central mechanism and molecular basis. *J. Therm. Biol.* 27:503–15
79. Heller HC, Colliver GW. 1974. CNS regulation of body temperature during hibernation. *Am. J. Physiol.* 227:583–89
80. Heller HC, Colliver GW, Beard J. 1977. Thermoregulation during entrance into hibernation. *Pflügers Arch.* 369:55–59
81. Heller HC, Poulson TL. 1970. Circannian rhythms—II. Endogenous and exogenous factors controlling reproduction and hibernation in chipmunks (*Eutamias*) and ground squirrels (*Spermophilus*). *Comp. Biochem. Physiol.* 33:357–83
82. Heller HC, Ruby NF. 2004. Sleep and circadian rhythms in mammalian hibernation. *Annu. Rev. Physiol.* 66:275–89
83. Hill VL, Florant GL. 2000. The effect of a linseed oil diet on hibernation in yellow-bellied marmots (*Marmota flaviventris*). *Physiol. Behav.* 68:431–37
84. Himms-Hagen J. 1985. Brown adipose tissue metabolism and thermogenesis. *Annu. Rev. Nutr.* 5:69–94
85. Hoo-Paris R, Sutter BCJ. 1980. Blood glucose control by insulin in the lethargic and arousing hedgehog (*Erinaceus europaeus*). *Comp. Biochem. Physiol. A* 66:141–43
86. Horwitz BA, Hamilton JS, Kott KS. 1985. GDP binding to hamster brown fat mitochondria is reduced during hibernation. *Am. J. Physiol. Regul. Integr. Comp. Physiol.* 249:R689–93
87. Horwitz BA, Smith RE, Pengelley ET. 1968. Estimated heat contribution of brown fat in arousing ground squirrels (*Citellus lateralis*). *Am. J. Physiol.* 214: 115–21
88. Huang SN, Morton ML. 1976. Seasonal changes in plasma proteins and lipids in the Belding's ground squirrels (*Spermophilus beldingi beldingi*). *Comp. Biochem. Physiol.* 54:239–43
89. Hudson JW, Wang LCH. 1979. Hibernation: endocrinologic aspects. *Annu. Rev. Physiol.* 41:287–303
90. Humphries MM, Thomas DW, Kramer DL. 2003. The role of energy availability in mammalian hibernation: a

cost-benefit approach. *Physiol. Biochem. Zool.* 76:165–79

91. Jameson EW, Mead RA. 1964. Seasonal changes in body fat, water, and basic weight in *Citellus lateralis*, *Eutamius speciosus*, *E. amoenus*. *J. Mamm.* 45:359–65
92. Kayser C. 1952. La dépense d'énergie des mammifères hibernants pendant toute la durée de l'hibernation. Recherches faites sur le spermophile (*Citellus citellus*). *Arch. Sci. Physiol.* 6:193–212
93. Kenagy GJ. 1987. Energy allocation for reproduction in the golden-mantled ground squirrel. *Symp. Zool. Soc. Lond.* 57:259–73
94. Kiell DJ, Millar JS. 1978. Growth of juvenile arctic ground squirrels (*Spermophilus parryii*) at McConnell River, N.W.T. *Can. J. Zool.* 56:1475–78
95. Klain GJ, Rogers GB. 1970. Seasonal changes in adipose tissue lipogenesis in the hibernator. *Int. J. Biochem.* 1:248–50
96. Klain GJ, Whitten BK. 1968. Plasma free amino acids in hibernation and arousal. *Comp. Biochem. Physiol.* 27:617–19
97. Klingenspor M. 2003. Cold-induced recruitment of brown adipose tissue thermogenesis. *Exp. Physiol.* 88:141–48
98. Kottinen A, Rajasalmi M, Sarajas HHS. 1964. Fat metabolism of the hedgehog during the hibernating cycle. *Am. J. Physiol.* 207:845–48
99. Krilowicz BL. 1985. Ketone body metabolism in a ground squirrel during hibernation and fasting. *Am. J. Physiol. Regul. Integr. Comp. Physiol.* 249:R462–70
100. Kronfeld-Schor N, Richardson C, Silvia BA, Kunz TH, Widmaier EP. 2000. Dissociation of leptin secretion and adiposity during prehibernatory fattening in little brown bats. *Am. J. Physiol. Regul. Integr. Comp. Physiol.* 279:R1277–81
101. Laurila M, Suomalainen P. 1974. Studies in the physiology of the hibernating hedgehog. 19. The changes in the insulin level induced by seasons and hibernation cycle. *Ann. Acad. Sci. Fenn. [Biol.]* 201:1–40
102. Lee TM, Pelz K, Licht P, Zucker I. 1990. Testosterone influences hibernation in golden-mantled ground squirrels. *Am. J. Physiol. Regul. Integr. Comp. Physiol.* 259:R760–67
103. Lee TM, Zucker I. 1991. Suprachiasmatic nucleus and photic entertainment of circannual rhythms in ground squirrels. *J. Biol. Rhythms* 6:315–30
104. Lyman CP. 1958. Oxygen consumption, body temperature and heart rate of woodchucks entering hibernation. *Am. J. Physiol.* 194:83–91
105. Lyman CP. 1963. Hibernation in mammals and birds. *Am. Scient.* 51:127–38
106. Lyman CP, Chatfield PO. 1955. Physiology of hibernation in mammals. *Physiol. Rev.* 35:403–25
107. Lyman CP, Willis JS, Malan A, Wang LCH. 1982. *Hibernation and Torpor in Mammals and Birds*. New York: Academic. 317 pp.
108. Mauer MM, Harris RB, Bartness TJ. 2001. The regulation of total body fat: lessons learned from lipectomy studies. *Neurosci. Biobehav. Rev.* 25:15–28
109. McArthur MD, Hanstock CC, Malan A, Wang LCH, Allen PS. 1990. Skeletal muscle pH dynamics during arousal from hibernation measured by ^{31}P NMR spectroscopy. *J. Comp. Physiol.* 160:339–47
110. McKeever S. 1964. The biology of the golden-mantled ground squirrel. *Ecol. Monogr.* 34:383–401
111. McKeever S. 1966. Reproduction in *Citellus beldingi* and *Citellus lateralis* in Northeastern California. In *Comparative Biology of Reproduction in Mammals*, ed. IW Rowland, Symp. Zool. Soc. (Lond.) 15:365–85. London: Academic
112. Michener GR. 1992. Sexual differences in over-winter torpor patterns of Richardson's ground squirrels in natural hibernacula. *Oecologia* 89:397–406
113. Milner RE, Wang LCH, Trayhurn P. 1989.

Brown fat thermogenesis during hibernation and arousal in Richardson's ground squirrel. *Am. J. Physiol. Regul. Integr. Comp. Physiol.* 256:R42–48
114. Mokrasch LC, Grady HJ, Grisolia S. 1960. Thermogenic and adaptive mechanisms in hibernation and arousal from hibernation. *Am. J. Physiol.* 199:945–49
115. Moreau-Hamsany C, Castex C, Hoo-Paris R, Kacemi N, Sutter B. 1988. Hormonal control of lipolysis from the white adipose tissue of hibernating jerboa (*Jaculus orientalis*). *Comp. Biochem. Physiol.* 91A:665–69
116. Morton, ML. 1975. Seasonal cycles of body weights and lipids in Belding's ground squirrels. *Bull. S. Calif. Acad. Sci.* 74:128–43
117. Morton ML, Sherman PW. 1978. Effects of a spring snowstorm on behavior, reproduction, and survival of Belding ground squirrels. *Can. J. Zool.* 56:2578–90
118. Mostafa N, Everett DC, Chou SC, Kong PA, Florant GL, Coleman RA. 1993. Seasonal changes in critical enzymes of lipogenesis and triacylglycerol synthesis in the marmot (*Marmota flaviventris*). *J. Comp. Physiol. B* 163:463–69
119. Mrosovsky N. 1974. Hypothalamic hyperphagia without plateau in ground squirrels. *Physiol. Behav.* 12:259–64
120. Mrosovsky N. 1975. The amplitude and period of circannual cycles of body weight in golden-mantled ground squirrels with medial hypothalamic lesions. *Brain Res.* 99:97–116
121. Mrosovsky N, Fisher KC. 1970. Sliding set points for body weight in ground squirrels during the hibernation season. *Can. J. Zool.* 48:241–47
122. Mrosovsky N, Powley TL. 1977. Set points for body weight and fat. *Behav. Biol.* 20:205–23
123. Nizielski SE, Billington CJ, Levine AS. 1989. Brown fat GDP binding and circulating metabolites during hibernation and arousal. *Am. J. Physiol. Regul. Integr. Comp. Physiol.* 257:R536–41
124. Ormseth OA, Nicolson M, Pelleymounter MA, Boyer BB. 1996. Leptin inhibits prehibernation hyperphagia and reduces body weight in arctic ground squirrels. *Am. J. Physiol. Regul. Integr. Comp. Physiol.* 271:R1775–79
125. Ortmann S, Heldmaier G. 2000. Regulation of body temperature and energy requirements of hibernating Alpine marmots (*Marmota marmota*). *Am. J. Physiol. Regul. Integr. Comp. Physiol.* 278:R698–704
126. Rauch JC. Behrisch HW. 1981. Ketone bodies: a source of energy during hibernation. *Can. J. Zool.* 59:754–60
127. Rayner DV, Trayhurn P. 2001. Regulation of leptin production: sympathetic nervous system interactions. *J. Mol. Med.* 79:8–20
128. Schwartz OA, Armitage KB, Van Vuren D. 1998. A 32-year demography of yellow-bellied marmots (*Marmota flaviventris*). *J. Zool. Lond.* 246:337–46
129. Smith RE, Horwitz BA. 1969. Brown fat and thermogenesis. *Physiol. Rev.* 49:330–425
130. Snapp BD, Heller HC. 1981. Suppression of metabolism during hibernation in ground squirrels. *Physiol. Zool.* 54:297–307
131. Speakman JR, Rowland A. 1999. Preparing for inactivity: how insectivorous bats deposit a fat store for hibernation. *Proc. Nutr. Soc.* 58:123–31
132. Squire TL, Lowe ME, Bauer VM, Andrew MT. 2003. Pancreatic triacylglycerol lipase in a hibernating mammal. II. Cold-adapted function and differential expression. *Physiol. Gen.* 16:131–40
133. Tahti H. 1978. Seasonal differences in O_2 consumption and respiratory quotient in a hibernator (*Erinaceus europaeus L.*). *Ann. Zool. Sci. Fenn. [Biol.]* 15:69–75
134. Tashima LS, Adelstein SJ, Lyman CP. 1970. Radioglucose utilization by active, hibernating, and arousing ground squirrels. *Am. J. Physiol.* 218:303–9

135. Thorp CR, Ram PK, Florant GL. 1994. Diet alters metabolic rate in the yellow-bellied marmot (*Marmota flaviventris*) during hibernation. *Physiol. Zool.* 67:1213–29
136. Tøien Ø, Drew KL, Chao ML, Rice ME. 2001. Ascorbate dynamics and oxygen consumption during arousal from hibernation in Arctic ground squirrels. *Am. J. Physiol. Regul. Integr. Comp. Physiol.* 281:R572–83
137. Tokuyama K, Galantino HL, Green R, Florant GL. 1991. Seasonal glucose uptake in marmots (*Marmota flaviventris*): the role of pancreatic hormones. *Comp. Biochem. Physiol.* 100A:925–30
138. Twente JW, Twente JA. 1965. Regulation of hibernating periods by temperature. *Proc. Natl. Acad. Sci. USA* 54:1058–61
139. Twente JW, Twente JA. 1967. Concentrations of d-glucose in the blood of *Citellus lateralis* after known intervals of hibernating periods. *J. Mamm.* 48:381–86
140. Twente JW, Twente J. 1978. Autonomic regulation of hibernation by *Citellus* and *Eptesicus*. In *Strategies in Cold: Natural Torpidity and Thermogenesis*, ed. LCH Wang, JW Hudson, pp. 327–73. New York: Academic
141. Twente JW, Twente J, Moy RM. 1977. Regulation of arousal from hibernation by temperature in three species of *Citellus*. *J. Appl. Physiol.* 42:191–95
142. van Dijk G. 2001. The role of leptin in the regulation of energy balance and adiposity. *J. Neuroendocrinol.* 13:913–21
143. Wang LCH. 1978. Energetic and field aspects of mammalian torpor: the Richardson's ground squirrel. In *Strategies in Cold: Natural Torpidity and Thermogenesis*, ed. LCH Wang, JW Hudson, pp. 109–46. New York: Academic
144. Wang P, Walter RD, Bhat B, Florant GL, Coleman RA. 1997. Seasonal changes in enzymes of lipogenesis and triacylglycerol synthesis in the golden-mantled ground squirrel (*Spermophilus lateralis*). *Comp. Biochem. Physiol.* 118B:261–67
145. Ward JM Jr, Armitage KB. 1981. Circannual rhythms of food consumption, body mass, and metabolism in yellow-bellied marmots. *Comp. Biochem. Physiol.* 69A:621–26
146. Whitten BK, Burlington RF, Posiviata MA. 1974. Temporal changes in amino acid catabolism during arousal from hibernation in the golden-mantled ground squirrel. *Comp. Biochem. Physiol.* 47A:541–46
147. Wilson BE, Deeb S, Florant GL. 1992. Seasonal changes in hormone sensitive and lipoprotein lipase mRNA concentrations in marmot white adipose tissue. *Am. J. Physiol. Regul. Integr. Comp. Physiol.* 262:R177–81
148. Wimsatt WA. 1969. Some interrelations of reproduction and hibernation in mammals. *Symp. Soc. Exp. Biol.* 23:511–49
149. Xia T, Mostafa N, Bhat BG, Florant GL, Coleman RA. 1993. Selective retention of essential fatty acids: the role of hepatic monoacylglycerol acyltransferase. *Am. J. Physiol. Regul. Integr. Comp. Physiol.* 265:R414–19
150. Zimny ML, Tyrone V. 1957. Carbohydrate metabolism during fasting and hibernation in the ground squirrel. *Am. J. Physiol.* 189:297–300
151. Zucker I. 2001. Circannual rhythms: mammals. In *Handbook of Behavioral Neurobiology*, Vol. 12: *Circadian Clocks*, ed. JS Takahashi, FW Turek, RY Moore, pp. 509–28. New York: Kluwer Acad./Plenum
152. Zucker I, Licht P. 1983. Seasonal variations in luteinizing hormone levels of gonadectomized male ground squirrels (*Spermophilus lateralis*). *Biol. Reprod.* 29:278–85

Annu. Rev. Nutr. 2005. 25:499–522
doi: 10.1146/annurev.nutr.25.050304.092708

First published online as a Review in Advance on February 18, 2005

DROSOPHILA NUTRIGENOMICS CAN PROVIDE CLUES TO HUMAN GENE-NUTRIENT INTERACTIONS

Douglas M. Ruden, Maria De Luca, Mark D. Garfinkel, Kerry L. Bynum, and Xiangyi Lu
Department of Environmental Health Sciences, University of Alabama at Birmingham, Alabama 35294; email: douglasr@uab.edu, mdeluca@uab.edu, mgarfinkel@ms.soph.uab.edu, kbynum@genetics.uab.edu, xlu@uab.edu

Key Words microarrays, proteomics, QTL analysis, longevity, epigenetics

■ **Abstract** Nutrigenomics refers to the complex effects of the nutritional environment on the genome, epigenome, and proteome of an organism. The diverse tissue- and organ-specific effects of diet include gene expression patterns, organization of the chromatin, and protein post-translational modifications. Long-term effects of diet range from obesity and associated diseases such as diabetes and cardiovascular disease to increased or decreased longevity. Furthermore, the diet of the mother can potentially have long-term health impacts on the children, possibly through inherited diet-induced chromatin alterations. *Drosophila* is a unique and ideal model organism for conducting nutrigenomics research for numerous reasons. *Drosophila*, yeast, and *Caenorhabditis elegans* all have sophisticated genetics as well as sequenced genomes, and researchers working with all three organisms have made valuable discoveries in nutrigenomics. However, unlike yeast and *C. elegans*, *Drosophila* has adipose-like tissues and a lipid transport system, making it a closer model to humans. This review summarizes what has already been learned in *Drosophila* nutrigenomics (with an emphasis on lipids and sterols), critically evaluates the data, and discusses fruitful areas for future research.

CONTENTS

INTRODUCTION

Nutrigenomics is a new discipline that examines nutrient-gene interactions on a genome-wide scale. Nutrigenomics is the intersection of three areas: health, diet, and genomics (Figure 1, see color insert). First, nutrition is a well-established field that involves the intersection of health and diet. Second, the intersection of diet and genomics is illustrated by the fact that improper diets are risk factors for disease (61, 63–66). New tools that take advantage of the numerous available whole-genome sequences to study diet-gene interactions include microarrays (transcriptomics), proteomics, metabolomics, and epigenomics. Microarrays can measure the changes in mRNA expression of every gene in the genome in a dose-dependent manner for a particular nutrient or drug. Proteomics measures the changes in the whole proteome, such as post-translational modifications. Metabolomics measures the changes in the entire metabolome, which is generally defined as metabolites with molecular weights less than 2000 Daltons, in a dose-dependent manner for a particular nutrient or drug. Epigenomics measures the changes in the epigenome, the histone post-translational modifications and DNA methylation pattern, in a dose-dependent manner for a particular nutrient or drug (for more information, see http://www.epigenome.org). Finally, the intersection of health and genomics relates to the identification of markers of aging, disease predisposition, and behavioral genomics.

The fruit fly *Drosophila* is ideally suited for conducting many types of nutrigenomics studies. For example, *Drosophila* has a fat body filled with adipocytes, and conserved metabolic and signaling pathways involved in fat metabolism, adipocyte development, and insulin signaling (6, 19–21). The major advantages of *Drosophila* as a model for nutrigenomics are its sophisticated genetics, small genome size, high fecundity, low cost, and short generation time. Genetic screens

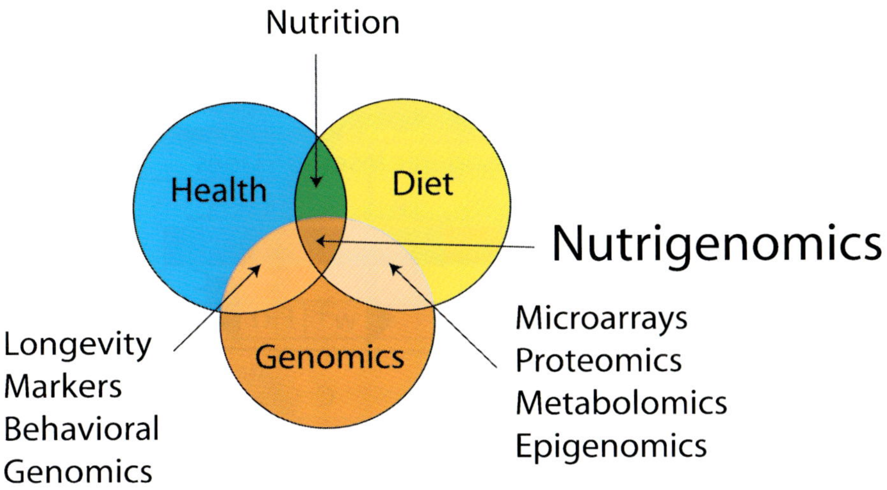

Figure 1 Venn diagram illustration of nutrigenomics as the intersection between health, diet, and genomics.

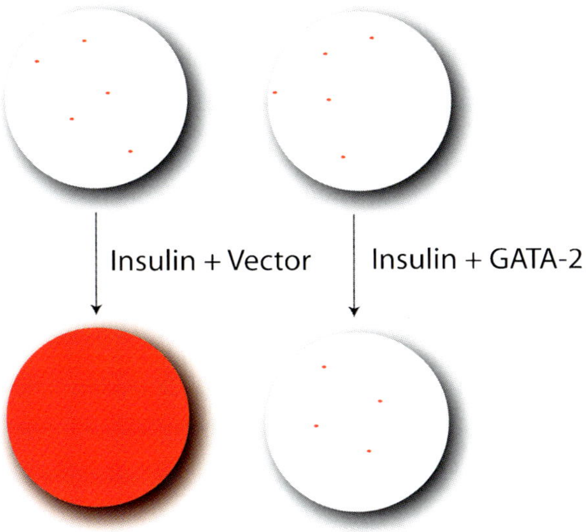

Figure 2 Verification that mammalian GATA-2 inhibits preadipocyte differentiation in a cell culture system. On the left, vector alone has no effect on differentiation of preadipocytes to adipocytes. The red color is Oil-Red-O staining of triglycerides. On the right, GATA-2 prevents differentiation of preadipocytes into adipocytes, as indicated by the lack of Oil-Red-O staining. Cartoon illustration of data from (127).

have already been conducted to isolate mutations and identify natural polymorphisms involved in triglyceride and metabolite levels. Isogenic deficiencies and other types of overlapping deficiencies have been generated that uncover more than 90% of the *Drosophila* genome (96). More than 50% of the genes in *Drosophila* already have been knocked out with transposition insertions and chemical-induced point mutations (for more information, see http://www.flybase.org). RNA microarrays and overlapping 1 kb tiling arrays have been developed to analyze gene expression changes and chromatin changes cause by altered genotypes and environments (116). Sophisticated proteomics analyses have been developed that can analyze global protein expression changes and post-translational modifications (4, 97). The challenge for the future is to use newly developed bioinformatics algorithms to combine all of these nutrigenomics approaches to provide clues to human gene-nutrient interactions (83).

Fruit flies have a life cycle that is very different from that of mammals, yet many developmental and cellular pathways are conserved. When the *Drosophila* genome sequence was initially released in early 2000, 177 out of 289 (~61%) human genes implicated in disease were found to have strong homologs or orthologs in the fly genome (107). Furthermore, two thirds of the genes implicated in human cancers have a counterpart in the fly genome (3). For example, entire signal transduction pathways are present in both organisms, including decapentaplegic (Dpp)/transforming growth factor-beta (TGF-β), Wingless/WNT, Toll/interleukin1 (IL1), Janus kinase/cytokine, Notch/Lin-12, Hedgehog (Hh), and the receptor tyrosine kinases and their intracellular adapter and serine-threonine kinase cascades (106). The insulin-signaling mechanisms in *Drosophila* are conserved with that of humans, as evidenced by the fact that human insulin activates the *Drosophila* insulin receptor (106). Mechanisms for regulating post-translational modification and trafficking of transcription factors from inert cytoplasmic forms to active nuclear forms are also conserved, as demonstrated by Cubitus interruptus (Ci)/Gli (controlled by Hh) and dorsal (dl)/nuclear factor kappa B (NFκB) [controlled by Toll/ interleukin 1(IL1)], among others. It is important to recall that many of the members of these pathways were first discovered by virtue of their mutant phenotypes in *Drosophila*, and further, that the genetic screens in which they were identified had nearly saturated the fly genome, leaving few to be discovered solely by genome sequence annotation (106).

The goals of this review are to summarize diverse types of nutrigenomics research already performed in *Drosophila* and to stimulate new research. Most of the publications in *Drosophila* nutrigenomics are in the subfield of caloric restriction and its effect on life-span extension. However, we only briefly mention caloric restriction research because several recent reviews have highlighted the contributions of model organisms to this field (9, 15, 28, 57). Instead, we focus on areas of nutrigenomics research that are less well studied, such as the genetics of triglyceride storage and steroid signaling, and the effects of dietary composition on longevity. We also promote new areas of studies in *Drosophila* that are poorly developed, such as the effects of diet on proteomics and metabolomics.

FORWARD GENETIC SCREENS FOR IDENTIFYING OBESITY GENES

Obesity is a multifactorial metabolic disorder that has both genetic and environmental components. Both human and mammalian model organism genetics have been used to identify genes that affect obesity (10). However, the identified genes that affect mammalian obesity represent a small fraction of obesity genes, so non-mammalian models need to be further developed (10). As discussed above, most of the human disease genes are present in the genome of *Drosophila* (107). Therefore, *Drosophila* genetic screens potentially could be used to identify candidate human disease genes that affect obesity.

Classical Genetic Screens

"Forward genetic screens" refer to classical genetic screens in which mutations in the genome are induced by a mutagen, and mutant organisms are analyzed for a particular phenotype. To our knowledge, no mutagenesis screen has been conducted in *Drosophila* with the specific purpose of looking for genes that affect obesity or triglyceride levels in *Drosophila*. However, quantitative trait loci (QTL) analyses and multigenerational selection experiments have been performed in *Drosophila* to determine the genetic basis for the natural variation in triglyceride levels (24, 25, 90). Also, mutations that affect lipid storage as secondary phenotypes were identified in massive screens for mutations that cause patterning defects in *Drosophila* embryos, such as those conducted in the early 1980s and before for which Edward Lewis, Eric Wieschaus, and Christiane Nüsslein-Volhard shared the 1995 Nobel Prize in Physiology or Medicine (67, 93, 139). In these classic embryonic patterning genetic screens, some mutations later have been shown to affect development of the fat body, the main lipid storage organ in larvae, as well as the development of other organs and tissues. For example, as described below and in the "Fat Body Development and Nutrient Signaling" section, Serpent was initially identified because it causes a defect in head involution during embryonic development (67), but later it was shown to be required also for fat body development (1, 2) and the immune response (99).

Serpent encodes a GATA transcription factor, a family of regulatory molecules that is conserved in mammalian cells (1, 2). The consensus DNA-binding sequence for Serpent and other GATA family members is 5′-(A/T)GATA(A/G)–3′ (41, 86, 102, 129). To determine whether mammalian GATA transcription factors have a conserved function in mammalian adipogenesis, Tong et al. (127) expressed GATA-2 and GATA-3, the family members that are expressed in adipocytes, in human 3T3-F442A preadipocytes and treated them with insulin for one week to stimulate differentiation (127). The adipocytes differentiated normally in the control "vector-alone" transfection, but constitutive GATA-2 and GATA-3 expression blocked adipocyte differentiation, as revealed by the absence of Oil-Red-O lipid staining (Figure 2, see color insert) (127). The authors concluded that downregulation of these transcription factors is required for terminal differentiation of adipocytes, which is consistent with the observation that GATA-2 and GATA-3 are downregulated in obese animals (127). These experiments demonstrate the usefulness of the *Drosophila* forward genetics to identify key mammalian candidate genes involved in adipocyte development. They also demonstrate that the adipocyte differentiation assay is a rapid means to validate candidate adipocyte genes that are first identified in *Drosophila* genetic screens (Figure 2).

The *Adipose* Gene

Another type of forward genetic screen is to survey a large population for natural variation in a phenotype or a spontaneous mutation in a gene. The $adipose^{60}$ (adp^{60}) mutation of *Drosophila* was isolated in 1960 from a natural population in Kaduna, Nigeria, and is, to our knowledge, the first example of a *Drosophila* genetic model for obesity (34, 35). In 1986, triglycerides, which serve as lipid stores, were shown to be increased by ~twofold in adp^{60} flies (121). The adp^{60} model is interesting because it demonstrates a balance between short-term fitness and long-term survival (34, 35). For example, adp^{60} flies are less fit when analyzed on flight-endurance tests (35). However, when well-fed adp^{60} flies are starved on a water-only diet, they significantly outlive wild-type flies, presumably because they utilize their larger fat reserves (34, 35, 55).

The *adp* gene was recently identified in *Drosophila* and shown to have a highly conserved mammalian cognate (55). Although the mammalian Adp cognate protein has not yet been demonstrated to have a similar function in mammalian models or in humans, it has a high degree of amino acid sequence homology throughout its structure with the mouse and human orthologs (55). One can argue that the *adp* variants in *Drosophila*, and similar types of natural polymorphisms in other genes, such as those that cause diabetes mellitus in humans, are maintained in populations that have unstable food resources. Unfortunately, as pointed out by Neel in 1962 (92), progress in eliminating famine has led to stable and unlimited food supplies in developed countries, so that the "thrifty genotype" now has detrimental effects. Because all natural populations of *Drosophila* have unstable food supplies, as did early human populations, the *Drosophila* genetic model promises to be of great use to identify further "thrifty genes."

REVERSE GENETIC SCREENS FOR IDENTIFYING OBESITY GENES

"Reverse genetics" refers to knocking out an already cloned candidate gene and then determining whether it has an expected phenotype. In this review, we call the knocking out of a single gene "reverse genetics," and the systematic knocking out of most or all of the genes in an organism a "reverse genetic screen." Examples of both types of knockout analyses are described below.

Perilipin Knockouts

Reverse genetics has recently been used to analyze the mechanism of lipid storage in *Drosophila*. Perilipins are proteins that surround and encapsulate lipids inside the cell, and *Drosophila* has two perilipin genes, *Lsd1* and *Lsd2* (87). By mobilizing a nearby transposable element to generate small deletions, two laboratories recently knocked out *Lsd2* in *Drosophila* to determine whether the mechanism for triglyceride storage is evolutionarily conserved (53, 122). As was found in mouse perilipin knockouts (119), *Drosophila* lacking one of the perilipin genes has a decrease in total triglyceride levels (53, 122). Kuhnlein's laboratory also made *Lsd2*-GFP transgenic flies and showed that this protein surrounds the lipid droplets in fat bodies (53). These studies demonstrate that components regulating homeostasis of lipid-based energy storage are evolutionarily conserved between invertebrates and vertebrates. The *Lsd2*-GFP transgenic flies will also be useful tools in future genetic screens to identify components that regulate the size and assembly of lipid droplets (53).

Whole-Genome Mutant Screens

In a reverse genetic screen, one constructs a panel of mutations in all or most of the cloned genes in an organism and then screens the collection of mutant organisms for a particular phenotype. The ultimate reverse genetic screen would be not only to knock out every gene in an organism, but also to determine the phenotype of each knockout line in a dose-dependent manner for a particular nutrient or drug. The closest to an ultimate screen was done in yeast, where site-specific recombination allowed the systematic knockout of every candidate gene in the organism (48, 140). The collection of knockouts is used by the yeast research community to systematically screen for a phenotype or to search for genetic interactions with other genes or pharmaceuticals (47, 49). A large-scale yeast genetic interaction screen identified a network containing 1000 genes and 4000 interactions by crossing mutations in 132 query genes into a set of deletion mutants and scoring the double-mutant progeny for growth defects (126). In this study, only 132 query genes were made double mutant for all of the other genes (126), but high-throughput technology should make it feasible to analyze the entire genome in this manner.

Whole-Genome RNA-Mediated Interference Screens

Although not yet conducted in whole *Drosophila* animals, a reverse genetic screen of most of the *Caenorhabditis elegans* genome for defects in lipid storage has been completed by Gary Ruvkun's laboratory (7). In this study, they used RNA-mediated interference (RNAi) to disrupt the expression of 16,757 *C. elegans* genes. They found 305 disruptions that lead to an increase in fat storage and 112 disruptions that lead to a decrease in fat storage. Some of the disruptions are in genes with conserved functions in mammalian cells, such as those in the insulin and serotonin-signaling pathways. However, most of the genes identified in this screen are conserved between mammals and worms, but have no known function in fat storage (7). Verification of the significance of the "pioneer genes" could be accomplished in the future by identifying novel adipocyte differentiation genes using the preadipocyte assay, described above, and by making knockout mice.

Although RNAi-type reverse genetic screens are not yet feasible in *Drosophila* because of the labor involved, RNAi screens knocking out 91% of the predicted fly genome have been performed using *Drosophila* tissue culture cell lines in Norbert Perrimon's laboratory (17). They analyzed cell growth and viability with an automated fluorescent assay that measures ATP levels and found that 438 RNAi constructs cause defects in these processes (17). Partial RNAi screens have also been performed in *Drosophila* cell lines by transfecting the cells with smaller collections of RNAi. For example, Lum and colleagues (75, 76) identified genes that affect the Hh-signaling pathway using a collection of 43% of the fly genome in cells containing an Hh-transcriptional reporter.

It would be extremely informative to conduct whole-genome RNAi screens with *Drosophila* adipocyte cell lines to identify genes involved in fat storage. Unfortunately, to our knowledge, *Drosophila* preadipocyte or adipocyte lines have not yet been developed. However, three recent reports have been published on large-scale RNAi-type screens in mammalian cells. Because long double-stranded RNA in mammalian cells induce the interferon response and shut down translation (40), short inverted RNAs (siRNAs) must be used in mammalian cells. The first large-scale siRNA screen in mammalian cells used the transfection of siRNAs targeted against 8000 individual genes to identify regulators of tumor necrosis factor-α signaling (142). The other two screens involved retroviral-expressed siRNA for 15,000 genes (10,000 human and 5000 mouse) and 8000 human genes (12, 95); the first screen identified modulators of proteosome function, whereas the second screen identified modulators of p53-induced apoptosis and cell cycle arrest (12, 95).

Whole-Genome Deficiency Screens

Whole-genome reverse genetic screens can also be performed in *Drosophila* using the large collection of existing mutations and deficiencies that have been generated in this organism over the past century (http://www.flybase.org). However, the extreme strain-to-strain variation in this collection makes them less useful for nutrigenomics research. Recently, Exelixis, Inc. has released to the *Drosophila* community a large collection of isogenic insertion lines and deficiencies that all have the same genetic background (96, 123). The Exelixis collection includes over 29,000 isogenic insertion lines that tagged or knocked out over 7200 different genes. The Exelixis isogenic deficiency collection, together with those generated by Kevin Cook and colleagues at Indiana University, includes 519 deficiencies that uncover 56% of the *Drosophila* genome (Figure 3, see color insert) (96, 123). Because these deficiencies generally uncover relatively small regions of the genome (100,000 to 300,000 base pairs), there is a lower chance of deleting multiple genes in the same pathway, which was a problem with previously generated deficiencies.

A type of experiment that could be conducted, for instance, would be to screen the isogenic deficiency lines for modulators of triglyceride levels. A secondary screen of genes uncovered by the deficiencies could be conducted by testing the isogenic insertion knockout lines that are uncovered by deficiencies that either raise or lower the triglyceride levels. Nonisogenic mutations in genes uncovered by the deficiencies can be made mostly isogenic by backcrossing the mutation to the nearest isogenic insertion line for 10 generations or more, as we described previously (46). Through this and similar types of experiments, the isogenic deficiency lines promise to be of great use in future nutrigenomics research. A caveat to performing screens using the isogenic deficiency lines is that single gene mutations often have very different phenotypes, depending on genetic backgrounds (see, for example, Reference 73). This suggests that focusing on a single isogenic strain will give some false negatives, and QTL-type approaches are valid and essential alternatives (24, 90).

PROTEIN-PROTEIN INTERACTION SCREENS

Two types of interaction screens are used to detect protein-protein interactions. The first type is the so-called two-hybrid screen, which is based on the first hybrid protein containing a DNA binding (DB) domain fused to one protein and an activating domain (AD) fused to a second protein (Figure 4, see color insert, top) (42). The second type of protein-protein interaction screen involves biochemical purification of interacting proteins. These two types of screens, and their relevance to nutrigenomics research, are described in this section.

Detecting Interactions Between Proteins with the Two-Hybrid Assay

In the two-hybrid assay, when both interacting hybrids are brought together in yeast cells, they activate expression of a reporter gene, such as β-galactosidase, which turns the yeast blue when grown on indicator plates containing X-GAL. Typically, if both hybrid proteins interact, they also activate expression of an prototrophic selection gene, such as for His3 or Leu2. Although not often used for this purpose, the two-hybrid assay can also potentially detect the effects of nutrients on protein-protein interactions (72). We note that endogenous GAL4 in yeast interacts with its repressor, GAL80, and that this repression is released when the sugar galactose is present in the medium. It is possible to transfect yeast with appropriate genes expressing enzymes that allow proteins to interact only when nutrients induce post-translational modifications, such as phosphorylation (72), mono-ubiquitin (18), mono-sumo (118), or O-GlcNAc (135–137). O-GlcNAc modification of proteins has been proposed to be a "nutrient sensor" (135–137), and the O-GlcNAc modifying enzymes, such as OGT and OGN, are conserved in *Drosophila* (http://www.flybase.org), but, to our knowledge, no laboratory has yet pursued this system in flies.

Genome-Wide Two-Hybrid Screens

In a classic two-hybrid screen, yeast cells containing the first DB-bait hybrid protein are transfected with a library of vectors that contain the AD-prey hybrid protein, where the "prey" is a library of random cDNAs (44). Proteins that interact with the "bait" are identified by colonies that are blue and grow on plates lacking histidine, for instance. Large-scale two-hybrid screens have recently been completed in yeast, *C. elegans*, and *Drosophila* (100). In the most extensive *Drosophila* two-hybrid screen (51), called interactive mating, a collection of DBs fused to full-length cDNAs for most of the genes from an organism is transfected, one at a time, into yeast cells. Next, a collection of ADs fused to the same collection of full-length cDNAs is transfected into yeast cells of the opposite mating type, again one at a time (44). Finally, robots are used to mate every AD-fusion protein containing yeast strain to every DB-fusion protein yeast strain (Figure 4, bottom). In the *Drosophila* large-scale screen conducted by CuraGen, Inc. and collaborators, 10,623 cDNA were screened against each other and a high-confidence refined map of 4679 proteins and 4780 interactions was produced (51). The authors noted that not all ($10{,}623^2$) possible interactions were analyzed, for several technical reasons (51). For example, a significant percentage of DB-fusion proteins activated transcription in the absence of the AD-fusion protein and therefore were not used further in the screen (51).

The results of the large-scale two-hybrid screens are of great use to the field of nutrigenomics. For example, one can find potential interacting proteins of a gene of interest by querying the CuraGen website, http://portal.curagen.com/. One could then test mutations in the candidate interacting proteins for similar phenotypes caused by mutations in the gene of interest (51).

Genome-Wide Protein Interaction Screens

The second type of interaction screen is based on a biochemical interaction in a test tube. In this screen, all of the proteins from a proteome are purified with an epitope tag and immobilized on a column. Next, whole cell extracts are added to the column, washed, and the bound proteins are eluted and identified with tandem mass spectrometric (MS/MS) approaches. So far, because of the incredible labor involved in this type of interaction screen, a biochemical interaction screen has only been published for a small subset of the *C. elegans* proteome (74), but yeast, *Drosophila*, and *Escherichia coli* proteomes are in progress. When this type of protein-protein interaction screen is fully developed in *Drosophila*, it could be used in nutrigenomics research to identify interactions that occur only in the presence of a particular nutrient, for example.

DROSOPHILA LESSONS CONCERNING STEROL BIOSYNTHESIS

Biosynthesis of a complex set of lipophilic signaling molecules, including steroids, isoprenoids, eicosanoids, and prostaglandins, among others, begins with stepwise enzymatic condensation of acetyl-CoA residues to form 3-hydroxy-3-methylglutaryl-CoA (HMG-CoA). The first committed step in the synthesis of the above lipophilic signaling molecules is catalyzed by HMG-CoA reductase to form mevalonate. Six enzymatic reactions then ensue to generate farnesyl diphosphate (Far-PP), which is the last molecule that serves as precursor for both steroids and isoprenoids. On the sterol branch, nine sequential enzymatic reactions convert Far-PP into cholesterol, which is the precursor of vitamin D3, various steroid hormones, and the bile acids that are the ultimate degradation products of sterols. Far-PP is also used to form geranylgeranyl-diphosphate (Ger-Ger-PP). Far-PP and Ger-Ger-PP can both be covalently attached to proteins, and serve as lipophilic tethers to retain these proteins in close apposition to cellular membranes. Far-PP and geranyl-PP are also precursors for terpenes, vitamins E and K, and, in plants, an extensive series of secondary metabolic pathways that generate (among other products) carotenoids.

Cholesterol Biosynthesis

Mammalian cells closely regulate the de novo biosynthesis of cholesterol in response to dietary uptake of cholesterol and the need to maintain proper membrane fluidity. A family of sterol-sensing proteins, including the endoplasmic reticulum (ER) sterol regulatory element binding protein (SREBP) cleavage-activating protein (SCAP), is involved in measuring sterol concentrations. When sterol concentrations are low, SCAP escorts the inactive form of SREBP from the ER to the Golgi, where proteolytic release of the bHLH-Zip domain of SREBP occurs (52, 108). The bHLH-Zip fragment of SREBP then translocates to the cell nucleus, where it acts as a transcription factor inducing expression of about 35 genes involved in unsaturated fatty acid biosynthesis and cholesterol biosynthesis including HMG-CoA reductase (58). Recently, Radhakrishnan and colleagues (101) showed that cholesterol directly binds SCAP, inducing a conformational change so that SCAP dissociates from the membrane-bound form of SREBP and instead binds to Insig proteins. The inability to escort membrane-bound inactive SREBP to Golgi when sterol concentrations have risen permits this transcription factor to be depleted from cell nuclei. In combination with ubiquitinylation and degradation of HMG-CoA reductase, cholesterol biosynthesis is downregulated both transcriptionally and post-transcriptionally, closing the feedback loop required for cholesterol homeostasis.

In contrast with mammalian cells, arthropods including insects such as *Drosophila* cannot synthesize cholesterol de novo from acetyl-CoA (103). In the case of *Drosophila* this metabolic inability was recently shown to be due to the absence from the genome of coding regions for seven enzymes in the sterol branch, including lanosterol synthase, which catalyzes the concerted cyclization reactions required to fabricate the four-fused-ring steroid nucleus, and 7-dehydrocholesterol reductase, which synthesizes the definitive cholesterol molecule (88). *Drosophila* is thus dependent upon provision of exogenous cholesterol or closely related sterols, and this dependency contributes to some of the ecological niches various *Drosophila* species inhabit.

Flies contain a single gene each for SCAP and SREBP (114). The subcellular localization, translocation, and proteolytic processing of these proteins are conserved between *Drosophila* and mammalian cells. Quite remarkably, though, SREBP proteolysis and nuclear translocation in *Drosophila* cultured cells is inhibited by palmitate levels rather than sterol levels (114), which operate through metabolic conversion of palmitate to phosphatidylethanolamine (36). Inactivation of either SREBP or SCAP in *Drosophila* cultured cells using RNA interference showed that these proteins are required for saturated fatty acid biosynthesis (114) rather than unsaturated fatty acid biosynthesis as found in mammals. Consistent with the severance of the association of cholesterol levels from HMG-CoA reductase activity, *Drosophila* transcription of the HMG-CoA reductase gene is not affected by inhibition of SREBP or SCAP activity (114). An interesting avenue for future research would be testing the SCAP/SREBp/palmitate network in flies fed different fatty acids, for example.

Ecdysone Biosynthesis

A principal use arthropods make of dietary cholesterol is for biosynthesis of the major molting hormone, 20-hydroxyecdysone (20-HE). This hormone is synthesized in the prothoracic glands during larval and pupal life, during which times it regulates growth and the onset of metamorphosis. In adult insects, 20-HE is additionally synthesized in ovaries, playing a crucial role in oogenesis. Maternal supplies of ecdysteroids are deposited into eggs; mobilization of these stores is required for successful completion of embryonic development. Akin to biosynthesis of steroid hormones such as testosterone, estradiol, and progesterone in mammals, arthropods synthesize 20-HE by mitochondrial cytochrome-P450 family members that catalyze position-specific hydroxylation reactions. Considerable recent progress has been made in cloning and characterizing the genes for the P450 enzymes from *Drosophila* (23, 26, 134) and for a putative cytosol-mitochondria cholesterol transporter (105) that has homology to the steroid acute-regulatory protein-related lipid transfer domain (115).

Sterols and Germ Cell Migration

Although *Drosophila* has deficits in the de novo cholesterol biosynthesis pathway, enzymes downstream of Far-PP required for prenylation of proteins and for isoprenoid biosynthesis are intact. These observations have led to an unexpected role for this pathway in the developing fly. In all animals, primordial germ cells form early during embryonic development and then migrate to somatic gonadal tissues before engaging in mitotic proliferation, gamete differentiation, and meiosis. In *Drosophila*, mutations that cause primordial germ cells to lose their way during migration and fail to arrive at the somatic gonad map to the genes encoding HMG-CoA reductase, farnesyl-diphosphate synthase (FPPS), geranylgeranyl-diphosphate synthase (GPPS), and the geranylgeranyl transferase type I (109). Ectopic expression of either FPPS or GPPS in the *Drosophila* embryonic nervous system is sufficient to cause germ cell migration to be inappropriately directed toward the nervous system, indicating a role for the isoprenoid pathway in synthesis of a germ cell chemoattractant. Application of either of two commonly prescribed statin drugs that inhibit HMG-CoA reductase activity caused similar defects in germ cell migration in developing zebra fish embryos, as did a drug inhibitor of geranylgeranyl-transferase activity but not of farnesyl-transferase activity (124). "Dietary" supplementation of drug-treated zebra fish embryos with farnesol, geranylgeraniol, or mevalonate, small metabolites downstream of the pharmacological blockades, partly restored germ cell migration (124). Thus, a role for isoprenoid pathway products, possibly a geranylgeranylated protein, in chemoattraction of germ cells is conserved between insects and vertebrates. These studies raise interesting questions regarding dietary and pharmacological interventions that perturb the mevalonate, sterol, or isoprenoid pathways.

DROSOPHILA STEROID RECEPTORS

The steroid receptor superfamily of transcription factors regulates diverse cellular processes, generally in response to binding of small lipophilic molecules. These lipophilic ligands are synthesized, for the most part, from the sterol and isoprenoid branches mentioned above. With the completion of various genome sequences it is possible to arrive at complete lists of superfamily members found in a variety of taxonomic groups and draw inferences about the evolutionary history of the superfamily in each lineage. Maglich and colleagues (77, 78) examined the then-available human, *Drosophila*, and nematode genome sequences for members of the steroid receptor superfamily. Although humans (and by extension, other mammals) contain about 50 functional steroid receptor family members, *Drosophila* contains only 21 steroid receptor family members.

Retinoid-X Receptor and Ecdysone Receptors

As is the case with vertebrate steroid receptors, *Drosophila* superfamily members come in three varieties: those that bind DNA as monomeric proteins, those that bind DNA as homodimers, and those that bind DNA as heterodimers partnered with the retinoid-X receptor (RXR). The molecular phylogenetic analysis of Maglich and colleagues (77, 78) enabled strong association of nine *Drosophila* steroid receptor superfamily members with their corresponding cognate, or orthologous, genes in human. For example, the *Drosophila* ultraspiracle (usp) gene, which encodes ultraspiracle (USP) protein, is the cognate of RXR. The *Drosophila* ecdysone receptor

(EcR) gene, which encodes ECR protein, is the cognate of vertebrate farnesoid-X receptor (FXR). Because of these cognate relationships and the critical importance of USP and ECR to *Drosophila* development, we shall use them as illustrations of the potential future directions of *Drosophila* nutrigenomics research.

First, and quite striking, *Drosophila* uses its EcR cognate as a 20-HE-activated regulator of development, whereas mammals use FXR as a bile-activated regulator of cholesterol metabolism. How the ligand-binding domains came to differ in binding specificity is an outstanding problem of structural biochemistry. More intriguing is how evolution in vertebrate and invertebrate lineages caused the deployment of the FXR/EcR cognates for such different roles. Perhaps the connection is nutritional regulation during development. If this is the case, then studying the nutrigenomics of EcR regulation should yield insights into FXR regulation.

Pathways Regulated by 20-Hydroxyecdysone

In *Drosophila* and other arthropods, larval-to-larval molting, the onset of metamorphosis (larval-to-pupal molting), adult emergence, and adult fertility are controlled principally by two hormones, 20-HE and juvenile hormone (JH). Whereas 20-HE, a steroid, stimulates molting, the nature of the molt is influenced by the presence of several structurally similar JHs, which are methyl-epoxy derivatives of farnesoate. Late in larval life, when JH and ecdysterone concentrations are low, ECR is cytosolic and binds heat-shock protein 90 (HSP90), a molecular chaperone, in an inactive complex. When the concentration of 20-HE rises, it binds to ECR, triggering dissociation from HSP90 (5). Ligand-bound ECR then binds to USP, translocates to the cell nucleus, binds DNA at specific sites, and recruits coactivator proteins that stimulate target gene transcription (5). ECR-USP activates several immediate-ecdysone-inducible genes in all tissues, whereas later-inducible genes are tissue- and developmental stage-specific (5). ECR-USP can also recruit corepressor proteins and inhibit target gene transcription in disparate tissues.

Ecdysone-regulated gene hierarchies have been studied by a variety of methods over the past three decades, most recently by microarrays (45, 85, 125, 138). Gene activation by ECR-USP can involve poly-ADP-ribosylation of histones (110), which has the effect of facilitating access to the chromatin by RNA polymerase II, and by recruitment of the histone H3-lysine-4-methyltransferase encoded by the *Drosophila* trithorax-related gene (113), among other mechanisms. If 20-HE and JH are both present in a cell-culture assay system, JH binds to the USP protein found in ECR-USP heterodimers (81). Ligand occupancy on USP stimulates the recruitment of transcriptional corepressor proteins, which results in a reduced ability of 20-HE to stimulate transcription of target genes. A similar finding was recently reported concerning human RXR agonists and their ability to prevent FXR from recruiting coactivators (69).

Endocrine Disruptors

Many insects are voracious herbivores, and numerous natural products have been isolated from plants that disrupt either ecdysone signaling or JH signaling and thus are lethal to the insects that consume them. Ecdysone antagonists from plants include oligostilbenes (84) and flavones (94). Ecdysone agonists include phytosteroids, such as makisterones (8), and nonsteroidal diacylhydrazines (32, 33). These natural products are being used to design, test, and eventually deploy novel insecticides. A growing body of molecular modeling, X-ray crystallographic, and structure-reactivity studies are being performed to take advantage of the evolutionary divergences among ECR and USP genes present in various insect taxonomic groups so as to minimize the harmful effects that synthetic insect endocrine disruptive agents have on beneficial insect species (13, 14). Likewise, X-ray structural studies have examined the correspondence between how the *Drosophila* ECR-USP heterodimer and the mammalian FXR-RXR each bind DNA sites (31).

In some crop plants, naturally occurring insect endocrine disruptors accumulate to high concentrations, and thus are nontrivial components of human diets. An important question, therefore, is the extent to which these phytoecdysteroids might act as ligands that bind either the human FXR and RXR cognates of insect ECR and USP, or perhaps other members of the human steroid receptor superfamily repertoire. Reviews of the literature indicate relatively little mammalian toxicity (32, 33). In contrast, there is good evidence of estrogenic effects of plant compounds (including, for example, genistein), and the recent computational discovery of a *Drosophila* ortholog of the vertebrate estrogen-receptor-related gene (77, 78) suggests that fly-derived assays may be useful in identifying natural ligands for this receptor and in determining whether plant products mimic (or antagonize) their effects.

OBESITY AND THE IMMUNE RESPONSE

Recent data have revealed a tight link between inflammation and metabolic conditions (27). The relevance of this relationship became evident upon the demonstration by Hotamisligil and colleagues (60) in 1993 that inflammatory pathways are critical in the mechanisms underlying insulin resistance and type 2 diabetes in mice. More recent data showed that human obesity is associated with a state of chronic inflammation characterized by abnormal production of cytokines, such as interleukin-6 and tumor necrosis factor-α, increased acute-phase reactants, such as C-reactive protein, and other stress-induced molecules (59). An interesting feature of the inflammatory response that emerges in the presence of obesity is that many of these alterations are initiated and reside within the adipose tissue (59). Recently, Hotamisligil (59) suggested that this tight relationship might be explained by evolutionarily conserved genetic pathways that regulate metabolic and immune functions by using common regulatory molecules.

Fat Body Development and Nutrient Signaling

It is interesting that the fat body in *Drosophila* functions not only in energy storage and intermediary metabolism but also in the innate immune response. Experimental results suggest that there is a close parallel between the molecular mechanisms functioning in the regulation of metabolic and immune functions in *Drosophila*. As discussed in the "Forward Genetic Screens for Identifying Obesity Genes" section, the developmental control of the *Drosophila* fat body specification, like mammalian white adipose tissue (127), is regulated by Serpent, a member of the GATA-binding family of transcription factors (56). Previously, Petersen and colleagues (99) had shown that Serpent regulates *Drosophila* immunity genes in the larval fat body. In particular, they reported that Serpent acts as a positive regulator in a GATA-dependent manner of the transcription of Cecropin A1 gene, which encodes for an antimicrobial peptide (99).

In an attempt to identify the mechanisms underlying nutrient signaling in *Drosophila*, Zinke et al. (143) used Affymetrix microarrays to identify genes regulated by starvation and sugar conditions. One of the genes that were regulated upon both conditions is *Thor* (143). Thor is a member of the 4E-binding protein (4E-BP) family, which in mammals has been defined as a critical regulator in a pathway that controls initiation of translation through binding eukaryotic initiation factor 4E. In accord with the studies in *Drosophila*, studies in mice have shown that the phosphorylation state of the 4E-BP1 changes in response to starvation and refeeding (117). In *Drosophila*, Thor also participates in host immune defense (11). The *Thor* promoter has the canonical nuclear factor-B and associated GATA recognition sequences that have been shown to be essential for immune induction, and becomes upregulated upon bacterial infection (11).

Dopamine and Serotonin

In mammals, the neurotransmitters norepinephrine, dopamine, and serotonin are well known to be involved in central energy balance circuits (111, 112). Dopamine and serotonin are also present in the central nervous system of insects. In *Drosophila* larvae, the presence of serotonergic nerves in several tissues involved in digestion, such as the pharyngeal muscles, the proventriculus, the midgut, and the ring gland, suggest that serotonin also modulates feeding behavior and neuroendocrine activity in this species (54, 89). In insects, dopamine acts as a neurotransmitter in the brain and as a precursor molecule in the synthesis of melanin used by the animal during the immune response. Notably, microarray expression studies have found that genes encoding for enzymes in the dopamine and serotonin pathways are upregulated following bacterial infection (30).

Fatty Acid–Binding Proteins

Recent data have shown that fatty acid–binding proteins, a family of cytoplasmic proteins, play an important role in transporting free fatty acids to various intracellular compartments, regulating cellular lipid metabolism and expression of inflammatory cytokines in mammals (16). Vierstraete and colleagues recently reported the results of two proteomic studies for the analysis of instantly released immune proteins in hemolymph of *Drosophila* third-instar larvae after challenge with lipopolysaccharide or pricking with sterile needles (132) and after induction with a suspension of Gram-positive bacteria or yeast (133). In both studies, the homologous *Drosophila* retinoid and fatty acid–binding protein was found to be significantly differentially expressed (132, 133). These findings highlight the notion that *Drosophila* is a powerful model to identify molecular pathways regulating both metabolic and immune functions.

HIGH-FAT DIET AND AGING STUDIES IN *DROSOPHILA*

In contrast to caloric restriction, which retards aging in *Drosophila* (43, 62, 79, 80, 104, 120, 141), and is not discussed in this review, the effects of saturated fats in the diet of *Drosophila* have been shown to play a role in the acceleration of aging in this species. However, the specific mechanism that is involved in promotion of aging has been difficult to identify. One of the first studies that attempted to make a connection between *Drosophila* diet and aging found that diets consisting of high fat and low carbohydrate concentrations would shorten, on average, the life span of *Drosophila* (39). This study, however, fell short of identifying the specific aging process or the multiple aging processes that were negatively affected by the consumption of fat. Instead, it laid the groundwork for future studies since some irreversible damage was sustained by the flies on a palmitic acid medium that was characteristic of an aging process.

Further studies of diet and aging in *Drosophila* focused on the fact that a greater stress was placed on older flies fed a high-fat diet than on flies fed a normal low-fat diet. Researchers began to look at metabolic parameters of aging *Drosophila* and went on to test the effects of a high-fat diet on these parameters (37). An interesting finding was that older flies consume more food than younger flies regardless of the diet they are fed. However, the increased consumption was greater in the flies fed a high-fat/low-carbohydrate diet. Further probing suggested that the efficiency of metabolism in *Drosophila* drops significantly with age. Therefore, the flies eat more to compensate for this impaired energy metabolism. It was also hypothesized that older flies are able to generate energy more efficiently from carbohydrates to obtain the needed energy to survive. This explained the greater stress seen in older flies on the high-fat diet mentioned above as well as in the first study. It also suggested that the shorter life span of flies on a high-fat diet could be attributed to this increased need for carbohydrates in energy metabolism.

Subsequent studies led researchers to conclude that some metabolite of fat must be the significant factor that links nutrition and aging (38). Still, the question remains as to what that metabolite could be. One suggestion is that a free-radical mechanism may be involved. Free radicals can be generated during normal fat metabolism as well as through hydrogen peroxide. Significant amounts of hydrogen peroxide are produced by peroxisomes during fat metabolism. Many other possibilities exist, however. In fact, very few studies other than CR have been done on the effects of diet on aging in *Drosophila*, and most of the studies that have been done were conducted more than 20 years ago. With the greater knowledge and improved technology we have today (especially in relation to genetics), we can further delve into solving for this unidentified mechanism of aging.

FUTURE PROSPECTS

Nutrigenomics, a subject of numerous recent reviews (22, 29, 50, 68, 70, 71, 82, 91, 98, 128, 130, 131), is an emerging field with great prospects for understanding the effect of nutrition on health and disease. Nutrigenomics requires a multidimensional understanding of how the diet affects gene expression, post-translational modifications of proteins, and changes in the chromatin. *Drosophila* is an ideal model to study nutrigenomics and, as outlined in this review, has already contributed a great deal to the field. Candidate pathways influenced by nutrients can be identified first in *Drosophila*, and later verified in mouse models and finally in humans. We hope that this review will stimulate more research in the field of *Drosophila* nutrigenomics.

ACKNOWLEDGMENTS

Work in the authors' laboratory is supported by NIH grants R01AA12276, R01GM63225, R01ES92133, R01CA105349, and R21ES11751 to D.M.R.; P50DK057301 to X.L.; and a UAB Center for Nutrient-Gene Interaction grant to M.D.G.

The *Annual Review of Nutrition* is online at http://nutr.annualreviews.org

LITERATURE CITED

1. Abel T, Bhatt R, Maniatis T. 1992. A *Drosophila* CREB/ATF transcriptional activator binds to both fat body- and liver-specific regulatory elements. *Genes Dev.* 6:466–80
2. Abel T, Michelson AM, Maniatis T. 1993. A *Drosophila* GATA family member that binds to Adh regulatory sequences is expressed in the developing fat body. *Development* 119:623–33
3. Adams MD, Celniker SE, Holt RA, Evans CA, Gocayne JD, et al. 2000. The genome sequence of *Drosophila melanogaster*. *Science* 287:2185–95
4. Aebersold R, Mann M. 2003. Mass spectrometry–based proteomics. *Nature* 422:198–207
5. Arbeitman MN, Hogness DS. 2000. Molecular chaperones activate the *Drosophila* ecdysone receptor, an RXR heterodimer. *Cell* 101:67–77
6. Arrese EL, Canavoso LE, Jouni ZE, Pennington JE, Tsuchida K, Wells MA. 2001. Lipid storage and mobilization in insects: current status and future directions. *Insect Biochem. Mol. Biol.* 31:7–17
7. Ashrafi K, Chang FY, Watts JL, Fraser AG, Kamath RS, et al. 2003. Genome-wide RNAi analysis of *Caenorhabditis elegans* fat regulatory genes. *Nature* 421:268–72
8. Baker KD, Warren JT, Thummel CS, Gilbert LI, Mangelsdorf DJ. 2000. Transcriptional activation of the *Drosophila* ecdysone receptor by insect and plant ecdysteroids. *Insect Biochem. Mol. Biol.* 30:1037–43
9. Barger JL, Walford RL, Weindruch R.

2003. The retardation of aging by caloric restriction: its significance in the transgenic era. *Exp. Gerontol.* 38:1343–51
10. Barsh GS, Schwartz MW. 2002. Genetic approaches to studying energy balance: perception and integration. *Nat. Rev. Genet.* 3:589–600
11. Bernal A, Kimbrell DA. 2000. Drosophila Thor participates in host immune defense and connects a translational regulator with innate immunity. *Proc. Natl. Acad. Sci. USA* 97:6019–24
12. Berns K, Hijmans EM, Mullenders J, Brummelkamp TR, Velds A, et al. 2004. A large-scale RNAi screen in human cells identifies new components of the p53 pathway. *Nature* 428:431–37
13. Billas IM, Iwema T, Garnier JM, Mitschler A, Rochel N, Moras D. 2003. Structural adaptability in the ligand-binding pocket of the ecdysone hormone receptor. *Nature* 426:91–96
14. Billas IM, Moulinier L, Rochel N, Moras D. 2001. Crystal structure of the ligand-binding domain of the ultraspiracle protein USP, the ortholog of retinoid X receptors in insects. *J. Biol. Chem.* 276:7465–74
15. Bitterman KJ, Medvedik O, Sinclair DA. 2003. Longevity regulation in *Saccharomyces cerevisiae*: linking metabolism, genome stability, and heterochromatin. *Microbiol. Mol. Biol. Rev.* 67:376–99
16. Boord JB, Fazio S, Linton MF. 2002. Cytoplasmic fatty acid–binding proteins: emerging roles in metabolism and atherosclerosis. *Curr. Opin. Lipidol.* 13:141–47
17. Boutros M, Kiger AA, Armknecht S, Kerr K, Hild M, et al. 2004. Genome-wide RNAi analysis of growth and viability in *Drosophila* cells. *Science* 303:832–35
18. Cagney G, Uetz P, Fields S. 2001. Two-hybrid analysis of the *Saccharomyces cerevisiae* 26S proteasome. *Physiol. Genomics* 7:27–34
19. Canavoso LE, Bertello LE, de Lederkremer RM, Rubiolo ER. 1998. Effect of fasting on the composition of the fat body lipid of *Dipetalogaster maximus*, *Triatoma infestans* and *Panstrongylus megistus* (*Hemiptera: Reduviidae*). *J. Comp. Physiol. B* 168:549–54
20. Canavoso LE, Jouni ZE, Karnas KJ, Pennington JE, Wells MA. 2001. Fat metabolism in insects. *Annu. Rev. Nutr.* 21:23–46
21. Canavoso LE, Wells MA. 2000. Metabolic pathways for diacylglycerol biosynthesis and release in the midgut of larval *Manduca sexta*. *Insect Biochem. Mol. Biol.* 30:1173–80
22. Chavez A, Munoz de Chavez M. 2003. Nutrigenomics in public health nutrition: short-term perspectives. *Eur. J. Clin. Nutr.* 57(Suppl. 1):S97–100
23. Chavez VM, Marques G, Delbecque JP, Kobayashi K, Hollingsworth M, et al. 2000. The *Drosophila* disembodied gene controls late embryonic morphogenesis and codes for a cytochrome P450 enzyme that regulates embryonic ecdysone levels. *Development* 127:4115–26
24. Clark AG. 1997. Stress and metabolic regulation in *Drosophila*. *EXS* 83:117–32
25. Clark AG, Keith LE. 1988. Variation among extracted lines of *Drosophila melanogaster* in triacylglycerol and carbohydrate storage. *Genetics* 119:595–607
26. Daborn PJ, Yen JL, Bogwitz MR, Le Goff G, Feil E, et al. 2002. A single p450 allele associated with insecticide resistance in *Drosophila*. *Science* 297:2253–56
27. Dandona P, Aljada A, Bandyopadhyay A. 2004. Inflammation: the link between insulin resistance, obesity and diabetes. *Trends Immunol.* 25:4–7
28. Das M, Gabriely I, Barzilai N. 2004. Caloric restriction, body fat and ageing in experimental models. *Obes. Rev.* 5:13–19
29. Davis CD, Milner J. 2004. Frontiers in nutrigenomics, proteomics, metabolomics and cancer prevention. *Mutat. Res.* 551:51–64
30. De Gregorio E, Spellman PT, Rubin GM, Lemaitre B. 2001. Genome-wide

analysis of the *Drosophila* immune response by using oligonucleotide microarrays. *Proc. Natl. Acad. Sci. USA* 98(22): 12590–95

31. Devarakonda S, Harp JM, Kim Y, Ozyhar A, Rastinejad F. 2003. Structure of the heterodimeric ecdysone receptor DNA-binding complex. *EMBO J.* 22:5827–40
32. Dinan L. 2001. Phytoecdysteroids: biological aspects. *Phytochemistry* 57:325–39
33. Dinan L, Savchenko T, Whiting P. 2001. On the distribution of phytoecdysteroids in plants. *Cell. Mol. Life Sci.* 58:1121–32
34. Doane WW. 1960. Developmental physiology of the mutant female sterile (2) adipose of *Drosophila melanogaster*. I. Adult morphology, longevity, egg production, and egg lethality. *J. Exp. Zool.* 145:1–21
35. Doane WW. 1960. Developmental physiology of the mutant female sterile (2) adipose of *Drosophila melanogaster*. II. Effects of altered environment and residual genome on its expression. *J. Exp. Zool.* 145:23–42
36. Dobrosotskaya IY, Seegmiller AC, Brown MS, Goldstein JL, Rawson RB. 2002. Regulation of SREBP processing and membrane lipid production by phospholipids in *Drosophila*. *Science* 296: 879–83
37. Driver CJ, Lamb MJ. 1980. Metabolic changes in ageing *Drosophila melanogaster*. *Exp. Gerontol.* 15:167–75
38. Driver CJ, Wallis R, Cosopodiotis G, Ettershank G. 1986. Is a fat metabolite the major diet-dependent accelerator of aging? *Exp. Gerontol.* 21:497–507
39. Driver CJI, Cosopodiotis G. 1979. The effect of dietary fat on longevity of *Drosophila melanogaster*. *Exp. Geront.* 14:95–100
40. Dykxhoorn DM, Novina CD, Sharp PA. 2003. Killing the messenger: short RNAs that silence gene expression. *Nat. Rev. Mol. Cell Biol.* 4:457–67
41. Evans T, Felsenfeld G. 1989. The erythroid-specific transcription factor Eryf1: a new finger protein. *Cell* 58: 877–85
42. Fields S, Song O. 1989. A novel genetic system to detect protein-protein interactions. *Nature* 340:245–46
43. Finch CE, Ruvkun G. 2001. The genetics of aging. *Annu. Rev. Genomics Hum. Genet.* 2:435–62
44. Finley RL Jr, Brent R. 1994. Interaction mating reveals binary and ternary connections between *Drosophila* cell cycle regulators. *Proc. Natl. Acad. Sci. USA* 91: 12980–84
45. Furlong EE, Andersen EC, Null B, White KP, Scott MP. 2001. Patterns of gene expression during *Drosophila* mesoderm development. *Science* 293:1629–33
46. Garfinkel MD, Sollars VE, Lu X, Ruden DM. 2004. Multigenerational selection and detection of altered histone acetylation and methylation patterns: toward a quantitative epigenetics in *Drosophila*. *Methods Mol. Biol.* 287:151–79
47. Giaever G. 2003. A chemical genomics approach to understanding drug action. *Trends Pharmacol. Sci.* 24:444–46
48. Giaever G, Chu AM, Ni L, Connelly C, Riles L, et al. 2002. Functional profiling of the *Saccharomyces cerevisiae* genome. *Nature* 418:387–91
49. Giaever G, Flaherty P, Kumm J, Proctor M, Nislow C, et al. 2004. Chemogenomic profiling: identifying the functional interactions of small molecules in yeast. *Proc. Natl. Acad. Sci. USA* 101:793–98
50. Gillies PJ. 2003. Nutrigenomics: the Rubicon of molecular nutrition. *J. Am. Diet. Assoc.* 103:S50–55
51. Giot L, Bader JS, Brouwer C, Chaudhuri A, Kuang B, et al. 2003. A protein interaction map of *Drosophila melanogaster*. *Science* 302:1727–36
52. Goldstein JL, Rawson RB, Brown MS. 2002. Mutant mammalian cells as tools to delineate the sterol regulatory element-binding protein pathway for feedback regulation of lipid synthesis. *Arch. Biochem. Biophys.* 397:139–48

53. Gronke S, Beller M, Fellert S, Ramakrishnan H, Jackle H, Kuhnlein RP. 2003. Control of fat storage by a *Drosophila* PAT domain protein. *Curr. Biol.* 13:603–6
54. Gruntenko N, Chentsova NA, Bogomolova EV, Karpova EK, Glazko GV, et al. 2004. The effect of mutations altering biogenic amine metabolism in *Drosophila* on viability and the response to environmental stresses. *Arch. Insect Biochem. Physiol.* 55:55–67
55. Hader T, Muller S, Aguilera M, Eulenberg KG, Steuernagel A, et al. 2003. Control of triglyceride storage by a WD40/TPR-domain protein. *EMBO Rep.* 4:511–16
56. Hayes SA, Miller JM, Hoshizaki DK. 2001. *Serpent*, a GATA-like transcription factor gene, induces fat-cell development in *Drosophila melanogaster*. *Development* 128:1193–200
57. Heilbronn LK, Ravussin E. 2003. Calorie restriction and aging: review of the literature and implications for studies in humans. *Am. J. Clin. Nutr.* 78:361–69
58. Horton JD, Shah NA, Warrington JA, Anderson NN, Park SW, et al. 2003. Combined analysis of oligonucleotide microarray data from transgenic and knockout mice identifies direct SREBP target genes. *Proc. Natl. Acad. Sci. USA* 100: 12027–32
59. Hotamisligil GS. 2003. Inflammatory pathways and insulin action. *Int. J. Obes. Relat. Metab. Disord.* 27(Suppl. 3):S53–55
60. Hotamisligil GS, Shargill NS, Spiegelman BM. 1993. Adipose expression of tumor necrosis factor-alpha: direct role in obesity-linked insulin resistance. *Science* 259:87–91
61. Hung T, Sievenpiper JL, Marchie A, Kendall CW, Jenkins DJ. 2003. Fat versus carbohydrate in insulin resistance, obesity, diabetes and cardiovascular disease. *Curr. Opin. Clin. Nutr. Metab. Care* 6:165–76
62. Inoue K, Fei YJ, Huang W, Zhuang L, Chen Z, Ganapathy V. 2002. Functional identity of *Drosophila melanogaster* Indy as a cation-independent, electroneutral transporter for tricarboxylic acid-cycle intermediates. *Biochem. J.* 367:313–19
63. Jenkins DJ, Kendall CW, Faulkner D, Vidgen E, Trautwein EA, et al. 2002. A dietary portfolio approach to cholesterol reduction: combined effects of plant sterols, vegetable proteins, and viscous fibers in hypercholesterolemia. *Metab. Clin. Exp.* 51:1596–604
64. Jenkins DJ, Kendall CW, Marchie A, Augustin LS. 2004. Too much sugar, too much carbohydrate, or just too much? *Am. J. Clin. Nutr.* 79:711–12
65. Jenkins DJ, Kendall CW, Marchie A, Faulkner DA, Wong JM, et al. 2003. Effects of a dietary portfolio of cholesterol-lowering foods vs lovastatin on serum lipids and C-reactive protein. *JAMA* 290:502–10
66. Jenkins DJ, Kendall CW, Marchie A, Jenkins AL, Augustin LS, et al. 2003. Type 2 diabetes and the vegetarian diet. *Am. J. Clin. Nutr.* 78:610S–16
67. Jurgens G, Wieschaus E, Nusslein-Volhard C, Kluding H. 1984. Mutations affecting the pattern of the larval cuticle in *Drosophila melanogaster*. II. Zygotic loci on the third chromosome. *Roux Arch. Dev. Biol.* 193:283–95
68. Kaput J, Rodriguez RL. 2004. Nutritional genomics: the next frontier in the postgenomic era. *Physiol. Gen.* 16:166–77
69. Kassam A, Miao B, Young PR, Mukherjee R. 2003. Retinoid X receptor (RXR) agonist-induced antagonism of farnesoid X receptor (FXR) activity due to absence of coactivator recruitment and decreased DNA binding. *J. Biol. Chem.* 278:10028–32
70. Kornman KS, Martha PM, Duff GW. 2004. Genetic variations and inflammation: a practical nutrigenomics opportunity. *Nutrition* 20:44–49
71. Labadarios D, Meguid MM. 2004. Nutrigenomics: unraveling man's constitution in relation to food. *Nutrition* 20:2–3

72. Lemmens I, Eyckerman S, Zabeau L, Catteeuw D, Vertenten E, et al. 2003. Heteromeric MAPPIT: a novel strategy to study modification-dependent protein-protein interactions in mammalian cells. *Nucleic Acids Res.* 31:e75
73. Leonard JR, Klocke BJ, D'Sa C, Flavell RA, Roth KA. 2002. Strain-dependent neurodevelopmental abnormalities in caspase-3-deficient mice. *J. Neuropathol. Exp. Neurol.* 61:673–77
74. Li S, Armstrong CM, Bertin N, Ge H, Milstein S, et al. 2004. A map of the interactome network of the metazoan *C. elegans*. *Science* 303:540–43
75. Lum L, Beachy PA. 2004. The Hedgehog response network: sensors, switches, and routers. *Science* 304:1755–59
76. Lum L, Yao S, Mozer B, Rovescalli A, Von Kessler D, et al. 2003. Identification of Hedgehog pathway components by RNAi in *Drosophila* cultured cells. *Science* 299:2039–45
77. Maglich JM, Sluder A, Guan X, Shi Y, McKee DD, et al. 2001. Comparison of complete nuclear receptor sets from the human, *Caenorhabditis elegans* and *Drosophila* genomes. *Genome Biol.* 2(8):RESEARCH0029
78. Maglich JM, Sluder AE, Willson TM, Moore JT. 2003. Beyond the human genome: examples of nuclear receptor analysis in model organisms and potential for drug discovery. *Am. J. Pharmacogenomics* 3:345–53
79. Magwere T, Chapman T, Partridge L. 2004. Sex differences in the effect of dietary restriction on life span and mortality rates in female and male *Drosophila melanogaster*. *J. Gerontol. A Biol. Sci. Med. Sci.* 59:3–9
80. Mair W, Goymer P, Pletcher SD, Partridge L. 2003. Demography of dietary restriction and death in *Drosophila*. *Science* 301:1731–33
81. Maki A, Sawatsubashi S, Ito S, Shirode Y, Suzuki E, et al. 2004. Juvenile hormones antagonize ecdysone actions through co-repressor recruitment to EcR/USP heterodimers. *Biochem. Biophys. Res. Commun.* 320:262–67
82. Mathers JC. 2004. The biological revolution—towards a mechanistic understanding of the impact of diet on cancer risk. *Mutat. Res.* 551:43–49
83. Mehta T, Tanik M, Allison DB. 2004. Towards sound epistemological foundations of statistical methods for high-dimensional biology. *Nat. Genet.* 36:943–47
84. Meng EC, Bourne HR. 2001. Receptor activation: What does the rhodopsin structure tell us? *Trends Pharmacol. Sci.* 22:587–93
85. Michaut L, Flister S, Neeb M, White KP, Certa U, Gehring WJ. 2003. Analysis of the eye developmental pathway in *Drosophila* using DNA microarrays. *Proc. Natl. Acad. Sci. USA* 100:4024–29
86. Miller JM, Oligino T, Pazdera M, Lopez AJ, Hoshizaki DK. 2002. Identification of fat-cell enhancer regions in *Drosophila melanogaster*. *Insect Mol. Biol.* 11:67–77
87. Miura S, Gan JW, Brzostowski J, Parisi MJ, Schultz CJ, et al. 2002. Functional conservation for lipid storage droplet association among Perilipin, ADRP, and TIP47 (PAT)-related proteins in mammals, *Drosophila*, and *Dictyostelium*. *J. Biol. Chem.* 277:32253–57
88. Moebius FF, Fitzky BU, Glossmann H. 2000. Genetic defects in postsqualene cholesterol biosynthesis. *Trends Endocrinol. Metab.* 11:106–14
89. Monastirioti M. 1999. Biogenic amine systems in the fruit fly *Drosophila melanogaster*. *Microsc. Res. Tech.* 45:106–21
90. Montooth KL, Marden JH, Clark AG. 2003. Mapping determinants of variation in energy metabolism, respiration and flight in *Drosophila*. *Genetics* 165:623–35
91. Muller M, Kersten S. 2003. Nutrigenomics: goals and strategies. *Nat. Rev. Genet.* 4:315–22

92. Neel JV. 1962. Diabetes mellitus: a "thrifty" genotype rendered detrimental by "progress"? *Am. J. Hum. Genet.* 14: 353–62
93. Nusslein-Volhard C, Wieschaus E, Kluding H. 1984. Mutations affecting the pattern of the larval cuticle in *Drosophila melanogaster*. I. Zygotic loci on the second chromosome. *Roux Arch. Dev. Biol.* 193:267–82
94. Oberdorster E, Clay MA, Cottam DM, Wilmot FA, McLachlan JA, Milner MJ. 2001. Common phytochemicals are ecdysteroid agonists and antagonists: a possible evolutionary link between vertebrate and invertebrate steroid hormones. *J. Steroid Biochem. Mol. Biol.* 77:229–38
95. Paddison PJ, Silva JM, Conklin DS, Schlabach M, Li M, et al. 2004. A resource for large-scale RNA-interference-based screens in mammals. *Nature* 428:427–31
96. Parks AL, Cook KR, Belvin M, Dompe NA, Fawcett R, et al. 2004. Systematic generation of high-resolution deletion coverage of the *Drosophila melanogaster* genome. *Nat. Genet.* 36:288–92
97. Patterson SD, Aebersold RH. 2003. Proteomics: the first decade and beyond. *Nat. Genet.* 33(Suppl.):311–23
98. Peregrin T. 2001. The new frontier of nutrition science: nutrigenomics. *J. Am. Diet. Assoc.* 101:1306
99. Petersen UM, Kadalayil L, Rehorn KP, Hoshizaki DK, Reuter R, Engstrom Y. 1999. Serpent regulates *Drosophila* immunity genes in the larval fat body through an essential GATA motif. *EMBO J.* 18:4013–22
100. Phizicky E, Bastiaens PI, Zhu H, Snyder M, Fields S. 2003. Protein analysis on a proteomic scale. *Nature* 422:208–15
101. Radhakrishnan A, Sun LP, Kwon HJ, Brown MS, Goldstein JL. 2004. Direct binding of cholesterol to the purified membrane region of SCAP: mechanism for a sterol-sensing domain. *Mol. Cell* 15:259–68
102. Rehorn KP, Thelen H, Michelson AM, Reuter R. 1996. A molecular aspect of hematopoiesis and endoderm development common to vertebrates and *Drosophila*. *Development* 122:4023–31
103. Roeske WR, Clayton RB. 1968. Behavior of sterols of insect muscle during homogenization and differential centrifugation. *J. Lipid Res.* 9:276–84
104. Rogina B, Helfand SL, Frankel S. 2002. Longevity regulation by *Drosophila* Rpd3 deacetylase and caloric restriction. *Science* 298:1745
105. Roth GE, Gierl MS, Vollborn L, Meise M, Lintermann R, Korge G. 2004. The *Drosophila* gene Start1: a putative cholesterol transporter and key regulator of ecdysteroid synthesis. *Proc. Natl. Acad. Sci. USA* 101:1601–6
106. Rubin GM, Lewis EB. 2000. A brief history of *Drosophila's* contributions to genome research. *Science* 287:2216–18
107. Rubin GM, Yandell MD, Wortman JR, Gabor Miklos GL, Nelson CR, et al. 2000. Comparative genomics of the eukaryotes. *Science* 287:2204–15
108. Sakai J, Rawson RB, Espenshade PJ, Cheng D, Seegmiller AC, et al. 1998. Molecular identification of the sterol-regulated luminal protease that cleaves SREBPs and controls lipid composition of animal cells. *Mol. Cell* 2:505–14
109. Santos AC, Lehmann R. 2004. Isoprenoids control germ cell migration downstream of HMGCoA reductase. *Dev. Cell* 6:283–93
110. Sawatsubashi S, Maki A, Ito S, Shirode Y, Suzuki E, et al. 2004. Ecdysone receptor-dependent gene regulation mediates histone poly(ADP-ribosyl)ation. *Biochem. Biophys. Res. Commun.* 320:268–72
111. Schwartz MW. 2001. Brain pathways controlling food intake and body weight. *Exp. Biol. Med.* 226:978–81
112. Schwartz MW, Woods SC, Seeley RJ, Barsh GS, Baskin DG, Leibel RL. 2003. Is the energy homeostasis system inherently biased toward weight gain? *Diabetes* 52:232–38

113. Sedkov Y, Cho E, Petruk S, Cherbas L, Smith ST, et al. 2003. Methylation at lysine 4 of histone H3 in ecdysone-dependent development of *Drosophila*. *Nature* 426:78–83
114. Seegmiller AC, Dobrosotskaya I, Goldstein JL, Ho YK, Brown MS, Rawson RB. 2002. The SREBP pathway in *Drosophila*: regulation by palmitate, not sterols. *Dev. Cell* 2:229–38
115. Stocco DM. 2000. The role of the StAR protein in steroidogenesis: challenges for the future. *J. Endocrinol.* 164:247–53
116. Sun LV, Chen L, Greil F, Negre N, Li TR, et al. 2003. Protein-DNA interaction mapping using genomic tiling path microarrays in *Drosophila*. *Proc. Natl. Acad. Sci. USA* 100:9428–33
117. Svanberg E, Ohlsson C, Hyltander A, Lundholm KG. 1999. The role of diet components, gastrointestinal factors, and muscle innervation on activation of protein synthesis in skeletal muscles following oral refeeding. *Nutrition* 15:257–66
118. Takahashi Y, Toh-e A, Kikuchi Y. 2001. A novel factor required for the SUMO1/Smt3 conjugation of yeast septins. *Gene* 275:223–31
119. Tansey JT, Sztalryd C, Gruia-Gray J, Roush DL, Zee JV, et al. 2001. Perilipin ablation results in a lean mouse with aberrant adipocyte lipolysis, enhanced leptin production, and resistance to diet-induced obesity. *Proc. Natl. Acad. Sci. USA* 98:6494–99
120. Tatar M, Bartke A, Antebi A. 2003. The endocrine regulation of aging by insulin-like signals. *Science* 299:1346–51
121. Teague BD, Clark AG, Doane WW. 1986. Developmental analysis of lipids from wild-type and adipose60 mutants of *Drosophila melanogaster*. *J. Exp. Zool.* 240:95–104
122. Teixeira L, Rabouille C, Rorth P, Ephrussi A, Vanzo NF. 2003. *Drosophila* Perilipin/ADRP homologue Lsd2 regulates lipid metabolism. *Mech. Dev.* 120:1071–81
123. Thibault ST, Singer MA, Miyazaki WY, Milash B, Dompe NA, et al. 2004. A complementary transposon tool kit for *Drosophila melanogaster* using P and piggyBac. *Nat. Genet.* 36:283–7
124. Thorpe JL, Doitsidou M, Ho SY, Raz E, Farber SA. 2004. Germ cell migration in zebrafish is dependent on HMGCoA reductase activity and prenylation. *Dev. Cell* 6:295–302
125. Toma DP, White KP, Hirsch J, Greenspan RJ. 2002. Identification of genes involved in *Drosophila melanogaster* geotaxis, a complex behavioral trait. *Nat. Genet.* 31:349–53
126. Tong AH, Lesage G, Bader GD, Ding H, Xu H, et al. 2004. Global mapping of the yeast genetic interaction network. *Science* 303:808–13
127. Tong Q, Dalgin G, Xu H, Ting CN, Leiden JM, Hotamisligil GS. 2000. Function of GATA transcription factors in preadipocyte-adipocyte transition. *Science* 290:134–38
128. Trayhurn P. 2003. Nutritional genomics—"nutrigenomics." *Br. J. Nutr.* 89:1–2
129. Tsai SF, Martin DI, Zon LI, D'Andrea AD, Wong GG, Orkin SH. 1989. Cloning of cDNA for the major DNA-binding protein of the erythroid lineage through expression in mammalian cells. *Nature* 339:446–51
130. van Ommen B. 2004. Nutrigenomics: exploiting systems biology in the nutrition and health arenas. *Nutrition* 20:4–8
131. van Ommen B, Stierum R. 2002. Nutrigenomics: exploiting systems biology in the nutrition and health arena. *Curr. Opin. Biotechnol.* 13:517–21
132. Vierstraete E, Verleyen P, Baggerman G, D'Hertog W, Van den Bergh G, et al. 2004. A proteomic approach for the analysis of instantly released wound and immune proteins in *Drosophila melanogaster* hemolymph. *Proc. Natl. Acad. Sci. USA* 101:470–75
133. Vierstraete E, Verleyen P, Sas F, Van den

Bergh G, De Loof A, et al. 2004. The instantly released *Drosophila* immune proteome is infection-specific. *Biochem. Biophys. Res. Commun.* 317:1052–60

134. Warren JT, Petryk A, Marques G, Jarcho M, Parvy JP, et al. 2002. Molecular and biochemical characterization of two P450 enzymes in the ecdysteroidogenic pathway of *Drosophila melanogaster. Proc. Natl. Acad. Sci. USA* 99:11043–48
135. Wells L, Hart GW. 2003. O-GlcNAc turns twenty: functional implications for post-translational modification of nuclear and cytosolic proteins with a sugar. *FEBS Lett.* 546:154–58
136. Wells L, Vosseller K, Hart GW. 2003. A role for N-acetylglucosamine as a nutrient sensor and mediator of insulin resistance. *Cell. Mol. Life Sci.* 60:222–28
137. Wells L, Whalen SA, Hart GW. 2003. O-GlcNAc: a regulatory post-translational modification. *Biochem. Biophys. Res. Commun.* 302:435–41
138. White KP, Rifkin SA, Hurban P, Hogness DS. 1999. Microarray analysis of *Drosophila* development during metamorphosis. *Science* 286:2179–84
139. Wieschaus E, Nusslein-Volhard C, Jurgens G. 1984. Mutations affecting the pattern of the larval cuticle in *Drosophila melanogaster*. III. Zygotic loci on the X chromosome and fourth chromosome. *Roux Arch. Dev. Biol.* 193:296–307
140. Winzeler EA, Shoemaker DD, Astromoff A, Liang H, Anderson K, et al. 1999. Functional characterization of the *S. cerevisiae* genome by gene deletion and parallel analysis. *Science* 285:901–6
141. Wood JG, Rogina B, Lavu S, Howitz K, Helfand SL, et al. 2004. Sirtuin activators mimic caloric restriction and delay ageing in metazoans. *Nature* 430:686–89
142. Zheng L, Liu J, Batalov S, Zhou D, Orth A, et al. 2004. An approach to genomewide screens of expressed small interfering RNAs in mammalian cells. *Proc. Natl. Acad. Sci. USA* 101:135–40
143. Zinke I, Schutz CS, Katzenberger JD, Bauer M, Pankratz MJ. 2002. Nutrient control of gene expression in *Drosophila*: microarray analysis of starvation and sugar-dependent response. *EMBO J.* 21:6162–73

Annu. Rev. Nutr. 2005. 25:523–47
doi: doi: 10.1146/annurev.nutr.25.050304.092704

First published online as a Review in Advance on April 7, 2005

THE COW AS A MODEL TO STUDY FOOD INTAKE REGULATION

Michael S. Allen and Barry J. Bradford
Department of Animal Science, Michigan State University, East Lansing, Michigan 48824; email: allenm@msu.edu, bradfo68@msu.edu

Kevin J. Harvatine
Department of Animal Science, Cornell University, Ithaca, New York 14853; email: kjh38@cornell.edu

Key Words cow, animal model, intake regulation, feeding behavior

■ **Abstract** Animal models have been invaluable for studying aspects of food intake regulation that for various reasons cannot be observed in humans. The dairy cow is a unique animal model because of an unrivaled energy requirement; its great drive to eat results in feeding behavior responses to treatments within the physiological range. Cows' docile nature and large size make them ideal for measuring temporal treatment effects because digestion and absorption kinetics and responses in endocrine systems, gene expression, metabolite pools and fluxes, and feeding behavior can be measured simultaneously. Thus, cows are important models to investigate interactions of short-term signals regulating food intake. Furthermore, different physiological states throughout the lactation cycle provide powerful models to study how short- and long-term signals interact to affect long-term energy status. The use of the cow as a model can lead to breakthroughs in understanding the complex interactions of signals regulating food intake.

CONTENTS

INTRODUCTION

The obesity epidemic in the United States and other developed countries has accentuated the importance of studying food intake regulation. Overweight and obese individuals are at increased risk of diseases such as diabetes, high blood pressure, high cholesterol, asthma, and arthritis (83). The proportion of overweight and obese adults in the United States is rising rapidly (35) and has a significant economic impact on the U.S. health care system (110). Although identification of individual satiety factors is progressing rapidly, food intake regulation is extremely complex, and immediate application of research results has been limited. Animal models are utilized to understand physiological and metabolic mechanisms that cannot be observed in human subjects owing to social influence, procedural invasiveness, or ethical limitations. Valuable animal models must provide one or more of the following advantages over human studies: (*a*) the possibility of invasive or repeated sampling with minimal interruption of feeding behavior; (*b*) accessibility of specific organs, portions of the brain, or sections of the gastrointestinal tract for infusion or biopsy; (*c*) existence of genetic polymorphisms or mutations in genes of interest for intake regulation. The use of any of the animal models to study human intake regulation requires the assumption that basic mechanisms controlling feeding behavior are conserved across species.

Rodent models are by far the most commonly used animal models for nutrition and metabolism experiments (42). Rodents require minimal housing facilities and are cost-effective because of their small size. Their extensive use in research provides a rich description of their physiological processes, and variation among strains is well documented and utilized experimentally. Rodent models are also amenable to transgenic manipulation and allow in vivo observation of the effects of gene deletion and overexpression. However, like all animal models, the rodent model has limitations in the study of food intake regulation. Regulatory mechanisms for food intake might be more closely conserved among humans and larger animals; divergence in mechanisms regulating energy intake likely occurred between small and large animals because of different evolutionary pressures (102). Speakman et al. (102) suggested that a system to regulate body mass within strict limits is more advantageous for small animals because they are less starvation-tolerant and have greater mass-dependent predation risk than large animals. Predation also caused rodents to evolve primarily nocturnal feeding behaviors, which may have resulted in further divergence in mechanisms regulating food intake compared with humans.

Rodent models have been invaluable in identifying mechanisms of intake and energy regulation such as the pathways involving leptin and agouti. However, human obesity is not caused by a malfunction of a single mechanism but is polygenic in nature (19). Research in bovine physiology has focused primarily on polygenic traits, making the cow a valuable biological model for studying complex human health issues such as obesity (43). In addition, the physiological states during the lactation cycle of the dairy cow may provide models that are relevant to conditions observed in humans, including hypophagia associated with stress, short-term regulation of hunger and satiety, and long-term regulation of energy homeostasis.

The use of animal models representing evolutionary clades distinct from rodents increases our ability to dissect the complex processes of food intake regulation that are conserved across many species. The objective of this chapter is to discuss the cow as such an alternate model. In the following sections, we provide background on the nutrition and physiology of the cow as it relates to strengths and limitations as a model for studying food intake regulation. We follow this with specific examples in which the cow has been used to study the effects of temporal pattern of fuel absorption on feeding behavior. We conclude by discussing the value of the different physiological states experienced within lactation cycles for studying the effects of interacting regulators of food intake.

STRENGTHS AND LIMITATIONS OF THE COW AS A MODEL

Lactating dairy cows are unique among animal models used to study food intake regulation for several reasons. They have extremely high energy requirements and marginal nutrient status, which makes them responsive to nutritional changes (Table 1); most energy is partitioned to milk, which is easily measured; they are docile and ideal for intensive measurements of digestion, metabolism, and behavior; and they cycle through different physiological states, greatly affecting energy balance on an annual basis (Figure 1). Few mammals have energy requirements that approach those of high-yielding dairy cows on a metabolic body-weight basis, and none that do have such requirements have been studied as extensively. Although there are very significant differences between fuels available to ruminants and humans because of pregastric fermentation, the basic mechanisms regulating food intake appear to be highly conserved across the species. In some respects, the cow is more similar to humans than is the rat. For instance, cows and humans are similar in respect to circadian eating patterns, ovulation cycles, gestation lengths, and the number of offspring per pregnancy. In addition, the bovine and human genomes seem to exhibit greater collinearity and sequence homology than do the mouse and human genomes (43).

Digestion and Metabolism

Ruminants, like other herbivores, consume diets that are higher in fiber and lower in fat than are diets of nonherbivores. In addition, nutrients absorbed differ markedly from those consumed because of fermentation by microbes in the rumen: organic

TABLE 1 Comparison of energy requirements and metabolic parameters of the cow, human, and rat

Parameter	Cow[a]	Human[b]	Rat[c]
Energy required, kcal d^{-1}	41,800	3081	170
Energy required, kcal $BW_{kg}^{-0.75}$	325	127	86
Maintenance energy, kcal d^{-1}	9270	1769	136
Maintenance energy, % of total	22	57	80
Activity, kcal d^{-1}	1030	1312	34
Milk production, kcal d^{-1}	31,500	—	—
Plasma glucose[d], mg dl^{-1}	55–64	90–130	110–130
Plasma insulin[d], μIU ml^{-1}	8–16	10–80	10–90
Hepatic gluconeogenesis, g glucose d^{-1}	3402	160[e]	2.15[e]

[a]Mature lactating cow: 100 days in lactation, 650 kg, producing 45 kg milk d^{-1} (3.5% fat), housed in individual stall. Energy requirements calculated from (87).

[b]70 kg man with moderate physical activity level, 30 years of age. Energy requirements calculated from (36).

[c]0.4 kg male rat in laboratory housing. Energy requirements calculated from (60).

[d]Typical daily range for fed subjects. Human and rat data from (114).

[e]Maximum rate in fasted subjects (63, 70).

matter (OM) is partially fermented to volatile fatty acids (VFAs; primarily acetic, propionic, and butyric); feed protein is partially degraded to amino acids and ammonia, which are incorporated into microbial protein of high biological value; and unsaturated fatty acids (FAs) are biohydrogenated and isomerized to varying degrees. The major fuels for cows are VFAs from ruminal and intestinal fermentation of OM, glucose from starch digestion in the small intestine (metabolized primarily to lactate by intestinal tissue), and nonesterified FAs (NEFAs) and amino acids absorbed from the gastrointestinal tract and mobilized from body reserves. More than 60% of absorbed amino acids are from microbial protein flowing from the rumen, with the remainder from feed protein escaping ruminal degradation. The large size of the digesta pool and its relatively slow passage from the rumen result in a more consistent absorption of nutrients in ruminants than in nonruminants. Rumen contents of high-producing dairy cows often exceed 100 kg (~15% dry matter), and passage rates of digesta are approximately 2%–4% h^{-1} for fiber, 10%–20% h^{-1} for starch, and 15%–20% h^{-1} for liquid.

Although differences in fuels between humans and cows might be considered a limitation of using cows as models to study food intake regulation, they are also a strength, providing us the opportunity to evaluate basic mechanisms regulating food intake that are conserved across species using very different fuels. This requires an understanding of comparative physiology and metabolism between the species. The physiology and metabolism of dairy cows has been extensively studied and is well documented (Table 1). One difference between cows and

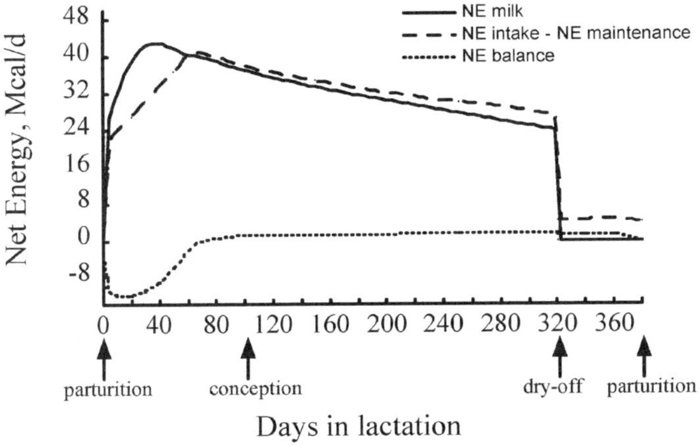

Figure 1 Graphical representation of energy balance through lactation for a mature 650 kg Holstein cow producing approximately 12,700 kg of milk in a 320-day lactation. Milk energy output exceeds net energy intake above the maintenance requirement of 10.3 Mcal day^{-1}, resulting in a large negative energy balance and mobilization of body energy reserves until ~60 days in lactation. The length of the lactation cycle (380 days in this example) is determined by time to conception, which is highly variable (100 days in this example) and gestation length (~280 days). Cessation of milking (dry-off) generally occurs approximately 60 days prior to the following parturition, but is also variable. Energy required for fetal growth increases throughout gestation, peaking at ~4 Mcal day^{-1} of net energy prior to parturition.

humans is that almost no glucose enters from the portal drained viscera in cows (95). Although many ruminant tissues preferentially utilize acetate rather than glucose (45), certain tissues require glucose, and large quantities are required for milk lactose production. As might be expected, the bovine liver functions primarily as a glucose factory. Hexokinase activity is very low in bovine liver (9) and gluconeogenic capacity is extremely high; net hepatic glucose release exceeded 3.5 kg d^{-1} for cows producing ~41 kg d^{-1} of milk (96). Propionate is the primary gluconeogenic substrate in ruminants, accounting for as much as 80% of glucose produced in lactating cows (104). Long-chain FAs (LCFAs) are a major source of energy in bovine liver, which has limited capacity for FA synthesis (45) or triglyceride export (31). As in rodent models, research in the physiology and metabolism of cows is progressing quickly with the use of genomics and this will likely lead to new approaches to study regulation of food intake. For example, the discovery of polymorphisms in the coding region of the leptin gene associated with differences in feed intake in cows (72) could provide a model to study leptin regulation of food intake. Recent sequencing of the bovine genome (86), coupled with the use of proteomics and metabolomics, is expected to further increase the pace of research in ruminant physiology and metabolism.

Energy Requirements and Physiological States

The mean milk yield of cows in the United States was more than 8500 kg year^{-1} in 2003, and it has increased by 16% over the past 10 years (111). Milk yield varies greatly among cows and across stage of lactation; individual cows have produced more than 30,000 kg of milk in a 365-day lactation, with a peak milk yield of over 90 kg d^{-1}. It is not uncommon for milk yield to exceed 60 kg d^{-1} for high-producing cows in early lactation, which requires synthesis of ~4.5 kg d^{-1} glucose [calculated using the formula of (29)] and 50 Mcal of net energy d^{-1} including ~10 Mcal d^{-1} for maintenance requirements of a 650-kg cow.

The dairy cow experiences multiple physiological states throughout a lactation cycle, including extended periods of negative and positive energy balance (Figure 1). Immediately before initiation of lactation, a short nonlactating period (~60 days) allows for mammary involution and ensures adequate nutrient availability for fetal growth and regeneration of mammary epithelial tissue. Around parturition, the cow experiences hypophagia, likely because of physiological stress and immune challenges at parturition. Peak milk synthesis often occurs within 40 days of parturition and imposes a large energy demand on the cow. This rapid increase in energy requirements cannot be matched by increased intake, so body reserves are mobilized. Maximum intake is reached 2–3 weeks following maximum milk yield, allowing a less negative energy balance. As milk production decreases later in lactation, the cow resumes a positive energy balance and begins to replenish body reserves. During the lactation cycle, the energy requirement varies severalfold, and nearly half of the cow's fat reserve may be lost and regained during a lactation (15).

Adaptation to Intensive Measurements

To study interactions between satiety mechanisms in vivo, measurements must be taken over time, often from different organs, with minimal interruption of feeding behavior. Cows thrive in individual stalls and their docile nature allows measurement of feeding behavior along with intensive measurements of site of digestion, fuel supply, and endocrine response. The extremely high energy requirement of lactating cows results in a strong drive to eat, which is maintained even during experimental interventions. We have developed a system to automatically record feed and water consumption, chewing behavior, and ruminal motility for 12 cows simultaneously (23) and to automatically collect blood and rumen fluid samples with minimal disturbance to the cow (2). This system allows continuous (integrated) sampling, pulse sampling as frequently as every 8 minutes, or pulse sampling triggered by behavioral events, without affecting feeding behavior. Behavioral events such as meal initiation have been used to automatically trigger infusion pumps to evaluate factors affecting satiety and hunger (20). In addition, we have demonstrated that needle biopsies of the liver can be collected over the course of a meal without significantly altering meal size ($P > 0.15$; M.S. Allen, unpublished results). These tissue samples as well as those from biopsy of adipose tissue and muscle can be used to measure temporal patterns of gene expression. Much larger biopsy samples can be taken for measurement of enzyme activity or for proteomic or metabolomic analysis.

Other groups have demonstrated proficiency in measuring portal flux and net liver flux of nutrients during voluntary meals in cattle (17), and in measuring gastric motility and digesta passage (67). Although cattle are not generally used for direct hypothalamic studies, sheep have been used for brain infusion work for years (51, 81), and the cow provides an equally good, albeit more expensive, model (3). In addition, nutrients may be supplied through intestinal or intravenous infusion to modify energy balance. Nutrients may be infused into the rumen, although abomasal or duodenal infusions allow more certain absorption of nutrients by avoiding metabolism by ruminal bacteria. Ruminal and duodenal cannulas may be maintained over multiple lactations without detrimental effects on the health of the animals; we have used groups of cows with both cannulas that averaged as much as 45 kg d^{-1} of milk (46). Abomasal infusion lines are easily placed by reaching through the rumen of a fistulated cow and feeding a catheter line through the reticular-omasal orifice. Although it is true that none of these methods is unique to the cow, the importance of using a large, docile animal with a strong drive to eat cannot be overemphasized. By combining several of these techniques, biologists have the opportunity to use the dairy cow to uncover many of the complex interactions between hormonal, metabolic, and sensory modulators of feeding behavior.

Measurement of Energy Status

In the lactating dairy cow, the large energy demand for lactation overwhelms the energy expended in physical activity. In contrast, physical activity greatly contributes to the energy expenditure of humans and other animals and thus has a large effect on their requirement for energy intake. Furthermore, exogenous infusions of the intake-regulating peptides ghrelin and agouti-related peptide decreased locomotor activity by 20% in rats (107). The large contribution of physical activity to total nonmaintenance energy expenditure and its modification by intake-regulating compounds demands that activity is measured and accounted for in understanding energy balance in humans and rodents at maintenance. Unfortunately, observation of physical activity and calculation of energy expended during physical activity is challenging and may lack accuracy (108). In comparison, observation of milk yield and composition allows convenient and accurate determination of the major portion of energy expenditure of cows. Milk yield is observed at least twice per day and the net energy required to produce milk can be calculated based on the yield of components. The maintenance energy requirement can be estimated from metabolic body size and is ~25% of the total energy requirement of a 650-kg cow producing 45 kg of milk d^{-1} (Table 1). Thus, the ability to more accurately account for the majority of the energy expended in the lactating cow provides an advantage for investigating maintenance of energy balance.

Retained energy is more difficult to measure for ruminants. Differences in body weight gain are difficult to detect because of a large variation in digesta weight relative to meals, and treatment bias can occur if treatments affect the weight of digesta. Ruminal empty body weight is a much more sensitive measure of body weight change and is observed as body weight after removal of ruminal contents through a fistula. Although change in body composition is difficult to assess without sacrificing animals, tissue energy gain can be estimated from change in body weight by assuming that changes occur primarily in adipose tissue.

TEMPORAL EFFECTS OF ABSORBED FUELS

Temporal patterns of fuel absorption and utilization affect food intake by altering meal size and frequency. Satiety factors that affect the length and size of meals include gut distension from the filling effect of foods and various physiological responses to absorbed fuels. Hunger, determined by sensory cues and clearance of fuels from the blood, affects the interval between meals and rate of food consumption. Pregastric fermentation affects the type and temporal pattern of absorption of fuels in ruminants, complicating the evaluation of their effects on feeding behavior. However, cannulation of the gastrointestinal tract allows determination of fuels available for absorption as well as the kinetics of digestion and absorption. Combined measurement of digestion kinetics and feeding behavior allows evaluation of responses to temporal absorption of fuels for different dietary treatments. Modification of feeding behavior by changes in kinetics of ruminal starch digestion and absorption of unsaturated FA are discussed in this section to demonstrate the potential contribution of temporal observations to our understanding of food intake regulation.

Regulation of Food Intake by Hepatic Oxidation of Fuels: Evidence in Ruminants

STARCH DIGESTION KINETICS AND FEEDING BEHAVIOR The rates of ruminal starch digestion and passage vary greatly across grains fed to ruminants and depend upon the type of cereal grain, conservation method, and processing (87). Ruminal digestion kinetics determine the site and extent of nutrient digestion, which can greatly affect the type and temporal pattern of fuels absorbed. Cereal grains that are highly digestible in the rumen can depress food intake of lactating cows; food intake was depressed nearly 3 kg DM d^{-1} ($\sim$13%) when more fermentable grains were substituted in diets of lactating cows in several studies reported in the literature (1). A recent experiment from our laboratory demonstrated that a more rapidly fermented starch source reduced meal size 17%, causing an 8% reduction in food intake despite a 10% decrease in intermeal interval (89). The more fermentable treatment nearly doubled the fractional rate of starch digestion in the rumen, increasing the contribution of VFA as a fuel at the expense of glucose from starch digestion in the small intestine.

Dynamic measures of fuel absorption and feeding behavior provide essential clues regarding the mechanism of diet-induced hypophagia. One possibility is that increased VFA production causes satiety by increasing the osmolality of rumen fluid during meals. Osmolality may stimulate satiety through osmoreceptors in the rumen wall (77) or the release of vasopressin, a hormone that can affect satiety (73), in response to water efflux from the blood to the rumen. Although mechanisms associated with osmolality likely contribute to satiety, changes in osmolality per se do not affect food intake. We reported that sodium chloride (NaCl) infused intraruminally at the onset of spontaneous meals decreased meal size 27% but did not affect daily food intake because intermeal interval decreased 31% compared with sham infusion (20). In that experiment, Na acetate and Na propionate decreased food intake compared with equimolar amounts of NaCl, primarily because of a greater intermeal interval, which indicates delayed hunger.

HYPOPHAGIC EFFECTS OF PROPIONATE Increasing ruminal starch fermentation increases propionate as a proportion of VFA absorbed in addition to increasing the amount of VFA produced (25). Hypophagic effects of propionate infusions have been documented extensively for ruminants (5, 30, 34, 58, 79, 82, 100). Propionate is more hypophagic than acetate or butyrate when infused into the portal vein of sheep (5), and infusion of propionate into the mesenteric veins of steers reduced feed intake, whereas acetate infused at similar rates did not (30). In the infusion study by Choi & Allen (20), propionate decreased dry matter intake compared with acetate by decreasing meal size, a finding that indicates increased satiety. Therefore, propionate likely causes satiety via mechanisms beyond those related to osmolality. Although propionate might be expected to decrease food intake compared with acetate because it has higher energy content, propionate linearly decreased metabolizable energy intake compared with acetate in lactating cows when infused intraruminally as iso-osmotic mixtures (91). As the proportion of propionate increased, the reduction in metabolizable energy intake from the diet exceeded that supplied from the infusate. Food intake was reduced primarily through a linear reduction in meal size from 2.5 to 1.5 kg DM as propionate increased from 0% to 100% of infusate. Meal frequency also tended to decrease linearly ($P = 0.08$), from 7.4 to 6.1 meals during the 12-h monitoring period, as propionate was increased. Therefore, propionate decreased energy intake compared with acetate by increasing satiety and possibly by decreasing hunger. Propionate also decreased food intake of dairy cows compared to iso-energetic infusions of VFA mixtures (58) or acetate (100). These studies suggest that hypophagic effects of propionate cannot be explained simply by the additional energy supplied as propionate. It is unlikely that animals consume feed to meet their energy requirements per se but rather have fuel-specific mechanisms regulating satiety and hunger.

MECHANISM FOR REGULATION OF INTAKE BY PROPIONATE The mechanism by which propionate regulates satiety is not fully understood. More than three decades ago, Baile (7) proposed that propionate receptors in the ruminal region of sheep might regulate food intake because propionate injections into the ruminal vein during spontaneous meals decreased food intake, but injections of larger amounts into the jugular vein did not. Subsequent research with nonruminants suggests that meals can be terminated by a signal carried from the liver to the brain via afferents in the vagus nerve that are affected by hepatic oxidation of fuels and generation of ATP (38, 75). The mechanism by which intracellular ATP concentrations affect the firing rate of the hepatic vagus has not been determined. Although it is possible that ATP-sensitive potassium channels are involved in signal initiation (39), adenosine-5′-monophosphate (AMP)-activated protein kinase (AMPK) is an emerging candidate. AMPK is activated in response to high AMP concentration (typically corresponding to low ATP concentration), and direct activation of AMPK in the hypothalamus increased food intake of rats (4). The ability of AMPK to phosphorylate ion channels and other proteins involved in signal transduction pathways provides a much broader range of possible mechanisms than does the ATP-sensitive potassium channel.

Regulation of food intake by propionate in ruminants is consistent with this proposed mechanism; propionate might decrease food intake of ruminants by stimulating oxidative metabolism in the liver (1). The liver is involved in regulation of intake by propionate because hypophagic effects of portal infusion of propionate were eliminated by splanchnic blockade with anesthetic, bilateral splanchnotomy, and hepatic vagotomy, as well as with total liver denervation in sheep (6). Of fuels metabolized by the ruminant liver, propionate is likely a primary satiety signal because its flux to the liver increases greatly during meals (18). While propionate is extensively metabolized by the ruminant liver, there is little net metabolism of acetate (95) because ruminant liver has high activity of propionyl CoA synthetase but not acetyl CoA synthetase (26, 97), thus explaining differences in hypophagic effects of infusions of propionate and acetate in ruminants.

Glucose is hypophagic in a variety of nonruminants (37), but intestinal and intravenous glucose infusions have not decreased energy intake of ruminants (1). The absence of effects of portal glucose infusion on food intake by sheep (8) casts doubt on the hypothesis that nutrient receptors in the portal vein mediate the hypophagic effects of glucose (54). Given that mechanisms regulating food intake are well conserved among mammals, it seems unlikely that highly specific receptors for glucose exist in rodents but not in cows. Rather, differences in hypophagic effects of glucose infusion observed between ruminants and nonruminants are likely because of differences in hepatic oxidation of glucose; liver hexokinase activity is low in ruminants compared with nonruminants (9), and in mature ruminants, hepatic removal of glucose appears to be negligible (103). Although the notion of fuel-specific receptors persists (54, 79) and the exact coding mechanisms of peripheral metabolic sensors that control food intake are not definitely known (98), this example is consistent with the hypothesis that feeding behavior is regulated by the hepatic oxidation of fuels. Further research with this animal model holds promise to test this hypothesis further.

HYPOPHAGIC EFFECTS OF PROPIONATE ARE VARIABLE Inconsistent effects of propionate infusion on food intake have led to doubts that VFAs per se are signals of satiety for ruminants (44). However, the partitioning of fuels among different tissues and between metabolic pathways affects food intake substantially (39). Propionate can be used for gluconeogenesis, which consumes ATP, or oxidized in the tricarboxylic acid (TCA) cycle as acetyl CoA, generating ATP. Therefore, the temporal pattern of oxidative metabolism in the liver is greatly altered by both propionate flux to the liver and fate of propionate within the liver (Figure 2). Insulin and glucagon are important for directing fuel partitioning, especially during meals. Decreased rate of gluconeogenesis when plasma glucose and insulin are high is expected to speed oxidation of propionate in the liver and cause satiety sooner. In support of this, the extent of hypophagia caused by propionate infusion increased linearly with plasma glucose concentration in dairy cows (90). Ruminants absorb little glucose during meals, and insulin responses to meals are less extreme than those of nonruminants. However, cephalic stimulation prompts insulin secretion in ruminants (52), and propionate (79) and butyrate (61) are insulin secretagogues. As a result, peripheral insulin concentrations increase substantially within and following major meals in lactating cows (Figure 3). Grovum (44) suggested that hypophagic effects of propionate are through insulin because propionate is an insulin secretagogue and insulin is a putative satiety hormone. However, hypophagic effects of propionate infusions have been observed without an increase in insulin (34, 41), and mechanisms exclusively involving insulin do not explain the elimination of hypophagic effects of portal infusions of propionate by hepatic denervation as discussed above.

In the previously mentioned study from our laboratory (89), more rapidly fermented starch decreased meal size, likely because propionate flux to, and oxidation in, the liver was higher during meals. More rapid increases in plasma insulin concentration during meals for the more fermentable starch treatment (89) likely increased fuel oxidation by inhibiting gluconeogenesis (88). Increased plasma insulin concentrations may have also contributed to increased hunger for this treatment by speeding clearance of fuels from the blood, especially following relatively smaller meals. This might explain inconsistent intake effects of peripheral insulin administration reported in the literature (50); although increased hepatic oxidation of fuels likely causes satiety, increased clearance of fuels from the blood is expected to cause hunger. The less fermentable starch source increased starch flux to the small intestine and likely increased lactate absorption because of glucose metabolism by intestinal tissues. Lactate stimulates hepatic oxidation to a lesser degree than propionate during meals because of the greater lag before lactate absorption and because hepatic extraction of lactate is much less than propionate (96). Hepatic extraction of lactate is probably lower because metabolism of lactate to pyruvate is thermodynamically unfavorable when cytosolic nicotinamide adenine dinucleotide redox potential is high.

These observations of the hypophagic effects of various fuels in ruminants strongly support the theory that hepatic oxidation of fuels contributes to the

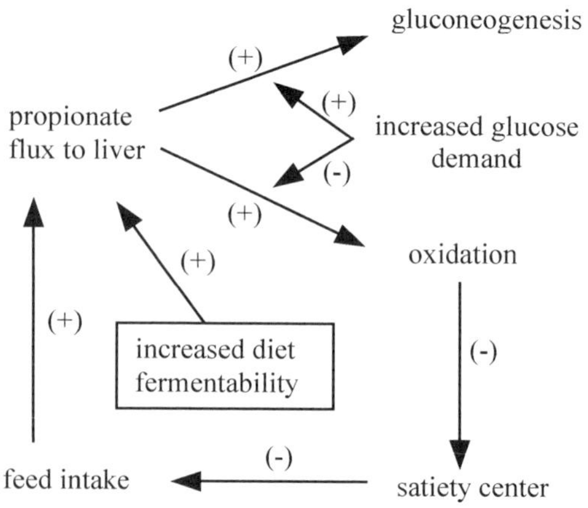

Figure 2 Model to demonstrate how propionate might affect satiety in ruminants. Propionate flux to the liver is affected by feed intake and diet fermentability and increases greatly during meals. Propionate can be used for gluconeogenesis, which consumes ATP, or oxidized in the tricarboxylic acid cycle as acetyl CoA, generating ATP. Supply of propionate to the liver relative to glucose demand should affect the temporal pattern of ATP (and AMP) concentration in the liver and is expected to affect satiety. When glucose demand is high, gluconeogenesis increases and less propionate is oxidized, resulting in greater meal size. When glucose demand is low, a greater fraction of propionate is oxidized, resulting in satiety and smaller meal size.

short-term regulation of food intake. The relative importance of hepatic oxidation of fuels likely varies with other factors such as physiological state, as discussed below.

Satiety from Dietary Unsaturated Fatty Acids

Fat sources are often added to diets of dairy cows with the goal of increasing energy intake to increase milk yield or energy balance. However, fat addition has had inconsistent effects on food intake of dairy cows, partly because of differences in fat sources. A meta-analysis of treatment means from the literature indicated diverse hypophagic effects of different fat supplements; within commonly fed rumen-protected fat sources, calcium salts of palm oil linearly decreased dry matter intake with increasing dietary concentration, whereas hydrogenated FA did not affect dry matter intake (1). Fat sources infused abomasally have different hypophagic effects depending upon source (28), and abomasal infusions have consistently demonstrated the hypophagic effect of unsaturated FA (17). Increasing the proportion of unsaturated LCFAs in rumen-protected fat sources linearly decreased food intake and tended to decrease digestible energy intake of lactating cows (47). Similar effects were reported in a study using human subjects, which indicated that polyunsaturated FAs were more hypophagic than monounsaturated or saturated FAs (76).

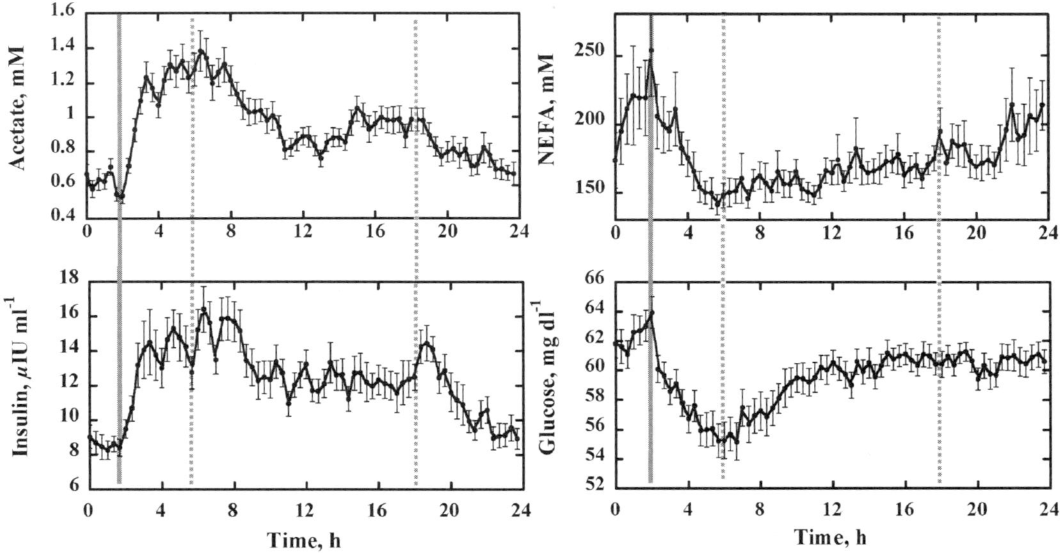

Figure 3 Diurnal variation in plasma insulin, glucose, nonesterified fatty acid (NEFA), and acetate concentration for cows in early to mid lactation offered feed ad libitum. Each data point represents means and standard errors of 32 observations (8 cows $\times$ 4 diets) and samples were taken every 20 minutes for 24 hours. Time 0 in the graph is when sampling began at noon; cows were fed once per day at 2 PM (*solid gray line*) and milked at 6 PM and 6 AM (*dashed gray lines*). The conditioned meal is typically the largest meal of the day for dairy cows fed ad libitum followed by 10 or more spontaneous meals (24). Plasma glucose and NEFA concentrations are affected by insulin and mirror its concentration in an opposite manner, whereas plasma acetate concentration is more dependent on absorption following meals and its temporal pattern is similar to that of insulin. (M. Oba & M.S. Allen, unpublished data)

FEEDING BEHAVIOR AND DIGESTION KINETICS Combined measurement of physiological responses with feeding behavior can provide important clues to unravel the mechanism by which unsaturated FAs depress food intake. Feeding supplemental fat can increase plasma NEFA concentration in lactating cows (21), and NEFAs are the primary source of FA oxidized in the liver of ruminants (31). The degree of FA oxidation in the liver is likely involved in the regulation of food intake (40, 74), and Friedman (39) suggested that fat that is oxidized is satiating, whereas fat that is stored is not satiating. Saturated FAs are not oxidized as fuels as rapidly as polyunsaturated FAs in humans (64) and might favor fat deposition over oxidation in rats (101). The depression of food intake with increasing unsaturated FA is consistent with expected differences in FA partitioning and hepatic oxidation. However, differences in hepatic metabolism do not explain the observed effects on feeding behavior and kinetics of digestion and passage as discussed below.

The reduction in food intake in lactating cows fed less saturated FA was through decreased meal size without a compensatory increase in meal frequency (47). Different effects of FA on meal size, and not intermeal interval, suggest that mechanisms other than hepatic oxidation are involved. The contribution of dietary FA to plasma NEFA within the course of a meal is likely small because passage of FA from the rumen of lactating cows is less than 10% h^{-1} (48), causing a lag prior to absorption. In addition, hepatic oxidation of NEFA is limited because insulin increases during meals (112), and propionate, which is rapidly absorbed during meals, inhibits ß-oxidation of FA by decreasing FA transport into mitochondria (62) and by decreasing activity of fatty acyl CoA dehydrogenase (31).

GUT PEPTIDE RELEASE DURING MEALS Gut-derived peptides have received increased attention in recent years for their potential role in meal-induced satiety. Although the contribution of dietary FA to plasma NEFA during a meal is small, flow of FA to the small intestine during a meal is adequate to stimulate release of gut peptides. Both fat and protein enhance expression and secretion of cholecystokinin (CCK), with serum concentrations peaking approximately 30 minutes after meal initiation in cows (22). Fasting quickly decreased plasma CCK concentration and refeeding gradually increased it in cows, with corresponding changes in duodenal CCK mRNA abundance (106). Blockade of CCK receptors by devazepide (MK-329) reduced the depression in food intake caused by a high-fat diet (22). CCK might affect satiety both by slowing gut motility (increasing gut distention and ruminal propionate production) and by acting directly on the nervous system.

INTERACTION OF GUT PEPTIDES AND PROPIONATE Gastrointestinal hormone signals may be integrated with metabolic signals at the level of peripheral nerves or the hypothalamus. Farningham and colleagues (33) investigated the interactions between CCK and propionate infusions in sheep during two-hour portal infusions. Simultaneous infusion of CCK and propionate decreased food intake 40%, but individual infusions at the same concentrations had no effect. The authors demonstrated that CCK receptors were present in vagal afferent nerves, which suggests that vagal signals initiated by hepatic oxidation of propionate may have been integrated with signals initiated by CCK receptors. Greater stimulation of CCK release for unsaturated fats (in the form of free FA and triglycerides) than for saturated fats (14) might explain the differences in their effects on satiety in the example above.

Hypophagic responses to propionate could also be amplified by other gut-derived hormones. Glucagon-like peptide 1 (GLP-1) is produced in the distal small intestine and is released in response to duodenal infusions of LCFAs and triglycerides in dairy cattle (17, 80). Dietary fat likely stimulates release of GLP-1, enhancing insulin secretion (56). Increased insulin concentrations alter hepatic metabolism, downregulating gluconeogenic pathways and likely directing a greater proportion of propionate toward oxidation. This effect, coupled with rapid liver uptake of propionate during a meal, likely promotes meal termination.

Determining the mechanisms behind diet-induced differences in food intake is complicated and difficult. These examples demonstrate that a change in concentration of any compound in response to a meal is not meaningful unless the timing of the change, the utilization of nutrients, and the organs affected are taken into account. Measurements to assess these factors are relatively easier to achieve in cows than in most other animal models.

INTERACTION OF IMMUNE RESPONSE, STRESS, AND NUTRITION

Hypophagia in the periparturient period is a significant problem in dairy cows, increasing the risk of metabolic diseases such as hepatic lipidosis and metabolic ketosis. Decreased food intake and negative energy balance can be observed as early as 10 days prior to parturition in cows, and intake declines precipitously at parturition and remains suppressed for at least 3–4 days postpartum (59). After more than a week of depressed intake, high-producing dairy cows are faced with a severe energy deficit, even as milk production continues to increase. The etiology of this periparturient hypophagia is not completely understood, and it provides an excellent case study for dissecting possible mediators of intake responses to physiological stress.

Hyperlipidemia in the Periparturient Period

Increased lipolysis in late gestation is likely an evolutionary adaptation to eliminate the mother's dependence on available food and to increase the FA concentration of milk for the first critical days of the neonate's life. However, because NEFAs are taken up by the ruminant liver in proportion to their concentration in plasma (31), lipid mobilization leads to extensive oxidation of FA in the liver. As discussed above, hepatic oxidation of FA may promote satiety and/or suppress hunger.

Therefore, lipid mobilization and hepatic oxidation of FA may inhibit feeding behaviors, widening the energy imbalance and promoting even more lipid mobilization.

Hyperlipidemia in the periparturient period is caused by a reduction in insulin sensitivity of adipose tissues combined with a reduction in plasma insulin concentration; plasma insulin concentrations decline prior to parturition with a nadir below 6 μIU ml^{-1} at four days postpartum (27). It is likely that lipolysis contributes to hypophagia rather than the reverse because plasma NEFA concentrations increase preceding periparturient hypophagia (113). Cytokines as well as growth hormone and other homeorhetic signals reduce insulin sensitivity and responsiveness and increase catecholamine responsiveness (16). These multiple metabolic changes result in plasma NEFA concentrations as much as tenfold higher in early lactation than during gestation (59).

Tissue sensitivity to insulin is decreased both at the onset of lactation (10) and during immune challenges (99), and evidence has emerged that implicates TNF-α in both situations. TNF-α concentrations were highly correlated with the degree of insulin resistance in both pregnant women (68) and postpartum dairy cows (92). Furthermore, blocking TNF-α activity by various means improves insulin sensitivity (57), whereas exogenous TNF-α infusion in cows induced a metabolic state similar to that observed during early lactation and bacterial infection (71). TNF-α and (or) other inflammatory response signals may be responsible for initiating insulin resistance in periparturient cows. However, adipose tissue is not completely unresponsive to insulin; administration of a low dose of insulin three days postpartum decreased plasma NEFA and hepatic triglyceride concentrations and increased food intake of dairy cows (50).

The implications of increased TNF-α production for food intake are not limited to altered insulin sensitivity in adipose tissue. Decreased gastric motility following TNF-α induction as reported in rats (53) would likely decrease food intake in high-producing cows, when physical fill is often the most limiting factor. Furthermore, TNF-α may decrease transcription and activity of PEPCK (55), which would likely dramatically impair gluconeogenic capacity in lactating cows. As discussed above, limiting the utilization of propionate for gluconeogenesis may increase its oxidation and limit meal size.

Hepatic Fatty Acid Oxidation Enhances Hypophagic Effects of Propionate

In early-lactation cows, a shortage of glucose precursors and increased FA oxidation in the liver leads to an abundance of NADH and a lack of TCA-cycle intermediates. This environment results in a buildup of the intracellular acetyl-CoA pool and export of ketone bodies. In this situation, hypophagic effects of propionate may be enhanced because propionate entry into the liver provides TCA-cycle intermediates that allow oxidation of acetyl-CoA. Oxidizing the pool of acetyl-CoA rather than exporting it dramatically increases ATP production and causes satiety, despite the use of propionate for glucose synthesis (90). Propionate infusion was less hypophagic when it increased plasma glucose concentration in mid-lactation cows, but that was not the case for early-lactation cows with higher plasma ketone concentrations (90).

Excessive mobilization of FA in late gestation or early lactation results in hepatic lipidosis and ketosis, and various treatments have been developed to decrease lipolysis, increase hepatic FA oxidation, or enhance FA export as VLDL. Among the most popular treatments for ketosis are oral drenches of glucogenic precursors, including propylene glycol and calcium propionate. Although both can theoretically increase plasma glucose and decrease plasma ketones by stimulating oxidation of acetyl CoA in the liver, their efficacy at doing so varies. Propylene glycol consistently decreases plasma NEFA concentrations and usually decreases plasma ketones, whereas calcium propionate does not (93). Propylene glycol is less hypophagic than propionate because it is converted to lactate and metabolized more slowly (69), and it is less likely to stimulate oxidation in the liver and cause satiety. Thus, calcium propionate may be a less-effective treatment for ketosis because it causes hypophagia by stimulating hepatic oxidation of fuels.

The interactions of stress response, metabolism, and intake regulation have profound human health impacts. Anorexia is experienced during trauma and disease and may prevent adequate nutrient intake (94), while insulin resistance is a prerequisite for metabolic syndrome (84). The periparturient dairy cow provides an excellent model for delineating the central versus metabolic effects of inflammatory response factors such as TNF-α. The condition known as fat cow syndrome (85) is an obvious choice to study the emerging links between obesity, stress, and insulin resistance. In addition, if the satiating effects of hepatic lipid oxidation can be demonstrated in bovines, the early-lactation cow will provide an interesting comparison for intake regulation in humans with hyperlipidemia.

ALTERATION OF MILK YIELD

Milk yield can be greatly altered by management practices such as frequency of milking (105) and length of photoperiod (109), endocrine factors such as growth hormone, thyroxin, and insulin (109), and specific nutrients, allowing the manipulation of fuel partitioning among tissues and evaluation of food intake responses. Homeorhetic signals such as growth hormone are associated with increased intake, yet there are apparently no direct mechanisms for these signals to increase intake (11, 49). However, these lactogenic agents do have a profound influence on metabolism during lactation, significantly increasing energy demand and altering nutrient partitioning. Direction of fuels to peripheral tissues during the postprandial period likely limits hepatic oxidation and delays satiety. This "nutrient pull" may also speed clearance of nutrients from the blood and promote hunger. Thus, homeorhetic signals may interact with dietary fuels to influence food intake.

Nutrient sparing may also provide insight into intake regulation. Intermediates of rumen FA biohydrogenation, including *trans*-10, *cis*-12 conjugated linoleic acid, decrease milk lipid synthesis in the dairy cow by up to 40% (12) via a coordinated downregulation of genes involved in milk fat synthesis (13). A significant decrease in milk fat synthesis representing a large decrease in energy requirement did not decrease energy intake commensurately, and increased body weight gain was observed (47). The ability to partition fuels in lactating cows provides an experimental model to observe the relationships between energy requirements and food intake.

INTERACTIONS OF SATIETY SIGNALS

It is broadly recognized that the various signals contributing to regulation of intake must be integrated and that this integration likely occurs in the central nervous system. However, the number of systems that are thought to act on hypothalamic control centers makes investigation of interactions a daunting task. The lactating dairy cow is an intriguing model for investigating the integration of signals regulating intake because it is possible to monitor pre- and postprandial changes in the gastrointestinal tract, blood, and liver. Most importantly, many of these observations can be made simultaneously and without interrupting normal feeding behaviors.

During mid-lactation, the large nutrient requirements for peak milk synthesis result in increased stimulation of feeding behavior. However, the high-fiber diets of ruminants require a long retention time in the rumen and increased ruminal fill may signal satiety through stimulation of tension receptors in the rumen wall, thereby limiting maximal energy intake (1). Given the existence of independent physical fill and fuel-responsive satiating mechanisms, rumen fill and nutrient metabolism may interact to alter food intake. Mbanya et al. (82) investigated the effects of rumen distention and ruminal infusions of acetate and propionate during three-hour treatments. Rumen distention, produced by inserting a balloon into the rumen of fistulated cows and inflating the balloon to a volume of 10 liters, did not independently alter food intake, nor did infusions of VFA. However, when balloon distention was combined with infusion of acetate, propionate, or both, feed intake was significantly depressed. This example indicates that peripheral satiety signals are additive and that the integrated signal must reach a threshold to cause satiety.

Although food intake decreases in late lactation, energy intake exceeds the diminishing energy requirements for milk production, allowing replenishment of body reserves (Figure 1). Regulation of food intake is accomplished through a variety of mechanisms, but signals derived from absorbed fuels, sensory stimulation, and gut peptides cannot regulate long-term energy balance. The continued drive to eat in late-lactation cows is likely mediated, in part, by low plasma leptin concentrations. Long-term energy balance is highly controlled (102), and the lipostatic theory proposed by Kennedy (66) describes an adiposity set point that drives regulation of energy intake, which is consistent with these observations. However, long-term signals coordinating energy balance clearly must function through modification of meal size and frequency. The integration of short- and long-term intake regulation is therefore an area of intense interest (49, 102, 115).

Short- and long-term regulatory mechanisms may interact in several ways. The primary mechanism may be that long-term signals alter the thresholds for response to short-term signals (1, 116). Hypophagia induced by intraperitoneal administration of CCK in rats was greatly increased by concomitant leptin administration, even though rats given only leptin showed no decrease in food intake (32). Similar interactions have been observed in rats treated with leptin and urocortin (65). Both studies provided evidence that integration of these signals occurred centrally. Hormones affecting food intake may also interact by altering the expression or secretion of other hormones. For example, insulin stimulates leptin secretion (78), whereas central leptin administration increases insulin secretion in fasted cows (3).

Clinical applications of findings involving the regulation of food intake have been elusive. One reason is that intake research has focused on individual mechanisms that can be demonstrated conclusively; however, physiological systems are inherently complex, with multiple layers of regulation. Interactions between hormonal, metabolic, and sensory regulators of food intake represent the next frontier of intake research. Use of the lactating cow model in various physiological states could provide valuable insights into these interactions.

CONCLUDING REMARKS

Nonconventional animal models such as the cow provide opportunities to study certain aspects of food intake regulation not possible with rodent models. Cows are unique among animal models to study food intake regulation because their extremely high energy requirements increase their drive to eat, because their docile nature and large size make them ideal for intensive measurements, and because they cycle through various physiological states throughout lactation. They are ideally suited to study interactions among short-term satiety signals affected by the temporal absorption of fuels because digesta flow, nutrient absorption, endocrine response, and feeding behavior can be measured simultaneously. Comparative ease of tissue sampling maximizes the potential for utilization of recent technological innovations for rapid and inexpensive measurement of gene expression and metabolite pools, which promises integrated information to unlock mechanisms regulating food intake. Wide-ranging physiological states throughout lactation and the ability to alter partitioning of fuels to tissues provides us the opportunity to study the interaction of long- and short-term signals, while natural or experimentally induced stimulation of stress and immune function in the cow may provide a valuable model to understand the interaction of stress, immune function, and intake. Future breakthroughs in understanding the multifactorial nature of food intake regulation may depend on alternative animal models such as the cow because of these unique advantages.

The *Annual Review of Nutrition* is online at http://nutr.annualreviews.org

LITERATURE CITED

1. Allen MS. 2000. Effects of diet on short-term regulation of feed intake by lactating dairy cattle. *J. Dairy Sci.* 83:1598–624
2. Allen MS, Oba M, Mooney CS. 2000. Automated system for collection of ruminal fluid and blood of ruminants. *J. Dairy Sci.* 83(Suppl. 1):288 (Abstr.)
3. Amstalden M, Garcia MR, Stanko RL, Nizielski SE, Morrison CD, et al. 2002. Central infusion of recombinant ovine leptin normalizes plasma insulin and stimulates a novel hypersecretion of luteinizing hormone after short-term fasting in mature beef cows. *Biol. Reprod.* 66:1555–61
4. Andersson U, Filipsson K, Abbott CR, Woods A, Smith K, et al. 2004. AMP-activated protein kinase plays a role in the control of food intake. *J. Biol. Chem.* 279:12005–8
5. Anil MH, Forbes JM. 1980. Feeding in sheep during intraportal infusions of short-chain fatty acids and the effect of liver denervation. *J. Physiol.* 298:407–14
6. Anil MH, Forbes JM. 1988. The roles of hepatic nerves in the reduction of food intake as a consequence of intraportal sodium propionate administration in sheep. *Q. J. Exp. Physiol.* 73:539–46
7. Baile CA. 1971. Metabolites as feedbacks for control of feed intake and receptor sites in goats and sheep. *Physiol. Behav.* 7:819–26
8. Baile CA, Forbes JM. 1974. Control of feed intake and regulation of energy balance in ruminants. *Physiol. Rev.* 54:160–214
9. Ballard FJ. 1965. Glucose utilization in mammalian liver. *Comp. Biochem. Physiol.* 14:437–43
10. Bauman DE, Currie WB. 1980. Partitioning of nutrients during pregnancy and lactation: a review of mechanisms involving homeostasis and homeorhesis. *J. Dairy Sci.* 63:1514–29
11. Bauman DE, Elliott JM. 1983. Control of nutrient partitioning in lactating ruminants. In *Biochemistry of Lactation*, ed. TB Mepham, pp. 437–68. Amsterdam/Lausanne/NY: Elsevier Sci.
12. Bauman DE, Griinari JM. 2003. Nutritional regulation of milk fat synthesis. *Annu. Rev. Nutr.* 23:203–27
13. Baumgard LH, Matitashvili E, Corl BA, Dwyer DA, Bauman DE. 2002. *trans*-10, *cis*-12 Conjugated linoleic acid decreases lipogenic rates and expression of genes involved in milk lipid synthesis in dairy cows. *J. Dairy Sci.* 85:2155–63
14. Beardshall K, Frost G, Morarji Y, Domin J, Bloom SR, Calam J. 1989. Saturation of fat and cholecystokinin release: implications for pancreatic carcinogenesis. *Lancet* 2:1008–10
15. Bell AW, Bauman DE. 1994. Animal models for the study of adipose regulation in pregnancy and lactation. *Adv. Exp. Med. Biol.* 352:71–84
16. Bell AW, Bauman DE. 1997. Adaptations of glucose metabolism during pregnancy and lactation. *J. Mammary Gland Biol. Neoplasia* 2:265–78
17. Benson JA, Reynolds CK. 2001. Effects of abomasal infusion of long-chain fatty acids on splanchnic metabolism of pancreatic and gut hormones in lactating dairy cows. *J. Dairy Sci.* 84:1488–500
18. Benson JA, Reynolds CK, Aikman PC, Lupoli B, Beever DE. 2002. Effects of abomasal vegetable oil infusion on splanchnic nutrient metabolism in lactating dairy cows. *J. Dairy Sci.* 85:1804–14
19. Challis BG, Yeo GS. 2002. Past, present and future strategies to study the genetics of body weight regulation. *Brief Funct. Genomic Proteomic* 1:290–304

20. Choi BR, Allen MS. 1999. Intake regulation by volatile fatty acids and physical fill. *S. Afr. J. Anim. Sci.* 29:40–41 (Abstr.)
21. Choi BR, Palmquist DL, Allen MS. 1997. Sodium mercaptoacetate is not a useful probe to study the role of fat in regulation of feed intake in dairy cattle. *J. Nutr.* 127:171–76
22. Choi BR, Palmquist DL, Allen MS. 2000. Cholecystokinin mediates depression of feed intake in dairy cattle fed high fat diets. *Domest. Anim. Endocrinol.* 19:159–75
23. Dado RG, Allen MS. 1993. Continuous computer acquisition of feed and water intake, chewing reticular motility, and ruminal pH of cattle. *J. Dairy Sci.* 76:1589–600
24. Dado RG, Allen MS. 1994. Variation in and relationships among feeding, chewing, and drinking variables for lactating dairy cows. *J. Dairy Sci.* 77:132–44
25. Davis CL. 1967. Acetate production in the rumen of cows fed either control or low-fiber, high-grain diets. *J. Dairy Sci.* 50:1621–25
26. Demigne C, Yacoub C, Remesy C, Fafournoux P. 1986. Propionate and butyrate metabolism in rat or sheep hepatocytes. *Biochim. Biophys. Acta* 875:535–42
27. Doepel L, Lapierre H, Kennelly JJ. 2002. Peripartum performance and metabolism of dairy cows in response to prepartum energy and protein intake. *J. Dairy Sci.* 85:2315–34
28. Drackley JK, Klusmeyer TH, Trusk AM, Clark JH. 1992. Infusion of long-chain fatty acids varying in saturation and chain length into the abomasum of lactating dairy cows. *J. Dairy Sci.* 75:1517–26
29. Elliot JM. 1976. The glucose economy of the lactating dairy cow. In *Proc. Cornell Nutr. Conf. Feed Manufact., Syracuse, New York*, pp. 59–66. Ithaca, NY: Cornell Univ.
30. Elliot JM, Symonds HW, Pike B. 1985. Effect on feed intake of infusing sodium propionate or sodium acetate into a mesenteric vein of cattle. *J. Dairy Sci.* 68:1165–70
31. Emery RS, Liesman JS, Herdt TH. 1992. Metabolism of long chain fatty acids by ruminant liver. *J. Nutr.* 122:832–37
32. Emond M, Schwartz GJ, Ladenheim EE, Moran TH. 1999. Central leptin modulates behavioral and neural responsivity to CCK. *Am. J. Physiol.* 276:R1545–49
33. Farningham DA, Mercer JG, Lawrence CB. 1993. Satiety signals in sheep: involvement of CCK, propionate, and vagal CCK binding sites. *Physiol. Behav.* 54:437–42
34. Farningham DA, Whyte CC. 1993. The role of propionate and acetate in the control of food intake in sheep. *Br. J. Nutr.* 70:37–46
35. Flegal KM, Carroll MD, Ogden CL, Johnson CL. 2002. Prevalence and trends in obesity among US adults, 1999–2000. *JAMA* 288:1723–27
36. Food Nutr. Board. 2002. *Reference Intakes for Energy, Carbohydrate, Fiber, Fat, Fatty Acids, Cholesterol, Protein, and Amino Acids (Macronutrients)*. Washington, DC: Natl. Acad. Press
37. Forbes JM. 1995. *Voluntary Food Intake and Diet Selection in Farm Animals*. Oxon, UK: CAB Int.
38. Friedman MI. 1995. Control of energy intake by energy metabolism. *Am. J. Clin. Nutr.* 62:1096–100S
39. Friedman MI. 1998. Fuel partitioning and food intake. *Am. J. Clin. Nutr.* 67:513–18S
40. Friedman MI, Tordoff MG, Ramirez I. 1986. Integrated metabolic control of food intake. *Brain Res. Bull.* 17:855–59
41. Frobish RA, Davis CL. 1977. Effects of abomasal infusions of glucose and propionate on milk yield and composition. *J. Dairy Sci.* 60:204–9
42. Gallaher DD. 1992. Animal models in human nutrition research. *Nutr. Clin. Pract.* 7:37–39
43. Gibbs R, Weinstock G, Kappes S, Schook

S, Skow L, Womack J. 2003. Bovine genomic sequencing initiative: cattle-izing the human genome. http://www.genome.gov/Pages/Research/Sequencing/SeqProposals/BovineSEQ.pdf
44. Grovum WL. 1995. Mechanisms explaining the effects of short chain fatty acids on feed intake in ruminants—osmotic pressure, insulin and glucagon. In *Ruminant Physiology: Digestion, Metabolism, Growth and Reproduction*, ed. WV Englehardt, S Leonhard-Marek, G Breves, D Geisecke, pp. 173–97. Stuttgart, Germany: Verlag
45. Hanson RW, Ballard FJ. 1967. The relative significance of acetate and glucose as precursors for lipid synthesis in liver and adipose tissue from ruminants. *Biochem. J.* 105:529–36
46. Harvatine KJ, Allen MS. 2003. Effects of rumen-inert fat saturation on feed intake, milk production, and plasma metabolites in lactating dairy cows. *J. Dairy Sci.* 86(Suppl. 1):148 (Abstr.)
47. Harvatine KJ, Allen MS. 2004. Effect of rumen-protected fatty acid saturation on feed intake and feeding and chewing behavior of lactating dairy cows. *J. Dairy Sci.* 87(Suppl. 1):309 (Abstr.)
48. Harvatine KJ, Allen MS. 2004. Kinetic model of rumen biohydrogenation: effects of rumen-protected fatty acid saturation on fractional rate of biohydrogenation and duodenal fatty acid flow in lactating dairy cows. *J. Dairy Sci.* 87(Suppl. 1):308 (Abstr.)
49. Havel PJ. 2001. Peripheral signals conveying metabolic information to the brain: short-term and long-term regulation of food intake and energy homeostasis. *Exp. Biol. Med. (Maywood)* 226:963–77
50. Hayirli A, Bertics SJ, Grummer RR. 2002. Effects of slow-release insulin on production, liver triglyceride, and metabolic profiles of Holsteins in early lactation. *J. Dairy Sci.* 85:2180–91
51. Henry BA. 2003. Links between the appetite regulating systems and the neuroendocrine hypothalamus: lessons from the sheep. *J. Neuroendocrinol.* 15:697–709
52. Herath CB, Reynolds GW, MacKenzie DD, Davis SR, Harris PM. 1999. Vagotomy suppresses cephalic phase insulin release in sheep. *Exp. Physiol.* 84:559–69
53. Hermann GE, Tovar CA, Rogers RC. 1999. Induction of endogenous tumor necrosis factor-alpha: suppression of centrally stimulated gastric motility. *Am. J. Physiol. Regul. Integr. Comp. Physiol.* 276:R59–68
54. Hevener AL, Bergman RN, Donovan CM. 1997. Novel glucosensor for hypoglycemic detection localized to the portal vein. *Diabetes* 46:1521–25
55. Hill MR, McCallum RE. 1992. Identification of tumor necrosis factor as a transcriptional regulator of the phosphoenolpyruvate carboxykinase gene following endotoxin treatment of mice. *Infect. Immun.* 60:4040–50
56. Holst JJ, Gromada J. 2004. Role of incretin hormones in the regulation of insulin secretion in diabetic and nondiabetic humans. *Am. J. Physiol. Endocrinol. Metab.* 287:E199–206
57. Hotamisligil GS. 2003. Inflammatory pathways and insulin action. *Int. J. Obes. Relat. Metab. Disord.* 27(Suppl. 3):S53–55
58. Hurtaud C, Rulquin H, Verite R. 1993. Effect of infused volatile fatty acids and caseinate on milk composition and coagulation in dairy cows. *J. Dairy Sci.* 76:3011–20
59. Ingvartsen KL, Andersen JB. 2000. Integration of metabolism and intake regulation: a review focusing on periparturient animals. *J. Dairy Sci.* 83:1573–97
60. Inst. Lab. Anim. Res. 1995. *Nutritional Requirements of Laboratory Animals*. Washington, DC: Natl. Acad. Press
61. Itoh F, Obara Y, Rose MT, Fuse H. 1998. Heat influences on plasma insulin and glucagon in response to secretogogues in non-lactating dairy cows. *Domest. Anim. Endocrinol.* 15:499–510

62. Jesse BW, Emery RS, Thomas JW. 1986. Control of bovine hepatic fatty acid oxidation. *J. Dairy Sci.* 69:2290–97
63. Jin ES, Jones JG, Merritt M, Burgess SC, Malloy CR, Sherry AD. 2004. Glucose production, gluconeogenesis, and hepatic tricarboxylic acid cycle fluxes measured by nuclear magnetic resonance analysis of a single glucose derivative. *Anal. Biochem.* 327:149–55
64. Jones PJ, Ridgen JE, Phang PT, Birmingham CL. 1992. Influence of dietary fat polyunsaturated to saturated ratio on energy substrate utilization in obesity. *Metabolism* 41:396–401
65. Kastin AJ, Pan W, Akerstrom V, Hackler L, Wang C, Kotz CM. 2002. Novel peptide-peptide cooperation may transform feeding behavior. *Peptides* 23:2189–96
66. Kennedy GC. 1953. The role of depot fat in the hypothalamic control of food intake in the rat. *Proc. R. Soc. Lond. B Biol. Sci.* 140:578–96
67. Kil SJ, Froetschel MA. 1994. Involvement of opioid peptides from casein on reticular motility and digesta passage in steers. *J. Dairy Sci.* 77:111–23
68. Kirwan JP, Hauguel-De Mouzon S, Lepercq J, Challier J-C, Huston-Presley L, et al. 2002. TNF-{alpha} Is a Predictor of Insulin Resistance in Human Pregnancy. *Diabetes* 51:2207–13
69. Kristensen NB, Danfaer A, Rojen BA, Raun BM, Weisbjerg MR, Hvelplund T. 2002. Metabolism of propionate and 1,2-propanediol absorbed from the washed reticulorumen of lactating cows. *J. Anim. Sci.* 80:2168–75
70. Kunert O, Stingl H, Rosian E, Krssak M, Bernroider E, et al. 2003. Measurement of Fractional Whole-Body Gluconeogenesis in Humans From Blood Samples Using 2H Nuclear Magnetic Resonance Spectroscopy. *Diabetes* 52:2475–82
71. Kushibiki S, Hodate K, Shingu H, Obara Y, Touno E, et al. 2003. Metabolic and lactational responses during recombinant bovine tumor necrosis factor-alpha treatment in lactating cows. *J. Dairy Sci.* 86:819–27
72. Lagonigro R, Wiener P, Pilla F, Woolliams JA, Williams JL. 2003. A new mutation in the coding region of the bovine leptin gene associated with feed intake. *Anim. Genet.* 34:371–74
73. Langhans W, Delprete E, Scharrer E. 1991. Mechanisms of vasopressin's anorectic effect. *Physiol. Behav.* 49:169–76
74. Langhans W, Scharrer E. 1987. Evidence for a vagally mediated satiety signal derived from hepatic fatty acid oxidation. *J. Auton. Nerv. Syst.* 18:13–18
75. Langhans W, Scharrer E. 1992. Metabolic control of eating. *World Rev. Nutr. Diet.* 70:1–67
76. Lawton CL, Delargy HJ, Brockman J, Smith FC, Blundell JE. 2000. The degree of saturation of fatty acids influences post-ingestive satiety. *Br. J. Nutr.* 83:473–82
77. Leek BF, Harding RH. 1975. Sensory nervous receptors in the ruminant stomach and the reflex control of reticulo-ruminal motility. In *Digestion and Metabolism in the Ruminant*, ed. IW McDonald, ACI Warner, pp. 60–76. Armidale, Australia: Univ. New Engl. Publ.
78. Leury BJ, Baumgard LH, Block SS, Segoale N, Ehrhardt RA, et al. 2003. Effect of insulin and growth hormone on plasma leptin in periparturient dairy cows. *Am. J. Physiol. Regul. Integr. Comp. Physiol.* 285:R1107–15
79. Leuvenink HG, Bleumer EJ, Bongers LJ, van Bruchem J, van der Heide D. 1997. Effect of short-term propionate infusion on feed intake and blood parameters in sheep. *Am. J. Physiol.* 272:E997–1001
80. Litherland NB, Thire S, Beaulieu AD, Reynolds CK, Benson JA, Drackley JK. 2005. Dry matter intake is decreased more by abomasal infusion of unsaturated free fatty acids than by unsaturated triglycerides. *J. Dairy Sci.* 88:632–43

81. Martin FH, Seoane JR, Baile CA. 1973. Feeding in satiated sheep elicited by intraventricular injections of CSF from fasted sheep. *Life Sci.* 13:177–84
82. Mbanya JN, Anil MH, Forbes JM. 1993. The voluntary intake of hay and silage by lactating cows in response to ruminal infusion of acetate or propionate, or both, with or without distension of the rumen by a balloon. *Br. J. Nutr.* 69:713–20
83. Mokdad AH, Ford ES, Bowman BA, Dietz WH, Vinicor F, et al. 2003. Prevalence of obesity, diabetes, and obesity-related health risk factors, 2001. *JAMA* 289:76–79
84. Moller DE, Kaufman KD. 2005. Metabolic syndrome: a clinical and molecular perspective. *Annu. Rev. Med.* 56:45–62
85. Morrow DA. 1976. Fat cow syndrome. *J. Dairy Sci.* 59:1625–29
86. Natl. Inst. Health. 2004. *Genbank*. http://www.ncbi.nih.gov/Genbank/
87. Natl. Res. Counc. 2001. *Nutritional Requirements of Dairy Cattle*. Washington, DC: Natl. Acad. Press
88. Newsholme EA, Dimitriadis G. 2001. Integration of biochemical and physiologic effects of insulin on glucose metabolism. *Exp. Clin. Endocrinol. Diabetes* 109(Suppl. 2):S122–34
89. Oba M, Allen MS. 2003. Effects of corn grain conservation method on feeding behavior and productivity of lactating dairy cows at two dietary starch concentrations. *J. Dairy Sci.* 86:174–83
90. Oba M, Allen MS. 2003. Extent of hypophagia caused by propionate infusion is related to plasma glucose concentration in lactating dairy cows. *J. Nutr.* 133:1105–12
91. Oba M, Allen MS. 2003. Intraruminal infusion of propionate alters feeding behavior and decreases energy intake of lactating dairy cows. *J. Nutr.* 133:1094–99
92. Ohtsuka H, Koiwa M, Hatsugaya A, Kudo K, Hoshi F, et al. 2001. Relationship between serum TNF activity and insulin resistance in dairy cows affected with naturally occurring fatty liver. *J. Vet. Med. Sci.* 63:1021–25
93. Overton TR, Waldron MR. 2004. Nutritional management of transition dairy cows: strategies to optimize metabolic health. *J. Dairy Sci.* 87:E105–19
94. Reid CL. 2004. Nutritional requirements of surgical and critically ill patients: Do we really know what they need? *Proc. Nutr. Soc.* 63:467–72
95. Reynolds CK. 1995. Quantitative aspects of liver metabolism in ruminants. In *Ruminant Physiology: Digestion, Metabolism, Growth and Reproduction*, ed. WV Englehardt, S Leonhard-Marek, G Breves, D Geisecke, pp. 351–72. Stuttgart, Germany: Verlag
96. Reynolds CK, Aikman PC, Lupoli B, Humphries DJ, Beever DE. 2003. Splanchnic metabolism of dairy cows during the transition from late gestation through early lactation. *J. Dairy Sci.* 86:1201–17
97. Ricks CA, Cook RM. 1981. Regulation of volatile fatty acid uptake by mitochondrial acyl CoA synthetases of bovine liver. *J. Dairy Sci.* 64:2324–35
98. Scharrer E. 1999. Control of food intake by fatty acid oxidation and ketogenesis. *Nutrition* 15:704–14
99. Seematter G, Binnert C, Martin JL, Tappy L. 2004. Relationship between stress, inflammation and metabolism. *Curr. Opin. Clin. Nutr. Metab. Care* 7:169–73
100. Sheperd AC, Combs DK. 1998. Long-term effects of acetate and propionate on voluntary feed intake by midlactation cows. *J. Dairy Sci.* 81:2240–50
101. Shimomura Y, Tamura T, Suzuki M. 1990. Less body fat accumulation in rats fed a safflower oil diet than in rats fed a beef tallow diet. *J. Nutr.* 120:1291–96
102. Speakman JR, Stubbs RJ, Mercer JG. 2002. Does body mass play a role in the regulation of food intake? *Proc. Nutr. Soc.* 61:473–87
103. Stangassinger M, Giesecke D. 1986. Splanchnic metabolism of glucose and

related energy substrates. In *Control of Digestion and Metabolism in Ruminants*, ed. LP Milligan, WL Grovum, A Dobson, pp. 347–66. Englewood Cliffs, NJ: Prentice Hall

104. Steinhour WD, Bauman DE. 1988. Propionate metabolism: a new interpretation. In *Aspects of Digestive Physiology in Ruminants*, ed. A Dobson, MJ Dobson, pp. 238–56. Ithaca, NY: Comstock Publ.
105. Stelwagen K. 2001. Effect of milking frequency on mammary functioning and shape of the lactation curve. *J. Dairy Sci.* 84:E204–11
106. Suominen AH, Glimm DR, Tedesco D, Okine EK, McBurney MI, Kennelly JJ. 1998. Intestinal nutrient-gene interaction: the effect of feed deprivation and refeeding on cholecystokinin and proglucagon gene expression. *J. Anim. Sci.* 76:3104–13
107. Tang-Christensen M, Vrang N, Ortmann S, Bidlingmaier M, Horvath TL, Tschop M. 2004. Central administration of ghrelin and agouti-related protein (83–132) increases food intake and decreases spontaneous locomotor activity in rats. *Endocrinology* 145:4645–52
108. Tou JCL, Wade CE. 2002. Determinants affecting physical activity levels in animal models. *Exp. Biol. Med.* 227:587–600
109. Tucker HA. 2000. Hormones, mammary growth, and lactation: a 41-year perspective. *J. Dairy Sci.* 83:874–84
110. US Dept. Health Hum. Serv. 2001. *The Surgeon General's call to action to prevent and decrease overweight and obesity.* Washington, DC: US GPO
111. USDA Natl. Agric. Stat. Serv. 2004. *Milk production.* http://www.usda.gov/nass/aggraphs/cowrates.htm
112. Vasilatos R, Wangsness PJ. 1980. Changes in concentrations of insulin, growth hormone and metabolites in plasma with spontaneous feeding in lactating dairy cows. *J. Nutr.* 110:1479–87
113. Vazquez-Anon M, Bertics S, Luck M, Grummer RR, Pinheiro J. 1994. Peripartum liver triglyceride and plasma metabolites in dairy cows. *J. Dairy Sci.* 77:1521–28
114. Westerterp-Plantenga MS, Fredrix E, Steffens AB. 1994. *Food Intake and Energy Expenditure.* Boca Raton, FL: CRC Press
115. Woods SC. 2004. Lessons in the interactions of hormones and ingestive behavior. *Physiol. Behav.* 82:187–90
116. Woods SC, Schwartz MW, Baskin DG, Seeley RJ. 2000. Food intake and the regulation of body weight. *Annu. Rev. Psychol.* 51:255–77

Annu. Rev. Nutr. 2005. 25:549–71
doi: 10.1146/annurev.nutr.24.012003.132254

First published online as a Review in Advance on May 4, 2005

THE ROLE OF ESSENTIAL FATTY ACIDS IN DEVELOPMENT

William C. Heird and Alexandre Lapillonne
Children's Nutrition Research Center, Department of Pediatrics, Baylor College of Medicine, Houston, Texas 77030-2600; email: wheird@bcm.tmc.edu

Key Words docosahexaenoic acid (DHA), arachidonic acid (ARA), neurodevelopmental outcome, visual acuity, long-chain polyunsaturated fatty acid (LC-PUFA)

■ **Abstract** The presence of docosahexaenoic acid (DHA) and arachidonic acid (ARA) in human milk but not in infant formula, coupled with lower plasma and brain lipid contents of DHA in formula-fed than in breast-fed infants and reports of higher IQ in individuals who were breast-fed versus formula-fed as infants, suggest that exogenous DHA (and ARA) may be essential for optimal development. Thus, since 1990, several studies have examined the impact of formulas containing DHA or DHA plus ARA on visual function and neurodevelopmental outcome. Some of these studies have shown benefits but others have not. These results leave largely unanswered the question of whether these fatty acids are beneficial for either the term or preterm infant. However, evidence that preterm infants might benefit is somewhat more convincing than that for term infants. Despite the limited evidence for efficacy, formulas supplemented with DHA and ARA are now available and appear to be safe.

CONTENTS

0199-9885/05/0714-0549$20.00

INTRODUCTION

Fatty acids are aliphatic monocarboxylicacids that may have multiple, but usually no more than six, double bonds (polyunsaturated fatty acids), one double bond (monosaturated fatty acids), or no double bonds (saturated fatty acids). Fatty acids other than the essential fatty acids (see below) can be synthesized endogenously; however, the major source is from dietary fat, which accounts for 25%–50% of the energy content of most diets. Triglycerides, which have three, usually different, fatty acid molecules esterified to a molecule of glycerol, are the major components of dietary fat. These are hydrolyzed in the intestinal lumen, the bulk of released fatty acids are reassembled within the enterocyte, and the reassembled triglycerides along with phospholipids, monoglycerides, diglycerides, and sterol esters are absorbed into the thoracic duct, eventually reaching the bloodstream, where they circulate primarily as components of the various lipoproteins. The remaining free fatty acids circulate bound to albumen.

Fatty acids have common names but also are identified by a "shorthand" system indicating their number of carbon atoms, their number of double bonds, and the site of the first double bond from the terminal methyl group of the molecule. For example, palmitic acid, a 16-carbon saturated fatty acid, is designated 16:0, and oleic acid, an 18-carbon monounsaturated fatty acid with its single double bond located between the ninth and tenth carbon from the methyl terminal, is designated 18:1ω9. Linoleic acid (18:2ω6) and α-linolenic acid (18:3ω3), both of which are 18-carbon polyunsaturated fatty acids, are designated 18:2ω6 and 18:3ω3, respectively. 18:2ω6 has two double bonds, the first between the sixth and seventh carbon from the methyl terminal, and 18:3ω3 has three double bonds, the first between the third and fourth carbon from the methyl terminal. Table 1 shows the common names as well as the shorthand designations of several common fatty acids. In this chapter, only the shorthand designations are used.

ESSENTIAL FATTY ACIDS

Fatty acids with double bonds at the ω6 and ω3 positions (e.g., 18:2ω6 and 18:3ω3) cannot be synthesized endogenously by the human species and, hence, must be provided in the diet. Both 18:2ω6 and 18:3ω3 are metabolized by the same series of desaturases and elongases to longer-chain, more unsaturated fatty acids. This pathway is outlined in Figure 1. As indicated, two desaturation-elongation cycles result in conversion of 18:2ω6 and 18:3ω3 to 22:4ω6 and 22:5ω3, respectively. Another elongation step converts these fatty acids to 24:4ω6 and 24:5ω3, which are then desaturated by Δ^6-desaturase to 24:5ω6 and 24:6ω3 and undergo partial β-oxidation, forming 22:5ω6 and 22:6ω3. This pathway was described in the early 1990s by Voss et al. (94). Whether there also is a Δ^4-desaturase step in which 22:4ω6 and 22:5ω3 are converted directly to 22:5ω6 and 22:6ω3, as formerly thought, is not clear. Involvement of the pathway described by Voss in formation

TABLE 1 Common names and numerical nomenclature of selected fatty acids

Common name	Numerical nomenclature
Caprylic acid	8:0
Capric acid	10:0
Lauric acid	12:0
Myristic acid	14:0
Palmitic acid	16:0
Stearic acid	18:0
Oleic acid	18:1ω9*
Linoleic acid	18:2ω6*
γ-Linolenic acid	18:3ω6
Dihomogamma-linolenic acid	20:3ω6
Arachidonic acid	20:4ω6
α-Linolenic acid	18:3ω3*
Eicosapentaenoic acid	20:5ω3
Docosahexaenoic acid	22:6ω3

*ω9, ω6, and ω3 are used interchangeably with n-9, n-6, and n-3.

of 20:4ω6 and 22:6ω3 from labeled 18:2ω6 and 18:3ω3, respectively, has been demonstrated in both infants (85) and adults (36).

Collectively, the longer-chain, more unsaturated fatty acids synthesized from 18:2ω6 and 18:3ω3 are referred to as long-chain (i.e., more than 18 carbons) polyunsaturated fatty acids (LC-PUFAs). Important metabolites of 18:2ω6 include 18:3ω6, 20:3ω6, and 20:4ω6. 20:5ω3 and 22:6ω3 are the most important metabolites of 18:3ω3. The parent fatty acids, 18:2ω6 and 18:3ω3, are found in storage lipids, cell membrane phospholipids, intracellular cholesterol esters, and plasma lipids. LC-PUFAs synthesized from these precursors, on the other hand, are found primarily in specific cell membrane phospholipids. 20:3ω6, 20:4ω6, and 20:5ω3 are immediate precursors of eicosanoids (42, 73) and compete with each other for the enzymes involved in eicosanoid synthesis. Each is converted to a different series of eicosanoids with different biological activities and/or functions.

18:2ω6 has been recognized as an essential nutrient for the human species for almost 75 years (12, 32). Symptoms of deficiency include poor growth and scaly skin lesions. Although the essentiality of 18:3ω3 was suspected for some time, it was not recognized as an essential nutrient until approximately 20 years ago. In animals, including primates, deficiency of this fatty acid results in visual and neurological abnormalities (3, 69, 70, 95). Neurological abnormalities also were observed in a human infant who had been maintained for several weeks on a parenteral nutrition regimen lacking 18:3ω3 (40) and in elderly nursing

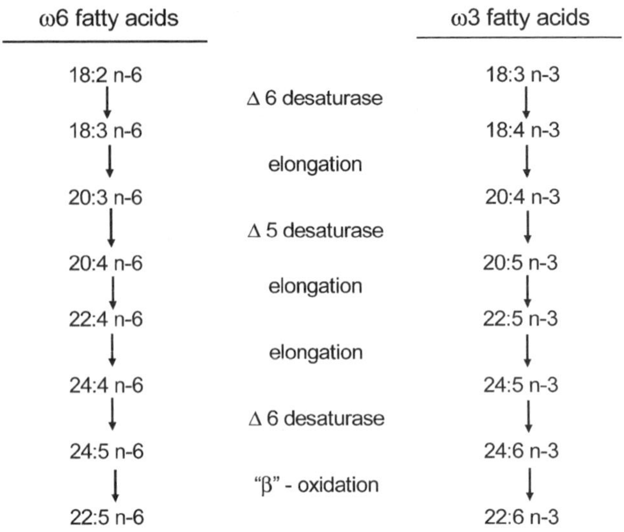

Figure 1 Metabolic pathways of $\omega6$ and $\omega3$ fatty acids.

home residents who were receiving intragastric feedings of an elemental formula with no 18:3ω3 (9). These symptoms were reversed by administration of 18:3ω3.

The clinical symptoms of ω6 fatty acid deficiency can be corrected by 18:2ω6, 18:3ω6, 20:3ω6, or 20:4ω6, and those of ω3 fatty acid deficiency can be corrected by 18:3ω3, 20:5ω3, or 22:6ω3. Whether 18:2ω6 and 18:3ω3 have specific functions that cannot be met by their metabolites is not clear.

The same series of enzymes that catalyze desaturation and elongation of ω6 and ω3 fatty acids also catalyze desaturation and elongation of ω9 fatty acids. The substrate preference of these enzymes is ω3, followed by ω6 and, finally, ω9; thus, competition between the ω9 fatty acids and either the ω6 or ω3 fatty acids is rare. However, if the concentrations of 18:2ω6 and 18:3ω3 are low, 18:1ω9 is readily desaturated and elongated to 20:3ω9 (eicosatrienoic acid). An elevated plasma ratio of this fatty acid to 20:4ω6, the triene/tetraene ratio, is a diagnostic index of ω6 fatty acid deficiency. A ratio of >0.4 was initially considered indicative of deficiency (38). However, since this ratio usually is <0.1, a ratio of >0.2 is now thought to be a more reasonable indicator. In the few documented cases of isolated 18:3ω3 deficiency in which it was measured, the triene/tetraene ratio was not elevated.

The minimum requirement for 18:2ω6 is thought to be from 2% to 4% of total energy intake (39). The minimum requirement for 18:3ω3 is less well defined but is thought to be about 1% of total energy intake (43). 18:2ω6 comprises about 15% to 20% of the total fatty acids of infant formulas available in the United States, and 18:3ω3 comprises 1.5% to 2%. Human milk contents of 18:2ω6 and 18:3ω3 are more variable than the contents in formulas. On average, 18:2ω6 comprises ~16%

of the total fatty acid content of the milk of U.S. women and 18:3ω3 comprises about 1% (51). Human milk also contains small amounts of a number of longer-chain, more unsaturated metabolites of both 18:2ω6 and 18:3ω3, including 20:4ω6 and 22:6ω3.

Maternal diet has a marked impact on the concentration of all fatty acids in human milk, particularly that of 22:6ω3. The concentration of this fatty acid in the milk of women consuming a typical North American diet is generally in the range of 0.1% to 0.3% of total fatty acids and the concentration of 20:4ω6 ranges from 0.4% to 0.6% (51). The milk of vegetarian women contains less 22:6ω3 than the milk of omnivorous women (81), whereas the milk of women whose dietary fish consumption is high, or who take ω3 fatty acid supplements, is higher than that of the typical North American woman (34, 48, 59). The 20:4ω6 content of human milk is less variable and appears to be less dependent on maternal intake of 20:4ω6, perhaps because the 18:2ω6 intake of most populations is relatively high.

Recent recommendations for the minimal content of 18:2ω6 in infant formulas range from 2.7% to 8% of total fatty acids, and those for the maximum content range from 21% to 35% of total fatty acids (26, 76). The recommendations for the minimum and maximum contents of 18:3ω3 in infant formulas are 1.75% and 4% of total fatty acids, respectively (76). To maintain a reasonable balance between the two fatty acids, it is further recommended that the 18:2ω6/18:3ω3 ratio should not be less than 5–6 nor more than 15–16 (26, 76). The term and preterm infant formulas currently available in the United States have 18:2ω6/18:3ω3 ratios of ~10 (see above). Formulas containing the LC-PUFAs 22:6ω3 and 20:4ω6 also are available for both term and preterm infants.

LONG-CHAIN POLYUNSATURATED FATTY ACIDS

The current interest in the role of LC-PUFAs in infant nutrition was precipitated by observations that plasma and erythrocyte lipid contents of these fatty acids, primarily 22:6ω3 and 20:4ω6, were lower in formula-fed than in breast-fed infants (14, 45, 52, 75). Since these fatty acids are present in human milk but not in formulas, the lower plasma and erythrocyte lipid content of these fatty acids in formula-fed infants was interpreted as indicating that infants cannot synthesize sufficient 22:6ω3 and 20:4ω6 to meet ongoing needs. Concurrent and earlier observations of better cognitive function of breast-fed versus formula-fed infants (55, 56, 67, 78) focused attention on the possibility that the lower cognitive function of formula-fed infants also might be related to inadequate intake of LC-PUFA. This, of course, ignores the many differences in education, socioeconomic status, etc., between women who choose to breast-feed versus formula-feed their infants that may have a greater impact on development than what the infant is fed. Further, of necessity, none of these observations are based on data from randomized, controlled trials, and attempts to control for differences in characteristics of mothers who choose to breast-feed versus formula-feed their infants either decreases or abolishes differences in cognitive function between breast-fed versus formula-fed infants.

The possibility that LC-PUFA intake may be necessary for optimal development is supported by the facts that 22:6ω3 and 20:4ω6 are the major ω3 and ω6 fatty acids, respectively, of neural tissues (18, 19, 62) and 22:6ω3 is the major fatty acid of retinal photoreceptor membranes (62). In addition, postmortem studies of infants who died suddenly during the first year of life (29, 47, 55) show that the cerebral content of 22:6ω3, but not 20:4ω6, is lower in formula-fed than in breast-fed term infants. In contrast, the 22:6ω3 content of the retina of breast-fed and formula-fed term infants does not differ (55), perhaps because the retinal content of 22:6ω3 reaches adult levels at approximately term, whereas the adult level of 22:6ω3 in cerebrum is not reached until approximately 2 years post-term (62). One of the postmortem studies showed that the cerebral 22:6ω3 content of infants fed a formula with a relatively high content of 18:3ω3 was higher than that of infants fed a formula with less 18:3ω3 (47). This finding is consistent with studies in piglets showing that an 18:3ω3 intake of at least 1.75% of total fatty acids is necessary to maintain normal brain levels of 22:6ω3 (1) and studies in infants showing a positive relationship between 18:3ω3 intake and the appearance of labeled 22:6ω3 in plasma following administration of labeled 18:3ω3 (84).

During pregnancy, LC-PUFAs are transported actively to the fetus from maternal plasma (4, 25). Thus, the infant who is born early in the third trimester of pregnancy receives less LC-PUFA prior to birth than does the infant who is born at term and is thought to have a higher LC-PUFA requirement. However, the daily accumulation of LC-PUFA in the developing central nervous system changes minimally between mid-gestation and 18–24 months of age (62), which suggests that the total daily LC-PUFA needs of preterm and term infants are likely to be similar. On the other hand, since preterm infants are smaller, their daily needs per kilogram, or per 100 kcal, are undoubtedly greater, particularly during early life.

Both term and preterm infants can convert 18:2ω6 to 20:4ω6 and 18:3ω3 to 22:6ω3 (17, 22, 80, 84, 92). This has been established by administering the precursor fatty acids labeled with stable isotopes of either carbon (^{13}C) or hydrogen (^{2}H) and serially measuring blood levels of the labeled precursors as well as labeled metabolites of each by gas chromatography/mass spectrometry. The studies of Sauerwald et al. (84, 85) and Uauy et al. (92), which included both term and preterm infants, suggest that the overall ability of preterm infants to synthesize LC-PUFA is at least equal to that of term infants. However, the amount of LC-PUFA synthesized is a function of both the rate of synthesis and the pool size of the precursor. Hence, the preterm infant's greater apparent rate of conversion of 18:2ω6 and 18:3ω3 to 20:4ω6 and 22:6ω3, respectively, may not be great enough to compensate for its smaller precursor pool. Additionally, there is considerable variability in apparent conversion among both preterm and term infants, including infants fed the same formulas. Further, measurement of the enrichment of 22:6ω3 and 20:4ω6 following administration of labeled precursors has been limited to plasma, which is only a fraction of the body pool of both the precursor and product fatty acids. Thus, since conversion as estimated from plasma enrichments may not be representative of conversion rates of other tissues, the amounts of LC-PUFA that either preterm or term infants can synthesize are not known.

The higher LC-PUFA content of the plasma lipids of breast-fed infants and infants fed formulas supplemented with LC-PUFA versus infants fed unsupplemented formulas support the concept that the amounts of LC-PUFA formed endogenously are less than the amounts provided by human milk or supplemented formulas. However, the extent to which the concentration of individual LC-PUFAs in plasma reflects the content of these fatty acids in tissues, particularly the brain, is not known. In piglets, the brain content of LC-PUFA is not correlated as highly with the content in plasma as is the content in erythrocytes, skeletal muscle, and liver (77). In contrast, one of the postmortem studies showed a weak, but statistically significant, correlation between brain and erythrocyte contents of 22:6ω3 (55). The correlation between the erythrocyte content of this fatty acid and its content in other tissues was not reported.

Studies in isolated cell systems suggest that 20:5ω3 and 22:5ω3 are transferred from plasma to astrocytes where they are converted to 22:6ω3, which, in turn, is transferred to neurons (5, 65, 66). Whether direct synthesis of 22:6ω3 within the central nervous system occurs in humans is not known, but at least one in vivo study in animals is compatible with this possibility (74).

Importance of Long-Chain Polyunsaturated Fatty Acids in Development

The findings discussed above, although far from definitive, are compatible with the possibility that failure to provide preformed LC-PUFA during early infancy, and perhaps longer, may compromise development of tissues/organs with a high content of these fatty acids, particularly 22:6ω3. However, the specific role(s) of LC-PUFA in normal development is (are) not clear (91, 54). It is known that these fatty acids affect gene transcription. They also may produce post-translational modifications. Moreover, many are precursors of eicosanoids that, in turn, modify a number of processes. These fatty acids also have other effects on signal transduction. Finally, the amount of these fatty acids in cell membranes can modify membrane fluidity, membrane thickness, and the microenvironment of the membrane as well as interactions between the fatty acid and membrane proteins. Such changes, in turn, can affect receptor function; in addition, the fatty acids may have direct effects on receptor function. Although the degree of unsaturation of membrane fatty acids affects fluidity, this effect is most marked by substituting a monounsaturated fatty acid or a fatty acid such as 18:2ω6 for a saturated fatty acid. In 22:6ω3 deficiency, 22:5ω6 replaces 22:6ω3 with little effect on fluidity. Possible mechanisms for the effects of LC-PUFAs have been reviewed recently by Uauy et al. (91) and by Lauritzen et al. (54).

Despite the lack of a clear mechanism of the role of LC-PUFAs in development, a number of studies over the past several years have focused on differences in visual acuity and neurodevelopmental indices between breast-fed and formula-fed infants as well as between infants fed LC-PUFA-supplemented and unsupplemented formulas. Since human milk contains a number of factors other than LC-PUFA that might affect visual acuity and/or neurodevelopmental indices, studies comparing breast-fed with formula-fed infants cannot help resolve the role of LC-PUFA in infant development. On the other hand, studies taking advantage of the natural variability in milk contents of LC-PUFA or enhanced variability secondary to maternal supplementation and, hence, differences in LC-PUFA intake of the recipient infants (31, 33, 46, 61) provide important insights. The following discussions of the effect of LC-PUFA intake on visual function and on cognitive/behavioral development are limited to findings from these types of studies and findings from studies in which LC-PUFA-supplemented formulas were compared with unsupplemented formulas.

Long-Chain Polyunsaturated Fatty Acid Intake and Visual Function

Early studies in rodents established the importance of $\omega 3$ fatty acids for normal retinal function (3, 95) and subsequent studies established this in primates (69, 70). More recently, studies have focused on the effect of $\omega 3$ fatty acids on retinal function and/or overall visual function of human infants. However, whereas the abnormal retinal/visual function of $\omega 3$ fatty acid–deficient animals clearly resulted from an inadequate intake of 18:3$\omega 3$ and were reversed by adding this fatty acid, the more recent studies in human infants have focused primarily on the effects of 22:6$\omega 3$ intake on retinal and/or visual function. Studies have been conducted in both term and preterm infants and have utilized both behaviorally based and electrophysiologically based methods for assessing visual function.

The most commonly utilized behaviorally based method for assessing visual acuity, the Teller Acuity Card procedure, is based on the innate tendency to look toward a discernible pattern rather than a blank field (23, 24, 64). This rapid measure of resolution acuity combines forced-choice and operant preferential looking procedures. The subject is shown a series of cards with stripes (gratings) of different widths on one side and a blank field on the other and his/her looking behavior is observed through a peephole in the center of the card. Cards with wider stripes are shown initially, followed by cards with progressively decreasing stripe widths. The subject's visual acuity is assumed to be the finest grating toward which he/she clearly looks preferentially (i.e., the finest grating that he/she is able to resolve).

The electrophysiologically based tests utilize visual evoked potentials (VEPs), which measure the activation of the visual cortex in response to visual information that is processed by the retina and transmitted to the visual cortex (88, 89). The presence of a reliable evoked response indicates that the stimulus information was resolved up to the visual cortex, where the response is processed. Use of VEPs to assess visual acuity requires measuring the electrical potentials of the visual cortex in response to patterns of contrast reversal with vertical square wave gratings or checkerboards. The frequency of the gratings or checkerboards is decreased from low (large) to high (small), and the visual acuity threshold is estimated by linear regression of the VEP amplitudes versus the frequency, or size, of the grating or checkerboard stimulus (71, 88). Data are recorded as the $\log_{10}$ of the minimum angle of resolution (logMAR), which is the smallest grating that results in a measurable amplitude. Thus, smaller logMAR values indicate better visual acuity. A rapid VEP method (sweep VEP) has been developed for use in infant populations (71).

The standard VEP also allows assessment of latency, or the time between presentation of a stimulus and the peak of the electrical potential. This reflects the rate of transmission of the stimulus and, hence, should be useful for assessing the effects of LC-PUFA (or other intervention). However, it has been used for this purpose by only a few investigators (10, 28, 49, 61, 93), perhaps because it does not provide a direct assessment of acuity.

Electroretinography, unlike the above procedures that measure the response of the entire visual system, measures only the activity of the retina (41, 68). However, this methodology is somewhat more invasive and time consuming than the other methods and has been used to assess effects of LC-PUFA in only a few studies (6, 89). The primary components of the electroretinogram generated in response to a flash of light are the a-wave, which is produced by hyperpolarization of the photoreceptor, and the b-wave, which reflects the subsequent activation of retinal neurons. Performance is quantified by parameters (41, 68) such as the threshold (the minimal intensity of light necessary to elicit a small amplitude), the implicit time or peak latency (the time from the presentation of a brief flash of light to the response peak), the maximal amplitude, and the sensitivity (the intensity of light that elicits a response of half the maximal amplitude).

Meta-analyses of data from studies using both behavioral and electrophysiological methods of assessment in both term and preterm infants have been reported (82, 83). Data from behaviorally based tests of visual acuity obtained in randomized studies of term infants fed 22:6ω3-supplemented versus unsupplemented formula show a statistically significant advantage of the supplemented formula at 2 months of age but not at other ages. Data from randomized studies utilizing electrophysiological methods of assessment in term infants fed 22:6ω3-supplemented versus unsupplemented formula showed no statistically significant advantages at any age (82).

A recently reported relatively large multicenter study (2), which was not included in the meta-analysis, showed no advantages of 22:6ω3 (0.14% of total fatty acids) plus 20:4ω6 (0.46% of total fatty acids) supplementation on visual acuity as assessed by the Teller Acuity Card procedure at 2, 4, 6, or 12 months of age. Whether inclusion of these additional data in a future meta-analysis will change the conclusions is not clear.

Recent studies of different designs also have shown an apparent relationship between 22:6ω3 intake and visual acuity measured by the Teller Acuity Card procedure. In one such study (46), term infants were breast-fed exclusively for at least three months following birth and then weaned to a standard formula. Visual acuity at 2 and 12 months of age was significantly correlated with the 22:6ω3 content of erythrocyte phosphatidylethanolamine at 2 months of age, but acuity at 4 and 6 months of age was not. In addition, infants with an erythrocyte phosphatidylethanolamine 22:6ω3 concentration >10.78 g/100 g at 2 months of age (i.e., the upper tertile) had significantly better acuity at 2 and 12 but not at 4 and 6 months of age than those with an erythrocyte phosphatidylethanolamine 22:6ω3 concentration <8.53 g/100 g at 2 months of age (i.e., the lowest tertile).

Birch et al. (8) recently reported results of a randomized controlled trial of supplemented (0.36% of total fatty acids as 22:6ω3 and 0.72% 20:4ω6) versus unsupplemented formula following near-exclusive breast-feeding (one feeding/day of formula allowed) for the first six weeks of life. Visual acuity of the two groups, measured by sweep VEP, was similar at enrollment, but that of the supplemented group was better at 17, 26, and 52 weeks of age. Random dot stereoacuity of the supplemented group also was better at 17 weeks of age but not at 26 and 52 weeks of age. Random dot stereopsis, which reflects processing in the visual cortex, is not present before 3 months of age and develops rapidly between 3 and 5 months of age. It is thought to be particularly sensitive to differences in maturation of the visual cortex between 3 and 5 months of age. If so and if adequate 22:6ω3 is necessary for optimal maturation, a dietary source of this fatty acid between 3 and 5 months of age (~12 and ~20 weeks) should enhance development of random dot stereopsis.

In a similar study, Hoffman et al. (35) assigned infants to the same formulas after 4 to 6 months (~16 to ~24 weeks) rather than 6 weeks of near-exclusive breast-feeding. Visual acuity of the supplemented group, assessed by sweep VEP, was better at 12 months of age but there was no difference in random dot stereoacuity between the two groups, presumably because the infants were still breast-fed during the period of rapid development of the visual cortex required for optimal stereopsis. Nonetheless, these findings suggest a possible need for 22:6ω3 beyond 4 to 6 months of age, the maximum duration of supplementation in most previous studies.

This possibility is further supported by another recent study by the same group of investigators (37). In this study, 6-month-old infants who had been primarily breast-fed were randomly assigned to either complementary foods that contained no 22:6ω3 or complementary foods with 22:6ω3-enriched egg yolk. Many in both groups continued breast-feeding, but this was not quantitated. The primary outcome variable was visual acuity assessed by sweep VEP at 12 months of age. Acuity of the control group improved from 0.49 log MAR at 6 months of age to 0.29 log MAR at 12 months of age, and that of the 22:6ω3-supplemented group improved from 0.48 log MAR at 6 months to 0.14 log MAR at 12 months of age, indicating a more rapid rate of retrieval and/or visual cortex maturation in the supplemented group. 22:6ω3 intake of the supplemented group from complementary foods was 83 mg/d and that of the control group was 0 mg/d. The 22:6ω3 content of erythrocyte lipids of the control group decreased by 21% between 6 and 12 months of age, whereas that of the supplemented group increased by 34%.

As observed in other studies (see above), VEP acuity of the total population at 12 months of age was significantly correlated with erythrocyte lipid 22:6ω3 content, further supporting the potential benefit of 22:6ω3 beyond 6 months of age.

Finally, a retrospective study of 435 children showed that stereoacuity was better at 3.5 years of age in children who had been breast-fed for at least four months than in those who had been formula-fed (97). Further, stereoacuity of the breast-fed infants at 3.5 years of age was greater in those whose mothers ate oily fish during pregnancy than in those whose mothers did not.

The aforementioned meta-analysis of data from randomized studies in preterm infants showed an advantage of 22:6ω3-supplemented versus unsupplemented formulas on both behaviorally based and electrophysiologically based measurements of visual acuity (83). Advantages with behaviorally based tests were apparent at 2 and 4 months post-term and advantages with electrophysiologically based measurements were apparent at 4 months post-term. A recent randomized, controlled trial in preterm infants (72), when analyzed according to intent to treat, showed no advantage of 22:6ω3 and 20:4ω6 supplementation (0.26% and 0.42% of total fatty acids, respectively, from birth to term, and then 0.16% and 0.42%, respectively, through the first year of life) on visual acuity at 2, 4, or 6 months of age as assessed by the Teller Acuity Card procedure or VEP. However, posthoc analysis showed that, in a subset of infants, there was an advantage of supplementation on acuity as assessed by sweep VEP at 6 but not at 4 months post-term. Another recent multicenter study in which supplemented (0.36% of total fatty acids as 22:6ω3 and 0.72% as 20:4ω6) versus unsupplemented formulas were fed to preterm infants for an average of ~28 days during hospitalization showed no effect on visual acuity at either 48 or 57 weeks postmenstrual age as assessed by the Teller Acuity Card procedure (44). Electrophysiological assessments were not performed. In yet another study (93) in which preterm infants were assigned randomly to receive a supplemented (0.34% and 0.70% of total fatty acids as 22:6ω3 and 20:4ω6, respectively, both from single cell oils) versus an unsupplemented formula until a corrected age of 6 months, visual acuity as assessed by the Teller Acuity Card procedure did not differ between groups at 3, 6, 12, or 24 months of age. VEP latency and amplitude of the two groups, assessed at 3 and 12 months of age, also did not differ (see below).

In apparent contrast to some of the findings discussed above, including the findings of the meta analyses (82, 83), recent Cochrane reviews of much, but not all, of the same data conclude that there are no consistent effects of LC-PUFA on visual acuity of either term (87) or preterm infants (86). In a review of most, but again not all, reported randomized controlled trials of supplemented versus unsupplemented formulas in both term and preterm infants in 2001, Gibson et al. (30) concluded that the evidence for a beneficial effect of LC-PUFA supplementation on visual function of preterm infants was "reasonably compelling," whereas the evidence of a beneficial effect on visual function of term infants was less so. Clearly, there is no consensus concerning the effect of LC-PUFA supplementation of either term or preterm infants on visual function. In part, this may be related to the fact that the studies reported to date have utilized different types as well as different durations of supplementation, making it difficult to reach a conclusion. An additional problem is the possibility that some infants might benefit from supplementation, whereas others receiving the same supplement may not.

Long-Chain Polyunsaturated Fatty Acids and Cognitive/Behavioral Development

Most studies addressing the cognitive/behavioral development of infants fed LC-PUFA-supplemented versus unsupplemented formulas have utilized the Bayley Scales of Infant Development, which are considered the gold standard for assessing global abilities of infants from birth to 42 months of age. They provide standardized indices of both mental (MDI) and psychomotor development (PDI). However, they are intended to distinguish between "normal" and "abnormal," not degrees of either. Thus, unless cognitive and/or psychomotor function as assessed by the Bayley Scales early in life is definitely abnormal, the relationship between these early scores and later function is poor (63).

The Fagan Test of Infant Intelligence (FTII) also has been used in several studies, either alone or in addition to the Bayley Scales. This test assesses novelty preference (27). The infant is shown a single stimulus (usually a face) for a standardized, age-based period, and then is shown this stimulus along with a novel one. If the infant has "learned" the original stimulus prior to the novelty test, the typical response is to look selectively toward the novel rather than the familiar image. Scores on this test during infancy are somewhat more predictive of later cognitive function than the Bayley MDI; however, its internal consistency (reproducibility), unlike that of the Bayley Scales, is relatively poor (21). Look duration during the familiarization and the paired comparison phases of the test also is a modest predictor of both concurrent performance on other tests during infancy and later tests of intelligence (21); shorter look durations during the familiarization phase predict better concurrent as well as later cognitive performance.

One or both of these tests has been used to evaluate the effect of LC-PUFA supplementation on cognitive/behavioral development. Some of these studies have shown advantages of LC-PUFA supplementation with both tests, some with one but not the other, and still others with neither. Available studies in term infants were reviewed in 1998 by an expert panel appointed by the Life Sciences Research Organization to assess the nutrient requirements for term infant formulas (76). The studies reviewed were criticized by consultants to the panel for including too few infants, failing to control adequately for confounding factors, failing to assess function at more than one age, failing to examine individual differences in development, and failing to follow the infants for a sufficiently long period (e.g., none of the studies available at that time included data beyond 1 year of age). Based partially on this critique, the panel did not recommend addition of LC-PUFA to term infant formulas but suggested that the issue be re-evaluated in about five years.

The randomized trials in term infants published since 1998 (2, 7, 57, 60) have not resolved many of these difficulties. The trials have differed with respect to the source of LC-PUFA supplementation, the duration of supplementation, the amounts of 22:6ω3 and 20:4ω6 supplementation, and the 22:6ω3/20:4ω6 ratio. There also were some differences in the 18:2ω6 and 18:3ω3 contents of the control and experimental formulas. The variance in Bayley MDI and PDI scores also varied among studies, being smallest in the one study that showed an advantage of 22:6ω3 and 20:4ω6 supplementation for the first 4 months of life on the Bayley MDI score at 18 months of age (7).

Fewer studies are available in preterm infants fed LC-PUFA-supplemented versus unsupplemented formulas, and these are subject to many of the same criticisms levied against the studies in term infants. The available data, including those from recently reported large, multicenter studies (20, 72), suggest that preterm infants may be more likely than term infants to benefit from supplementation. However, it is important to note that this conclusion is based on posthoc analyses of data from selected groups of the study populations (e.g., infants who received only the assigned formula rather than the assigned formula plus breast milk; infants who weighed less than 1250 g at birth; infants whose parents were English speaking). Analysis of the data according to how the infants were randomized shows few differences in any outcome variable among groups. The study of van Wezel-Meijler et al. (93) showed no difference in scores on the Dutch version of the Bayley Scales of Infant Development between preterm infants who were assigned to receive supplemented (0.34% and 0.70% 22:6ω3 and 20:4ω6, respectively) versus unsupplemented formulas through 6 months corrected age (see below). This was true at 12 and 24 as well as at 3 and 6 months of age.

A few methods other than the Bayley Scales and the FTII have been used to assess the effects of LC-PUFA on cognitive/behavioral development. For example, Willats et al. (96) found that term infants assigned to a formula supplemented with both 22:6ω3 and 20:4ω6 versus an unsupplemented formula had better visual habituation scores at 4 months of age and performed better on a means-end problem-solving test at 10 months of age. The supplemented group not only had more intentional solutions to items of this test but also scored higher than those assigned to the control formula, findings that have been related to higher intelligence quotient scores later in childhood.

Innis et al. (46), studying breast-fed term infants with a range of 22:6ω3 and 20:4ω6 as well as 18:2ω6 and 18:3ω3 intakes and, hence, a range of plasma and erythrocyte lipid 22:6ω3 and 20:4ω6 contents, found no statistically significant relationships between infant 22:6ω3 and 20:4ω6 status at 2 months, when all infants were exclusively breast-fed, and scores on an object-search test at either 6 or 12 months of age. There also was no statistically significant relationship at either 6 or 12 months of age between infant 22:6ω3 or 20:4ω6 status at 2 months of age and novelty preference, Bayley MDI, or Bayley PDI scores. However, there was a positive relationship between ability to discriminate non-native retroflex and phonetic contrasts at 9 months of age and the 22:6ω3 content of plasma phospholipid as well as erythrocyte phosphatidylethanolamine at 2 months of age. This finding was interpreted by the investigators to indicate more rapid language development in those with higher plasma and erythrocyte lipid levels of 22:6ω3 at 2 months of age.

Two other studies of the effect of maternal 22:6ω3 supplementation and, hence, intake of 22:6ω3 by the breast-feeding infant are relevant. Gibson et al. (31) supplemented breast-feeding mothers with varying amounts of 22:6ω3 and achieved breast milk 22:6ω3 concentrations ranging from 0.1%–1.7% of total fatty acids and, hence, a wide range in 22:6ω3 content of infant plasma lipids. Although there was no relationship between the 22:6ω3 content of milk or infant plasma lipids and VEP acuity at either 12 or 16 weeks of age, Bayley MDI scores were weakly correlated with milk 22:6ω3 content at 12 but not at 24 months of age.

In a somewhat similar study, Jensen et al. (50) assigned breast-feeding mothers to receive 22:6ω3 ($\sim$250 mg/d as an algal-derived triglyceride) or a control oil containing no 22:6ω3 for the first 4 months postpartum. At 4 months of age, plasma phospholipid 22:6ω3 content of infants whose mothers had received 22:6ω3 was approximately 50% higher than that of infants whose mothers received the control oil, but there was no difference in visual acuity between the two groups at either 4 or 8 months of age, whether assessed by sweep VEP or the Teller Acuity Card procedure. There also was no difference between groups in scores on a variety of neurodevelopmental tests at either 12 or 18 months of age. However, at 30 months of age, the mean Bayley PDI of the group whose mothers received 22:6ω3 was eight points higher than that of the group whose mothers received the control oil ($p < 0.01$). There was no statistically significant difference in mean Bayley MDI between the two groups at 30 months of age. Nor was there a statistically significant relationship between either PDI or MDI scores at 30 months of age and plasma phospholipid 22:6ω3 content at 4 months of age.

Helland et al. (33), examining the effect of supplementing women with either cod liver oil ($\sim$1.2 g/d of 22:6ω3 and 0.8 mg/d of 20:5ω3) or corn oil from week 18 of pregnancy until 3 months after delivery, found that children whose mothers received cod liver oil scored higher at 4 years of age on the Mental Processing Composite of the Kaufman Assessment Battery for Children (106.4 $\pm$ 7.4; n = 48) than children whose mothers received corn oil (102.3 $\pm$ 11.3; n = 36). In a multiple regression model, maternal 22:6ω3 intake during pregnancy was the only variable related significantly to the mental processing scores of the children at 4 years of age.

In a somewhat similar study, Malcolm et al. (61) assigned pregnant women to fish oil (n = 50) or control oil capsules (n = 50) from week 15 of pregnancy through term. The fish oil capsules provided about 200 mg 22:6ω3 per day. Although the 22:6ω3 content of maternal erythrocytes at birth was $\sim$50% higher in the supplemented group, the 22:6ω3 content of umbilical cord erythrocytes did not differ between the two groups and there was no difference in erythrocyte 22:6ω3 contents between groups at either 50 or 66 weeks postconceptional age. However, infants with higher erythrocyte 22:6ω3 content at birth had shorter pattern-evoked VEP latencies at 50 and 66 weeks postconceptional age than those with lower erythrocyte 22:6ω3 content at birth. This finding suggests more rapid nerve conduction.

Long-Chain Polyunsaturated Fatty Acids and Other Aspects of Central Nervous System Development

The effects of LC-PUFA supplementation of infant formulas on other aspects of brain function and/or development also have been examined. Three studies showed no effects of 22:6ω3-supplemented versus unsupplemented formulas on brain auditory evoked potentials of preterm infants (10, 28, 91). In one of these studies (10), supplemented infants had peripheral nerve conduction that was slower than that of infants fed human milk but not slower than that of infants fed the control formula.

Another recent study (11) investigated the effect of supplemented (0.3% of total fatty acids, by weight, as 22:6ω3 and 0.45% as 20:4ω6 from a mixture of egg yolk, tuna oil, and a fungal oil) versus unsupplemented formula during the first 2 months of life on the quality of the infants' general movements at 3 months of age as assessed from videotapes made at that time. The quality of general movements is thought to be useful for evaluating the overall quality of brain function in young infants. The unsupplemented group had mildly abnormal general movements significantly more often than did either the supplemented group or a breast-fed group that was studied concurrently (31%, 19%, and 20%, respectively); however, the frequency of "normal optimal" movements did not differ between supplemented and unsupplemented groups (18% and 21%, respectively) but was less in both than was the frequency observed in the breast-fed group (34%).

Only one study has examined the effect of LC-PUFA supplementation on structural brain development (93). In this study, preterm infants were assigned randomly to receive either a standard formula ($n = 20$) or a formula supplemented with 0.34% and 0.70% of total fatty acids as 22:6ω3 and 20:4ω6, respectively ($n = 22$), both from single cell oils, until a corrected age of 6 months (preterm formula until weight reached 3000 g and a term formula thereafter). Brain structural development, assessed by magnetic resonance imaging at 3 and 12 months corrected age, did not differ between groups at either age. This method essentially assesses the degree of myelination and, in this study, neither global myelination nor myelination of the cerebral visual system differed between groups. This may not be surprising since the LC-PUFA content of myelin is low. However, myelin deposition is dependent on close interaction among neurons, their axons, and their oligodendrocytes, all of which are rich in LC-PUFA. Thus, myelination is thought to reflect the functional maturity of all these components.

Effects of Long-Chain Polyunsaturated Fatty Acids on Growth

The observation in the early 1990s that preterm infants assigned to a formula supplemented with fish oil (0.3% of total fatty acids as 20:5ω3 and 0.2% as 22:6ω3) weighed less and had a lower weight-for-length at various times during the first year of life than did infants assigned to an unsupplemented formula (13) has generated considerable concern. In this study, weight at 12 months corrected age correlated with plasma phospholipid 20:4ω6 content at various times during the first year of life (15). A less marked effect on growth was observed subsequently by the same investigators in preterm infants fed a formula supplemented with low-20:5ω3 fish oil versus an unsupplemented formula (16). In this study, there was no correlation between 20:4ω6 status and growth, but there was a correlation between weight at some ages and the plasma phospholipid ratio of 20:4ω6/22:6ω3.

Interestingly, a smaller study, also conducted in the early 1990s, did not show differences in growth between supplemented and unsupplemented preterm infants, although the supplemented group received even more of a similar fish oil (90). However, the duration of this study may not have been sufficient to permit detection of weight differences.

Ryan et al. (79) observed lower rates of growth in preterm male, but not female, infants fed a formula supplemented with low-20:5ω3 fish oil (0.2% of total fatty acids as 22:6ω3) versus a control formula from shortly before hospital discharge until 59 weeks postmenstrual age (PMA). In this study, as in most studies in which 20:4ω6 is not supplemented, plasma phospholipid 20:4ω6 content of the supplemented group was lower through 59 weeks PMA, but there was no statistically significant correlation between plasma phospholipid 20:4ω6 content and any aspect of growth. Rather, rates of increase in both weight and length of male infants were inversely correlated with plasma phospholipid 22:6ω3 content.

A lower weight at 4 months of age also was observed in term infants fed formulas with a 18:2ω6:18:3ω3 ratio of ~4 versus ~40 and, in this study, weight at 4 months of age was correlated with plasma phospholipid 20:4ω6 content (49).

More recently, Innis et al. (46), studying infants who were breast-fed exclusively for the first 3 months of life, reported a statistically significant inverse correlation between erythrocyte phosphatidyl choline and phosphatidyl ethanolamine contents of 22:6ω3 and weight at 6 but not at 12 months of age. There was no statistically significant relationship between 22:6ω3 or 20:4ω6 contents of plasma lipids and size at any age.

In contrast to these observations of a possible adverse effect of ω3 fatty acids on growth, Innis et al. (44) reported a more rapid rate of growth in preterm infants fed a formula supplemented with both 22:6ω3 (0.33% of fat as an algal oil) and 20:4ω6 (0.6% of fat as a fungal oil) versus a formula supplemented with only 22:6ω3 (0.34% of fat as an algal oil) or infants fed an unsupplemented formula for at least 28 days prior to hospital discharge and followed until 57 weeks PMA. Another recent study [so far reported only as an abstract (20)] also showed a positive growth effect of formulas supplemented with both 22:6ω3 and 20:4ω6 either as single cell oils or a mixture of fish and fungal oils (20). In this study, weight of preterm infants fed the formula supplemented with single cell oils was greater than that of the control infants from 66 through 118 weeks PMA and equal to that of breast-fed term infants at 118 weeks PMA. Length of this group also was greater at 79 and 92 weeks PMA than that of either the control group or the group supplemented with fish and fungal oil and equal to that of the breast-fed term infants by 79 weeks PMA.

The reason(s) for an inhibitory effect of ω3 fatty acids or, perhaps, a stimulatory effect of ω6 fatty acids on growth are not clear (53). Possibilities that have been suggested include inhibition of desaturation and elongation of 18:2ω6 to 20:4ω6 by the ω3 fatty acids, inhibition of eicosanoid synthesis from 20:4ω6 by the intake of preformed 20:5ω3 or endogenous synthesis of 20:5ω3 from a moderately high intake of 18:3ω3, and effects of ω3 and ω6 fatty acids on transcription of genes controlling lipolysis and lipogenesis.

SUMMARY

The LC-PUFAs 22:6ω3 and 20:4ω6 are the major ω3 and ω6 fatty acids, respectively, in the developing central nervous system, and 22:6ω3 comprises 30%–40% of the fatty acid content of photoreceptor membranes. Hence, both are thought to be needed for optimal development of the brain and retina. Both fatty acids are present in human milk and the content of both, particularly 22:6ω3, are lower in the plasma and erythrocyte membranes as well as the brain of formula-fed in comparison with breast-fed infants. Moreover, some but by no means all studies of the effects of these fatty acids on neurodevelopmental as well as visual outcomes suggest that provision of preformed 22:6ω3 and 20:4ω6, particularly the former, may be beneficial. Hence, these fatty acids are often considered conditionally indispensable nutrients.

Both term and preterm infants can synthesize 22:6ω3 and 20:4ω6 from their respective precursors, 18:3ω3 and 18:2ω6; however, the amounts synthesized are difficult to quantitate. Furthermore, although intake of 18:2ω6 (which is usually high) has little effect on plasma lipid content of 20:4ω6, even a relatively high intake of 18:3ω3 does not result in a plasma lipid content of 22:6ω3 equal to that of breast-fed infants. Many studies, therefore, have examined visual and neurodevelopmental outcomes of infants fed unsupplemented formulas versus formulas supplemented with either 22:6ω3 or both 22:6ω3 and 20:4ω6. Some of these studies have shown advantages of supplementation, particularly for preterm infants, but roughly an equal number have not. An intriguing and logical explanation for these discrepant findings is that the rates of endogenous synthesis and, hence, the requirements of 22:6ω3 vary considerably from infant to infant. However, until rates of endogenous synthesis can be more accurately quantitated than is currently possible, this potential reason for the discrepancies among studies must remain theoretical. Finally, considering the generally satisfactory outcomes of infants fed unsupplemented formulas, any advantage of 22:6ω3 (or 22:6ω3 plus 20:4ω6) supplementation is likely to be subtle and possibly not detectable by currently available methods of assessment.

Formulas containing 22:6ω3 and 20:4ω6 are now available throughout the world and, regardless of their efficacy, appear to be safe. Although some studies have suggested that ω3 fatty acids may inhibit growth, most have shown no effects on growth, and recent studies suggest that supplementation of formulas with 22:6ω3 and 20:4ω6 may enhance growth of preterm infants. Current studies focus on possible long-term effects of supplementation during early life as well as possible benefits of supplementation during pregnancy and lactation and beyond the first 4 to 6 months of life, when infants are either breast-fed or fed supplemented formulas.

The *Annual Review of Nutrition* is online at http://nutr.annualreviews.org

LITERATURE CITED

1. Arbuckle LD, MacKinnon MJ, Innis SM. 1994. Formula 18:2 (n-6) and 18:3 (n-3) content and ratio influence long-chain polyunsaturated fatty acids in the developing piglet liver and central nervous system. *J. Nutr.* 124:289–98
2. Auestad N, Halter R, Hall RT, Blatter M, Bogle ML, et al. 2001. Growth and development in term infants fed long-chain polyunsaturated fatty acids: a double-masked, randomized, parallel, prospective, multivariate study. *Pediatrics* 108:372–81
3. Benolken RM, Anderson RE, Wheeler TG. 1973. Membrane fatty acids associated with the electrical response in visual excitation. *Science* 182:1253–54
4. Berghaus TM, Demmelmair H, Koletzko B. 1998. Fatty acid composition of lipid classes in maternal and cord plasma at birth. *Eur. J. Pediatr.* 157:763–68
5. Bernoud N, Fenart L, Benistant C, Pageaux JF, Dehouck MP, et al. 1998. Astrocytes are mainly responsible for the polyunsaturated fatty acid enrichment in blood-brain barrier endothelial cells in vitro. *J. Lipid Res.* 39:1816–24
6. Birch DG, Birch EE, Hoffman DR, Uauy RD. 1992. Retinal development in very-low-birth-weight infants fed diets differing in omega-3 fatty acids. *Invest. Ophthalmol. Vis. Sci.* 33:2365–76
7. Birch EE, Garfield S, Hoffman DR, Uauy R, Birch DG. 2000. A randomized controlled trial of early dietary supply of long-chain polyunsaturated fatty acids and mental development in term infants. *Dev. Med. Child Neurol.* 42:174–81
8. Birch EE, Hoffman DR, Castañeda YS, Fawcett SL, Birch DG, Uauy RD. 2002. A randomized controlled trial of long-chain polyunsaturated fatty acid supplementation of formula in term infants after weaning at 6 wk of age. *Am. J. Clin. Nutr.* 75:570–80
9. Bjerve KS, Fischer S, Alme K. 1987. Alpha-linolenic acid deficiency in man: effect of ethyl linolenate on plasma and erythrocyte fatty acid composition and biosynthesis of prostanoids. *Am. J. Clin. Nutr.* 46: 570–76
10. Bougle D, Denise P, Vimard F, Nouvelot A, Penneillo MJ, Guillois B. 1999. Early neurological and neuropsychological development of the preterm infant and polyunsaturated fatty acids supply. *Clin. Neurophysiol.* 110:1363–70
11. Bouwstra H, Dijck-Brouwer DA, Wildeman JA, Tjoonk HM, van der Heide JC, et al. 2003. Long-chain polyunsaturated fatty acids have a positive effect on the quality of general movements of healthy term infants. *Am. J. Clin. Nutr.* 78:313–18
12. Burr GO, Burr MM. 1929. A new deficiency disease produced by the rigid exclusion of fat from the diet. *J. Biol. Chem.* 82:345–67
13. Carlson SE, Cooke RJ, Werkman SH, Tolley EA. 1992. First year growth of preterm infants fed standard compared to marine oil n-3 supplemented formula. *Lipids* 27:901–7

14. Carlson SE, Rhodes PG, Ferguson MG. 1986. Docosahexaenoic acid status of preterm infants at birth and following feeding with human milk or formula. *Am. J. Clin. Nutr.* 44:798–804
15. Carlson SE, Werkman SH, Peeples JM, Cooke RJ, Tolley EA. 1993. Arachidonic acid status correlates with first year growth in preterm infants. *Proc. Natl. Acad. Sci. USA* 90:1073–77
16. Carlson SE, Werkman SH, Tolley EA. 1996. Effect of long-chain n-3 fatty acid supplementation on visual acuity and growth of preterm infants with and without bronchopulmonary dysplasia. *Am. J. Clin. Nutr.* 63:687–89
17. Carnielli VP, Wattimena DJ, Luijendijk IH, Boerlage A, Degenhart HJ, Sauer PJ. 1996. The very low birth weight premature infant is capable of synthesizing arachidonic and docosahexaenoic acids from linoleic and linolenic acids. *Pediatr. Res.* 40:169–74
18. Clandinin MT, Chappell JE, Leong S, Heim T, Swyer PR, Chance GW. 1980. Extrauterine fatty acid accretion in infant brain: implications for fatty acid requirements. *Early Hum. Dev.* 4:131–38
19. Clandinin MT, Chappell JE, Leong S, Heim T, Swyer PR, Chance GW. 1980. Intrauterine fatty acid accretion rates in human brain: implications for fatty acid requirements. *Early Hum. Dev.* 4:121–29
20. Clandinin M, Van Aerde J, Antonson D, Lim D, Stevens K, et al. 2002. Formulas with docosahexaenoic acid (DHA) and arachidonic acid (ARA) promote better growth and development scores in very-low-birth-weight (VLBW) infants. *Pediatr. Res.* 51:187–88 (Abstr.)
21. Colombo J. 1997. Individual differences in infant cognition: methods, measures, and models. In *Developing Brain and Behaviour*, ed. J Dobbing, pp. 339–85. London: Academic
22. Demmelmair H, von Schenck U, Behrendt E, Sauerwald T, Koletzko B. 1995. Estimation of arachidonic acid synthesis in full-term neonates using natural variation of ^{13}C content. *J. Pediatr. Gastroenterol. Nutr.* 21:31–36
23. Dobson V. 1983. Clinical applications of preferential looking measures of visual acuity. *Behav. Brain Res.* 10:25–38
24. Dobson V, Teller DY. 1978. Visual acuity in human infants: a review and comparison of behavioral and electrophysiological studies. *Vision Res.*18:1469–83
25. Dutta-Roy AK. 2000. Transport mechanisms for long-chain polyunsaturated fatty acids in the human placenta. *Am. J. Clin. Nutr.* 71:315–22S
26. ESPGAN Committee on Nutrition. 1991. Comment on the content and composition of lipids in infant formulas. *Acta. Paediatr. Scand.* 80:887–96
27. Fagan JF III, Singer LT. 1983. Infant recognition memory as a measure of intelligence. *Adv. Infancy Res.* 2:31–78
28. Faldella G, Govoni M, Alessandroni R, Marchiani E, Salvioli GP, et al. 1996. Visual evoked potentials and dietary long chain polyunsaturated fatty acids in preterm infants. *Arch. Dis. Child* 75:F108–12
29. Farquharson J, Cockburn F, Patrick WA, Jamieson EC, Logan RW. 1992. Infant cerebral cortex phospholipid fatty acid composition and diet. *Lancet* 340:810–13
30. Gibson RA, Chen W, Makrides M. 2001. Randomized trials with polyunsaturated fatty acid interventions in preterm and term infants: functional and clinical outcomes. *Lipids* 36:873–83
31. Gibson R, Neumann M, Makrides M. 1997. Effect of increasing breast milk docosahexaenoic acid on plasma and erythrocyte phospholipid fatty acids and neural indices of exclusively breast-fed infants. *Eur. J. Clin. Nutr.* 51:578–84
32. Hansen AE, Steward RA, Hughes G, Soderhjelm L. 1962. The relation of linoleic acid to infant feeding. *Acta Paediatr.* 51(Suppl. 137):1–41
33. Helland IB, Smith L, Saarem K, Saugstad OD, Drevon CA. 2003. Maternal supplementation with very-long-chain n-3 fatty

acids during pregnancy and lactation augments children's IQ at 4 years of age. *Pediatrics* 111:e39–44 http://www.pediatrics.org
34. Henderson RA, Jensen RG, Lammi-Keefe CJ, Ferris AM, Dardick KR. 1992. Effect of fish oil on the fatty acid composition of human milk and maternal and infant erythrocytes. *Lipids* 27:863–69
35. Hoffman DR, Birch EE, Castañeda YS, Fawcett SL, Wheaton DH, et al. 2003. Visual function in breast-fed term infants weaned to formula with or without long-chain polyunsaturates at 4 to 6 months: a randomized clinical trial. *J. Pediatr.* 142:669–77
36. Hoffman DR, DeMar JC, Heird WC, Birch DG, Anderson RE. 2001. Impaired synthesis of DHA in patients with X-linked retinitis pigmentosa. *J. Lipid Res.* 42:1395–401
37. Hoffman DR, Theuer RC, Castaneda YS, Wheaton DH, Bosworth RG, et al. 2004. Maturation of visual acuity is accelerated in breast-fed term infants fed baby food containing DHA-enriched egg yolk. *J. Nutr.* 134:2307–13
38. Holman RT. 1960. The ratio of trienoic: tetraenoic acids in tissue lipids as a measure of essential fatty acid requirement. *J. Nutr.* 70:405–10
39. Holman RT, Caster WO, Wiese HF. 1964. The essential fatty acid requirement of infants and the assessment of their dietary intake of linolenate by serum fatty acid analysis. *Am. J. Clin. Nutr.* 14:70–75
40. Holman RT, Johnson SB, Hatch RF. 1982. A case of human linolenic acid deficiency involving neurological abnormalities. *Am. J. Clin. Nutr.* 35:617–23
41. Hood DC, Birch DG. 1990. The a-wave of the human electroretinogram and rod receptor function. *Invest. Ophthalmol. Vis. Sci.* 31:2070–81
42. Innis SM. 1991. Essential fatty acids in growth and development. *Prog. Lipid Res.* 30:39–103
43. Innis SM. 1993. Fat. In *Nutritional Needs of the Preterm Infant*, ed. RC Tsang, A Lucas, R Uauy, S Zlotkin, pp. 65–86. Baltimore, MD: Williams & Wilkins
44. Innis SM, Adamkin DH, Hall RT, Kalhan SC, Lair C, et al. 2002. Docosahexaenoic acid and arachidonic acid enhance growth with no adverse effects in preterm infants fed formula. *J. Pediatr.* 140:547–54
45. Innis SM, Akrabawi SS, Diersen-Schade DA, Dobson MV, Guy DG. 1997. Visual acuity and blood lipids in term infants fed human milk or formulae. *Lipids* 32:63–72
46. Innis SM, Gilley J, Werker J. 2001. Are human milk long-chain polyunsaturated fatty acids related to visual and neural development in breast-fed term infants? *J. Pediatr.* 139:532–38
47. Jamieson EC, Abbasi KA, Cockburn F, Farquharson J, Logan RW, Patrick WA. 1994. Effect of diet on term infant cerebral cortex fatty acid composition. *World Rev. Nutr. Diet.* 75:139–41
48. Jensen CL, Maude M, Anderson RE, Heird WC. 2000. Effect of docosahexaenoic acid supplementation of lactating women on milk total lipid, and maternal and infant plasma phospholipid fatty acids. *Am. J. Clin. Nutr.* 71(Suppl.):292–99S
49. Jensen CL, Prager TC, Fraley JK, Chen H, Anderson RE, Heird WC. 1997. Effect of dietary linoleic/alpha-linolenic acid ratio on growth and visual function of term infants. *J. Pediatr.* 131:200–9
50. Jensen CL, Voigt RG, Prager TC, Zou YL, Fraley JK, et al. 2005. Effects of maternal docosahexaenoic acid (DHA) supplementation on visual function and neurodevelopment of breast-fed infants. *Am. J. Clin. Nutr.* In press
51. Jensen RG. 1999. Lipids in human milk. *Lipids* 34:1243–71
52. Jørgensen MH, Hernell O, Lund P, Holmer G, Michaelsen KF. 1996. Visual acuity and erythrocyte docosahexaenoic acid status in breast-fed and formula-fed term infants during the first four months of life. *Lipids* 31:99–105
53. Lapillonne A, Clarke SD, Heird WC.

2003. Plausible mechanisms for effects of long-chain polyunsaturated fatty acids on growth. *J. Pediatr.* 143:S9–16
54. Lauritzen L, Hansen HS, Jorgensen MH, Michaelsen KF. 2001. The essentiality of long chain *n*-3 fatty acids in relation to development and function of the brain and retina. *Prog. Lipid Res.* 40:1–94
55. Lucas A, Morley R, Cole TJ. 1998. Randomised trial of early diet in preterm babies and later intelligence quotient. *Br. Med. J.* 317:1481–87
56. Lucas A, Morley R, Cole TJ, Gore SM, Lucas PJ, et al. 1990. Early diet in preterm babies and developmental status at 18 months. *Lancet* 335:1477–81
57. Lucas A, Morley R. 1999. Efficacy and safety of long-chain polyunsaturated fatty acid supplementation of infant-formula milk: a randomised trial. *Lancet* 354:1948–54
58. Makrides M, Neumann MA, Byard RW, Simmer K, Gibson RA. 1994. Fatty acid composition of brain, retina, and erythrocytes in breast- and formula-fed infants. *Am. J. Clin. Nutr.* 60:189–94
59. Makrides M, Neumann MA, Gibson RA. 1996. Effect of maternal docosahexaenoic acid (DHA) supplementation on breast milk composition. *Eur. J. Clin. Nutr.* 50: 352–57
60. Makrides M, Neumann MA, Simmer K, Gibson RA. 2000. A critical appraisal of the role of dietary long-chain polyunsaturated fatty acids on neural indices of term infants: a randomized, controlled trial. *Pediatrics* 105:32–38
61. Malcolm CA, McCulloch DL, Montgomery C, Shepherd A, Weaver LT. 2003. Maternal docosahexaenoic acid supplementation during pregnancy and visual evoked potential development in term infants: a double blind, prospective, randomised trial. *Arch. Dis. Child. Fetal Neonatal Ed.* 88:F383–90
62. Martinez M. 1992. Tissue levels of polyunsaturated fatty acids during early human development. *J. Pediatr.* 120:S129–38
63. McCall RB, Mash CW. 1997. Long-chain polyunsaturated fatty acids and the measurement and prediction of intelligence (IQ). In *Developing Brain and Behaviour*, ed. J Dobbing, pp. 295–338. London: Academic
64. McDonald MA, Dobson V, Sebris SL, Baitch L, Varner D, Teller DY. 1985. The acuity card procedure: a rapid test of infant acuity. *Invest. Ophthalmol. Vis. Sci.* 26: 1158–62
65. Moore SA. 1993. Cerebral endothelium and astrocytes cooperate in supplying docosahexaenoic acid to neurons. *Adv. Exp. Med. Biol.* 331:229–33
66. Moore SA, Yoder E, Murphy S. 1991. Astrocytes, not neurons, produce docosahexaenoic acid (22:6ω3) and arachidonic acid (20:4ω6). *J. Neurochem.* 56:518–24
67. Morrow-Tlucak M, Haude RH, Ernhart CB. 1988. Breastfeeding and cognitive development in the first 2 years of life. *Soc. Sci. Med.* 26:635–39
68. Naka KI, Rushton WAH. 1966. S-potentials from colour units in the retina of fish (cyprindae). *J. Physiol.* 185:536–55
69. Neuringer M, Connor WE, Lin DS, Barstad L, Luck S. 1986. Biochemical and functional effects of prenatal and postnatal ω3 fatty acid deficiency on retina and brain in Rhesus monkeys. *Proc. Natl. Acad. Sci. USA* 83:4021–25
70. Neuringer M, Connor WE, Van Petten C, Barstad L. 1984. Dietary omega-3 fatty acid deficiency and visual loss in infant Rhesus monkeys. *J. Clin. Invest.* 73:272–76
71. Norcia AM, Tyler CW. 1985. Spatial frequency sweep VEP: visual acuity during the first year of life. *Vision Res.* 25:1399–408
72. O'Connor DL, Hall R, Adamkin D, Auestad N, Castillo M, et al. 2001. Growth and development in preterm infants fed long-chain polyunsaturated fatty acids: a prospective, randomized controlled trial. *Pediatrics* 108:359–71

73. Oliw E, Gramström E, Änggärd E. 1983. The prostaglandins and essential fatty acids. In *Prostaglandins and Related Substances*, ed. C Pace-Asciak, E Gramström E, pp. 1–19 Amsterdam: Elsevier
74. Pawlosky RJ, Denkins Y, Ward G, Salem N Jr. 1997. Retinal and brain accretion of long-chain polyunsaturated fatty acids in developing felines: the effects of corn oil–based maternal diets. *Am. J. Clin. Nutr.* 65: 465–72
75. Ponder DL, Innis SM, Benson JD, Siegman JS. 1992. Docosahexaenoic acid status of term infants fed breast milk or infant formula containing soy oil or corn oil. *Pediatr. Res.* 32:683–88
76. Raiten DJ, Talbot JM, Waters JH. 1998. LSRO report: assessment of nutrient requirements for infant formulas. *J. Nutr.* 128:2059–93S
77. Rioux FM, Innis SM, Dyer R, MacKinnon M. 1997. Diet-induced changes in liver and bile but not brain fatty acids can be predicted from differences in plasma phospholipid fatty acids in formula- and milk-fed piglets. *J. Nutr.* 127:370–77
78. Rogan WJ, Gladen BC. 1993. Breastfeeding and cognitive development. *Early Hum. Dev.* 31:181–93
79. Ryan AS, Montalto MB, Groh-Wargo S, Mimouni F, Sentipal-Walerius J, et al. 1999. Effect of DHA-containing formula on growth of preterm infants to 59 weeks postmenstrual age. *Am. J. Hum. Biol.* 11: 457–87
80. Salem N Jr, Wegher B, Mena P, Uauy R. 1996. Arachidonic and docosahexaenoic acids are biosynthesized from their 18-carbon precursors in human infants. *Proc. Natl. Acad. Sci. USA* 93:49–54
81. Sanders TAB, Reddy S. 1992. The influence of a vegetarian diet on the fatty acid composition of human milk and the essential fatty acid status of the infant. *J. Pediatr.* 120:S71–77
82. SanGiovanni JP, Berkey CS, Dwyer JT, Colditz GA. 2000. Dietary essential fatty acids, long-chain polyunsaturated fatty acids, and visual resolution acuity in healthy fullterm infants: a systematic review. *Early Hum. Dev.* 57:165–88
83. SanGiovanni JP, Parra-Cabrera S, Colditz GA, Berkey CS, Dwyer JT. 2000. Meta-analysis of dietary essential fatty acids and long-chain polyunsaturated fatty acids as they relate to visual resolution acuity in healthy preterm infants. *Pediatrics* 105: 1292–98
84. Sauerwald T, Hachey DL, Jensen CL, Chen H, Anderson RE, Heird WC. 1996. Effect of dietary α-linolenic acid intake on incorporation of docosahexaenoic and arachidonic acids into plasma phospholipids of term infants. *Lipids* 31:S131–35
85. Sauerwald TU, Hachey DL, Jensen CL, Chen H, Anderson RE, Heird WC. 1997. Intermediates in endogenous synthesis of C22:6ω3 and C20:4ω6 by term and preterm infants. *Pediatr. Res.* 41:183–87
86. Simmer K, Cochranes Neonatal Group. 2001. Long-chain polyunsaturated fatty acid supplementation in preterm infants. *Cochrane Database Syst. Rev.* 2: Entire issue
87. Simmer K, Cochrane Neonatal Group. 2001. Long-chain polyunsaturated fatty acid supplementation in infants born at term. *Cochrane Database Syst. Rev.* 3: Entire issue
88. Sokol S, Hansen VC, Moskowitz A, Greenfield P, Towle VL. 1983. Evoked potential and preferential looking estimates of visual acuity in pediatric patients. *Ophthalmology* 90:552–62
89. Uauy R, Birch E, Birch D, Peirano P. 1992. Visual and brain function measurements in studies of n-3 fatty acid requirements of infants. *J. Pediatr.* 120:S168–80
90. Uauy R, Hoffman DR, Birch EE, Birch DG, Jameson DM, Tyson JE. 1994. Safety and efficacy of omega-3 fatty acids in the nutrition of very-low-birth-weight infants: soy oil and marine oil supplementation of formula. *J. Pediatr.* 124:612–20

91. Uauy R, Hoffman DR, Peirano P, Birch DG, Birch EE. 2001. Essential fatty acids in visual and brain development. *Lipids* 36:885–95
92. Uauy R, Mena P, Wegher B, Nieto S, Salem N Jr. 2000. Long chain polyunsaturated fatty acid formation in neonates: effect of gestational age and intrauterine growth. *Pediatr. Res.* 47:127–35
93. van Wezel-Meijler G, van der Knaap MS, Huisman J, Jonkman EJ, Valk J, Lafeber HN. 2002. Dietary supplementation of long-chain polyunsaturated fatty acids in preterm infants: effects on cerebral maturation. *Acta Paediatr.* 91:942–50
94. Voss A, Reinhart M, Sankarappa S, Sprecher H. 1991. The metabolism of 7,10,13,16,19-docosahexaenoic acid to 4,7,10,13,16,19-docosahexaenoic acid in rat liver is independent of a 4-desaturase. *J. Biol. Chem.* 266:19995–20000
95. Wheeler TG, Benolken RM. 1975. Visual membranes: specificity of fatty acid precursors for the electrical response to illumination. *Science* 188:1312–14
96. Willats P, Forwyth JS, DiModugno MK, Varma S, Colvin M. 1998. Effect of long-chain polyunsaturated fatty acids in infant formula on problem solving at 10 months of age. *Lancet* 352:688–91
97. Williams C, Birch EE, Emmett PM, Northstone K. 2001. Avon Longitudinal Study of Pregnancy and Childhood (ALSPAC) Study Team. 2001. Stereoacuity at age 3.5 y in children born full-term is associated with prenatal and postnatal dietary factors: a report from a population-based cohort study. *Am. J. Clin. Nutr.* 73:316–22

Subject Index

B

G

N

Q

T

Cumulative Indexes

CONTRIBUTING AUTHORS, VOLUMES 21–25

CHAPTER TITLES, VOLUMES 21–25

Proteins, Peptides, and Amino Acids

Vitamins

Nutrition and Metabolic Regulation

Genetics and Molecular Biology

Clinical Nutrition

Nutritional Anthropology

Nutritional Microbiology

Nutritional Pharmacology and Toxicology

Public Health Nutrition

Comparative Nutrition

Special Topics